SECOND EDITION

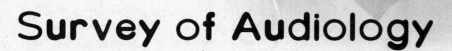

Survey of Audiology

Fundamentals for Audiologists and Health Professionals

David A. DeBonis

The College of Saint Rose
Sunnyview Hospital and Rehabilitation Center

Constance L. Donohue

The College of Saint Rose

D1517847

PEARSON

Boston New York San Francisco
Mexico City Montreal Toronto London Madrid Munich Paris
Hong Kong Singapore Tokyo Cape Town Sydney

Executive Editor and Publisher: *Stephen D. Dragin*
Editorial Assistant: *Katie Heimsoth*
Marketing Manager: *Kris Ellis-Levy*
Editorial-Production Service: *Omegatype Typography, Inc.*
Composition Buyer: *Linda Cox*
Manufacturing Buyer: *Linda Morris*
Electronic Composition: *Omegatype Typography, Inc.*
Cover Administrator: *Kristina Mose-Libon*

For related titles and support materials, visit our online catalog at www.ablongman.com.

Between the time website information is gathered and then published, it is not unusual for some sites to have closed. Also, the transcription of URLs can result in typographical errors. The publisher would appreciate notification where these errors occur so that they may be corrected in subsequent editions.

ISBN-13:   978-0-205-53195-0
ISBN-10:   0-205-53195-4

Library of Congress Cataloging-in-Publication Data

DeBonis, David A.
  Survey of audiology : fundamentals for audiologists and health professionals / David A. DeBonis and Constance L. Donohue.—2nd ed.
      p. cm.
  Includes bibliographical references and index.
  ISBN-13: 978-0-205-53195-0 (pbk.)
  ISBN-10: 0-205-53195-4 (pbk.)
  1. Audiology.
    [DNLM: 1. Audiology—methods. 2. Hearing Disorders—diagnosis. 3. Rehabilitation of Hearing Impaired.   WV 270 D287s 2008]   I. Donohue, Constance L. II. Title.
  RF290.D43 2008
  617.8—dc22

                                                                2007018279

Printed in the United States of America

10 9 8 7 6   11

This book is dedicated to . . .

Dr. Charleen Bloom, of The College of St. Rose,
for introducing us to the field of Communication Disorders
and for inspiring us;

Our fathers, Ted DeBonis and John LaPosta,
for instilling in us the value
of education; and,

Joe Donohue for his unwavering support, patience,
good humor, and home cooking.

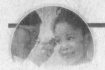

About the Authors

David DeBonis is associate professor and chair of the Communication Sciences and Disorders Department at the College of Saint Rose. He has his master's degree in audiology from Pennsylvania State University and his doctorate in educational psychology from the State University of New York at Albany. David has over twenty years of clinical experience and over ten years of college teaching experience. He has co-authored articles in *Topics in Language Disorders* and the *Journal of Attention Disorders*. His areas of interest include pediatric audiological assessment, auditory processing disorders, self-regulation, and research methods.

Connie Donohue is an audiologist and an adjunct faculty member at the College of Saint Rose, where she has taught in the Communication Sciences and Disorders program since 1991. She also provides audiological and auditory processing evaluations in the Pauline K. Winkler Speech and Hearing Clinic at Saint Rose. Connie received her master's degree in audiology and hearing impairment from Northwestern University. Since 1998, she has worked in state government, including seven years at the New York State Department of Health, where she helped establish and implement the statewide Newborn Hearing Screening Program.

Contents

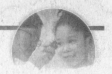

4 Pure Tone Testing 79

5 Speech Audiometry 125

6 Physiological Assessment of the Auditory System 169

7 Disorders of the Auditory System   233

8 Pediatric Audiology   281

12 Helping Individuals with Hearing Loss   429

Preface

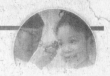

As audiologists, we have had the wonderful good fortune of working in challenging and stimulating settings in which we have met a wide variety of clients with various audiometric and personal profiles. We have interacted with a range of clients from newborn babies to those who had celebrated their 100th birthdays; from clients whose hearing losses were a mild inconvenience to those whose hearing losses altered their lives forever; from clients who enjoyed the support and guidance of family and friends to those who had to deal with their hearing loss alone.

These invaluable human interactions created in us a sense of what the practice of audiology is and what it is not. It is not just about ears or hearing. It is about people and it is about communication. It is also about people's temperaments, their outlooks, and their beliefs; it is about their families and support systems.

After years of day-to-day clinical work, we both were given the opportunity to teach audiology to undergraduate and graduate students. As is often the case, through teaching, we learned a lot. One thing that we learned was that few audiology textbooks addressed adequately the more humanistic domains of audiological care. Students would often ask why a certain topic that we had discussed in class was not included in their text. Also, we learned that students were relying heavily on our notes but were reading the text only infrequently. They also were not using their text as a reference in later classes.

From our teaching we also learned that students in speech–language pathology programs often felt that the issues addressed in their textbooks were, in large part, not relevant to them. In fact, students often could not find in their texts information to help them understand their scope of practice, responsibilities, or contributions as members of a team of professionals helping individuals with hearing loss. In short, these students often felt "left out" of the audiology class.

Based on these rich clinical and teaching experiences, we decided to write an audiology text that would accomplish several things. First, it would maintain the scientific rigor that many of the texts on the market already had. Second, it would include ongoing discussion of the complex humanistic themes that are critical to providing audiological care in the real world. In fact, the text unambiguously defines audiology as a scientific and humanistic discipline. Third, it would specifically address the relevance of audiology concepts, practices, and data to speech–language pathologists and individuals in other health professions. Finally, the text would be written in a way that was consistent with our teaching style: in understandable language and with extensive use of examples and cases. In this edition, we sought to maintain these elements and update certain topics that had undergone change.

Of course, we hope that this text will be well received by students and will make their experiences in audiology classes more rewarding. However, our hope for this text extends beyond that. We also hope that this text will foster greater understanding among future audiologists that the humanistic themes that undoubtedly emerge in the real-world practice of audiology must be considered an important part of our work; that attending to these human factors is critical to our success as audiologists.

We welcome feedback from our readers regarding this text. Feel free to contact us at ddebonis@nycap.rr.com or cdonohue@nycap.rr.com.

New to This Edition

The second edition of this text includes more detailed information regarding the profession of audiology and some of the related professional organizations about which students should know. Information about recent changes in training is also addressed. In Chapter 6, we added information about the use of Stacked ABR testing to identify smaller acoustic tumors; we also reorganized the chapter to facilitate understanding. In Chapter 7 we integrated many audiograms into the text and added photos and illustrations of specific pathologies of the ear. We also added a major section on assessment and management of balance disorder, reflecting the growing interest in this area. In Chapter 9 we added updated information on multicultural issues, and in Chapter 10 we added some current information on screening and referring students for (central) auditory processing testing. Chapter 12 includes some major new information on digital hearing aids and wireless technology, as well as updates on surgically implanted hearing aids and adult aural rehabilitation. New detailed information is also included about speech coding strategies for cochlear implant users and implant/hearing aid arrangement options. New information has also been added on the two main tinnitus treatment approaches, as has research about otoprotection and hair cell regeneration.

Supplements

To help you get the most out of *Survey of Audiology*, we have provided useful supplements for instructors and students:

- **Instructor's Manual and Test Bank.** A teacher's tool, this manual provides a wealth of ideas and activities designed to help instructors teach the course. Each chapter includes content summaries and outlines, key terms, discussion questions, topic launchers, suggested readings, and a variety of test questions, including multiple choice items, fill-in-the-blank items, true/false items, and essay questions.
- **Companion Website.** This website provides a comprehensive collection of tools and activities that will help students study more effectively and can take them beyond the book. It includes learning objectives, practice tests, web links, and flash cards. Visit www.ablongman.com/debonis2e.

Acknowledgments

We wish to thank numerous individuals for their support in developing this text. First, we thank again the four individuals to whom this text is dedicated. Writing the dedication was perhaps the easiest part of this project, because of the opportunities and support provided by these individuals. We appreciate the support of our families, colleagues, and friends, who encouraged us along the way. We would especially like to thank Anthony Cacace for his technical assistance.

The contributions of several peer reviewers were invaluable in the process of shaping and refining the manuscript to optimize its benefit to students and professionals alike: Flint A. Boettcher, University of South Alabama; Jeff Brockett, Idaho State University; Gerald Church, Central Michigan University; and Karen S. Helfer, University of Massachusetts.

We thank our executive editor, Steve Dragin. Steve's skillful management of this project allowed us to maintain our original themes while broadening our scope to meet the needs of a wider audience of readers. We also thank Katie Heimsoth for her fine efforts on behalf of this text.

We thank our clients for providing us with a rich variety of clinical experiences and interactions, which led us to a deeper understanding of the dynamic connections between the science and humanism of our profession. Similarly, our students, through their questions, comments, and insights, have reinforced the need to address audiology in the larger context of the field of communication disorders and to put this information on paper. We thank them for this.

Audiology as a Scientific, Collaborative, and Humanistic Discipline

AFTER COMPLETING THIS CHAPTER, YOU SHOULD BE ABLE TO:

1. Define *audiology* and support the statement that it is a scientific and humanistic discipline.
2. Define and differentiate between *speech–language pathologist* and *audiologist.*
3. Support the argument that scientific knowledge alone does not adequately prepare audiologists to meet client needs.
4. Describe consultative and collaborative models of interaction that foster humanism in clinical practice.
5. Understand the components of an educational program designed to facilitate the human dimensions of clinical care.
6. Identify three organizations for hearing and speech clinicians.

Audiology, as a scientific discipline, is the study of hearing and hearing disorders. **Audiologists** are individuals who "provide comprehensive diagnostic and rehabilitative services for all areas of auditory, vestibular, and related disorders" (ASHA, 2004). The national organization that certifies audiologists and **speech–language pathologists** in the United States is the American Speech-Language-Hearing Association (ASHA, 2004).

Not only is the **scope of practice** in audiology broad, the particular knowledge base that could theoretically be required for a given audiologist in a clinical audiology setting is also vast. Consider the clinical audiologist working in a medical facility who is required to carry out:

- Comprehensive audiological evaluations
- **Auditory brainstem testing** for both site of lesion and hearing estimation purposes
- Intraoperative monitoring
- **Otoacoustic emission** testing
- **Electronystagmography**

2

•

Chapter 1
Audiology as
a Scientific,
Collaborative,
and Humanistic
Discipline

- **Vestibular** rehabilitation
- **Cochlear implant** programming
- Hearing aid dispensing using state-of-the-art programmable and digital products
- Dispensing of **assistive listening devices**

This combination of responsibilities represents a range of technical and decision-making skills that speaks to the ever-growing complexity of the field of audiology and to the need for audiologists to have a firm foundation of scientific knowledge in order to collect and interpret competently the data generated from these activities.

Because most audiologists, regardless of their type of practice, find themselves in settings in which their knowledge base must be expansive and in which learning is an ongoing process (in order to remain current with technological advances), the profession of audiology is currently undergoing a dramatic reconfiguration of its training programs, moving to the clinical doctorate as the entry-level degree. Also, state licensure boards in many states across the country have passed continuing education requirements for audiologists as a way of ensuring that this process of ongoing education takes place.

Further examination of the Scope of Practice in Audiology (ASHA, 2004) reveals that scientific knowledge alone does not adequately prepare the audiologist. Audiology is also a humanistic discipline, and because of this audiologists must acquire knowledge that goes beyond that involved in the collection and interpretation of scientific data. As noted in the Scope of Practice, audiologists provide their services "across the entire age span from birth through adulthood; to individuals from diverse language, ethnic, cultural, and socioeconomic backgrounds; and to individuals who have multiple disabilities" (ASHA, 2004, p. 1). The Scope of Practice also notes that audiologists are engaged in counseling for psychosocial adjustment to hearing loss to persons with hearing loss and their caregivers/families.

This challenge that audiology services be provided to diverse individuals and that such services address the psychosocial aspects of hearing loss requires audiologists to assess and use the human elements of their interactions with clients to do their work competently and ethically. In order to work effectively with a diversity of individuals, audiologists must have some broad understanding and comfort with the range of characteristics that make up human beings. People differ not only in their age, ability, and cultural background but also in such variables as temperament, motivation, ability to change, family dynamic, and reaction to hearing loss. Integrating these factors into our scientific knowledge effectively requires not only specialized knowledge and understanding of people, but also an increased understanding of ourselves.

Although audiology is both a scientific and a humanistic endeavor, the humanistic aspect of our field has received less attention and perhaps some resistance by professionals in our field. This is not unlike the struggle in the field of medical education. According to Novak, Epstein, and Paulsen (1999), "as medical knowledge and effective remedies have multiplied, the science of curing has overshadowed the art of healing" (p. 516). The authors add that restoring the balance between technology and healing requires such things as ongoing communication, words of reassurance, and affirmation, and that when these things are provided to patients, "the greatest satisfaction of clinical care" can result (p. 517).

Peters and colleagues (2000) investigated the long-term effects of an innovative, problem-solving, and humanistic-based curriculum on medical students in preclinical training programs at Harvard Medical School. The program was designed specifically to promote knowledge of basic sciences combined with competency in integrating psychosocial and humanistic elements of patient care. Measured during medical school, during residency, and in private practice, students exposed to the innovative curriculum continued to function differently than a similar group who received the traditional curriculum, even ten years later. Specifically, the experimental group members were much more likely to choose low-technology, socially oriented careers (e.g., psychiatry, primary care) in which human interactions would be the focus. These students also viewed ongoing medical education as a means to solve patient problems. Students in the traditional curriculum were more likely to choose positions with less direct patient contact and viewed lifelong learning as a way to build a larger scientific knowledge base.

Despite research, widespread dissatisfaction among consumers of health care, and repeated recognition that "there is more to medical practice than hard science" (Maheux, 1990, p. 41), few clients believe that the day-to-day practice of medicine has been moved toward a more humanistic approach. Novak and colleagues (1999) identify three possible reasons. One is that it is easier to teach facts and protocols than to facilitate problem solving using the numerous and complex variables of real human interaction. Also, many of the calls for curricular change have been addressed in a very peripheral fashion, relegating "soft" courses to low-priority status. And finally, much of a medical student's clinical exposure is with physicians who, in an effort to be "efficient," rarely move beyond the technical aspects of cases and therefore do not model these humanistic dimensions.

The parallels between the struggles in the field of medical education and the current status of audiology should be noted and are an opportunity for us to learn. Audiology, like the medical field, is experiencing an explosion of technology that demands our time and cognitive energy in order for us to remain current and provide our clients with the most up-to-date service possible. Much of the continuing education coursework that is currently available to professionals is designed to meet this need to maintain an ever-broadening scientific base of knowledge. For training programs, this technology explosion means that decisions will have to be made regarding how much of each of these areas can reasonably be covered in the classroom. Just as has occurred in the medical field, this decision-making process may lead to cursory coverage of the "soft" areas involving interpersonal aspects of client care.

Also, as noted above, failure to maintain some reasonable balance between the science and humanity of our field can result in dissatisfaction for our clients and for ourselves as clinicians. Many, like Robinson (1991), believe that audiology is clearly moving toward technical management and away from human management. This is indeed unfortunate, because "as audiologists we come into our own when we begin to face the challenge of caring for our patients and their families through an ongoing interpersonal dialogue, the kind of dialogue that can only emerge within a positive, well-developed relationship with our patients" (Clark, 1994, p. 2).

The Profession of Audiology

What Is an Audiologist?

According to the American Speech-Language-Hearing Association (ASHA, 2004), an audiologist is a professional who works to promote healthy hearing, communication competency, and quality of life across the life span. This is achieved by working to

4

•

Chapter 1
Audiology as
a Scientific,
Collaborative,
and Humanistic
Discipline

prevent hearing loss whenever possible, by screening individuals for hearing loss, and by assessing and treating individuals for disorders of hearing and balance. As needed, audiologists provide hearing aid and cochlear implant services, including equipment dispensing, follow-up services, and counseling.

The important work of the audiologist is performed for all clients, regardless of their race, age, gender, religion, ethnicity, or sexual orientation. The practice of audiology is guided by scope of practice documents offered by both ASHA (2004) and the American Academy of Audiology (AAA, 2004).

Education, Training, and Credentials

At one time, the educational requirements to become an audiologist were met with a bachelor's degree. This changed to a master's degree and remained in place for many years until the decision was made in the late 1980s that audiology would be a doctorate-level profession. In order for this to occur, programs offering master's degrees in audiology had to transition to the new doctoral programs, which began to appear in the mid-1990s. These programs are typically three to four years in length and require more intensive study so that audiologists are better prepared to meet the challenges of an expanding scope of practice.

The specific degree that students now earn is a clinical doctorate in audiology, designated as Au.D. Currently, seventy universities in the United States offer this degree and more than 2,000 audiologists have one. This degree is different from the traditional Ph.D., which prepares individuals to pursue the important work of conducting research in audiology.

In addition to their educational training, in most states audiologists are also required to be licensed or registered to practice. In order to maintain this credential, they are also often required to document the continuing education work they have done. Some states also require separate registration to dispense hearing aids. These requirements are in place to ensure that an individual practicing as an audiologist has the necessary education and training to serve the public. Other countries often have different requirements.

ASHA and AAA

Two very important organizations that must be highlighted in this discussion of the profession of audiology are ASHA and AAA. ASHA has been involved in creating standards for educational training programs in speech–language pathology and audiology and for clinical practice for over fifty years. Although ASHA remains a powerful force in the profession, many audiologists now view AAA as their professional organization—one that is uniquely able to provide them with the support and professional identity they need. Currently, more than 10,000 audiologists are members of AAA, which was founded in 1988.

Professional Organizations

National, state, and local speech and hearing associations are an important source of information about the past, present, and future direction of the profession of audiology. These organizations also afford professionals and students an opportunity to network and learn from one another. Table 1.1 contains the names, Web sites, and descriptions of several organizations relevant to hearing and speech professionals and those interested in learning more about the professions of audiology and/or speech–language pathology.

The Work of Audiologists

Audiology is a dynamic and rewarding profession, and the work done by audiologists impacts individual lives in positive and important ways. As students studying audiology, perhaps for the first time, consider the following scenarios and imagine that you are the audiologist portrayed.

TABLE **1.1** **Hearing and Speech Professional Organizations**

Group	Web Site (Uniform Resource Locator)	Description/Mission
American Speech-Language-Hearing Association	www.asha.org	ASHA is the professional, scientific, and credentialing association for more than 123,000 members and affiliates who are audiologists, speech–language pathologists, and speech, language, and hearing scientists.
American Academy of Audiology	www.audiology.org	With more than 10,000 members, the American Academy of Audiology is the world's largest professional organization of, by, and for audiologists.
American Auditory Society	www.amauditorysoc.org	The primary aims of the society are to increase knowledge and understanding of the ear, hearing, and balance; disorders of the ear, hearing, and balance, and preventions of these disorders; and habilitation and rehabilitation of individuals with hearing and balance dysfunction.
Educational Audiology Association	www.edaud.org	The Educational Audiology Association is an international organization of audiologists and related professionals who deliver a full spectrum of hearing services to all children, particularly those in educational settings.
		The mission of EAA is to act as the primary resource and active advocate for its members through its publications and products, continuing educational activities, networking opportunities, and other professional endeavors.
Academy of Doctors of Audiology (formerly the Academy of Dispensing Audiologists)	www.audiologist.org	The Academy of Doctors of Audiology, founded in 1976 as the Academy of Dispensing Audiologists, provides valuable resources to the private practitioner in audiology and to other audiology professionals who have responsibility for the concerns of quality patient care and business operation.

6
•
Chapter 1
Audiology as
a Scientific,
Collaborative,
and Humanistic
Discipline

- A 3-month-old child is referred to you due to concerns that a hearing loss might exist. The parents are filled with anxiety about the possible hearing loss. After performing your testing, you report to the parents that the child's hearing is within normal limits.
- Three months after having identified a 4-year-old with a moderate hearing loss and fitting him with two hearing aids, you receive a call from his speech–language pathologist reporting substantial gains in the child's vocabulary and articulation skills.
- A 6-year-old with almost no useable hearing in either ear has had a surgical procedure (cochlear implantation) to improve her access to speech. You activate the device and call her name. For the first time, she turns her head toward the speech signal. Her parents are overjoyed.
- An elderly resident of a nursing home appears confused and unresponsive. Your testing reveals wax blockage in each ear. You refer him to the physician who removes the wax. The resident is now able to engage with others.
- You are a research audiologist working on a treatment for cochlear hearing loss and you discover a substance that is effective in certain animals. You apply for funding to study if it would work in human adults.

Audiology as a Humanistic Discipline

In order to avoid the imbalance that has hindered the medical field in becoming a true helping profession, audiology must be viewed as a humanistic discipline. To define **humanism** in audiology, we paraphrase Branch and colleagues (2001) and define it as the audiologist's "attitudes and actions that demonstrate interest in and respect for the patient and that address the patient's concerns and values" (p. 1967). Table 1.2, adapted from Branch et al. (2001), summarizes the broad categories that might be included in educating students and professionals in the humanistic aspects of audiology.

Listening

A few of these broad themes should be highlighted. Note that, through both verbal and nonverbal means, the clinician collects information about factual matters as well as about the client's emotional state. The audiologist listens actively when clients share information about their emotional response, understanding that listening can be part of the healing process for the client. In addition, the audiologist attempts to evoke such information because ultimately this insight will assist in the process of diagnosis and rehabilitation. A humanistic audiologist recognizes her role as not only providing content counseling in the form of factual information, but also engaging with the client, and the client's parent/family, in support counseling as clients adjust to the life changes resulting from their communication disorder.

In addition, the audiologist uses his or her observational skills to uncover information that the client might not readily discuss and to probe for greater understanding. The audiologist also observes family interactions, and understands that the family, as well as the other important people in the client's life, will play an important role in any effort to reduce the degree of communication deficit.

TABLE 1.2   Content of Educational Program to Facilitate the Human Dimensions of Clinical Care

Social Amenities
Greeting the patient
Introducing team members
Asking clients for permission, when appropriate

Verbal Communication Skills
Gathering information using open-ended and closed questions, active listening, and obtaining psychosocial information
Eliciting, clarifying, and attending to patients' emotions, beliefs, concerns, and expectations
Providing client education and facilitating behavioral change
Monitoring tone and pace of voice

Nonverbal Communication Skills
Position, including maintaining appropriate eye contact, placing oneself at the same level as the client, including client in clinical discussions
Monitoring facial expressions

Observational Skills
Client's verbal and nonverbal communications and communication styles
Client's unspoken reactions to difficult information
Client's family and social interactions
Colleague's communication and decision-making skills

Humanistic Care
Attending to the patient with respect as a unique individual
Providing care in the context of the client's values, history, needs, beliefs, abilities, culture, and social network
Providing care in the context of what is meaningful for the client
Providing humane care at the time of transitions, such as loss of functional status
Being honest and genuine regarding how one portrays oneself to the client
Respecting client confidentiality
Collaborating with clients, family members, and other professionals as a means of meeting the clients' needs effectively
Making use of various nonpaternalistic models of clinician–client interactions for purposes of fostering the client's independence and self-regulation

Self-Awareness
Being aware of the emotions that are evoked in the context of a client interaction
Being aware of the communication skills that one has used
Being aware of one's values, beliefs, history, needs, and culture
Being aware of how the above aspects of self-awareness affect one's interaction with and care of the client
Being aware of the "ego" that can be involved in assuming the role of the "expert"
Using this information to improve one's care of the client and achieve mutual benefit

Source: Adapted from Branch, W., Kern, D., Haidet, P., Weissmann, P., Gracey, C. F., Mitchell, G., & Inui, T. (2001). The patient–physician relationship. Teaching the human dimension of care in clinical settings. *Journal of the American Medical Association, 286*(9), 1067–1074. Copyright 2001, American Medical Association. All rights reserved.

8

•

Chapter 1
Audiology as
a Scientific,
Collaborative,
and Humanistic
Discipline

Clients as Individuals

Humanistic care that is provided to the client must be done in the context of the client's values, beliefs, history, needs, abilities, culture, and social network. This recognition that humanistic care is contextualized is critical to providing service that addresses the individual needs of clients, rather than forcing prescribed procedures and protocols on clients. Only when humanistic audiology is practiced can information about the particular client be integrated into the diagnostic and rehabilitation process.

Consider a 6-year-old child who, due to medical problems, has a history of traumatizing experiences when brought for medical treatment. Certainly, this history should be considered carefully when making decisions about the type of testing that will be used and the sequence in which those tests will be performed. Although most 6-year-olds may be able to participate in the audiological assessment in a certain standard manner, a humanistic approach requires that every effort be made to be flexible in approach in order to meet the needs of individuals.

Next, consider an adult who is severely physically impaired, having limited use of his upper extremities. An audiologist who assumes, because of the presenting physical characteristics, that the client will not be able to participate actively in the diagnostic assessment is not providing humanistic care. It is only in viewing this client as a unique person that the audiologist learns that physical limitations do not automatically imply cognitive deficits.

Transitions

Another very important consideration of humanistic care has to do with the audiologist's handling of transitions such as the loss of functional status. For audiologists, especially those with experience in the field, loss of hearing is a common occurrence and one that typically can be managed successfully. However, humanistic care requires us to make every effort to understand hearing loss from a client's perspective. Individuals who have hearing loss often react to their loss in ways that may seem disproportionate to us. Empathy and insight reveal that when a client learns that she has a hearing loss, concerns about future "losses" or sadness about previous "losses" may be generated. One illustrative example is an elderly gentleman who, upon learning that he had a considerable hearing loss in each ear, began to grieve for the loss of his wife, who had died three years earlier.

Self-Awareness

Self-awareness on the part of the audiologist is another requirement of a humanistic education. This refers primarily to clinicians developing an understanding of their own values, beliefs, history, and needs and how these can influence emotional responses evoked in their interactions with clients. Just as it is critical in a humanistic approach to audiology to acknowledge that we are providing services to individuals, it is equally important to acknowledge that we, as care providers, are individuals with our own unique traits. Only through this self-understanding are we able to use our own uniqueness for the benefit of the client–clinician relationship.

Consider an audiologist whose client is a 1-year-old deaf male, both of whose parents are individuals who have normal hearing. Upon making the diagnosis, the audiologist provides a range of options to the family, covering a continuum from auditory/oral to total communication to manual approaches. The parents, who have a history of deafness in the family, indicate that they have chosen to pursue the use of sign language and immersion into the deaf culture at this time. Other parents in a similar situation might opt for high-powered hearing aids and consideration of cochlear implantation. All of these parties—the audiologist and the parents—are influenced by their own personal backgrounds and beliefs during the decision-making process. The self-aware clinician is comfortable with and respects the choices made by parents regarding their child's communication.

Roles of an Audiologist

The above case and the issue of self-awareness raise the very important related issue in humanistic care involving role identification on the part of the audiologist. Some audiologists derive personal gratification from being an expert and often adopt a paternalistic style with their clients, in which they diagnose the problem and then determine the solution. Ylvisaker and Feeney (1998), in their discussion of various models of client–clinician relationships, refer to this model as the surgeon–patient model or the medical model. Another paternalistic model is the teacher–student model, in which the clinician identifies deficiencies in the client's knowledge or skills and then attempts to remediate these deficiencies. Neither of these two paternalistic models is consistent with a humanistic approach to client care.

Audiologists and other clinicians who adopt a humanistic approach to their work are likely to be guided well by one of the following two nonpaternalistic models. In the consultant–client model, the audiologist views himself not as one who determines goals but as one who assists clients in achieving their own self-determined goals. Similarly, the counselor–client model involves empowering the client to move beyond personal obstacles in the pursuit of personal goals. Each of these two models calls for audiologists to be honest in how they portray themselves to clients and to recognize that consultants can only facilitate independence and self-regulation when clients assume responsibility for their own management.

Collaboration

A logical outgrowth of audiologists assuming roles that are not authoritative is that their work becomes collaborative. As audiologists become familiar with techniques to collaborate with their clients in a supportive and empowering manner, they also develop the ability and appreciate the value of collaborating with other professionals, family members, and significant others in the client's life. This approach has far-reaching benefits for professionals, clients, and their families. For example, when a child is newly identified with hearing loss, the number and complexity of issues to be addressed can be daunting. Once the work is shared among the child's caregivers, health care providers, and parents, the process becomes manageable and parents find themselves with the necessary tools and support to make informed decisions about their child's care. Taking this a step further, parents and clients ultimately develop the inner resources and practical information to manage challenges that inevitably arise both in the short term and in the long term.

10

•

Chapter 1
Audiology as
a Scientific,
Collaborative,
and Humanistic
Discipline

Advocates of collaboration are many, and, in the work of the speech and language pathologist, collaboration has become the norm. Speech and language pathologists routinely work with reading specialists, preschool teachers, elementary education teachers, and special education teachers on a range of skills, including preliteracy skills, social skills, and behavior management. These services are now routinely offered in various "push-in," inclusive delivery models. In medical settings, speech–language pathologists are often part of a multidisciplinary team that includes an occupational therapist, physical therapist, psychologist, social worker, and physician.

Collaboration between a speech–language pathologist and an audiologist is a special partnership that should be highlighted for students in training because of the obvious and important links between the two disciplines. Audiologists who foster this collaboration understand that speech–language pathologists can provide a wealth of information about clients that can be used to make the diagnostic process much more efficient and reliable. In addition, healthy collaboration between speech–language pathologists and audiologists requires that reports be written so that meaningful interpretation of the data can occur.

For example, a speech–language pathologist is working with a client with a hearing impairment on speech intelligibility due to articulation errors. An audiologist providing the speech–language pathologist with information that specifically addresses what speech sounds the client does and does not have auditory access to will directly affect the pathologist's work and is evidence of the power of collaboration.

Furthermore, Ylvisaker and Feeney (1998) have long advocated the use of collaboration in both the diagnostic and the helping phases of their work with individuals who have traumatic brain injury (TBI). The authors note that collaboration is valuable in diagnostics because it increases the number and types of observations that can be made. Also, including a variety of individuals in the diagnostic process increases the likelihood that these same people will be engaged in the intervention stage. Further, when important people in the life of the client are included, they are able to maximize the value of natural opportunities that may arise for the client to practice new skills.

For instance, an elderly woman was in the process of obtaining new hearing aids. Her daughter had accompanied her for all of the audiology visits and was an integral part of the assessment and fitting process. One day the client and her daughter stopped in to a busy restaurant. When asked where they would like to sit, the client responded that they had no preference. The daughter then asked her mother, "Mom, do you remember what we discussed the other day at the audiologist's?" The client, remembering the discussion regarding the negative effects of background noise, then requested a seat in the quieter section of the room. As Ylvisaker and Feeney (1998) point out, helping individuals with disabilities often requires some change in everyday routines. This includes change on the client's part, as well as on the part of other people involved in those routines.

When humanistic audiology is at its finest, our efforts to collaborate may reach what Ylvisaker and Feeney (1998) call a "new level" in which professionals "embrace a vision of themselves not as experts who have a profoundly important contribution to make, but as experts who work in collaboration, who learn through collaboration, and who empower others through collaboration" (p. 247).

To balance this discussion, students of audiology and seasoned clinicians must also be aware of certain realities involved in providing audiological/hearing health care in the twenty-first century. For example, increased medical care costs combined with shrinking reimbursement from public and private sources have forced clinicians to add clients to their caseloads to maintain revenue. The practice of audiology has not escaped the growing trend to "do more with less," and this trend makes efforts to provide humanistic care more challenging. It also makes it necessary for professionals to be aware of sources of funding and the workings of third-party reimbursement. Although assisting clients with these matters can be part of humanistic care, audiologists may become overwhelmed with these issues, which can interfere with providing direct audiological services. Another reality is that, despite progress toward making audiology an autonomous profession, in some settings, the audiologist's role is more consistent with that of a technician than a professional.

Considering these ideas, students of audiology require exposure to both the technical and humanistic aspects of this discipline. We hope that this philosophy of practicing audiology is evident throughout this introductory text for students of speech–language pathology, audiology, and related fields. For example, in the chapters on acoustics of sound and disorders of the auditory system, we present the required technical material, which is then applied directly to clinical practice. This establishes the important connections for the student that learning audiological concepts is only the first step in the process; using the concepts to make clinical decisions is the next step. Finally, the information must be synthesized in a humanistic framework in the service of clients.

Other chapters lend themselves readily to this humanistic approach. The chapters on pediatric audiology and special populations present a broad view of the individual client and provide methods for establishing client-specific protocols for assessment. Numerous case examples reinforce this approach. Similarly, the chapter on helping individuals with hearing loss emphasizes the need to blend both technology and humanistic services (e.g., counseling and collaboration with other disciplines) to maximize the effectiveness of our aural rehabilitation efforts.

A separate chapter on auditory processing disorders is included in this text in response to the many requests we have received from colleagues in speech–language pathology and related disciplines. This is consistent with a humanistic approach, recognizing that collaboration with other professions is vital to serving the diverse and complex needs of clients in the twenty-first century.

Recommendations for the Future

As the discipline of audiology moves forward to this new level of academic training, the ever-expanding base of scientific knowledge in our field will require ongoing efforts to maintain rigor in preparing students to use this information for the welfare of their clients. However, we must recognize that our field can only achieve the level of client satisfaction, clinician satisfaction, and respect that we seek by integrating technical, scientific, and humanistic knowledge.

Audiology cannot be a purely data-driven or technology-driven discipline; it must also be a client-driven one. This requires that students learn that our ability to collect and meaningfully interpret data is intimately linked to our knowledge of the client. This knowledge includes both audiological and nonaudiological factors. In addition, our

12
•
Chapter 1
Audiology as
a Scientific,
Collaborative,
and Humanistic
Discipline

presentation of data to clients is influenced by our own internal beliefs and values, as well as by those of the client. Balancing the scientific and humanistic aspects of audiology will require that our instructional materials, our curriculum, and our student clinical experiences begin to reflect this blending of science and humanity. Although the process will be challenging, we are encouraged by feedback from students in communication disorders that reveals not only an awareness of the imbalance between scientific and humanistic aspects of our work but also an understanding of creative approaches that would improve our service delivery system.

The ASHA Code of Ethics (ASHA, 2003) states that the welfare of the clients should be held "paramount" and that we are obligated to use "every resource . . . to ensure that high-quality service is provided" (p. 1). Audiology is both a scientific and humanistic endeavor, which represents our very best effort to achieve this purpose.

In closing, we cite Van Hecke (1994) on a woman with hearing loss: "First remember that you are dealing with another human being. I have found that audiologists tend to retreat behind their technology and testing machinery. The majority of them have made me feel like a walking audiogram. Ten percent of an audiological exam is taken up with making contact with the client and ninety percent with testing and billing. I think these proportions should be reversed, or at least made equitable" (p. 94). The effort to balance these proportions should begin today.

REFERENCES

American Academy of Audiology (AAA). (2004). Audiology: Scope of practice. Accessed March 7, 2007, from www.audiology.org/publications/documents/practice

American Speech-Language-Hearing Association (ASHA). (2003). Code of ethics (revised). *ASHA Supplement, 23,* 13–15.

American Speech-Language-Hearing Association. (2004). Scope of practice in audiology. *ASHA Supplement, 24,* in press.

Branch, W., Kern, D., Haidet, P., Weissmann, P., Gracey, C. F., Mitchell, G., & Inui, T. (2001). The patient–physician relationship. Teaching the human dimension of care in clinical settings. *Journal of the American Medical Association, 286*(9), 1067–1074.

Clark, J. (1994). Audiologists' counseling purview. In J. Clark & F. Martin (Eds.), *Effective counseling in audiology: Perspectives and practice* (pp. 1–15). Englewood Cliffs, NJ: Prentice Hall.

Maheux, B. (1990). Humanism in medical education: A study of educational needs perceived by trainees of three Canadian schools. *Academic Medicine, 65*(1), 41–45.

Novak, D., Epstein, M., & Paulsen, R. (1999). Toward creating physician-healers: Fostering medical students' self-awareness, personal growth, and well-being. *Academic Medicine, 74*(5), 516–520.

Peters, A., Greenberger-Rosovosky, R., Crowder, C., Block, S., & Moore, G. (2000). Long-term outcomes of the new pathway program at Harvard medical school: A randomized controlled trial. *Academic Medicine, 75*(5), 470–479.

Robinson, D. (1991). Universities and aural rehabilitation: In search of tigers. *Audiology Today, 3*(1), 22–23.

Van Hecke, M. (1994). Emotional responses to hearing loss. In J. Clark & F. Martin (Eds.), *Effective counseling in audiology: Perspectives and practice* (pp. 92–115). Englewood Cliffs, NJ: Prentice Hall.

Ylvisaker, M., & Feeney, T. (1998). *Collaborative brain injury intervention: Positive everyday routines.* San Diego: Singular.

chapter 2

Acoustics of
Sound and Preliminary
Clinical Application

AFTER COMPLETING THIS CHAPTER, YOU SHOULD BE ABLE TO:

1. Define the term *sound*.
2. Illustrate on a waveform the following aspects of sound: amplitude, frequency, wavelength, and period.
3. Describe the key features of the logarithmic decibel scale.
4. Use the appropriate formula to convert dynes/square centimeter (dynes/cm²) to decibels sound pressure level (dB SPL).
5. Interpret basic audiograms, including the relationship between air conduction and bone conduction.
6. Compare and contrast the air and bone conduction pathways.
7. Understand the difference between conductive and sensorineural hearing loss.
8. Define the terms *noise* and *reverberation* and describe their roles in classroom speech understanding.

Because hearing is the perception of sound, it makes sense that an audiology text includes some extensive information about sound. Many students are somewhat intimidated by the topic of acoustics, partly because of its abstract nature and partly because it involves some mathematical formulas. Thus, this chapter presents this information in a logical, step-by-step manner, using numerous illustrative examples. Students should also be aware that much of the trepidation that may surround this topic is truly unwarranted.

In addition to being somewhat intimidated by the topic of acoustics, students often view this material as not directly related to what they need to know to perform competently as audiologists and speech–language pathologists. Nothing could be further from the truth. With this in mind, we address two broad topics for which the acoustics of sound serves as the foundation: reading audiograms and environmental acoustics. Applying acoustics information to the understanding of these concrete topics will give readers a greater sense of how the acoustics of sound are relevant to their professional knowledge and clinical practice.

14

Chapter 2
Acoustics of
Sound and
Preliminary
Clinical
Application

What Is Sound?

Sound is a type of energy. This energy is the result of pressure waves that are the product of force being applied to a sound source.

Think of a guitar string as the sound source and the degree to which you pluck it as the force. When you do so, you create a disturbance of air molecules. More specifically, the sound produced is the result of the compression and rarefaction of molecules in the air through which they are traveling.

In order for sound to be created, there first must be some source of **vibration,** which refers to the back and forth motion of an object. Vibrating guitar strings or vibrating vocal folds are examples. Second, the energy created by this vibration must then be applied to and create a disturbance in a medium. Although in audiology we are concerned almost exclusively with the medium of air, sound can occur in other mediums as long as they have mass and are elastic.

Elasticity is an important concept. Think about what happens when you squeeze a tennis ball very hard. It temporarily changes shape but then is restored to its original shape. Air molecules have the same characteristic; they attempt to move back to their original positions after they have been displaced. However, as they attempt to do this, an opposing force called inertia comes into play. **Inertia,** described by Sir Isaac Newton, refers to the tendency of an object to remain in its current motion state. So, moving air molecules tend to want to remain in motion. This results in air molecules moving beyond their original resting positions and then displacing other adjacent air molecules.

Although we cannot see them, we are surrounded by innumerable air molecules that are constantly moving in a random manner. This movement is known as **Brownian motion.** For the purpose of our discussion of sound waves, ignore this constant movement of air particles momentarily and assume that each air particle has a relatively fixed resting position.

So, some force is applied to a sound source and as a result groups of molecules are pushed together and pulled apart repeatedly. When the molecules are close together, this is the **compression** (or condensation) part of the wave, which creates high pressure in the atmosphere. When the molecules are far apart, this is the **rarefaction** part of the wave, which creates low pressure. This series of compressions and rarefactions, which occurs over time and is depicted in Figure 2.1, creates what we refer to as pressure waves. Fortunately, the human eardrum is very sensitive to pressure changes, which constitute sound.

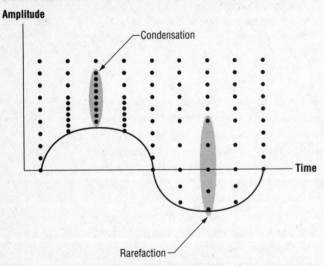

FIGURE **2.1** **Disturbance of particles in a medium during the production of simple sound.**

Source: Donald F. Fucci & Norman J. Lass. *Fundamentals of Speech Science.* Published by Allyn & Bacon, Boston, MA. Copyright © 1997 by Pearson Education. Reprinted by permission of the publisher.

Compression & Rarefraction = pressure wave

Sound can be represented on a number of different displays, including waveforms, spectra, and spectrograms. **Waveforms** represent sound with amplitude on the vertical axis and time on the horizontal axis. Figure 2.1 is an example of a waveform. Spectral analysis provides a representation of sound with amplitude on the vertical axis and frequency on the horizontal axis. This is shown in Figure 2.2. Note that the vertical line in the middle of the graph represents a middle-frequency sound with a high amplitude. **Spectrograms** provide an excellent way to display speech sounds because they show frequency, intensity, and time. In this case, frequency is on the vertical axis, time is on the horizontal axis, and the degree of darkness of the tracing reflects the intensity of the sound. Figure 2.3 shows a spectrogram of a vowel sound. In this chapter, waveforms are used to illustrate particular acoustic concepts.

Once you understand that pressure waves create sound, note that air molecules do not actually move through the air. Rather, the waves created by the particle movement travel. Furthermore, the type of waves relevant to this discussion of sound traveling in the air is longitudinal. In **longitudinal waves,** the air molecules move parallel to the direction of the wave motion. Contrast this information with a different type of wave—**transverse waves**—in which the motion of the molecules is perpendicular to the direction of the wave motion.

Now imagine a field of wheat blowing in the wind. The grains of wheat move in the same direction as the wind, illustrating that with longitudinal waves the waves and the molecules move in the same direction.

Picture a swimming pool. You throw a pebble into the water, creating a hole. Water from the surrounding area fills in this hole, and a circular trough is created around the original hole. The circular waves created by this action move out, away from the pebble. Now picture a float that is in the pool. What does it do in response to these waves? It moves up and down. So, in the case of transverse waves, the waves and the molecules of the mass are not moving in the same direction—the waves are moving out and the molecules are moving up and down. Examine Figure 2.4, which illustrates the wave and molecule movement.

Simple Sound

Now that you have a very basic understanding of the nature of sound, note the important distinction between simple and complex sound. **Simple sound** is a sound that has all of its energy at one frequency, creating a pure tone. Simple sounds are very rare and are created by tuning forks and pure tone audiometers. **Complex sounds,** on the other hand, have energy at more that one frequency and include, for example, the sound created by the human voice, musical instruments, and the heater in the corner of the room.

In this section we examine some important characteristics of sound, using simple sound displays. The simplest kind of sound wave motion that can occur in a medium is **sinusoidal motion.**

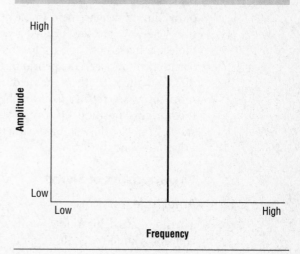

FIGURE **2.2** **Spectrum of a middle-frequency pure tone with high intensity.**

16

Chapter 2
Acoustics of
Sound and
Preliminary
Clinical
Application

FIGURE **2.3** **Spectrogram of a vowel sound.**

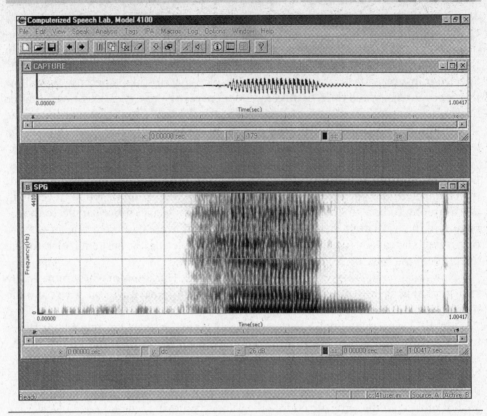

As shown in Figure 2.5, sinusoidal motion, also called **simple harmonic motion,** is illustrated by placing a sheet of paper beneath a clock pendulum and tracing the resulting movement. The pendulum will (1) go from its resting position to a point of maximum displacement in one direction; (2) return to its point of rest and go through it to a point of maximum displacement in the opposite direction; and (3) return to its resting position. The wave created is called a **sine wave.** Think back to the earlier discussion of air molecule movement and notice the connections between that information and simple harmonic motion. As the pendulum moves from rest to maximum displacement in one direction, the particles in the medium become compressed. As the pendulum begins to move toward its resting position, the air particles, which are elastic, attempt to return to their original position. Of course, the particles overshoot this position and are now in a state of rarefaction. As noted earlier, this series of compressions and rarefactions comprise the sound disturbance.

Characteristics of Sound

Amplitude

The sine wave helps us to simplify some important concepts related to sound. The first concept is amplitude. Although there are various ways to define amplitude, one useful

FIGURE 2.4 **Demonstration of transverse wave motion.**

First, a hole in the water is created by a pebble (A). Next, water flows to fill in the hole, producing a trough (B). When water flows to fill in the first trough, a second trough is created (C). A cork on the surface of the water moves up and down in a circular motion, but the waves created in the water are moving out, not up and down.

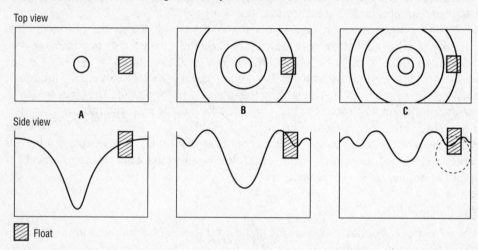

Top view

Side view

Float

FIGURE 2.5 **Sinusoidal motion recorded on paper.**

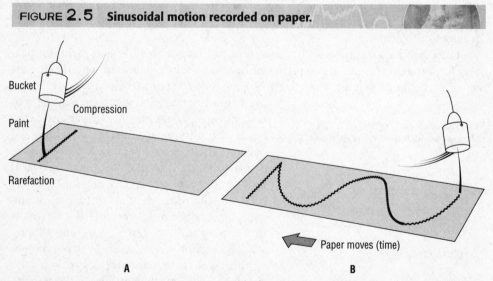

Bucket

Compression

Paint

Rarefaction

Paper moves (time)

A   B

18

•

Chapter 2
Acoustics of
Sound and
Preliminary
Clinical
Application

definition of **peak amplitude** is the maximum displacement of the particles in a medium. In the illustration of a sine wave in Figure 2.6, amplitude is the distance from the baseline to the point of maximum displacement on the wave. Amplitude determines the intensity of a sound and is related to the force with which the original particle disturbance was created. Clap your hands lightly (with little force) and you create a small disturbance and a quiet sound. Clap your hands with great force and the resulting sound has greater amplitude and greater intensity.

At this point it is important to make a distinction between the objective term **intensity** and the subjective term **loudness.** Because the maximum displacement of particles is quantifiable and not open to different interpretation, intensity is viewed as objective. Loudness, on the other hand, is a subjective experience involving the judgment and perception of the listener regarding the intensity of the sound. Although the judgments a person makes about loudness typically do include intensity information, they also include other perceptions. The loudness level that you deem perfect for your car radio might be judged by someone else as obnoxiously loud. Why? Because loudness is subjective. We will encounter other examples of subjective and objective aspects of sound as our discussion continues.

The Decibel (dB)

The development of the telephone created a need to describe and measure the magnitude of the sound produced. The unit of measure chosen was the bel, named after Alexander Graham Bell, who not only invented the telephone but also was an educator of hearing-impaired children. In our field today, the unit of measure for intensity most commonly used is the **decibel (dB)**, which is one-tenth of a bel.

Keep in mind that the amplitude of sound can be expressed as sound power or sound pressure. In our field, sound pressure is most commonly used, in part because most of the measuring devices used (e.g., microphones) are sensitive to pressure. Dealing with sound pressure is also helpful for students as they think of sound as pressure striking the eardrum.

The decibel scale is logarithmic in nature, not linear. This has two main implications for our discussion. The first is that, rather than all units of measurement being the same size, each unit is larger than the preceding unit. One of the advantages of using a logarithmic scale is that it compresses the very wide range of sound pressures capable of being heard by the human ear (a ratio of 10 million:1 between the highest tolerable sound pressure and the sound pressure that can just be heard) into a more manageable scale ranging from 140 to 0 dB. Interestingly, this feature of sound compression is similar to what the normally functioning auditory system does with sound.

The second implication of using a logarithmic scale is that the decibel scale has no absolute zero. In other words, 0 dB is an intensity value and is *not* the absence of sound. This means that 0 dB **sound pressure level**

FIGURE **2.6**   **Sine wave illustrating amplitude.**

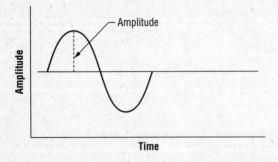

(SPL) is a starting point for sound pressure with reference to human hearing ability. For example, think about temperature. If it is 0 degrees outside, does this 0 mean the absence of temperature? Of course not. Now, think of a linear system. You go to the bank to inquire about your checking account balance. You are told that you have a balance of $0. We all know that on this linear scale, zero certainly does mean the absence of money.

Another important point about decibels is that they are always represented as a ratio between the sound pressure (or sound power) at hand and some referent sound pressure. For purposes of human hearing, and for this discussion, the reference used for sound pressure is 0.0002 **dyne**/square centimeter, abbreviated dyne/cm^2, or 0 dB SPL. (Some texts use 20 micropascals, abbreviated μPa). This is approximately the smallest amount of sound pressure that will cause the eardrum to vibrate in the average adult human. Another reference for decibel measurements that students of acoustics will encounter is a power reference. This decibel scale is also logarithmic; however, a different referent is used. Power measurements are expressed in **watts** (**W**) and recorded as dB IL (intensity level). This reference is commonly encountered, for example, when working with electrical systems or equipment.

One other reference that is important to audiologists is dB HL (hearing level). Hearing level is commonly used on audiograms, and dB HL refers to the decibel reading on the audiometer dial. An HL referent is used because the human ear is not equally sensitive to all frequencies. In other words, different amounts of sound pressure are needed to create 0 dB HL. By converting to an HL scale, plotting of standard audiograms is made more straightforward. These principles will be further explained in this chapter and in Chapter 4.

Logarithms

You may remember from high school math that a logarithm is a number expressed as an exponent, and a **logarithmic scale** is a measurement scale based on exponents of a base number. The exponent refers to the number of times a base number is multiplied by itself. In a base-10 system, the log of 1,000 is 3 because $1,000 = 10 \times 10 \times 10$ or 10 to the 3rd power. What, then, is the log of 10,000? The log of 10,000 is 4, because $10,000 = 10 \times 10 \times 10 \times 10$ or 10 to the 4th power. Students are usually very relieved to learn that in a base-10 system, which is very common in acoustics, the log of a number is equal to the number of zeros appearing after the 1.

Table 2.1 summarizes logarithmic values that will be useful to us as we convert dynes/square centimeter to dB SPL or watts/square centimeter (W/cm^2) to dB IL. The reason for these conversions is to demonstrate the principles described about the decibel, and to introduce the commonly used and convenient decibel scale. Note also in Table 2.1 that the log of 1 is 0.

At this point let's examine the formula we use to convert force, in dynes per square centimeter, to decibels sound pressure (dB SPL). The formula is

$$\text{dB SPL} = 20 \times \log\left(\frac{\text{output pressure}}{\text{referent pressure}}\right)$$

In this formula, 20 (a constant) is multiplied by the log of the relationship (ratio) between the pressure that is of interest (output pressure) and the referent pressure (also a

TABLE 2.1 Ratios, Logarithms, and Outputs for Determining Number of Decibels with Intensity and Pressure References

A Ratio	B Log	C Intensity Outputs (I_o) cgs (W/cm²)	C Intensity Outputs (I_o) SI (W/m²)	D dB IL*	E Equal Amplitudes	F dB SPL†	G Pressure Outputs (P_o) cgs (dyne/cm²)	G Pressure Outputs (P_o) SI (µPa)
1:1	0	10^{-16}	10^{-12}	0	Threshold of Audibility	0	.0002	$20.0(2 \times 10^1)$
10:1	1	10^{-15}	10^{-11}	10		20	.002	$200.0(2 \times 10^2)$
100:1	2	10^{-14}	10^{-10}	20		40	.02	$2,000.0(2 \times 10^3)$
1,000:1	3	10^{-13}	10^{-9}	30		60	.2	$20,000.0(2 \times 10^4)$
10,000:1	4	10^{-12}	10^{-8}	40		80	2.0	$200,000.0(2 \times 10^5)$
100,000:1	5	10^{-11}	10^{-7}	50		100	20.0	$2,000,000.0(2 \times 10^6)$
1,000,000:1	6	10^{-10}	10^{-6}	60		120	200.0	$20,000,000.0(2 \times 10^7)$
10,000,000:1	7	10^{-9}	10^{-5}	70		140	2000.0	$200,000,000(2 \times 10^8)$
100,000,000:1	8	10^{-8}	10^{-4}	80				
1,000,000,000:1	9	10^{-7}	10^{-3}	90				
10,000,000,000:1	10	10^{-6}	10^{-2}	100				
100,000,000,000:1	11	10^{-5}	10^{-1}	110				
1,000,000,000,000:1	12	10^{-4}	10^{-0}	120				
10,000,000,000,000:1	13	10^{-3}	10^{1}	130				
100,000,000,000,000:1	14	10^{-2}	10^{2}	140	Threshold of Pain			

*The number of dB with an intensity reference ($I_R = 10^{-12}$ W/m²) uses the formula dB (IL) $= 10 \times \log(I_o/I_R)$.

†The number of dB with a pressure reference ($P_R = 20$ µPa) uses the formula dB (SPL) $= 20 \times \log(P_o/P_R)$.

Source: F. N. Martin & J. G. Clark. *Introduction to Audiology.* 9e. Published by Allyn & Bacon, Boston, MA. Copyright © 2006 by Pearson Education. Reprinted by permission of the publisher.

constant). The logic here is that a determination of how intense a given output pressure is, in dB SPL, must be made by comparing that pressure to the smallest amount of sound pressure that will create a just-detectable sound in the average adult human who has normal hearing. If the output pressure is much greater than the referent pressure, the dB value will be large. However, if the output pressure is close to the referent pressure, the dB value will be small.

Let's use the following calculations of SPL to practice using the formula and to demonstrate the three important features of the decibel.

What is the dB SPL value if the output pressure is 2 dynes/cm^2? Because the output pressure is considerably greater than the referent pressure, the resulting dB value should be large. Using the formula, we find that

$$\text{dB SPL} = 20 \times \log\left(\frac{\text{output pressure}}{\text{referent pressure}}\right)$$

$$= 20 \times \log\left(\frac{2 \text{ dynes/cm}^2}{0.0002 \text{ dynes/cm}^2}\right)$$

$$= 20 \times \log 10,000$$

$$= 20 \times 4$$

$$= 80$$

In the next example, assume that the output pressure is 0.2 dyne/cm^2. Because this value is closer to the referent pressure, what do you predict about the dB SPL value? It will be smaller than in the first example. Using the formula, we find:

$$\text{dB SPL} = 20 \times \log\left(\frac{\text{output pressure}}{\text{referent pressure}}\right)$$

$$= 20 \times \log\left(\frac{0.2 \text{ dyne/cm}^2}{0.0002 \text{ dyne/cm}^2}\right)$$

$$= 20 \times \log 1,000$$

$$= 20 \times 3$$

$$= 60$$

Now assume that the output pressure is 0.02 dyne/cm^2. Because this value is even closer to the referent pressure, what do you predict about the dB SPL value? It will be smaller than in the preceding examples. Using the formula, we find:

$$\text{dB SPL} = 20 \times \log\left(\frac{\text{output pressure}}{\text{referent pressure}}\right)$$

$$= 20 \times \log\left(\frac{0.02 \text{ dyne/cm}^2}{0.0002 \text{ dyne/cm}^2}\right)$$

$$= 20 \times \log 100$$

$$= 20 \times 2$$

$$= 40$$

22

•

Chapter 2
Acoustics of
Sound and
Preliminary
Clinical
Application

The preceding examples not only serve to illustrate the use of the formula, they also demonstrate the first principle of the decibel as a logarithmic scale: each unit is larger than the preceding unit. Notice that although the dB SPL values calculated (40, 60, and 80 dB) differ by 20 dB, the respective pressure ratios are 100:1, 1,000:1, and 10,000:1. As noted earlier, this feature of a logarithmic scale allows us to compress the very wide range of sound pressures capable of being heard by the human ear into a more manageable scale.

Let's now assume that our output pressure is the same as our referent pressure. The pressure of interest to us is 0.0002 dyne/cm^2. Of course, you are already predicting a very small dB value because the pressure against the eardrum is the same as the referent pressure and we know that the referent is the smallest amount of sound pressure that will create a just-detectable sound in the average adult human who has normal hearing. Using the formula, we find:

$$dB\ SPL = 20 \times \log\left(\frac{\text{output pressure}}{\text{referent pressure}}\right)$$

$$= 20 \times \log\left(\frac{0.0002\ \text{dyne/cm}^2}{0.0002\ \text{dyne/cm}^2}\right)$$

$$= 20 \times \log 1$$

$$= 20 \times 0$$

$$= 0$$

As noted earlier, the log of 1 is 0, and because any number multiplied by 0 is 0, the dB SPL value when the absolute and referent pressures are equal is 0 dB. In other words, 0 dB is the point on the decibel scale at which the sound pressure against the eardrum is the same as the smallest amount of sound pressure that will create a just-detectable sound in the average adult human who has normal hearing.

In view of the above information, is it possible for someone to hear at −5 or −10 dB? Based on our discussion, the answer is yes. Remember that the referent used in the dB SPL formula is the smallest amount of sound pressure that will create a just-detectable sound in the average adult human who has normal hearing. Because the referent is an average value, some individuals detect sound at even softer levels than this referent. These individuals detect sound when the pressure against the eardrum is less than the referent pressure. This same principle applies if one is dealing with sound power and working in watts per square centimeter.

Similarly, formulas allow us to convert power, in watts per square centimeter, to decibels **intensity level** (dB IL). Specifically,

$$dB = 10 \times \log\left(\frac{\text{Wo}}{\text{Wr}}\right)$$

where

Wo = watts per cm^2 (power) output

Wr = watts per cm^2 (power) reference

The agreed-upon intensity-level reference is 10^{-16} W/cm^2. As was the case during our
discussion of sound pressure level, when the output (power) is the same as the referent, or when Wo = Wr, the ratio of the reference to the output is 1 and, since the logarithm of 1 is 0, the decibel output in this case is 0 dB IL. Again, 0 dB does not mean the absence of sound or the absence of power. It means that the power output of the system is the same as the reference being used for measuring the decibel. For additional instruction on this topic, consult the work of Charles I. Berlin (1970).

Frequency

Before defining frequency, it is necessary to define a cycle. A **cycle of a sound wave** is defined as air molecule movement from rest to maximum displacement in one direction, back to rest, and then to maximum displacement in the other direction. More simply, a cycle is one compression and one rarefaction of a sound wave. This concept of cycle is important because frequency is defined as the number of cycles of vibration completed during a time period. In acoustics that time period is typically one second (1 sec).

On the sine wave in Figure 2.7, note that the greater the number of cycles that occur in 1 sec, the higher the frequency; the fewer the cycles occurring in 1 sec, the lower the frequency. The **period of a sound wave** is the time required to complete one cycle of vibration of a sound wave. Logically, the greater the number of cycles occurring in 1 sec, the smaller the amount of time each cycle can take. Therefore, frequency and period have an inverse relationship. Low-frequency sounds have greater (longer) periods;

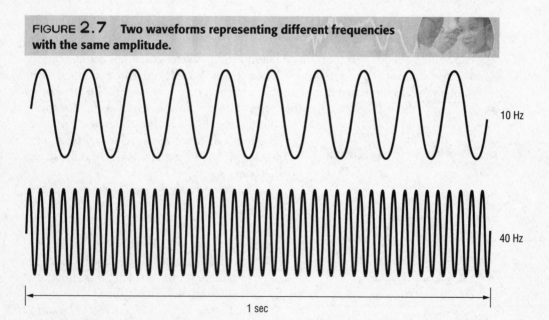

FIGURE **2.7** **Two waveforms representing different frequencies with the same amplitude.**

10 Hz

40 Hz

1 sec

24

•

Chapter 2
Acoustics of
Sound and
Preliminary
Clinical
Application

high-frequency sounds have smaller (shorter) periods. The formula expressing this relationship between period and frequency is

$$\text{Period} = \left(\frac{1}{\text{frequency}}\right)$$

As noted in our discussion of intensity and loudness, there are both subjective and objective aspects to sound. **Frequency** is an objective measure that is determined by the number of cycles over time. **Pitch** is the psychological correlate to frequency and, although a person's judgment about the pitch of an acoustic event is related to the stimuli's frequency, it is also influenced by other factors, such as the listener's experience, the intensity of the signal, and whether the sound is perceived as pleasant.

The unit of measure for frequency is the **hertz (Hz)**, named after the German physicist, H. R. Hertz (1857–1894), whose work on electromagnetic waves contributed to the development of the radio. The former unit of measure for frequency was cycles per second (cps), refering to the definition of frequency as cycles per second.

Velocity

We noted at the beginning of this chapter that one of the requirements for sound is that the energy created by vibration be applied to and create a disturbance in a medium. The speed at which sound travels through this medium is **velocity**. We also noted earlier that for our purposes air is the medium of interest. The average speed of sound in air, which may be described in feet, meters, or centimeters, is approximately 1,130 feet per second (ft/sec), 340 meters per second (m/sec), or 34,000 centimeters per second (cm/sec). Other factors that influence the velocity of sound in a medium include elasticity, density, and temperature.

Wavelength

The concept of velocity is important to determining wavelength, often denoted by the Greek letter lambda (λ) and sometimes denoted by w. **Wavelength** can be defined as the length of a wave, as measured from an arbitrary point on a sine wave to the same point on the next cycle of the wave. Another way to describe wavelength is the distance a sound wave travels in one cycle. Because wavelength is a distance measure, it is typically expressed in feet or meters. Figure 2.8 illustrates this concept.

The formula for determining wavelength is

$$w = \frac{v}{f}$$

where v refers to velocity of sound in air and f refers to the frequency. The relationship between frequency and wavelength is illustrated by the following two calculations.

What is the wavelength (in feet) of a sound whose frequency is 250 Hz?

FIGURE 2.8   Sine wave illustrating wavelength.

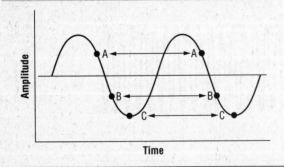

$$w = \frac{v}{f}$$

$$= \frac{1,130 \text{ ft/sec}}{250 \text{ Hz}}$$

$$= 4.52 \text{ ft}$$

What is the wavelength (in feet) of a sound whose frequency is 8,000 Hz?

$$w = \frac{v}{f}$$

$$= \frac{1,130 \text{ ft/sec}}{8,000 \text{ Hz}}$$

$$= .14 \text{ ft}$$

It should be clear from these calculations that low-frequency sounds have longer wavelengths and high-frequency sounds have shorter wavelengths. This is related to our discussion later in this chapter of classroom acoustics and speech perception. Sounds that have shorter wavelengths are less likely to travel around surfaces and are more likely to be missed by the listener. Hearing the low-frequency rumble of speech from another room is an example of the robustness of low-frequency sounds. Unfortunately, it is the high frequencies, not the lows, that carry most of the meaning in our language.

Despite their acoustic disadvantages, the low frequencies do carry important information for speech understanding. A summary of the information carried in the frequencies important for hearing and understanding speech is presented in Table 2.2.

Phase

Phase may be described as an air molecule's location at a given point in time during displacement, relative to the degrees of a circle. A sine wave in compression, with maximum displacement, corresponds to the 90-degree point on the circle. Likewise, a sine wave in rarefaction, with maximum displacement, corresponds to the 270-degree point on the circle.

It is possible for two sine waves of the same frequency and intensity to be in phase or out of phase with one another. When the compression and rarefaction of two sound waves are in exact agreement, the sound waves are said to be in phase with one another. Sound waves that are out of phase have air molecules that begin at different locations from one another.

Although phase differences are much less important to auditory perception than other aspects of sound (e.g., frequency, intensity, time), phase can provide information about the starting point of sounds. Figure 2.9 demonstrates two simple sounds that differ only in their starting points. If two simple sounds of *identical* frequency and phase are combined (i.e., begin at exactly the same location), a 6-dB increase in sound intensity will occur. For example, consider two radios each set at 60 dB, and on the same radio station, placed side by side. We would expect a doubling of sound

26

•

Chapter 2
Acoustics of
Sound and
Preliminary
Clinical
Application

TABLE **2.2** **Speech Cues Available by Frequency**

Frequency	Cues
125 Hz	F0 of most adult male voices
250 Hz	Voicing cues F0 of most female and child voices Low harmonics of adult male voices Nasal murmur (F1 of /m/, /n/, and /ng/) F1 of high back and high front vowels, /u/, / ℧/; /I/, /ɪ/
500 Hz	Primary cues on manner of production, most consonants Harmonics of most voices F1 and T1 of most vowels Noise bursts of plosives in back vowel contexts T1 of the semivowels (glides) /w/ and /j/ F1 of the liquids (glides) /l/ and /r/
1,000 Hz	Additional cues on manner of consonant production Harmonics of most voices T1 of the liquids (glides) /l/ and /r/ F2 of nasal consonants, /m/, /n/, /ng/ F2 and T2 of back and central vowels, /u/, / ℧/, / ɔ/, /a/; /ə/, /ɚ/ Noise bursts of most plosives T2 of the semivowels (glides) /w/ and /j/
2,000 Hz	Primary cues on place of consonant production Additional cues on manner of consonant production Harmonics of most voices F2 and T2 of most voices F2 and T2 of front vowels, /i/, /ɪ/, /ɛ/, /æ/ Noise bursts of most plosives and affricates Turbulent noise of fricatives /sh/, /f/, and /th/
4,000 Hz	Secondary cues on place of consonant production Upper range of harmonics for most voices F3 and T3 of most vowels Noise bursts of plosives and affricates Turbulent noise of voiced and unvoiced fricatives
8,000 Hz	Turbulent noise of all fricatives and affricates

F0: fundamental frequency (lowest frequency of a sound).

F1: first formant frequency; generally associated with the space behind the tongue or pharyngeal cavity; formant frequencies are dependent on the length of the individual's vocal tract.

F2: second formant frequency; generally associated with the space in front of the tongue or oral cavity.

T1: formant transition (shift in frequency resulting from changing tongue position).

T2 and T3: formant transitions.

F3: third formant frequency.

Source: Adapted from Ferrand, C. T. (2001). *Speech science: An integrated approach to theory and clinical practice* (pp. 162–164). Boston: Allyn & Bacon.

FIGURE **2.9**   **Two sine waves that are out of phase.**

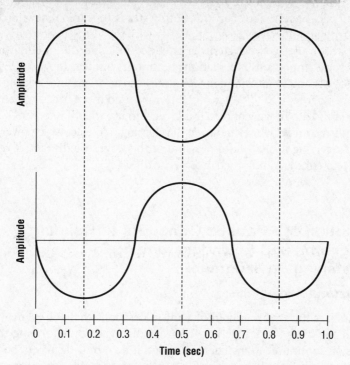

Source: Donald F. Fucci & Norman J. Lass. *Fundamentals of Speech Science.* Published by Allyn & Bacon, Boston, MA. Copyright © 1997 by Pearson Education. Reprinted by permission of the publisher.

pressure to occur, resulting in an output of 66 dB. More commonly, because sounds are not perfectly in phase with one another, the increase in sound pressure is approximately 3 dB. If two identical sounds that are 180 degrees out of phase (i.e., begin at directly opposite points) are presented simultaneously, they will cancel each other out, resulting in silence.

A Word about Units of Measure

It is very important that students develop the habit of using the correct units of measure when dealing with information about acoustics, because the interpretation of a numeric value is changed dramatically by the unit of measure. For example, the decibel level of a given signal is determined not only by the numeric value but also by what follows that value. Is the decibel scale SPL, IL, HL, or sensation level (SL)? Because clinical audiology makes considerable use of the HL scale, many of the values in this book will have that referent; but you must pay attention to units of measure. Units of measure cannot be assumed.

28
•
Chapter 2
Acoustics of
Sound and
Preliminary
Clinical
Application

To assist in developing a better understanding of units of measure, remember that two different metric systems are used: the MKS and cgs systems. Although the MKS system is generally preferred in acoustics, both systems appear in the research literature. Because students should have a basic familiarity with the terms associated with each system, a comparison of the two systems is provided in Table 2.3. In addition, Table 2.4 summarizes some important information about units of measure.

Speaks (1992) notes that although technically the term *intensity level* should be used only when the referent is 10^{-16} W/cm^2, the term is used more broadly than that, as has been done in this text. In view of this, it is critical to use the dB referent (e.g., SPL, HL) to avoid confusion and misinterpretation. If referring to the acoustic power of a sound, use dB IL; if referring to the sound pressure of the wave, use dB SPL; if referring to a sound level referenced to audiometric zero, use dB HL.

Application of Acoustic Concepts to Reading Audiograms and to Understanding the Listening Environment

How to Interpret Audiograms

The audiogram is the key to numerous clinical decisions that will be made as clients/patients and clinicians work together toward reducing or ameliorating the effects of hearing loss on communication. The **audiogram** is a graphic display of an individual's hearing levels or, more specifically, his or her hearing thresholds. It contains information about responses to simple sounds (pure tones). In this section we will focus on interpreting the symbols for responses to tones typically presented on an audiogram, relating this information to the acoustics of sound previously discussed, and beginning to consider the potential impact of various audiometric profiles on communication.

Understanding the information contained in an audiogram enables clinicians not only to use the information to their clients' advantage, but also to request additional

TABLE 2.3 Comparison of Units of Measure Used in the MKS and cgs Metric Systems

Unit	MKS	cgs
Length	meter (m)	centimeter (cm)
Mass	kilogram (kg)	gram (g)
Time	second (sec)	second (sec)
Force	newton (N)	dyne
Pressure	newton per meter squared (N/m^2) or pascal (Pa)	dyne/cm^2
Sound intensity (dB IL)	Reference is W/cm^2	
Sound pressure (dB SPL)	Reference is 20 µPa	Reference is 1 dyne/cm^2

29

•

Application of
Acoustic Concepts
to Reading
Audiograms and to
Understanding the
Listening
Environment

TABLE 2.4 Summary of Important Terms/Units of Measure Related to the Acoustics of Sound

newton (N): Unit of measure of force (a push or a pull; the product of mass and acceleration) in the MKS system. The force required to accelerate a mass of one kilogram from a velocity of 0 meters per second to a velocity of 1 meter per second in 1 second of time.

dyne: Unit of measure of force in the cgs system. The force required to accelerate a mass of 1 gram (g) from a velocity of 0 centimeters per second to a velocity of 1 centimeter per second in 1 second of time. One newton equals 100,000 dynes.

pressure: Amount of force per unit area. Unit of measure is the newton per square meter (N/m^2) or dynes/centimeter squared or pascals (Pa). When the referent is 20 micropascals (μPa) we refer to dB SPL. $1 Pa = 1 N/m^2 = 10 dynes/cm^2$.

bel: Named after Alexander Graham Bell; measure of relative sound intensity (based on a referent); a logarithmic scale.

decibel (dB): one-tenth of a bel.

dB SPL (sound pressure level): Relative intensity of a sound based on a referent intensity of dynes per square centimeter. Sound pressure level can also be referenced to 20 micropascals (μPa)

dB IL (intensity level): Relative intensity of a sound based on a referent intensity of watts per square centimeter (W/cm^2).

watt (W): Unit of measure of power.

dB HL (hearing level): Level of sound in decibels referenced to audiometric zero. Used regularly in audiometry.

hertz (Hz): Unit of measure for frequency, the rate at which vibratory motion occurs; the number of cycles occurring in one second. Former unit of measure was cycles per second (cps).

Source: Speaks (1992).

information that may influence therapeutic approaches when the need arises. The audiogram is a graph designed to record a person's hearing levels for frequencies that are important for hearing and understanding speech. These frequencies fall between 125 Hz (male voicing fundamental frequency) and 8,000 Hz (upper limits of voiceless fricatives such as /s/ and /θ/ [voiceless "th"]). Average conversational speech is typically at 20–50 dB HL when presented from a distance of 3 ft in a quiet setting. Hearing levels that fall within the normal range allow the listener access to these speech sounds. In addition, the audiogram provides a graphic representation of reduced access to important speech sounds in individuals who have hearing loss. As such, it is a very important tool for both the audiologist and the speech–language pathologist.

Frequency and Intensity

Figure 2.10 shows the standard graph, or audiogram, used to record hearing test results. Frequency is across the top of the audiogram, beginning with 125 Hz (a relatively low

30

Chapter 2
Acoustics of
Sound and
Preliminary
Clinical
Application

FIGURE **2.10** **Sample audiogram with symbols.**

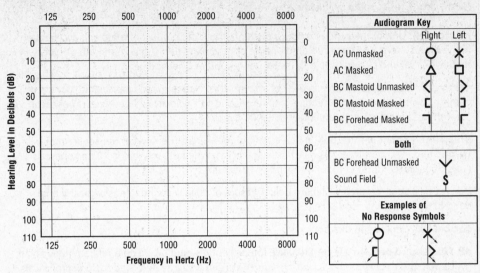

Source: ASHA (1990). Reprinted by permission.

frequency containing fewer cycles per second) and ending with 8,000 Hz (a relatively high frequency containing a greater number of cycles per second). The intensity of the sound is labeled on the left side of the audiogram, in decibels, with 0 dB HL (a relatively soft sound) on the top and 110 dB HL (a relatively intense sound) on the bottom. When symbols are recorded on the audiogram, this is a representation of the softest sound (in dB HL) the individual hears for each of the frequencies tested. In other words, we have recorded the **thresholds,** or levels at which an individual "barely hears" the sound, for a variety of frequencies.

Recall that a decibel is a logarithmic measure that represents a ratio between a given sound pressure and a reference sound pressure. In the case of the audiogram, the reference used is **hearing level (HL)**, and dB HL means the decibel reading on the audiometer dial. Another important point is that for each of the frequencies across the top of the audiogram, audiometric zero (or 0 dB HL) represents a different amount of sound pressure. As you will note in Table 2.5, 45 dB SPL is required to create movement of the eardrum in the average person at 125 Hz, but only 10 dB of sound pressure is required at 3,000 Hz if TDH-39 earphones are used. Rather than deal with these different sound pressure values—all of which represent threshold at different frequencies—the audiometer represents threshold, regardless of the frequency, as 0 dB. This means that an audiometer set to 0 dB at 125 Hz produces 45 dB SPL at the eardrum, but an audiometer set to 0 dB at 3,000 Hz delivers only 10 dB. If the audiogram uses a different referent, such as sound pressure level or dB SPL, the graph looks different and categorizing the degree of hearing loss is less straightforward. In addition, regarding the various

31

•

Application of
Acoustic Concepts
to Reading
Audiograms and to
Understanding the
Listening
Environment

TABLE 2.5 **Standard Output Levels for 0 dB HL for Various Earphones**

Frequency in Hz	Supra-Aural Earphones			Insert Earphones (HA-1 Coupler)
	IEC 60318-3	TDH-39	TDH-49/50	
125	45.0	45.0	47.5	26.5
250	27.0	25.5	26.5	14.5
500	13.5	11.5	13.5	6.0
1,000	7.5	7.0	7.5	0.0
2,000	9.0	9.0	11.0	2.5
3,000	11.5	10.0	9.5	2.5
4,000	12.0	9.5	10.5	0.0
6,000	16.0	15.5	13.5	−2.5
8,000	15.5	13.0	13.0	−3.5
Speech	20.0	19.5	20.0	12.5

Source: Excerpted from ANSI S3.6-2004 American National Standard Specification for Audiometers, © 2004 with the permission of the Acoustical Society of America, 35 Pinelawn Road, Suite 114E, Melville, NY 11747.

amounts of sound pressure required at different frequencies to arrive at 0 dB HL, significantly greater sound pressure is needed at lower frequencies. Thus, the audiometer has a more limited output at lower frequencies, sometimes only reaching 70 or 75 dB HL at the lowest test frequency.

Before we look at the various categories of hearing loss and scales for defining the degree of hearing loss and the symbols that represent test results for the right and left ears, the following useful frames of reference should be remembered. First, the closer the symbols on the audiogram are to 0 dB HL (the top of the audiogram), the better the individual's hearing. Second, the intensity level of *average* conversational speech is approximately 50 dB HL. Since this is an average, some speech sounds will be softer than this level and others will more intense. The softer sounds (e.g., voiceless "th" is approximately 20 dB HL) are of particular importance, because even a mild degree of hearing loss can render them inaudible. These frames of reference will be important as you read various illustrations and case examples, linking the foundation in acoustics, interpreting audiograms, and considering the effects of various hearing levels/degrees of hearing loss on communication. In keeping with this approach to audiogram interpretation, audiograms throughout this text will represent the right and left ears on the same graph, using separate symbols for each ear, consistent with the American Speech-Language-Hearing Association (ASHA) conventions (ASHA, 1990). This reflects a more comprehensive and integrated view of the individual's auditory status and his or her communicative needs, compared to a system used by some audiologists, in which data from each ear are recorded on separate graphs.

32
•
Chapter 2
Acoustics of
Sound and
Preliminary
Clinical
Application

Fundamental Pathways of Sound

Air Conduction

Figure 2.11 is a very basic diagram of the ear with a sample of the structures of each of the three sections of the ear: the outer, middle, and inner ears. The sound wave, produced by some disturbance of air molecules, is picked up by the pinna and carried to the ear canal. As shown in Figure 2.11, these two structures are part of the outer ear. The sound hits the eardrum, which is a structure that borders the outer and middle ears. As the eardrum vibrates, it carries sound into the middle ear space and across the three smallest bones of the body, called the ossicles. The third ossicle, called the stapes, fits directly into the oval window, which is the entrance point to the inner ear. As the stapes rocks in and out of the oval window, fluid in the inner ear moves, and this movement of fluid (in ways that are not completely understood) causes us to hear. Because of special neurons in the inner ear, sound is carried from the cochlea to the brainstem.

The process just described, in very basic terms, is the **air conduction pathway** of sound. Note that the sound travels through all three sections of the ear. This is the normal route of hearing, and the most efficient method of hearing for most people because it makes use of all of the structures of the auditory system, which are designed to help us to hear.

FIGURE **2.11**   **Primary pathway of sound for air conduction.**

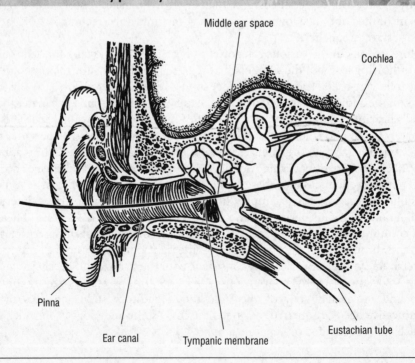

Middle ear space

Cochlea

Pinna

Ear canal

Tympanic membrane

Eustachian tube

Any disorder or pathology at any place in the pathway can affect air conduction hearing. So, any problem in the outer, middle, or inner ear can affect hearing by air conduction. Let's examine a few examples. One of the most common problems audiologists see is wax that builds up in the ear canal. What will happen as the sound travels down the ear canal of a person who has wax in his ear? The sound will become either partially or completely blocked, and the person may experience hearing loss. What about a person who has a hole (also referred to as a perforation) in one eardrum? As the sound strikes the eardrum, the vibration of the drum can be affected by the hole, depending on its size and location, and this can create hearing loss. Finally, what happens to the college student who listens to very loud music regularly through headphones? This can damage part of the cochlea, which is located in the inner ear, and once again can cause hearing loss. It should be clear at this point what the air conduction pathway is and that pathology at any point in the air conduction system can create hearing loss.

Bone Conduction

We have just described the air conduction pathway as sending sound to the inner ear by way of the outer and middle ears. The **bone conduction pathway** largely bypasses the outer and middle ears, and sends the sound directly to the inner ear. As noted in Figure 2.12, the sound wave does not pass through the ear canal and does not vibrate the eardrum or the ossicles of the middle ear space. Instead, through subtle vibration of the bones of the skull, the sound is sent directly to the cochlea, which is part of the inner ear.

FIGURE **2.12**   **Pathway of sound for bone conduction.**

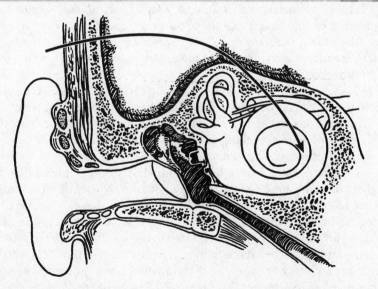

Note: Secondary effects of the middle ear on bone conduction results are not shown.

34

•

Chapter 2
Acoustics of
Sound and
Preliminary
Clinical
Application

Unlike air conduction, this is not the normal route of sound, and for most individuals it is not the most efficient method of hearing. In fact, it takes considerably more energy to stimulate the cochlea directly through the bones of the skull than via the normal air conduction route. The impact of this on bone conduction testing will be discussed in Chapter 4.

As stated earlier, any problem in the auditory system can potentially affect air conduction hearing. In view of the pathway that bone conduction takes, is this also true of bone conduction? In order to answer this question, let's examine the same examples discussed previously. The first example was wax in the ear canal; bone conduction hearing would not be affected by this, because the sound would not be sent down the ear canal. Similarly, a hole in the eardrum would not affect bone conduction hearing because the sound would not hit the eardrum. Taking this a step further, any problem in the outer or middle parts of the auditory system should not have a significant effect on bone conduction hearing. What about the college student who has damaged the cochlea due to noise exposure? Hearing by bone conduction *would* be affected by this, because the problem lies in the inner ear.

Air and Bone Conduction Relationships

One of the most important diagnostic tools for audiologists is to compare the results of air and bone conduction testing in order to determine whether the hearing loss is in the outer/middle ear system or in the inner ear system. Air conduction is tested with the client wearing earphones (testing the entire auditory system), and bone conduction is tested with the person wearing a bone vibrator (testing only the inner ear and, for the most part, bypassing the outer and middle ears) to isolate the sensorineural component. By comparing air conduction with bone conduction findings, an audiologist gains essential diagnostic information. Figures 2.13, 2.14, and 2.15 present basic graphs on which air and bone results have been plotted. Note that frequency is represented across the top (the *x* axis) of the graph and intensity is plotted from top to bottom (the *y* axis). These terms will be described in greater detail in Chapter 4, but for now let's examine the graphs and the air and bone conduction findings to learn the relationships between them.

Figure 2.13 is the client who has wax in the ear canal. Although ideally a client with wax in the ear canal would have this addressed prior to having his hearing tested, for the purposes of this discussion, assume that this was not the case. Note that the air conduction responses are not falling within the normal region. This is consistent with what we said earlier: air conduction can be affected by pathology in any part of the auditory system. By looking at just the air conduction findings, the audiologist knows that the client has some hearing loss but does not know whether that hearing loss is in the outer/middle ear system or in the inner ear system. However, when we compare air conduction with bone conduction, it becomes clear that the problem lies in the outer/middle ear system because bone conduction is unaffected by the problem. Note that this is the same pattern that is obtained in Figure 2.14 for the client who has a hole in her eardrum, because once again bone conduction is not influenced by problems in the outer or middle ears. The fact that Figures 2.13 and 2.14 are the same also illustrates that a comparison of air and bone conduction testing does not tell the audiologist what

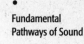

FIGURE 2.13   Air–bone relationship for client with wax blockage (a form of outer ear pathology).

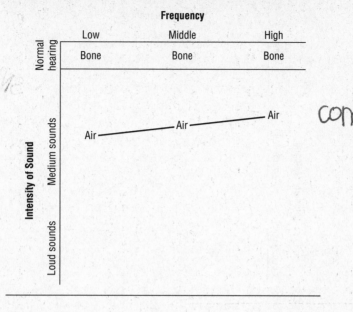

conductive

FIGURE 2.14   Air–bone relationship for client with a hole in the eardrum (a form of middle ear pathology).

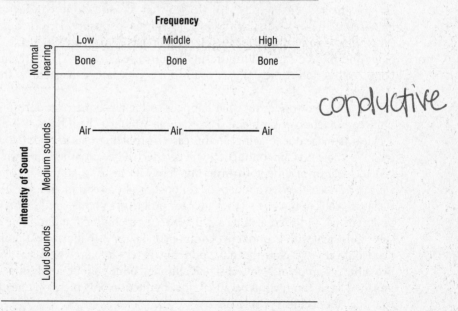

conductive

36
•
Chapter 2
Acoustics of
Sound and
Preliminary
Clinical
Application

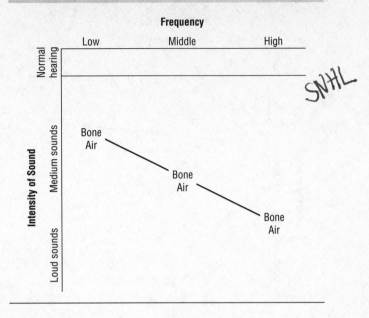

FIGURE **2.15** **Air–bone relationship for client with history of noise exposure (a form of inner ear pathology).**

the specific disorder is, but gives general information about the presence of a gap or a difference between air conduction and bone conduction hearing, with the gap (or difference) representing the conductive component. This relationship between air and bone conduction results also provides information about which part or parts of the ear are affected. In Figure 2.15, we see that air and bone conduction are equally impaired in this individual with a history of noise exposure. This is consistent with our earlier discussion because for this client, who has damage to her cochlea, bypassing the outer and middle ears will not result in improved hearing. Equally impaired air and bone conduction scores (i.e., no air–bone gap) are consistent with an inner ear disorder.

You may be wondering what happens to the air–bone relationship if a person has some combination of problems. For example, what if a client has wax buildup and some cochlear damage due to aging? In this case, a problem exists in both the outer and inner ears. We know that air conduction will be affected because there are two problems, wax and cochlear involvement, that can interfere with hearing, so the air conduction results will not be normal. What about bone conduction? Bone conduction will be affected by the cochlear problem but not by the outer ear problem, so bone conduction results will also be abnormal, and there will be a gap between air conduction and bone conduction results, consistent with a conductive component. Figure 2.16 illustrates the air–bone pattern that would emerge. Note that air conduction is very impaired because of the effect of the two different problems. Note also that although bone conduction is impaired, it is not as impaired as air conduction because bone conduction only picks up one of the two problems (i.e., the cochlear problem).

FIGURE 2.16   Air–bone relationship for client with combined wax blockage and cochlear damage.

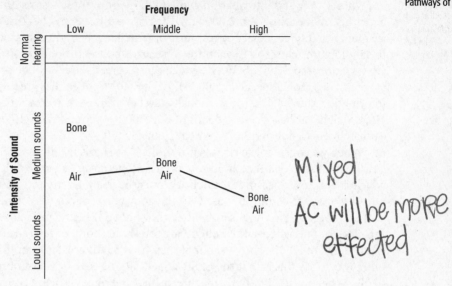

Mixed
AC will be more
effected

Symbols Used for Air Conduction

In addition to the previously discussed graph of frequency and intensity, audiograms contain a key including symbols and an explanation of what the symbols represent. These symbols will now replace the Air and Bone symbols that were just used in this chapter. Commonly used symbols are shown in Figure 2.17. For a more exhaustive discussion of the standards for audiometric symbols, refer to ASHA (1990). As you can see from the figure, the convention is to use a circle (O) to represent the right ear and a cross (X) to represent the left ear. These symbols are used to record the responses to sound obtained while the individual wears earphones. Sound traveling through earphones enters the auditory system and affects the entire auditory pathway (outer, middle, and inner ears), as discussed previously. In other words, sound introduced through earphones to the auditory system travels via air conduction, so the symbols O and X represent responses to air-conducted sounds for the right and left ears, respectively. Responses to signals presented via air conduction (the Os and Xs on the audiogram) correspond to the degree of hearing or hearing loss an individual possesses. Traditionally, the symbols for the right ear were recorded in red and the symbols for the left ear were recorded in blue. With the increased use of copy machines, facsimilies, and other technology, the use of

FIGURE 2.17   Audiogram key.

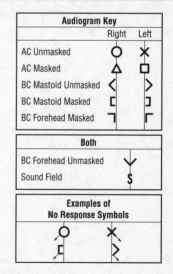

Source: ASHA (1990). Reprinted by permission.

38

•

Chapter 2
Acoustics of
Sound and
Preliminary
Clinical
Application

two colors is less common, but this system is particularly useful when students are learning how to record and interpret audiograms.

Look at the responses plotted for the right and left ears for the frequency 2,000 Hz in Figure 2.18. What information can you draw from these test results? Which ear has better hearing sensitivity at 2,000 Hz? The right ear has better hearing sensitivity at the frequency of interest, since the response obtained for the right ear is closer to the top of the audiogram (closer to 0) than the left-ear response. If the intensity level of average conversational speech is 50 dB HL, which ear has greater access to the components of average conversational speech at 2,000 Hz? Again, the right ear has greater access to speech information at 2,000 Hz. If the intensity level of average conversational speech is 50 dB HL, the right ear has access to 35 dB of our 2,000-Hz sound (50 – 15 dB), while the left ear has access to only 5 dB of sound at 2,000 Hz (50 – 45 dB).

When we consider the client's threshold as the basis for discussion of sound intensity, we are using that threshold as a point of reference. As you will learn, the decibel, which is a unit of measure of intensity, must have a referent and there are numerous referents that are commonly used. In the above discussion, we considered the client's access to speech based on his individual threshold of hearing in each ear at 2,000 Hz. In this case, for the right ear, the individual's threshold (point of reference) is 15 dB and the input signal of 50 dB (conversational speech) is 35 dB greater than this threshold. Another way to say this is that the input signal (50 dB) is 35 dB **sensation level (SL)** or 35 dB SL. When we see 35 dB SL, this means that the signal is being considered relative to the client's own threshold. Assume that the input signal remains at 50 dB and the client's threshold is now 20 dB. What is the sensation level of the input signal? It is 30 dB SL.

FIGURE 2.18 **Air conduction thresholds at 2,000 Hz indicating normal hearing sensitivity in the right ear and a hearing loss in the left ear.**

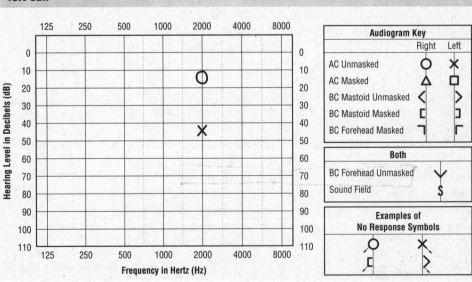

Degrees of Hearing Loss

The audiogram is a record of an individual's hearing levels for frequencies from 125 to 8,000 Hz. As stated previously, responses to air-conducted stimuli provide us with the degree of hearing sensitivity or hearing loss. Once hearing levels are recorded, it is clinically useful to consider whether they are in the range of normal hearing sensitivity. Hearing levels recorded outside the normal range represent degrees of hearing loss on a continuum from mild to profound. For adults, the following categories are typically used to classify the degree of hearing or hearing loss present (Bess and Humes, 1995):

−10 to 25 dB HL	normal range
26 to 40 dB HL	mild hearing loss
41 to 55 dB HL	moderate hearing loss
56 to 70 dB HL	moderately severe hearing loss
71 to 90 dB HL	severe hearing loss
91+ dB HL	profound hearing loss

For children, the classification of degree of hearing loss differs somewhat, recognizing that even a slight loss of hearing sensitivity can have a significant effect on a young child who is acquiring language. With this in mind, for young children we believe hearing levels should be categorized as follows:

−10 to 15 dB HL	normal range
16 to 25 dB HL	slight hearing loss
26 to 40 dB HL	mild hearing loss
41 to 55 dB HL	moderate hearing loss
56 to 70 dB HL	moderately severe hearing loss
71 to 90 dB HL	severe hearing loss
91+ dB HL	profound hearing loss

As Haggard and Primus (1999) point out, classification systems such as those above provide a "systematic way to measure and classify the degree of hearing loss" (p. 83). They further state that numerous systems have been developed, largely to assist clinicians in the process of counseling individuals regarding their hearing loss and associated implications for communication. Haggard and Primus (1999) studied parents' perceptions of the degree of difficulty associated with three of the categories of childhood hearing loss above—slight, mild, and moderate. In general, there was a discrepancy between the standard terminology and the degree of difficulty perceived by the parents, so that, for example, a mild hearing loss as conventionally measured and described was termed "serious" or "handicapping" in many instances. The potential mismatch between the terms used to categorize degrees of hearing loss and the perceived communication deficit imposed by the hearing loss should be kept in mind during audiogram interpretation, to avoid minimizing the potential effect of the hearing loss on communication.

Many authorities in the field of audiology now believe that the term *mild hearing loss* is confusing, especially when applied to children. The thresholds on the audiogram may fall into the mild range, but the effects on the child in real-world environments can be great. It is the responsibility of the audiologist and speech–language pathologist to

40
•
Chapter 2
Acoustics of
Sound and
Preliminary
Clinical
Application

educate others about this potential pitfall. Numerous factors in addition to the audiogram itself come into play during interpretation of test results. These considerations will be addressed more fully in Chapter 12, concerning management of hearing loss. They include, but are not limited to, the patient's age, lifestyle, hobbies, and vocation/occupation.

Symbols Used for Bone Conduction

Responses to pure tone stimuli presented by bone conduction are represented on the audiogram by "carats": < for the right ear and > for the left ear. The placement of these symbols on the audiogram is the opposite of what you might expect: the left-ear symbol for bone conduction is recorded to the right of the line for the test frequency on the audiogram; and conversely, the right-ear symbol for bone conduction is recorded to the left of the line for the frequency of interest on the audiogram. This makes more intuitive sense if you think of facing the patient/client and consider where the signal is being routed, as shown in Figure 2.19.

These symbols < and > are used to record the responses to sound obtained while the individual wears a bone conduction vibrator. Sound traveling in this manner (via bone conduction) enters the auditory system through the skull and affects the inner ear directly (bypassing the outer and middle ears), as discussed previously. In other words, sound introduced through the bone vibrator to the auditory system travels via bone conduction, so the symbols < and > represent responses to bone-conducted sounds for the right and left ears, respectively.

While responses to air-conducted signals indicate the degree of hearing loss, responses to bone-conducted signals provide insight regarding the *type* of hearing loss present. The type of hearing loss (sometimes referred to as the *nature* of the hearing loss) will fall into one of three categories: conductive, sensorineural, or mixed. It should also be noted that a given ear might have more than one type of hearing loss, as some of the examples that follow will illustrate. The type or nature of hearing loss is determined by comparing the test results obtained by air conduction with those obtained by bone conduction.

In an **audiogram showing conductive hearing loss,** the air conduction results are outside the normal hearing range and the bone conduction results are within the range of normal hearing, as shown in Figure 2.20. The resulting audiometric pattern contains an "air–bone gap," reflecting normal hearing sensitivity via bone conduction (or when the inner ear receives the signal directly) compared with abnormal hearing sensitivity when the signal must travel through the entire auditory system (outer, middle, and inner ears). An air–bone gap is defined as a difference, in decibels, between thresholds obtained by air conduction and thresholds

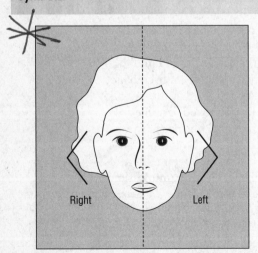

FIGURE 2.19 **Depiction of a face and ears as a method for remembering the correct use of right and left unmasked bone conduction symbols.**

Right   Left

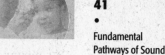

FIGURE 2.20 Mild conductive hearing loss (air–bone gap) in the right ear at 2,000 Hz.

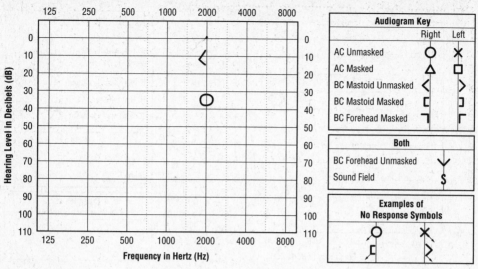

obtained by bone conduction at a particular frequency in an ear. This audiometric pattern is consistent with a problem in the outer and/or middle ear systems. Not infrequently, conductive hearing losses may be reduced or resolved through some type of medical or possibly otological management.

In an **audiogram showing sensorineural hearing loss,** the air and bone conduction results are similar to each other (or the same) and both air and bone conduction results are outside the normal range. An example of results consistent with sensorineural hearing loss appears in Figure 2.21. Because both air and bone conduction results in this case are abnormal to the same degree, we can conclude that the site of auditory dysfunction is in the inner ear, involving the cochlea and/or eighth cranial nerve. Sensorineural hearing loss is usually permanent, and management efforts typically include the use of hearing aids/amplification, along with other devices and strategies that are discussed in Chapter 12. In general, when testing adults, an air–bone gap of 10 dB HL or less is not considered clinically significant (i.e., is not consistent with a significant conductive component in the hearing loss). For young children, however, an air–bone gap of 10 dB HL may be significant. In either case, consideration is also given to results of middle ear analysis (tympanometry) and other tests as appropriate when the type of hearing loss is being determined. This will be discussed further in Chapter 6.

As the name implies, a hearing loss that is mixed in nature includes both conductive and sensorineural elements, and an air–bone gap is present. In an **audiogram showing mixed hearing loss,** neither the air conduction threshold nor the bone conduction threshold is in the normal hearing range. This situation is shown in Figure 2.22. This audiometric pattern indicates that dysfunction exists in both the conducting portion of the auditory system (outer and/or middle ear) and the sensorineural portion

42

Chapter 2
Acoustics of
Sound and
Preliminary
Clinical
Application

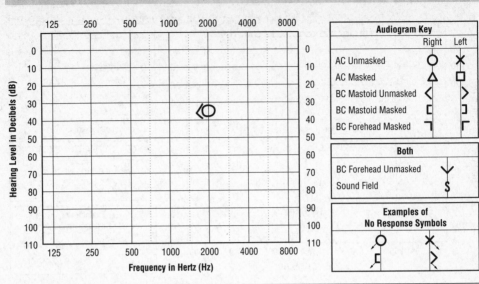

FIGURE **2.21**   **Mild sensorineural hearing loss in the right ear at 2,000 Hz.**

of the auditory system (inner ear). Management considerations for a mixed hearing loss may be two-pronged, including medical or otological intervention to address the outer and/or middle ear (conductive) component of the hearing loss and amplification/aural rehabilitation to address the remaining sensorineural hearing loss.

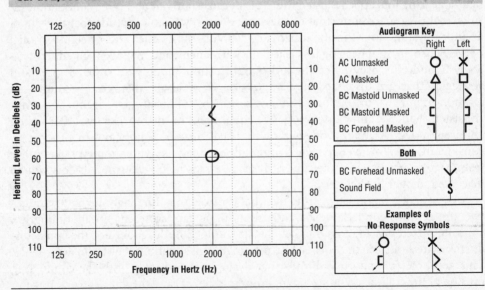

FIGURE **2.22**   **Moderately severe mixed hearing loss in the right ear at 2,000 Hz.**

It is not unusual to find asymmetrical hearing levels when comparing the right and left ears during audiometric testing/audiological evaluation. In instances where a sufficient difference exists when hearing thresholds by air conduction (in the test ear) are compared to hearing thresholds by bone conduction (in the non-test ear), it becomes necessary to employ masking to ensure that the better ear is not participating in the responses from the poorer ear. In other words, if the signal presented to the poorer ear is sufficiently intense, and the hearing in the opposite ear is good enough, it is possible for the intense signal to "cross over" via the bones of the skull to the good ear. Masking helps us to establish that the measured response is a true reflection of the hearing sensitivity of the test (poorer) ear and not influenced by participation from the non-test (better) ear. Masking may be required during either air or bone conduction testing. In audiology, **masking** is defined as "noise used in an attempt to eliminate the participation of one ear while the opposite ear is being tested" (Nicolosi, Harryman, & Krescheck, 1989, p. 159). Different types of sounds are used during masking, depending on the stimulus.

In addition to the symbols used for recording unmasked air and bone conduction results, Figure 2.17, the audiogram key, also contains the symbols [and], which are used to record results obtained during bone conduction testing when masking has been employed to isolate the test ear from the non-test ear. As in the case of unmasked bone conduction, the symbol recorded to the right of the line reflects the status of the left inner ear (cochlea) and was obtained with masking in the right ear. The symbol recorded to the left of the line reflects results from the right inner ear and was obtained with masking in the left ear. At this point you should be able to examine Figure 2.23 and should know the following:

FIGURE 2.23 **Left masked bone conduction testing revealing the type of loss in the left ear to be sensorineural.**

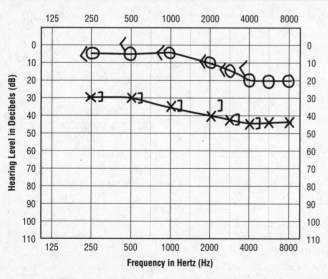
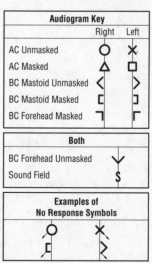

44
•

Chapter 2
Acoustics of
Sound and
Preliminary
Clinical
Application

- Assuming the client is an adult, the right ear hearing is within normal limits and has no gap between air and bone conduction.
- A mild to moderate hearing loss exists in the left ear.
- Because of the absence of air–bone gaps in the left ear, the type of loss is sensorineural.
- The left bone conduction responses, recorded using the masked symbol (]), were obtained with masking in the right ear.

Symbols Used for Masked Air Conduction Testing

Closer inspection of the symbols for air conduction testing will reveal additional symbols: a triangle for the right ear (Δ) and a box (□) for the left ear. As already stated, in instances in which a sufficient difference exists when hearing thresholds by air conduction (in the test ear) are compared to hearing thresholds by bone conduction (in the non-test ear), it becomes necessary to deliver masking noise to the non-test ear, so that the non-test ear does not "participate" in the test or contribute to the response of the test ear. In other words, the masking noise is used to occupy or "block out" the non-test ear.

Figure 2.24 shows the air conduction results obtained for the right ear at 1,000 Hz when masking was used to eliminate the participation of the non-test (left) ear. At this point, you should understand the following based on the symbols recorded on the audiogram:

- Hearing sensitivity is within normal limits in the left ear.
- The use of masking was necessary at 1,000 Hz.

FIGURE **2.24** **Use of masking for both air and bone conduction testing of the right ear.**

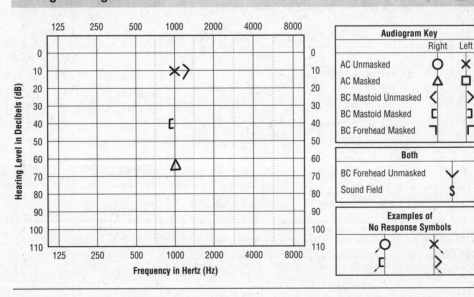

- When the right ear air conduction threshold at 1,000 Hz was being established, masking noise was delivered to the left (non-test) ear.
- Masking was also necessary to establish the right ear bone conduction response at 1,000 Hz.
- The type of the right ear hearing loss is mixed because there is an air–bone gap *and* the bone conduction masked threshold is not in the normal range.

Mastery of the symbols for air and bone conduction and knowledge of the degrees and types of hearing loss form the foundation for understanding audiological case management. For example, if the type of hearing loss is conductive, a referral to a physician will likely be made. If the type of hearing loss is sensorineural and the degree sufficient, recommendations will most likely include consideration of amplification. In addition to awareness of these more general aspects of audiological case management, speech–language pathologists and other professionals working with an individual with a hearing loss should understand how the audiogram and the information it contains relates to something called the "average speech spectrum."

Work published by French and Steinberg in 1947 discussed the characteristics of speech, hearing, and noise in relation to recognition of speech sounds by the ear. Much of the work reported in this paper was based on earlier work done at Bell Laboratoies. Researchers' interests in this topic stemmed in part from the need to determine what components of speech were critical to speech intelligibility so those components could be transmitted efficiently over a speech communication system such as the telephone. Factors related to the intelligibility of speech included the loudness of the signal reaching the ear, as well as effects of echoes, reverberation, and unwanted (masking) noise.

To be complete, audiogram interpretation must include not only the type (or nature) and degree of the hearing loss present, but also the probable impact of those findings on understanding speech. Looking at the frequency–intensity information of familiar sounds in Figure 2.25, consider the specific speech sounds carried by the lower frequencies and those carried by the higher frequencies. While this visual representation is a useful tool for counseling purposes, speech–language pathologists and audiologists should also be familiar with the more detailed relationships between frequency and acoustic cues for speech perception summarized earlier in Table 2.2.

The concept of the "average speech spectrum" was described by French and Steinberg (1947). They recognized that speech is a succession of sounds varying rapidly over time in both intensity and frequency. In addition, for listeners to understand a speech signal, the signal must reach the ear with sufficient intensity. They further recognized that vowels as a group tend to be lower in frequency and higher in intensity, while consonants are higher in frequency and lower in intensity. Tests called articulation tests were conducted to study the relative importance of the contributions of speech components in different frequency regions to the intelligibility of speech. For calculation purposes, the frequency range was divided into "bands" and the bands were weighted to reflect the differential contribution of lower and higher frequencies to speech intelligibility. The resulting **articulation index (AI)**, now more commonly referred to as the **audibility index,** that was derived from these calculations is a number ranging from 0.0 to 1.0 and reflects the degree to which the total speech signal is audible to the listener.

46
•
Chapter 2
Acoustics of
Sound and
Preliminary
Clinical
Application

FIGURE **2.25** **Frequency spectrum of familiar sounds plotted on an audiogram.**

Shaded area represents the "speech banana" that contains most of the sound elements of spoken speech.

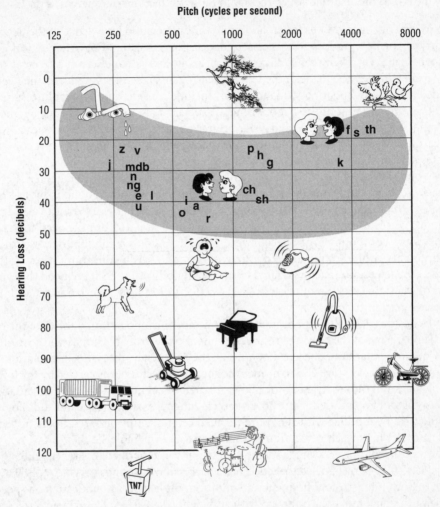

Source: Northern, J., & Downs, M. (2002). *Hearing in children* (5th ed.). New York: Lippincott, Williams & Wilkins. Reprinted by permission.

The audibility index is a useful construct as we look at audiograms and consider what part of the average speech spectrum is (or is not) audible to a listener. The audiogram is a graphic display of an individual's hearing levels, or, more specifically, his or her hearing thresholds. It contains information about responses to simple sounds (pure tones). In this section, we will focus on interpreting the symbols for responses to tones typically presented on an audiogram, relating this information to the acoustics of sound previously discussed, and beginning to consider the potential impact of various audiometric profiles on communication.

A visual representation of the audibility index (AI) is found in Figure 2.26. When speech is presented at a conversational intensity level (50 dB HL) to an individual with normal hearing sensitivity, that individual has access to all of the sounds contained in the "average speech spectrum." For individuals with hearing loss, access to the average speech spectrum will be compromised depending on the degree and configuration of the hearing loss. A variation on this theme is the speech intelligibility index (SII), a measure ranging from 0.0 to 1.0, that is strongly related to a person's ability to understand speech (Hornsby, 2004). The SII is also a way of measuring the proportion of speech cues that are audible to and usable for a listener. An SII of 0.0 means that none of the speech information is available in a setting, whereas an SII of 1.0 suggests that all of the speech cues are available and usable to the listener. Clinically, audiologists continue to use the audibility index, but the SII will most likely gain favor over time. We will revisit this concept in Chapter 12 when we cover assessment of benefit from amplification relative to improved access to speech sounds and improved speech understanding.

Begin to think about the implications of partial or absent auditory cues for communication in general. This information on audibility of the speech signal will be expanded in other chapters and is a critical link between diagnostics and rehabilitation. Familiarity with these concepts forms a foundation for providing communication assistance to individuals with hearing loss and their families for audiologists, speech–language pathologists, and members of other professional disciplines who encounter individuals with hearing loss.

Environmental Acoustics

Audiologists and speech–language pathologists are regularly faced with the unfortunate reality that, despite increased awareness over the years, hearing loss remains a hidden impairment and its effects are regularly overlooked. As we continue to work to educate others about the serious effects of hearing loss, we must address another reality: it is not hearing loss alone that can interfere with an individual's ability to understand incoming speech and language information. A poor acoustic environment can add distortion to or subtract information from the original acoustic signal, resulting in deterioration of the message and misinterpretation by the listener. Although this can be problematic for all listeners, the resulting difficulty may be compounded for individuals who have hearing loss, developmental disabilities, learning disabilities, or for whom English is a second language (ASHA, 1995).

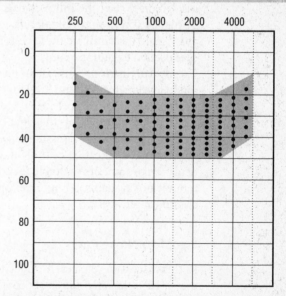

FIGURE **2.26**   **Count-the-dots audiogram form.**

Source: Mueller, G., & Killion, M. (1990). An easy method for calculating the articulation index. *The Hearing Journal, 45*(9), 14–17. Reprinted by permission.

48

•

Chapter 2
Acoustics of
Sound and
Preliminary
Clinical
Application

Acoustics is the study and science of sound and sound perception. Because most of the research regarding acoustics and speech perception involves school environments, that is the emphasis of this discussion. Despite this, you should keep in mind that these issues apply to a broad range of environments.

Noise and Its Measurement

Noise is often the first factor that students mention when asked what factors contribute to poor acoustic environments. When asked to give an example of noise, students often mention radio static or the sound of the heater in the classroom. Certainly these are fine examples, but as clients with hearing aids will tell you emphatically, speech can be considered noise if it interferes with what you are trying to understand. As you are talking on the telephone to a friend, the chatter of someone else in the next room is considered noise. In fact, a very helpful definition, for the purposes of this chapter, is to describe **noise** as any unwanted sound.

What is it about this unwanted sound that makes it problematic for people to understand speech? In general, noise blocks out or masks the high-frequency sounds in our language. These sounds are usually the consonants and are typically (but not always) weak in energy. Try saying the unvoiced "th" (θ) sound, as in the word *thumb*, loudly. It is not really possible, because this sound is weak. The same is true for many of the consonants, including *s, sh, t,* and *k.* Noise, on the other hand, tends to be intense and can easily cover (mask) these weaker sounds. Also, noise often contains considerable low-frequency energy. The tendency for low-frequency energy to mask high-frequency sounds is referred to as the upward spread of masking.

Importantly, the high-frequency sounds are the sounds that carry the meaning in our language. Say the following words aloud: *shoe, too, chew,* and *stew.* If the high-frequency consonant information was removed, it would be very difficult, if not impossible, to discriminate these words. The vowel sound would not give us the acoustic cues needed to gain meaning.

Measurement of noise in an environment is accomplished using a device called a sound level meter. A **sound level meter** is an electronic instrument that measures the intensity of sound in decibels (dB). Most sound level meters have three scales, and all have a microphone to pick up the signal being measured. One of the scales, the A scale, is particularly suited for assessing noise in the environment that may be harmful to hearing. Another application of the sound level meter might be to determine whether a particular environment is suitable for conducting hearing screening when a sound-treated room is not available. Sound level meters are also used to assess the amount of noise in classroom settings.

Signal-to-Noise Ratio

In this discussion of speech understanding, it would, of course, be incorrect to imply that noise is the only source of problems. The level of the speech is also a factor. Anyone who has attended a lecture given by a speaker who, even without a microphone, could be heard clearly in the back of the auditorium, knows that the effects of environmental noise can be minimized by increasing the level of the speech signal. Also, research suggests that when in the presence of increasing background noise, speakers tend to increase their vocal intensity in an effort to compensate for the negative effects of noise. Although this may be somewhat helpful to the listener, the positive effects on speech understanding are noted only when the speaker and listener are very close to each other.

The difference in decibels between the level of the signal (usually speech) and the level of the background noise is referred to as the **signal-to-noise (S/N) ratio**. As you will note in the following examples, the calculation is not really a ratio, but a subtraction of the smaller value from the larger value. (We hope that the signal is the larger value, but this is not always the case.) This simple yet important concept will be mentioned in several places throughout the text.

Now let's calculate some signal-to-noise ratios. If the level of the signal is 60 dB and the level of the noise is 50 dB, what is the signal-to-noise ratio? If you answered 10 dB you are correct. What if the signal is 50 dB and the noise is 60 dB? That is a signal-to-noise ratio of −10 dB. Now, what would the values of the signal and noise have to be in order to create a signal-to-noise ratio of 0 dB? They would each have to be of the same intensity level. It should be clear at this point that when the level of the signal exceeds the level of the noise, the signal-to-noise ratio is positive. When the level of the noise exceeds the level of the signal, the signal-to-noise ratio is negative. When the two values are the same, the ratio is 0 dB.

Before examining noise levels of classrooms, remember that the effects of noise on speech understanding are in part related to the listener's language skills and experience. A favorite example of this concept is on a train going to New York City. Because the public announcement system can be very unclear, the announcement of the train's next stop is sometimes nothing more than a combination of static and vowels. Despite this, passengers who travel that route regularly respond immediately to the announcement. Inexperienced passengers, on the other hand, panic because the message was too distorted to understand.

This example should give you some insight into the effects of noise on children. Children are much less able than adults to "fill in" missing information because they do not have the linguistic or experiential base to do so. Children are more dependent than adults on the clarity of the signal. In fact, research indicates that children with normal hearing typically require better signal-to-noise ratios than normal-hearing adults to achieve the same level of speech understanding. To take this one step further, think about the considerable negative effects of noise on a young child who also has a language impairment or a fluctuating conductive hearing loss.

With this background information in mind, let's examine the noise levels and resulting signal-to-noise ratios found by researchers in typical classrooms. Ideally, because of the known negative effects of noise on speech understanding, the signal-to-noise ratio in the typical classroom in the United States would be very favorable. An examination of the data in Table 2.6 suggests that this is not the case.

Across five different studies from 1965 to 1988, the signal-to-noise ratios in classrooms ranged from −7 dB to +5 dB. These ratios would rapidly worsen, of course, if the distance between the child and the speaker increased. In fact, according to the inverse square law (which typically applies at distances of 6 ft or less), as the distance between the speaker and listener is doubled, the sound pressure level (i.e., intensity of speech) decreases by 6 dB. So, if the signal-to-noise ratio is 6 dB at 3 ft, it becomes 0 dB at 6 ft because the intensity of the signal has decreased by 6 dB.

Individuals who have hearing loss are already likely to be missing the consonant sounds in our language, which, as mentioned previously, are the meaning carriers.

50
•
Chapter 2
Acoustics of
Sound and
Preliminary
Clinical
Application

TABLE 2.6   **Summary of Studies Examining Classroom Signal-to-Noise Ratios**

Study	Signal-to-Noise Ratio (dB)
Sanders (1965)	+1 to +5
Paul (1967)	+3
Blair (1977)	−7 to 0
Markides (1986)	+3
Finitzo-Hieber (1988)	+1 to +4

Source: Crandell, C., & Smaldino, J. (2000). Classroom acoustics for children with normal hearing and with hearing impairment. *Language, Speech and Hearing Services in Schools, 31*(4), 362–370. Reprinted by permission.

When noise takes away even more of this important acoustic information, the listener's ability to understand becomes even more compromised.

Research suggests that the minimum signal-to-noise ratio for classrooms of normal-hearing students should be +6 to +12 dB; for students who have hearing loss the ratio should be at least +15 dB. In order for all students to have appropriate acoustical environments, ASHA (2005) recommends a minimum signal-to-noise ratio of +15 dB in educational settings.

Knecht and colleagues (2002) analyzed the noise levels in thirty-two unoccupied elementary classrooms and discovered that only four rooms had background noise below the 35 dB(A) level recommended by the American National Standards Institute (ANSI). Only one room met the stricter criterion of 30 dB(A) set by ASHA. The authors also note that several of the classrooms located in newer schools met the ANSI noise standard. This is encouraging because it suggests that the requirements can be met with appropriate construction planning and design. Also, it was noted that none of the classrooms that had the heating, ventilating, or air conditioning system on during measurement of noise met the criterion. This suggests that a priority when building new schools will be to find heating/cooling systems that operate with less noise than most current systems.

Reverberation

As serious as the problem of noise is, it is rarely the only problem that exists in classroom settings. Because of the predominance of reflective surfaces such as walls, desks, bookcases, and windows, the speech signal that is directed to the students bounces off these surfaces, remains in the acoustic environment, and distorts new information being presented.

To quantify the extent of this problem, **reverberation time** can be measured. This is the amount of time it takes for a sound to decrease by 60 dB once the original sound has been terminated. The greater the reverberation time, the longer the old information is bouncing around the room and the greater is the potential distortion of new information.

Recommended reverberation times for classrooms depend on the size of the room. In general, however, for students who have normal hearing, a reverberation time of

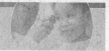

TABLE **2.7** **A Summary of Studies Examining Classroom Reverberation Times**

Study	Reverberation Time (sec)
Kodaras (1960)	0.4 to 1.1
Nabalek and Pickett (1974)	0.5 to 1.0
McCroskey and Devenes (1975)	0.6 to 1.0
Bradley (1986)	0.39 to 1.2
Crandell and Smaldino (1994)	0.35 to 1.2

Source: Crandell, C., & Smaldino, J. (2000). Classroom acoustics for children with normal hearing and with hearing impairment. *Language, Speech and Hearing Services in Schools, 31*(4), 362–370. Reprinted by permission.

0.6 sec should not be exceeded (ANSI, 2002). For children who have hearing loss, reverberation times should not exceed 0.5 to 0.6 sec. Table 2.7 summarizes actual reverberation times in classrooms for five different studies. Note that reverberation times range from 0.35 to 1.2 sec. ASHA guidelines are stricter than those of ANSI and recommend no greater than a 0.4-sec reverberation time (ASHA, 2005).

The ANSI recommendation of maximum permissible reverberation time of 0.6 sec was exceeded by 13 of the 32 classrooms studied by Knecht and colleagues (2002); the ASHA recommendation of maximum reverberation time of 0.4 sec was achieved by only six classrooms. Finally, based on the finding that all classrooms with ceilings of 10 feet or less met the reverberation requirement, the researchers suggest that lower ceilings in classrooms may be helpful.

For purposes of discussion, we have addressed noise and reverberation separately. Logically, these two variables typically occur together in the real world. Together, they have a combined negative effect on speech perception that is greater than the effect of the two factors added together. Specific strategies to deal with noise and reverberation will be addressed in Chapter 12. You may have also noted that different standards exist regarding sound and its measurement. While ASHA provides guidance for practicing clinicians, state and federal regulations generally rely on the standards of ANSI.

ANSI is a private, nonprofit organization made up of technical specialists, manufacturers, and consumers that administers and coordinates the use of standards in a wide variety of fields. These include audiology, medicine, the automotive industry, telecommunications, and electronics. In audiology, for example, ANSI has standards regarding calibration of audiometers (ANSI, 2004), the maximum amount of noise that can be present in a room that is used for hearing testing, and how to measure the characteristics of hearing aids. Standards are important because they facilitate communication among different groups, can lead to improved quality of products that are put on the market, and can provide consumers with increased confidence regarding the quality of the products that they purchase or that are used as part of their care.

The International Organization for Standardization (ISO) is a worldwide federation of national standards bodies from approximately 140 countries. This organization

52

•

Chapter 2
Acoustics of
Sound and
Preliminary
Clinical
Application

also develops standards, many of which are quite similar to those produced by ANSI. The ISO stresses the importance of international standards to promote the efficient exchange of goods among countries, as well as to facilitate the exchange of ideas around the world.

CHAPTER SUMMARY

This chapter presented the physics of sound, considering characteristics of sound such as frequency and intensity. These concepts are a foundation for discussing audiograms and the symbols typically recorded on an audiogram. Following audiogram interpretation, the chapter presented information on environmental acoustics. The concept of the audibility index was also introduced. This information is critical to audiologists, whose primary role and responsibility is the provision of accurate diagnostic information and direction/recommendations for audiological management. Understanding the relationships among acoustics, the audiogram, and the communication implications of different types and degrees of hearing loss is the responsibility of not only the audiologist but also the speech–language pathologist and other professionals working on interdisciplinary teams with individuals with hearing loss.

QUESTIONS FOR DISCUSSION

1. What key points regarding the decibel are illustrated by using the formula

$$\text{dB SPL} = 20 \times \log\left(\frac{\text{output pressure}}{\text{referent pressure}}\right)?$$

2. List five applications that can be made to clinical work using acoustic principles described in this chapter.
3. Describe the two primary factors that can negatively influence room acoustics. List ways to improve room acoustics.
4. Using Air and Bone symbols, draw audiograms for each of the following conditions:
   • Middle ear disease
   • Inner ear hearing loss
   • Combination of middle ear and inner ear difficulties

RECOMMENDED READING

Berlin, C. I. (Revised, 1970). Programmed instruction on the decibel in clinical audiology, Kresge Hearing Research Laboratory of the South, prepared with the Information Center for Hearing, Speech, and Disorders of Human Communication, The Johns Hopkins Medical Institutions, Baltimore, MD 21205.

Fucci, D., & Lass, N. (1999). *Fundamentals of speech science*. Boston: Allyn & Bacon.

Mueller, G., & Killion, M. (1990). An easy method for calculating the articulation index. *The Hearing Journal, 45*(9), 14–17.

Mullin, W., Gerace, W., Mestre, J., & Velleman, S. (2002). *Fundamentals of sound with application to speech and hearing*. Boston: Allyn & Bacon.

American National Standards Institute (ANSI). (2002). Acoustic standards for U.S. classrooms. ANSI S12-60-2002. New York: Author.

American National Standards Institute (ANSI). (2004). Specifications for audiometers. ANSI S3.6-2004. New York: Author.

American Speech-Language-Hearing Association (ASHA). (1990, April). Guidelines for audiometric symbols. *ASHA, 32*(Suppl. 2), 25–30.

American Speech-Language-Hearing Association (ASHA). (1995). Guidelines for acoustics in educational environments. *ASHA, 37*(Suppl. 14), 15–19.

American Speech-Language-Hearing Association (ASHA). (2005). Guidelines for addressing acoustics in educational settings. Available at: www.asha.org/members/deskrefjournals/deskref/default

Berlin, C. I. (Revised, 1970). Programmed instruction on the decibel in clinical audiology, Kresge Hearing Research Laboratory of the South, prepared with the Information Center for Hearing, Speech, and Disorders of Human Communication, The Johns Hopkins Medical Institutions, Baltimore, MD 21205.

Bess, F., & Humes, L. (1995). *Audiology: The fundamentals.* Baltimore: Williams & Wilkins.

Crandell, C., & Smaldino, J. (2000). Classroom acoustics for children with normal hearing and with hearing impairment. *Language, Speech and Hearing Services in Schools, 31*(4), 362–370.

Ferrand, C. T. (2001). *Speech science: An integrated approach to theory and clinical practice* (pp. 162–224). Boston: Allyn & Bacon.

French, N. R., & Steinberg, J. C. (1947). Factors governing the intelligibility of speech sounds. *Journal of the Acoustical Society of America, 19*(1), 90–119.

Fucci, D., & Lass, N. (1999). *Fundamentals of speech science.* Boston: Allyn & Bacon.

Haggard, R. S., & Primus, M. A. (1999). Parental perceptions of hearing loss classification in children. *American Journal of Audiology, 8,* 83–92.

Hornsby, B. (2004). The speech intelligibility index: What is it and what's it good for? *The Hearing Journal, 57*(10), 10–17.

Knecht, H., Nelson, P., Whitelaw, G., & Feth, L. (2002). Background noise levels and reverberation times in unoccupied classrooms: Predictions and measurements. *American Journal of Audiology, 11,* 65–71.

Martin, F., & Clark, J. (2003). *Introduction to audiology* (8th ed.). Boston: Allyn & Bacon.

Mueller, G., & Killion, M. (1990). An easy method for calculating the articulation index. *The Hearing Journal, 45*(9), 14–17.

Nicolosi, L., Harryman, E., & Kresheck, J. (1989). *Terminology of communication disorders: Speech-language-hearing* (3rd ed.). Baltimore: Williams & Wilkins.

Northern, J. L., & Downs, M. P. (2002). *Hearing in children* (5th ed.). Baltimore: Williams & Wilkins.

Speaks, C. (1992). *Introduction to sound: Acoustics for the hearing and speech sciences.* San Diego: Singular Publishing Group.

chapter 3

Anatomy and Physiology of the Auditory System

AFTER COMPLETING THIS CHAPTER, YOU SHOULD BE ABLE TO:

1. Describe the structure and understand the function of the outer, middle, and inner ears.
2. Describe the structure and understand the function of the acoustic reflex arc.
3. Compare and contrast characteristics of inner and outer hair cells.
4. Define fundamental neurological terms.
5. Describe the structure and function of the central auditory system.

This chapter presents the anatomy and physiology of the auditory system. In Chapter 2 we introduced two different pathways of sound that are used in audiology: air conduction and bone conduction. These are relevant to our discussion of anatomy and physiology because these pathways introduce the basic structures of the auditory system and they also introduce the two routes for getting sound to the inner ear. In addition, knowledge of air and bone conduction pathways is related to the discussion in Chapter 2 regarding how to read audiograms.

Anatomy and Physiology of the Peripheral Auditory System

Although the treatment of the auditory system that follows is more detailed than the very basic description in Chapter 2, it is nonetheless basic in that it does not provide in-depth information about any of the topics. This discussion of anatomy and physiology is intended to provide a working knowledge of the auditory system as a foundation for further study in advanced courses, as well as to support understanding of subsequent chapters of this text.

One of the questions that emerges when deciding how best to present information about anatomy and physiology is whether to discuss anatomy (structure) and physiology (function) separately or to combine them. An advantage of combining them is that separating this information can seem artificial; how do we talk meaningfully about a structure without also talking about its function? A disadvantage of combining anatomy and physiology is that understanding how the auditory system operates can become lost in the details involved in learning the system's anatomy.

To address this dilemma, anatomy and physiology are combined and periodic summaries of the physiology of the auditory system are provided to give the student a clear sense of the process of hearing at different stages. We begin with the peripheral auditory system, which is made up of the outer, middle, and inner ears and the eighth cranial nerve.

The Outer Ear

The outer ear consists primarily of two structures: the **pinna** (also referred to as the auricle) and the ear canal (also referred to as the **external auditory canal** or external auditory meatus). These structures are depicted in Figures 3.1 and 3.2. The pinna, or external ear, is made up of cartilage covered with skin and has characteristic folds, or landmarks, as Figure 3.1 shows. At one time, the pinna was seen as mostly cosmetic, meaning it was not believed to have much of a role in hearing. We now know that the pinna does, in fact, have a minor role in hearing. First, the pinna's resonant frequency occurs at approximately 1,500 Hz, meaning that sounds in that frequency region are naturally enhanced. In addition, you may have seen a person cup his hand over his pinna in an effort to improve his hearing. What he is actually doing is increasing the surface area over which sound can be collected, which results in a small advantage in sound collection.

In addition to the role of the pinna as a sound collector, it also makes important contributions to same-side **localization.** When you hear the word *localization* you may think of babies learning to do left/right localization. They turn to the left or to the right as they seek out the source of sound. They do this, in part, because they have two ears

FIGURE **3.1**   **Human pinna and its landmarks.**

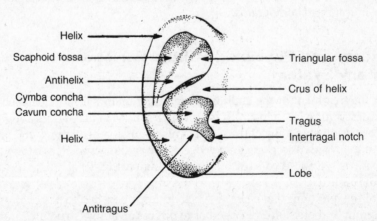

Source: F. N. Martin & J. G. Clark. *Introduction to Audiology,* 9e. Published by Allyn & Bacon, Boston, MA. Copyright © 2006 by Pearson Education. Reprinted by permission of the publisher.

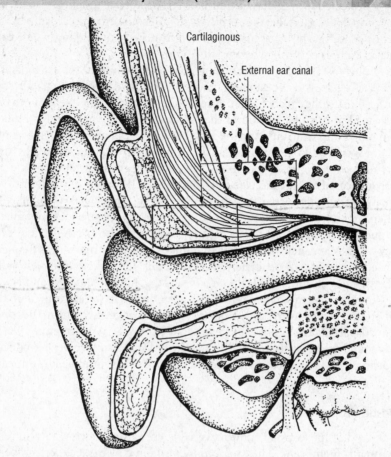

Cartilaginous

External ear canal

1/3 = cartilage
2/3 = bone.

Source: J. L. Northern. *Hearing Disorders,* 3e. Published by Allyn & Bacon, Boston, MA. Copyright ©
1996 by Pearson Education. Reprinted by permission of the publisher.

that are separated by their head. As they mature, they are also able to determine that a
particular sound is on their right side and above them versus being on their right side
and below them. This more sophisticated type of localization is related to the way the
sound wave impacts the various unique cartilaginous features of the pinna illustrated in
Figure 3.1. Sounds coming from different locations impact the pinna at slightly different times, thereby providing different acoustic cues to the listener about the location of
the sound.

The first one-third of the external auditory canal is made of cartilage and, in fact,
that cartilage is continuous with the cartilage of the pinna. The inner two-thirds of the
ear canal, the osseous or bony portion, course through part of the temporal bone of the
skull. The place where the cartilaginous and osseous portions of the external auditory
canal meet is called the **osseocartilaginous junction.** The ear canal has a number of
important functions, one of which is simply to direct sound waves to the eardrum.

Another role of the external auditory canal is to situate the eardrum deep into the skull so that it is protected from external trauma. This protective function also explains the bend that most ear canals take; they typically do not course to the eardrum in a straight fashion, but curve sharply, keeping the eardrum tucked out of danger. The eardrum's location also ensures controlled temperature and humidity.

One of the most important and misunderstood functions of the ear canal is to produce wax (also referred to as **cerumen**). Wax is the result of sebaceous glands, located in the first one-third of the canal, that produce an oily substance called sebum. Wax and hair follicles located in this first section of the ear canal help to repel foreign bodies (both living and nonliving) from entering the ear. Despite the valuable role that wax plays and the frequent warnings to patients not to "put anything into your ear smaller than your elbow," many people consider wax to be "dirty" and aggressively attempt to remove it. The consequences of this are discussed in Chapter 7 on disorders of the auditory system.

Perhaps the most important role of the external auditory canal is that of a resonator tube. When sound travels down the ear canal, some of the frequencies contained in that complex auditory signal will match the natural frequency (also referred to as the resonant frequency) of the ear canal. The sounds that match, or nearly match this frequency, will be enhanced or amplified. Fortunately, in most adults, the resonant frequency of the ear canal is between 2,700 and 3,400 Hz, which means that high-frequency sounds will be increased. The enhancement in the sound pressure delivered to the eardrum is on the order of 10–20 dB, and results from the combination of resonance effects from the concha (the bowl-shaped part of the pinna) and ear canal (Libby & Westermann, 1988). High-frequency sounds are crucial to our understanding of speech information, and it is clearly to our advantage as listeners that these sounds are naturally amplified by our ear canal.

The Middle Ear

At the very end of the external auditory canal is the eardrum, which is also referred to as the **tympanic membrane.** The eardrum is considered by most experts to be the borderline structure between the outer and middle ears. Like any drum, the eardrum is stiff, and this particular drum vibrates easily in response to sound pressure that hits it. An overview of the structures of the middle ear is found in Figure 3.3, which illustrates the position of the eardrum.

The eardrum is made of three layers, the first of which consists of the same type of skin that is found in the bony portion of the ear canal. The next layer of the eardrum consists of fibrous connective tissue. It is this tissue that accounts for the eardrum's ability to vibrate so well. The third layer of the drum is made up of mucous membrane. In addition, the part of the eardrum making up the largest surface area is referred to as the **pars tensa** because of its stiff nature. Similar to a drum, the largest area of the eardrum vibrates maximally due to the presence of fibrous tissue. The superior part of the eardrum, where no fibrous tissue exists, is referred to as the **pars flaccida** and vibrates minimally. The pars flaccida is also referred to as Schrapnell's membrane. Refer to Figure 3.3 for a depiction of these areas. Note that you can tell whether the eardrum being viewed is the right eardrum or the left eardrum by checking which way the handle, or **manubrium,** of the malleus is pointing. In the right ear, the malleus points toward "1 o'clock" and in the left ear, the malleus points toward "11 o'clock."

FIGURE 3.3   Lateral view of a tympanic membrane.

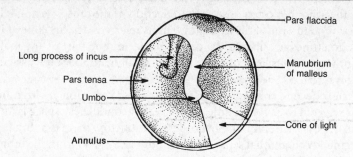

Source: F. N. Martin & J. G. Clark. *Introduction to Audiology,* 9e. Published by Allyn & Bacon, Boston, MA. Copyright © 2006 by Pearson Education. Reprinted by permission of the publisher.

When talking about the eardrum, it is convenient to divide it into four quadrants. Figure 3.4 shows a right eardrum divided into four quadrants. This makes it easier to discuss either landmarks or potential abnormalities that may be observed when viewing the eardrum.

Another feature of the eardrum is that it is semitransparent, which means that to some extent we can usually see through it into the middle ear space. This process of

FIGURE 3.4   Four quadrants of tympanic membrane.

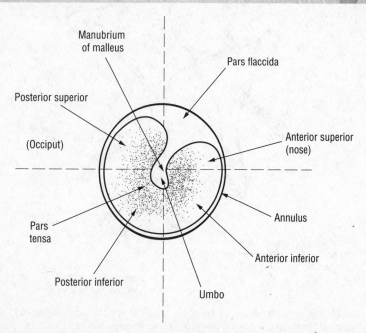

examining the eardrum and the middle ear is most commonly done by directing a light, from an instrument called an **otoscope,** into the ear canal toward the eardrum. When this is done, the examiner often observes a reflection of the otoscope's light in the anterior and inferior quadrants of the eardrum. This is referred to as the **cone of light.** In addition, it is sometimes possible to see the manubrium, the part of the malleus that is embedded into the fibrous layer of the eardrum. An illustration of the **ossicular chain** is found in Figure 3.5.

Immediately beyond the eardrum lies an air-filled space lined with mucous membrane that is referred to as the middle ear space. The middle ear space is an irregularly shaped cavity that has several notable borders. On the top, there is a thin layer of bone called the **tegmen tympani** that separates the middle ear cavity from the brain. The floor of the middle ear cavity, called the **fundus tympani,** is a thin plate of bone that separates the middle ear from the jugular bulb. Posteriorly, the middle ear space is bordered by the **mastoid,** which contains pneumatized bone (bone containing air pockets).

As already noted, suspended in this middle ear space are the three smallest bones in the body, referred to collectively as the **ossicles.** The malleus, which is the first of the three middle ear bones, is embedded directly into the fibrous portion of the eardrum. So, as the drum vibrates in response to sound, this vibration is carried to the malleus, which then transfers it to the incus and then to the stapes.

FIGURE **3.5** **The ossicular chain.**

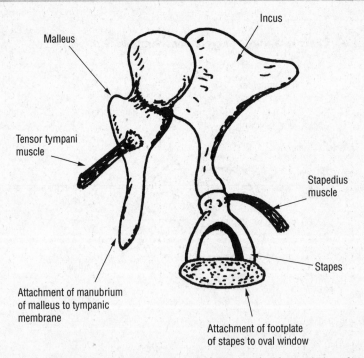

Source: The Speech Sciences, 1st edition, by Kent. © 1998. Reprinted with permission of Delmar Learning, a division of Thomson Learning: www.thomsonrights.com. Fax 800-730-2215.

We noted previously that the middle ear space is air-filled. This is true under normal conditions, but many of you may know of young children whose middle ears become fluid-filled due to some type of middle ear pathology. Although this will be discussed later in the section on middle ear disorders, it is important to point out that the middle ear contains an opening for a structure that contributes significantly to keeping the middle ear healthy. This structure is the **Eustachian tube,** which leads to the nasopharynx. This tube is normally closed, and opens regularly throughout the day when we yawn, chew, or swallow, in order to keep the pressure in the middle ear space the same as the atmospheric pressure. If these two pressures become unequal, a "plugged up" feeling can result, and over time middle ear fluid and even a ruptured eardrum can occur. In addition, faulty Eustachian tube function makes the middle ear an inefficient sound carrier.

Before proceeding to the inner ear, brief mention should be made of the role of the middle ear as an *impedance-matching device.* The word *impedance,* which is covered in Chapter 6, refers to opposition to the flow of energy; in this discussion we are referring to opposition to sound that would result if the sound waves traveled directly from the air-filled ear canal to the fluid-filled inner ear. The change in the media through which the sound is traveling (air to fluid) would result in a significant decrease in sound intensity (approximately 30 dB) if the middle ear were not constructed to compensate for this. In other words, the middle ear is uniquely designed to enhance the signal intensity that would have been lost due to the impedance mismatch created by the change from an air medium to a fluid medium.

Let's discuss briefly the three primary means by which the middle ear enhances the intensity of sounds. First, when sound is collected over a large surface area and then directed to a smaller surface area, an increase in sound pressure results. This principle applies when we collect sound pressure over the large surface area of the eardrum and then deliver it to the much smaller surface area of the stapes footplate, which is positioned in the oval window. It is estimated that an enhancement of as much as 23 dB is created due to this eardrum/stapes footplate relationship.

Second, the tympanic membrane has a curved shape that results in greater movement (displacement) on the curved aspects and less displacement nearer the manubrium. The end result of this is an increase in the force transmitted through the middle ear.

Third, as sound travels from the malleus to the much longer incus, the difference in lengths between these ossicles sets up a lever-type action that results in a small increase in sound pressure. To understand this, think about what happens when you change a tire. You place the very short part of the jack under your car and you direct pressure to the long handle. By doing so, you are able, with relatively little effort, to raise up your car. This same principle applies to sound traveling across the ossicles and enhances the signal intensity that would have been lost due to attenuation by the inner ear fluid. It is estimated that this lever action provides a boost of approximately 2.4 dB to the signal.

Middle Ear Muscles

This section would not be complete without including two important muscles that are found in the middle ear: the **stapedius muscle** and the **tensor tympani muscle.** The stapedius muscle originates in the posterior (mastoid) wall of the middle ear and attaches to the neck of the stapes bone. During loud acoustic stimulation, the stapedius muscle contracts, causing changes in middle ear impedance. These changes are measurable and are discussed further in Chapter 6 in the context of middle ear analysis and acoustic reflex testing. The tensor tympani attaches to the manubrium of the malleus and contracts in response to nonauditory stimulation such as a jet of air in the external auditory canal or eye. Both of these muscles respond reflexively and bilaterally.

The Acoustic Reflex Arc

As noted above, presentation of loud sounds to either ear results in contraction of the stapedius muscles in both middle ears; the resultant muscle contraction is called the acoustic reflex. This section includes the anatomy and physiology of the acoustic reflex arc.

There are both **ipsilateral** (same-side) and **contralateral** (opposite side) **acoustic reflex** pathways. The pathways involved in the acoustic reflex arc have been studied in animal models and are not fully understood in humans. Figure 3.6 shows the ipsilateral and contralateral acoustic (stapedius) reflex pathways. There are two ipsilateral and two contralateral acoustic reflex pathways. The acoustic reflex arc is complicated because the ipsilateral pathways differ from the contralateral pathways and each of the two ipsilateral and contralateral pathways differ from each other. The ipsilateral and contralateral

FIGURE 3.6 Schematic of the ipsilateral and contralateral acoustic reflex pathways.

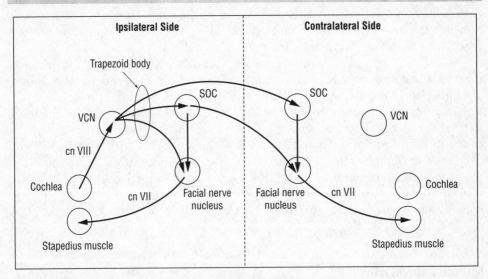

Note: SOC refers to the superior olivary complex. VCN refers to the ventral cochlear nucleus.

Source: Gelfand, S. (2002). The acoustic reflex. In *Handbook of Clinical Audiology,* J. Katz, Ed., New York: Lippincott, Williams & Wilkins, p. 206.

pathways contain a series of **synapses** as the stimulation travels from the beginning of the reflex arc (the ventral cochlear nucleus) to its final destination (the stapedius muscle).

The ipsilateral synapses include the eighth nerve, the ventral cochlear nucleus and the ipsilateral facial (seventh) nerve nucleus, and the stapedius muscle. The contralateral synapses include the ipsilateral superior olivary complex, the contralateral facial nerve nucleus, the seventh facial nerve, and the contralateral stapedius muscle. The two ipsilateral and two contralateral pathways are described below. It may be helpful to refer to Figure 3.6 as the pathways are reviewed.

Ipsilateral Acoustic Reflex Pathways
1. From eighth nerve to ventral cochlear nucleus (VCN) to facial (seventh) nerve nucleus to stapedius muscle on same side as stimulated cochlea.
2. From eighth nerve to VCN to ipsilateral superior olivary complex (medial superior olive) to facial (seventh) nerve nucleus on same side to motor neurons of seventh (facial) nerve to ipsilateral stapedius muscle. In some cases, trapezoid bodies are involved.

Contralateral Acoustic Reflex Pathways
1. From eighth nerve to ipsilateral VCN to ipsilateral superior olivary complex, then crossing over to the contralateral facial (seventh) nerve nucleus. Note that the point of crossover is the superior olivary complex.
2. From eighth nerve to ipsilateral VCN to contralateral superior olivary complex, to contralateral facial (seventh) nerve nucleus.

Now the stimulation has reached the seventh nerve nucleus in the contralateral pathway. From here, for *both* contralateral pathways, the motor portion of the reflex arc goes from the facial nerve nucleus along the seventh cranial (facial) nerve to the stapedius muscle in the ear opposite the stimulation (the contralateral ear). This information is the foundation for interpretation of acoustic reflex patterns, an essential part of the clinical diagnostic audiologic process, as discussed in Chapter 6.

The Inner Ear

As we begin our discussion of the inner ear, it is important to remember that much less is understood about the inner ear compared to the outer and middle ears. There are a few reasons for this. First, because of the inner ear's location deep in the petrous portion of the temporal bone of the skull, it cannot be easily visualized. Further, the actual structure of the inner ear is so complicated that it is referred to as a **labyrinth,** which is a maze of interconnecting chambers. Also, unlike the outer and middle ears, which can be viewed by microscopes, examination of the inner ear requires sophisticated imaging techniques. In addition, the outer and middle ears are comparatively simple systems that make use of a number of acoustic principles that are well understood (the lever principle, resonance, etc.). If one wanted to, one could construct an outer/middle ear system using basic materials that would simulate the function of the various structures (tubes, a drum, etc.). Creating an inner ear system would be far more challenging because this system takes the mechanical energy of the middle ear and creates complicated fluid movements, which result in electrochemical and then neurological activity that allows the brain to receive auditory information.

Because of the complicated nature of the inner ear and because experts are continually refining their understanding of this system, the information that follows makes use of theories and hypotheses about the probable role of the structures of the inner ear in the hearing process. Before we discuss the inner ear and hearing, let's make brief mention of the other important role of the inner ear: maintaining balance.

The Vestibular System

The part of the inner ear that is directly beyond the oval window (where the stapes footplate rocks in and out) is called the **vestibule** of the inner ear and is filled with a fluid

FIGURE **3.7** **Illustration of the vestibular (semicircular canals, utricle, saccule) and auditory (cochlea) portions of the inner ear.**

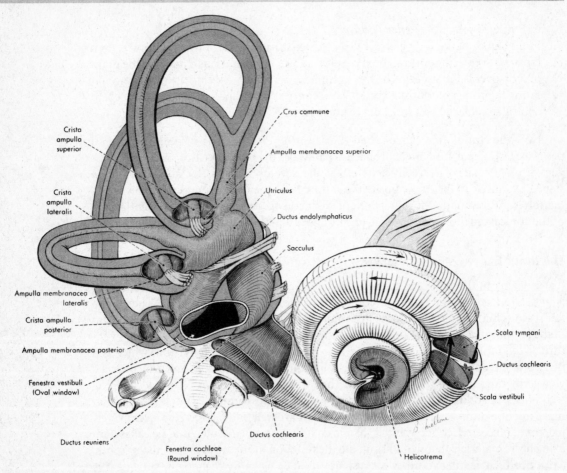

Crus commune

Crista ampulla superior

Ampulla membranacea superior

Crista ampulla lateralis

Utriculus

Ductus endolymphaticus

Sacculus

Ampulla membranacea lateralis

Crista ampulla posterior

Ampulla membranacea posterior

Scala tympani

Ductus cochlearis

Fenestra vestibuli (Oval window)

Scala vestibuli

Ductus reuniens

Ductus cochlearis

Fenestra cochleae (Round window)

Helicotrema

Source: Abbott Laboratories. *An atlas of some pathological conditions of the eye, ear, and throat.* Abbott Park, IL: Author. Reprinted by permission.

called **perilymph.** This part of the inner ear contains the structures that deal with a person's balance. Any client who has experienced a balance disorder will attest to the importance of a properly functioning balance system. Located in the vestibule are membranous sacs, referred to as the **utricle** and the **saccule.** These sacs, although surrounded by perilymph, contain a fluid called **endolymph.** These two fluids differ in composition primarily in the mix of potassium/sodium that they contain. Arising from the utricle is a series of canals, referred to as the **semicircular canals.** These canals contain endolymph and are surrounded by perilymph. Each canal contains an enlarged area called an **ampulla.** The ampullae contain **cristae,** which are sense organs for balance. Together, the utricle, saccule, and the semicircular canals respond, through fluid movement, to changes in the body that require maintenance of balance. Most experts believe that the utricle and saccule respond to linear movements such as going up and down in an elevator and that the semicircular canals respond to angular changes, such as tilting your head to one side. Refer to Figure 3.7 for illustrations of the structures of the vestibular system. Further reference is made to the anatomy and physiology of the balance mechanism in the section on inner ear disorders in Chapter 7, in which examples of disorders of balance are provided.

The Cochlea

Moving beyond the vestibular portion of the inner ear, we are now ready to discuss the **cochlea,** which contains the sense organ for hearing, the **organ of Corti.** Students should remember that the cochlea is a snail-shaped organ that is carved into the temporal bone. Because of this, Venema (2006) states that analyzing the cochlea would be like wanting to study a hole in the ground by trying to dig it out. In order to get around some of these difficulties, it has become common for audiology instructors and textbook authors to "unroll" the cochlea. This is done in Figure 3.8, where we see three primary chambers called *scala.* The uppermost chamber, the *scala vestibuli,* lies immediately beyond the oval window and is so named because of its closeness to the

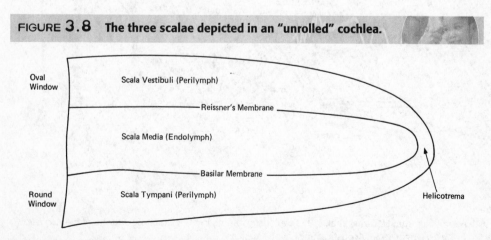

FIGURE **3.8** **The three scalae depicted in an "unrolled" cochlea.**

vestibule. The lowermost chamber is the *scala tympani,* which terminates at the round window. Both the scala vestibuli and the scala tympani are filled with perilymph, and this fluid is continuous by way of the *helicotrema,* which is located at the top (apex) of the cochlea.

In the middle of the scala vestibuli and scale tympani lies the most important chamber, referred to as the **scala media** or the *cochlear duct.* Note in Figure 3.9 that the scala media, which contains endolymph, is separated from the scala vestibuli by *Reissner's membrane* and from the scala tympani by the **basilar membrane.** Note also that located on the basilar membrane is the organ of Corti, which is the end organ of hearing. These structures, the basilar membrane and the organ of Corti, are critical in the process of hearing and will now be discussed in detail.

As we discuss the basilar membrane, remember that although we have, for discussion purposes, unrolled the cochlea (and therefore also the basilar membrane), it

FIGURE 3.9 **Cross section of the central portion of the cochlear cavity.**

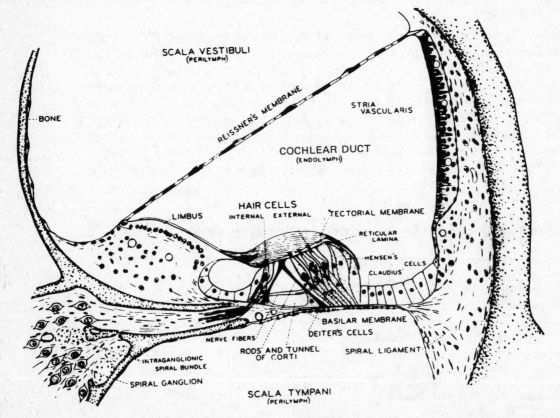

Source: Reprinted with permission from H. Davis, et al. (1953). Acoustic trauma in the guinea pig. *Journal of the Acoustical Society of America, 25,* 1180. Copyright 1953, Acoustical Society of America.

**FIGURE 3.10   Unrolled cochlea (longitudinal section) depicting
basilar membrane from base to apex.**

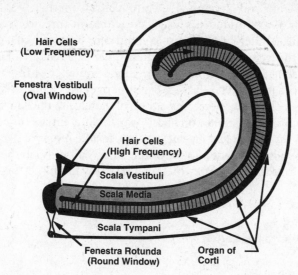

Hair Cells
(Low Frequency)

Fenestra Vestibuli
(Oval Window)

Hair Cells
(High Frequency)

Scala Vestibuli

Scala Media

Scala Tympani

Fenestra Rotunda
(Round Window)

Organ of
Corti

Source: Donald F. Fucci & Norman J. Lass. *Fundamentals of Speech Science.* Published by Allyn & Bacon,
Boston, MA. Copyright © 1997 by Pearson Education. Reprinted by permission of the publisher.

actually runs the length of the snail-shaped cochlea from the base of the cochlea (lowest portion) to the apex (uppermost portion). This is illustrated in Figure 3.10. One very important fact about the basilar membrane is that its width is not uniform, ranging from 0.08 to 0.16 mm at the base and from 0.42 to 0.65 mm at the apex. Also, the apical portion of the basilar membrane tends to move more freely and be less stiff; the basal end tends to be stiffer. In order to help us understand some implications of this information to the act of hearing, let's stop for a minute and think about a guitar. What happens when you pluck the fatter string of a guitar, compared to the thinner, tauter string? The fatter string produces a lower-frequency sound and the thinner string produces a higher-frequency sound. Although we do not completely understand how this works in the inner ear, it appears clear that the characteristics of the basilar membrane have a direct bearing on our ability to perceive different frequencies of sound. Specifically, high-frequency sounds excite the base of the cochlea and low-frequency sounds excite the apex. Logically, low frequencies travel farther up the cochlea compared to high frequencies, which are processed much closer to the oval window. The fact that different frequencies result in different points of displacement of the basilar membrane is referred to as the **tonotopic** organization of the cochlea.

We noted previously that located on the basilar membrane is the organ of Corti. This is a very important structure in part because it contains rows of outer and inner hair cells that differ in shape and function. Attached to the top of outer hair cells are cilia (small hairs), and some of these cilia are embedded into the **tectorial membrane.**

Take a look at Figure 3.11 and note that the tectorial membrane overhangs the organ of Corti. One way for students to remember the tectorial membrane is to remember that in Latin *tectum* means "roof." The tectorial membrane, then, is the roof that hangs over the organ of Corti and has embedded into it cilia from the outer hair cells. There are approximately 12,000 outer hair cells configured in three rows throughout the length of the cochlea. Inner hair cells also contain cilia, but these cilia do not make direct contact with the tectorial membrane. These inner hair cells are in a single row and total approximately 3,500. The combined (bilateral) number of inner and outer hair cells totals approximately 30,000. Table 3.1 summarizes the characteristics of the outer and inner hair cells, their functions, and effects of damage to the hair cells on hearing.

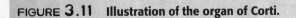

According to Brownell (1996), one basic way to differentiate outer and inner hair cell function is to say that the inner hair cells are, for the most part, *afferent,* meaning that they carry sound information to the brain. Outer hair cells, on the other hand, are *efferent,* which means that they carry messages from the brain (i.e., brainstem) back to

---

FIGURE 3.11   Illustration of the organ of Corti.

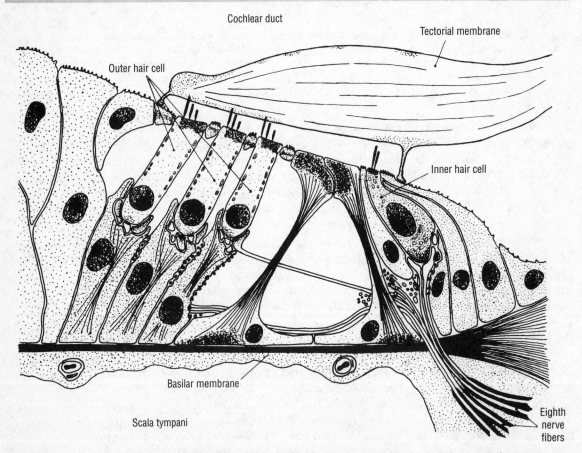

Source: Jerry L. Northern. *Hearing Disorders,* 3e. Published by Allyn & Bacon, Boston, MA. Copyright © 1996 by Pearson Education. Reprinted by permission of the publisher.

the cochlea. Also, outer hair cells have a role in enabling the inner hair cells to sense soft incoming sounds.

Now, back to our more general discussion of the organ of Corti, the basilar membrane, and the tectorial membrane. As the stapes rocks in and out of the oval window, fluid moves in the inner ear. Specifically, fluid moves in the form of a traveling wave

---

TABLE 3.1 Characteristics of Outer and Inner Cochlear Hair Cells

Outer Hair Cells	Inner Hair Cells
Approximately 12,000 in each cochlea; cylindrical in shape (Yost, 1994).	Approximately 3,500 in each cochlea; rounded or flasklike in shape (Yost, 1994).
Do make contact with the bottom of the tectorial membrane.	Do not make contact with the tectorial membrane.
Communicate mostly through the olivocochlear bundle, which begins at the right and left superior olivary complexes, runs alongside the afferent fibers of the eighth nerve, and ends at the outer hair cells (Brownell, 1996).	Communicate mostly with the eighth nerve fibers and terminate at the lower brainstem.
Are mostly efferent (take information from the brain back to the cochlea). The messages from the brain directs them to either stretch or shrink.	Are mostly afferent; that is, they send information to the brain (Brownell, 1996).
Are stimulated by soft sounds.	Are stimulated by incoming sounds of 40 to 60 dB SPL.
Help inner hair cells sense soft sounds by amplifying them. Soft incoming sounds cause outer hair cells to shrink, which pulls the tectorial membrane closer to the tips of the inner hair cells (Killion, 1997).	Once they are closer to the tectorial membrane, the inner hair cells can be bent and can send sound to the brain.
A second role is to alter the physical properties of the basilar membrane in order to make the peak of the traveling wave sharper, which improves the ability to discriminate different frequencies (Brownell, 1996).	
Are usually damaged before inner hair cells (Willott, 1991).	
Damage typically results in losses in the 40–60-dB HL range (Berlin, 1994).	Losses greater than 60 dB, most likely involve outer and inner hair cell damage.
Presbycusis and long-term noise-induced hearing loss (Engstrom & Engstrom, 1988) are believed to cause damage to these hair cells.	Impact noise may cause both outer and inner hair cell damage (Killion, 1997).
Damage may result in difficulty understanding speech in noise	Damage often results in difficulty understanding speech in quiet and in noise due to reduction of sound from ear to the brain.

Source: Venema (2006).

(discussed shortly) and causes movement of fluid in the scala media. Because the basilar and tectorial membranes have different points of attachment to neighboring structures, movement of fluid results in simultaneous movement of the basilar and tectorial membranes but in different directions. This causes a bending and shearing of hair cells as depicted in Figure 3.12. This shearing triggers an electrochemical reaction, which transmits information to auditory neurons that are attached to the hair cells.

These auditory nerve fibers leave the cochlea and course through a central bony pillar of the cochlea called the **modiolus**. The cell bodies of these neurons cluster and form the spiral ganglion, as shown in Figure 3.9. As they exit the modiolus, these neurons form the cochlear branch of the auditory nerve. The cochlear branch joins the vestibular

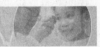

FIGURE **3.12** **Depiction of the shearing of outer hair cells caused by movement of the basilar and tectorial membranes.**

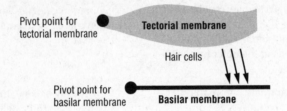

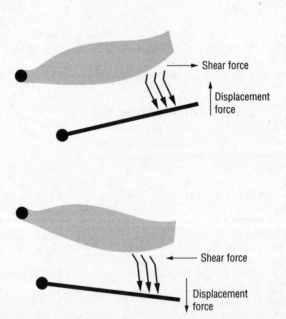

Source: Willard R. Zemlin. *Speech and Hearing Science.* Published by Allyn & Bacon, Boston, MA. Copyright © 1998 by Pearson Education. Adapted by permission of the publisher.

branch of the auditory nerve, coursing through the internal auditory canal. Interestingly, the tonotopic characteristic of the cochlea is also noted in the eighth cranial nerve. Nerve fibers from the base of the cochlea (high frequencies) form the outer part of the auditory nerve; fibers from the apex (low frequencies) form the middle of the nerve.

Summary of Physiology of Hearing from the Outer Ear to the Inner Ear

Before proceeding to the central auditory system, let's use what you have just learned to recap the hearing process from sound traveling in the air to it reaching the eighth cranial nerve.

A sound wave is produced and is picked up by the pinna, which is a sound collector. The pinna directs the wave down the ear canal and as this occurs, an increase in sound pressure also occurs, resulting from the difference in surface area between the larger pinna and smaller canal. Those components of the sound wave that are close to the resonant frequencies of the canal (approximately 2,700 to 3,400 Hz) are amplified. Sound pressure then hits the eardrum, a pressure-sensitive structure, which vibrates and passes this vibration along to the malleus, which is embedded into the fibrous portion of the eardrum. Because the malleus is continuous with the incus and stapes, vibrations of the drum and malleus are transferred across the ossicular chain. The stapes footplate lies directly in the oval window, which is the entrance point to the inner ear. As sound travels through this middle ear system it is amplified significantly, due, in part, to the difference in area (size) between the eardrum and the oval window and the lever system set up by the difference in the lengths of the malleus and incus.

As the stapes rocks in and out of the oval window, a "traveling wave" of fluid is set up in the inner ear, which moves from the base of the cochlea to the apex. For sounds that are higher in frequency, maximum displacement of the basilar membrane occurs near the basal end of the cochlea; for lower-frequency sounds, maximum displacement occurs closer to the apex of the cochlea. This is illustrated in Figure 3.13. So, along with

FIGURE **3.13** **Diagram of a traveling wave produced by a 200-Hz tone.**

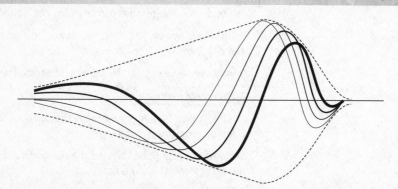

Source: Jerry L. Northern. *Hearing Disorders,* 3e. Published by Allyn & Bacon, Boston, MA. Copyright © 1996 by Pearson Education. Reprinted by permission of the publisher.

the tectorial membrane, movement of the basilar membrane results in shearing of hair cells. This shearing triggers electrochemical reactions that are picked up by auditory neurons and carried to the eighth cranial nerve.

Anatomy and Physiology of the Central Auditory System

Before considering the anatomy and physiology of the central auditory system, a brief review of basic neurological terms is provided in Table 3.2.

Just as the **central nervous system** (CNS) consists of the brainstem, spinal cord, and brain, the central auditory system involves those brainstem and brain structures responsible for directing signals from the peripheral auditory system to the cerebral cortex. It is important that you realize that, in addition to transmitting signals, a critical aspect of the process of hearing is the coding of auditory parameters, such as frequency, intensity, and time. These are the essential acoustic cues for speech perception, and although this process is begun in the peripheral auditory system (e.g., frequency is coded by the tonotopic arrangement of the cochlea), it must be maintained and enhanced in the central auditory system.

TABLE 3.2   Review of Basic Neurological Terms

Term	Definition
Central nervous system (CNS)	Consists of spinal cord and brain; receives sensory impulses from the peripheral nervous system (PNS) and sends motor impulses to the PNS.
Peripheral nervous system (PNS)	Consists of the cranial and spinal nerves; peripheral nerves transmit impulses to move the muscles of the body; conducts information to and from the CNS.
Neuron	Specialized cells of the nervous system; responsible for transmitting, receiving, and processing impulses; includes cell body plus extensions such as axons and dendrites.
Synapse	Point where two nerve cells meet, at the junction of axon and dendrite.
Ganglia	Bundles of nerve cells in the peripheral nervous system.
Neural firing	Activation of neural cells.
Axon	Conduct nerve impulses away from the cell body; another term for "away from" is efferent.
Dendrite	Conduct nerve impulses toward the cell body; another term for "toward" is afferent.
Myelin	A fatty insulating sheath that forms around nerve fiber; facilitates rapid, efficient transfer of nerve impulses.

How does this transmission and coding of auditory information occur? Depicted in Figure 3.14 are the **auditory nuclei** that make up much of the central auditory system. These nuclei, which are often referred to as relay stations, are the site of a series of synapses, and it is through this neuronal communication that the central auditory system makes its contribution to auditory perception.

By most accounts, the central auditory system begins with the **cochlear nuclei**, which are bundles of nerves located on the brainstem at the junction of the pons and the medulla. It is believed that all fibers from the eighth cranial nerve terminate at the cochlear nuclei. Because basal fibers terminate in a different part of the cochlear nuclei than apical fibers, the tonotopic nature of the auditory system is maintained. Beyond the cochlear nuclei, some fibers (ipsilateral) remain on their original side of the brainstem, while other fibers (contralateral) cross over (*decussate*) to the other side. Because of the

FIGURE 3.14 Illustration of peripheral and central auditory system pathways.

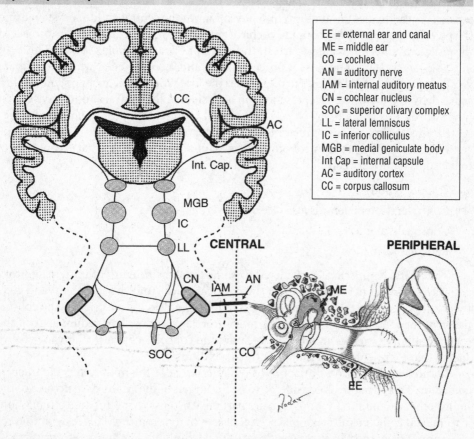

EE = external ear and canal
ME = middle ear
CO = cochlea
AN = auditory nerve
IAM = internal auditory meatus
CN = cochlear nucleus
SOC = superior olivary complex
LL = lateral lemniscus
IC = inferior colliculus
MGB = medial geniculate body
Int Cap = internal capsule
AC = auditory cortex
CC = corpus callosum

Source: Musiek, F., & Baran, J. *The Auditory System: Anatomy, Physiology, and Clinical Correlates.* Published by Allyn & Bacon, Boston, MA. Copyright © 2007 by Pearson Education. Reprinted by permission of the publisher.

predominance of contralateral fibers in the auditory system, auditory stimulation of one ear is represented more predominantly on the cortex of the opposite side. This concept of crossing over and contralateral dominance applies to other nervous system activity as well.

Use of contralateral fibers by the central nervous system is important for a number of reasons. First, opportunities for accurate perception of auditory information by a listener are enhanced by the redundancy created by the multiple overlapping pathways of the auditory system. Second, for the more peripheral aspects of the auditory system (e.g., outer ear, middle ear, inner ear), there is greater involvement of ipsilateral fibers; conversely, for the more central aspects of the auditory system, there is greater involvement of contralateral fibers. Also, the type of stimuli being processed by the listener is a factor. Simple stimuli (e.g., pure tones) are processed more peripherally; more complex auditory tasks (e.g., listening to speech in a background of noise) are processed using more central pathways.

Central Auditory Pathways

This section addresses the anatomy and physiology of the central auditory system using the preceding framework. From the cochlear nuclei, most of the nerve fibers project to the ipsilateral and contralateral parts of the **superior olivary complex (SOC).** This is an important relay station because it processes time and intensity cues, which contribute greatly to localization abilities. Further, this is the first point in the relay system where a signal delivered to one ear is represented on both sides of the central auditory system. In other words, this is the first instance of binaural representation of a monaurally presented signal. Also, because different nuclei within the superior olivary complex process high and low frequencies, tonotopicity is maintained. The fibers that do not project to the superior olivary complex may ascend to the:

Trapezoid body

Contraleral lateral lemniscus

Contralateral inferior colliculus

Reticular formation

The **lateral lemniscus** is considered by some to be the primary brainstem auditory pathway, receiving nerve fibers from the cochlear nuclei and the ipsilateral and contralateral portions of the superior olivary complex. Evidence also supports the continuance of the tonotopicity noted at the previous relay stations. This redundancy of the central auditory system is an important feature and contributes to our ability to perceive speech that is presented in less than optimal conditions.

Located in the section of the brainstem referred to as the midbrain is the **inferior colliculus.** This structure is considered to be the largest of the auditory structures of the brainstem and contains neurons that are particularly sensitive to binaural stimulation. The inferior colliculus also exhibits a great degree of tonotopicity. This relay station receives input from most of the fibers of the lateral lemniscus and lower auditory areas.

The last subcortical auditory relay station is the **medial geniculate body,** located in the thalamus. This structure receives most of its fibers from the ipsilateral inferior colliculus and some from the lateral lemniscus. Like the inferior colliculus, the medial geniculate body contains neurons that are sensitive to binaural stimulation and like much of the auditory system is characterized by a tonotopic nature. From the medial geniculate body, nerve fibers course through a special tract to the **cerebral cortex,** carrying a variety of auditory information, including auditory discrimination cues.

Before discussing the cerebral cortex, at least brief mention should be made of the **reticular formation,** a "diffusely organized area" comprised of nuclei and tracts that form the central portion of the brainstem. This formation interacts with the auditory system through its connections to the spinal cord and cerebrum. Evidence suggests that the reticular formation prepares the cortex to respond to incoming auditory information and that it may have an important role in selective attention.

The cerebral cortex is the final auditory area in the process of auditory perception. The cerebrum is the largest part of the brain and consists of the lobes of the brain. The cortex refers to the uppermost surface of the brain. The specific areas of auditory reception are located in the temporal lobes in *Heschl's gyrus,* as depicted in Figure 3.15. Evidence suggests that this area is capable of decoding information about frequency, intensity, and time. Regarding frequency, research has suggested that different parts of Heschl's gyrus are responsive to low- and high-frequency stimulation. Further, similar to the eighth cranial nerve, intensity for lower-intensity signals appears to be coded in the primary auditory cortex based on the rate of neural firing. Research regarding the coding of timing cues suggests that different neurons in the auditory cortex respond to the onset of sound compared to the cessation of sound and other neurons respond to the presence of sound. Neurons in the primary auditory cortex are also sensitive to timing cues involving interaural phase differences that contribute to localization abilities. Finally, it is important to note that although there is evidence that specific areas of the brain are responsible for certain auditory functions, there is also evidence that the auditory pathways are complex and

FIGURE **3.15 Lobes of the brain, including location of Heschl's gyrus.**

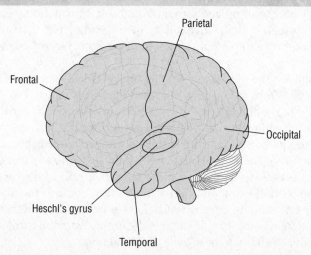

redundant. The question of the degree to which the language/auditory processing centers in the brain are focused or diffuse remains unanswered.

Summary of the Physiology of Hearing from the Eighth Cranial Nerve to the Cerebral Cortex

Recall from our previous discussion that auditory neurons attached to the hair cells leave the cochlea and course through a central bony pillar of the cochlea called the modiolus. The cell bodies of these neurons cluster and form the spiral ganglion. As they exit the modiolus, these neurons form the cochlear branch of the auditory nerve. The cochlear branch joins the vestibular branch of the auditory nerve (whose fibers innervate the utricle, saccule, and semicircular canals), coursing through the internal auditory canal. The auditory nerve extends from the internal canal and attaches to the brainstem at the *cerebellopontine angle,* which is the junction of the cerebellum, medulla, and the pons.

Fibers from the eighth cranial nerve terminate at the cochlear nuclei, with basal and apical fibers terminating at different places in order to maintain the tonotopic arrangement of the auditory system. From the cochlear nuclei, fibers project to a variety of relay stations, including the superior olivary complex, which uniquely processes time and intensity cues used for localization. Some fibers from the cochlear nuclei extend to the trapezoid body, the lateral lemniscus, the inferior colliculus, and the reticular formation.

The continuance of tonotopicity is noted at the lateral lemniscus, which receives fibers from both the cochlear nuclei and the superior olivary complex. Most of the fibers of the lateral lemniscus and lower auditory areas extend to the inferior colliculus, located in the midbrain. Here, tonotopicity is maintained and coding for binaural stimulation occurs.

The medial geniculate body, the last subcortical auditory relay station, is located in the thalamus and receives fibers from the inferior colliculus and the lateral lemniscus. Like the inferior colliculus, information regarding tonotopicity and binaural stimulation are coded here. Also, information regarding auditory discrimination is carried to the cerebral cortex. At the cerebral cortex, information is directed to Heschl's gyrus, where tonotopicity is maintained and information regarding intensity and timing cues is represented. Once coding here is completed, this information is directed to *Wernicke's area* of the temporal lobe. This is the receptive language center of the brain.

In this section on the central auditory system, we have focused on the pathway directing information from the cochlea to the brain. This is referred to as the ascending auditory pathway or the afferent pathway. An efferent or descending pathway also exists, which connects the auditory cortex with the lower brain centers and the cochlear hair cells. Although this pathway is far from completely understood, it appears that the olivocochlear bundle, located in the pons, is an important structure and that it has two tracts. Fibers from one of these tracts extend to the inner hair cells of the cochlear and fibers from the other tract to the outer hair cells. In addition, some of the fibers of the olivocochlear bundle extend to the cochlear nuclei. It has been suggested that because the efferent auditory system is able to regulate signals coming from the cochlea, it may play an important role in our ability to hear in background noise.

This examination of the structures of the auditory system and how the process of hearing works forms an important foundation for further exploration of audiological evaluation and management.

CHAPTER SUMMARY

This chapter presented the anatomy and physiology of the auditory system, including the outer, middle, and inner ear structures and their function. You learned about the pinna, or external ear, which collects sound; the impedance-matching function of the middle ear; and the complex system of fluid movement and electrochemical events that take place in the inner ear. Transmission of sound through the auditory system is tonotopic. In the cochlea, the displacement of the basilar membrane at the basal end transmits high-frequency sounds; low-frequency sounds are transmitted at the apical end. Bending and shearing of hair cells results in stimulation of auditory neurons and directs impulses to the eighth cranial nerve.

Important central auditory pathways were reviewed. The cochlear and vestibular branches of the eighth cranial nerve, which travel through the internal auditory canal and attach to the brainstem at the cerebellopontine angle (CPA) were noted. An important juncture, the cochlear nucleus, where auditory nerve fibers terminate, was discussed. Finally, you learned about the various relay stations to which cochlear fibers project, including the superior olivary complex (SOC), where cues for localization are processed, and the trapezoid body (TB), lateral lemniscus (LL), inferior colliculus (IC), and the reticular formation (RF). The medial geniculate body (MGB), the last subcortical relay station, receives fibers from the IC and LL. From here, information regarding auditory discrimination is carried to the cerebral cortex, where Heschl's gyrus is located. Heschl's gyrus maintains information about tonotopicity and is where timing and intensity cues are represented.

QUESTIONS FOR DISCUSSION

1. Discuss tonotopicity relative to the peripheral and central auditory systems.
2. How does redundancy in the auditory system help us hear in adverse listening conditions?
3. Discuss the contribution of the external ear to hearing and speech perception.
4. Describe the role of the middle ear in sound transmission through the peripheral auditory system.
5. Compare and contrast the inner and outer hair cells; discuss their relative contributions to the process of hearing.

RECOMMENDED READING

Anson, B. J., & Donaldson, J. A. (1973). *Surgical anatomy of the temporal bone and ear* (2nd ed.). Philadelphia: Saunders.

Berlin, C. (1998). *The efferent auditory system: Basic science and clinical applications.* New York: Delmar Thomson Learning.

Jahn, A., & Santos-Sacchi, J. (2001). *Physiology of the ear.* New York: Delmar Thomson Learning.

Zemlin, W. (1998). *Speech and hearing science: Anatomy and physiology* (4th ed.). Boston: Allyn & Bacon.

REFERENCES

American Speech-Language-Hearing Association (ASHA). (1995, March). Position statement and guidelines for acoustics in educational settings. *ASHA, 37*(Suppl. 14), 15–19.

Berlin, C. (1994). When outer hair cells fail, use correct circuitry to stimulate their function. *The Hearing Journal, 47*(4), 43.

Brownell, W. (1996). Outer hair cell electromotility and otoacoustic emissions. In C. Berlin (Ed.), *Hair cells and hearing aids* (pp. 3–28). San Diego: Singular.

Davis, H., Bensen, R., Covell, W., Fernandez, C., Goldstein, R., Katuki, Y., Legouix, J., McAuliffe, D., & Tasaki, I. (1953). Acoustic trauma in the guinea pig. *Journal of the Acoustical Society of America, 25*(6), 1180–1189.

Engstrom, H., & Engstrom, H. (1988). *The ear.* Uppsala, Sweden: Widex.

Fucci, D. N., & Lass, N. J. (1999). *Fundamentals of speech science.* Boston: Allyn & Bacon.

Gelfand, S. (2002). The acoustic reflex. In J. Katz (Ed.), *Handbook of clinical audiology* (p. 206). New York: Lippincott, Williams & Wilkins.

Killion, M. (1997). The SIN report: Circuits haven't solved the hearing-in-noise problem. *The Hearing Journal, 50*(10), 28–34.

Libby, E., & Westermann, S. (1988). Principles of acoustic measurement and ear canal resonances. In R. Sandlin (Ed.), *Handbook of hearing aid amplification: Volume 1. Theoretical and technical considerations* (pp. 165–220). San Diego: Singular.

Martin, F. N., & Clark, J. G. (2006). *Introduction to audiology* (9th ed.). Boston: Allyn & Bacon.

Musiek, F., & Baran, J. (2007). *The auditory system: Anatomy, physiology, and clinical correlates.* Boston: Allyn & Bacon.

Northern, J. L. (1996). *Hearing disorders* (3rd ed.). Boston: Allyn & Bacon.

Venema, T. (2006). *Compression for clinicians.* San Diego: Singular.

Willott, J. (1991). *Aging and the auditory system: Anatomy, physiology and psychophysics.* San Diego: Singular.

Yost, W. (1994). *Fundamentals of hearing: An introduction* (3rd ed.). San Diego: Academic Press.

chapter 4

Pure Tone Testing

AFTER COMPLETING THIS CHAPTER, YOU SHOULD BE ABLE TO:

1. Define *pure tones* and describe their unique role in hearing assessment.
2. Define *calibration* and describe its importance to hearing assessment.
3. Describe the components and function of a two-channel diagnostic audiometer.
4. Explain procedures for obtaining and recording pure tone air and bone conduction thresholds.
5. Determine when to use masking during air and bone conduction testing for specific audiometric profiles.
6. Describe some of the major pitfalls to be avoided in obtaining accurate pure tone thresholds.

Recall from Chapter 2 that **pure tones** are defined as signals consisting of only one frequency of vibration. You may also recall that pure tones do not exist in nature and are produced by tuning forks and audiometers. Many of you probably remember having your hearing screened in school by the school nurse or speech–language pathologist, who used an audiometer and asked you to respond when you heard the pure tones of various frequencies. These same tones are commonly used in screening the hearing ability of people of all ages, from preschoolers to the elderly. They are also a very important part of comprehensive audiological assessment performed by audiologists, who identify the softest level at which the patient can just barely hear tones of various frequencies. This chapter discusses pure tone testing used as part of a comprehensive audiological assessment (i.e., threshold testing). Even though such comprehensive assessment is part of the audiologist's scope of practice, speech–language pathologists need to understand the results of pure tone testing and use this information for planning and implementing speech and language therapy. Further, the scope of practice of the speech–language pathologist does include use of pure tones for screening purposes. Screening is discussed in Chapter 11.

Relationship between Pure Tones and Perception of Speech Sounds

One of the questions that students commonly ask is why pure tones are such an important part of hearing assessment. After all, we typically listen to **complex sounds,** consisting of more than one frequency, such as speech or music, not pure tones. One of the answers to this question lies in the nature of hearing loss and in the definition of pure tones noted above. Hearing loss typically does not affect all frequencies equally. In fact, the most common type of age-related hearing loss, called *presbycusis*, typically affects the high frequencies to a greater degree than the low frequencies. Individuals who have noise-induced hearing losses often have normal low-frequency hearing, with considerable impairment in the high frequencies. Because complex stimuli, such as speech or music, are made up of multiple frequencies, when an individual responds to them, it is not clear which parts of the signal (i.e., which frequencies) have been heard. Did the person hear the entire range of frequencies or just some portion of it? And if it is the latter, which specific frequencies did she hear? So, complex stimuli are not the most efficient type of stimuli to separate those frequencies that an individual hears normally from those that are impaired. Because pure tones consist of only one frequency of vibration, they are ideally suited to this task.

In addition, pure tones are related to speech. Each of the speech sounds in our language (called *phonemes*) is associated with a particular frequency region. In general, vowels and nasals tend to be lower in frequency and stop consonants and fricatives tend to be higher in frequency. Because the high frequencies carry the most critical information for speech intelligibility in our language, individuals who have high-frequency hearing loss are at risk for misunderstanding words, especially if those words are similar sounding (e.g., *suit* versus *shoot*).

Recall that in Chapter 2 we referred to an audiogram of familiar sounds. This audiogram is based on what many refer to as the "speech banana," because the energy concentration created by the various speech sounds in our language takes the form of a banana. You may also recall that the "speech banana" contains less energy in the very low and very high frequencies. Figure 4.1 illustrates this. Note that there are two lines that serve as the boundaries for this speech banana. These represent the lower and upper ranges of the intensity of speech when it is presented at conversational levels. When this speech banana is superimposed on an audiogram of a client's pure tone thresholds, the informed reader is quickly able to determine which aspects of speech are acoustically available to this client. While numerous factors (age of onset of hearing loss, age of identification of hearing loss, use of assistive technology, etc.) influence how an individual with hearing loss may perform, information about access to speech sounds does provide a foundation for the audiologist and speech–language pathologist to work from.

Recall the audibility (articulation) index introduced in Chapter 2. Mueller and Killion (1990) proposed an **articulation index (AI)** audiogram based on 100 dots as shown in Figure 4.2. The placement of the dots is based on knowledge of those frequencies that are most important to speech perception. Note, for example, that there is a concentration of dots in the range 1,000–3,000 Hz, and far fewer dots between 250 and 500 Hz and above 4,000 Hz. According to Mueller and Killion, the articulation (audibility) index is calculated by counting the dots that fall above (i.e., are more intense than) the client's thresholds. Referring now to Figure 4.3, note that a total of 26 dots are above the client's thresholds, resulting in an articulation (audibility) index of 0.26. The closer the AI is to 1.0, the better, because an AI of 1.0 means that the energy contained in conversational speech is acoustically accessible to the listener.

FIGURE **4.1** **Audiogram with conversational speech spectrum.**

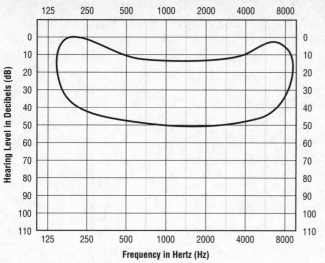
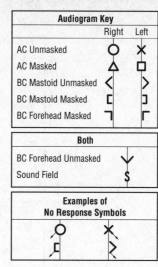

FIGURE **4.2** **Count-the-dots audiogram denoting critical areas for speech perception.**

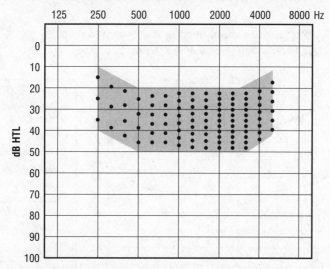

Source: Mueller, G., & Killion, M. (1990). An easy method for calculating the articulation index. *The Hearing Journal, 45*(9), 14–17. Reprinted by permission.

FIGURE **4.3** **Mild to moderately severe bilateral sensorineural hearing loss recorded on a count-the-dots audiogram.**

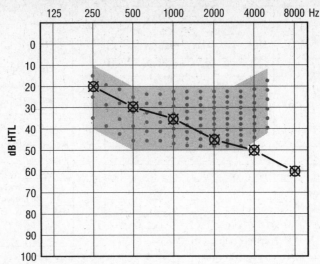

The previous discussion of the relationship between access to information at various frequencies and access to speech sounds is related directly to understanding how hearing loss affects speech and language. Let's now examine two pure tone audiograms that illustrate this concept.

The audiogram in Figure 4.4 is of a client who has a profound hearing loss. When viewing the client's pure tone thresholds at various frequencies relative to the average speech

FIGURE **4.4** **Profound bilateral hearing loss recorded on an audiogram with conversational speech spectrum.**

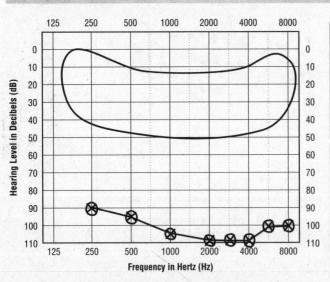
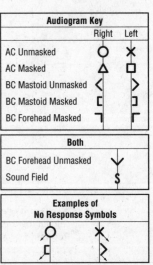

spectrum, or speech banana, it is immediately apparent that without the use of some type of amplification (e.g., hearing aids, FM auditory trainer), this client will not have access to conversational speech information. As a result, the client may have impaired articulation because he will be unable to hear the acoustic models of sound produced by those around him. In addition, without clearly hearing the speech sounds of our language, the client will have great difficulty uncovering the rules of language to which individuals with normal hearing are exposed auditorally. Language rules can also affect articulation and phonology, as well as the use of grammar or syntax. Vocabulary development, which occurs in part by a process of attaching labels (heard over and over) to specific referents in the environment, will also be disrupted. Chapter 12 includes information about amplification and how it can be helpful to individuals who have hearing loss. For now, it will suffice to say that even with well-fitted amplification or other technology, speech and language development will likely be affected by this degree of hearing loss. One consequence of this is that individuals who are deaf may choose to use American Sign Language (ASL) rather than oral English as their primary means of communication. This is discussed further in Chapter 9.

Figure 4.5 is an audiogram showing a mild to moderate high-frequency hearing loss bilaterally. The client is a child who was born with this loss and who was not identified as having a hearing loss until age 2 years. The pure tone thresholds are superimposed on the average speech spectrum. In addition, consistent with the audiogram of familiar sounds illustrated in Chapter 2, Figure 2.25, the specific phonemes associated with each frequency are included. Knowledge of the specific phonemes associated with various frequencies is important because, unlike clients who have virtually no access to speech sounds, these clients will have access to certain sounds but will miss others. For example, vowels, semivowels, and nasals will be heard by these children because of their normal hearing in the low to

FIGURE 4.5 **Mild to moderate bilateral high-frequency hearing loss recorded on an audiogram with a depiction of the primary intensity and frequency of speech sounds found in normal conversational speech.**

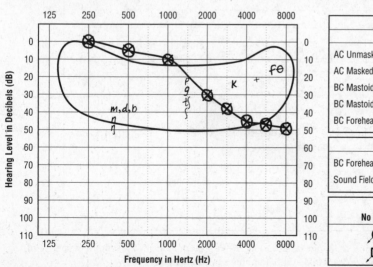

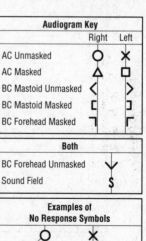

middle frequencies. They also will have access to the suprasegmental aspects of speech, such as rising and falling intonation patterns. The child whose audiogram is displayed in Figure 4.5 is not likely to have access to the weaker, high-frequency consonants, which will negatively affect not only articulation abilities but also vocabulary and morphology. The words *fail* and *sail* differ by only one phoneme, and because this child does not have access to weak high-frequency phonemes, she may mishear words, confuse them, and have greater difficulty developing vocabulary at the same rate as normally hearing children. Further, looking at this child's audiogram, consider morphological development. When adults model morphology by saying "Look, one book and two books," what might this child hear? Rather than hearing two different words that model morphology, the child is likely to hear only the initial /b/ phoneme followed by the vowel each time. The same is true for the words *walk* and *walked*. Although in written form the past tense is communicated by adding "ed," acoustically this is the weak, high-frequency /t/ phoneme. This information is essential to those working with the child on speech–language development as well as others on the child's educational team. Another way to visualize this information is provided in Figure 4.6.

The Audiometer

It is important to examine those parts of the audiometer that allow us to perform pure tone testing. The **audiometer** is the device that generates the pure tone signals used in testing hearing. A typical audiometer is shown in Figure 4.7. Figure 4.8 summarizes the

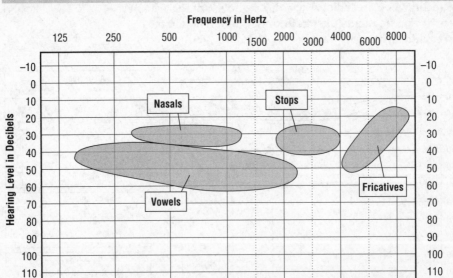

FIGURE 4.6 Frequency/intensity distribution of categories of speech sounds superimposed on an audiogram.

Source: Olsen, W., Hawkins, D., & Van Tasell, D. (1997). Representations of the long-term spectra of speech. *Ear and Hearing, 8*(45), 1003–1085. Reprinted by permission.

FIGURE 4.7 An audiometer.

85
•
The Audiometer

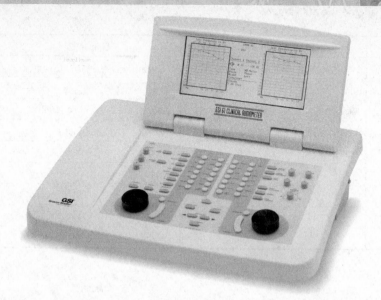

Source: Courtesy of Grason-Stadler, a division of VIASYS Healthcare. Used with permission.

major functions of an audiometer that are needed to conduct audiological evaluations. Note first that the audiometer depicted in Figure 4.8 has two channels. The purpose of a two-channel audiometer is that the audiologist can deliver the auditory stimuli (e.g., pure tones, speech) to one ear, while at the same time sending a different stimulus to the opposite ear (e.g., **masking** a competing stimulus). Because many audiologists use channel 1 of the audiometer to deliver the primary stimulus, let's begin with channel 1.

Note that channel 1 selections include "Stimulus" and "Transducer." The options for stimulus include tone, microphone, tape, and compact disc, and obviously we would select tone to present pure tones. A **transducer** is a device that converts one form of energy to another (e.g., earphone, microphone) and options here include phone, bone, or speaker. Whenever possible, the audiologist attempts to present pure tones through the earphones because this allows assessment of the right ear separate from the left ear. If pure tones are presented through speakers (referred to as **sound field testing**) information is being collected about the better ear (if there is one), but separate right and left ear information is not obtained. Sound field testing is often used in testing young children, individuals who will not tolerate earphones, and when validating the benefit of hearing aids. Sound field applications will be discussed in subsequent chapters.

Bone conduction testing is carried out by choosing the bone transducer, which directs the signal to the bone oscillator. The concept of bone conduction, introduced in Chapter 2, will be expanded in this chapter.

Now that we have reviewed our options for the stimuli and the transducer, note the selection for routing. This option includes left, right, and left/right. This allows us to direct the stimulus to either the right or left earphone or speaker, or to both simultaneously.

FIGURE **4.8** **Schematic of the primary components of the control panel of a diagnostic audiometer.**

FM	Channel 1		Channel 2	
Pulsed	*Stimulus*	*Transducer*	*Transducer*	*Stimulus*
	Tone	Phone	Phone	Tone
	Microphone	Bone	Bone	Microphone
	Tape A	Speaker	Speaker	Tape A
	Tape B			Tape B
		Routing	*Routing*	
		Left	Left	Narrow Bands of Noise
		Right	Right	Speech Noise
		Left/Right	Left/Right	White Noise

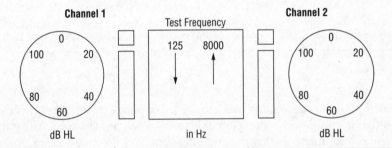

When testing bone conduction, these left and right designations do not apply, because bone conduction signals are picked up by the better cochlea. Bone conduction will be addressed in detail later in the chapter.

Next note the hearing level dial located in the front of the audiometer. Sometimes referred to as the **attenuator dial** (because attenuation refers to reduction in sound energy), this allows the audiologist to increase or decrease the intensity of the signal. Adjacent to the hearing level dial is the interrupt bar. Depression of this bar introduces the pure tone signal to the specific transducer. Finally, the test frequency selection, which includes up and down arrows, allows the audiologist to increase or decrease the test frequency.

Calibration

When the accuracy of the output of some measuring instrument is checked, the instrument is being calibrated. **Calibration** is an important process in our field because audiologists and speech–language pathologists regularly use equipment to generate data regarding the status of some aspect of the client's communication ability. Examples include use of the visi-pitch, nasometer, and the audiometer. When equipment is used in this way, clinicians should consider the underlying relationship between the data generated using that equipment and their client's communication status.

Let's use an example to illustrate. Imagine that you are on a diet. After two weeks of discipline and sticking to your program you step on the scale and find, to your surprise and disappointment, that you have gained 2 pounds. Is it possible that despite the numbers on the scale you have actually lost weight? Yes, if the scale is out of calibration. If, for example, the relationship between 1 pound of weight and the movement of the needle on the scale has become flawed, the data will be erroneous. Even small errors in calibration can be problematic. If for every pound a person weighs the scale registers 1.2 pounds, a 140-pound person would register a weight of 168 pounds. Recall from Chapter 2 that the dial reading on the audiometer uses the reference HL (hearing level). You may also recall that 0 dB HL on the audiometer represents different amounts of sound pressure at different frequencies. This is due to the fact that the eardrum's sensitivity varies with frequency. It takes more sound pressure to create eardrum vibration in the low frequencies compared to the higher frequencies.

In the next section, we discuss the amount of sound pressure required to produce the desired intensity level during audiological testing. We should also note that the standards used to specify standard output levels are different depending on the particular earphone that is being used in the testing process. TDH-39, TDH-49, and TDH-50 are three types of **supra-aural earphones,** or earphones that rest on the outside of the pinna. **Insert earphones,** also called insert receivers, fit directly into the external auditory canal.

ANSI (S3.6-2004) standard output levels for 0 dB HL, which were summarized in Chapter 2 (Table 2.5), are also included in this chapter in Table 4.1. These values serve as the basis for our understanding of calibration. In order to know that the audiometer

TABLE **4.1** **Standard Output Levels for 0 dB HL for Various Earphones**

Frequency in Hz	Supra-Aural Earphones			Insert Earphones (HA-1 Coupler)
	IEC 60318-3	TDH-39	TDH-49/50	
125	45.0	45.0	47.5	26.5
250	27.0	25.5	26.5	14.5
500	13.5	11.5	13.5	6.0
1,000	7.5	7.0	7.5	0.0
2,000	9.0	9.0	11.0	2.5
3,000	11.5	10.0	9.5	2.5
4,000	12.0	9.5	10.5	0.0
6,000	16.0	15.5	13.5	−2.5
8,000	15.5	13.0	13.0	−3.5
Speech	20.0	19.5	20.0	12.5

Source: Excerpted from ANSI S3.6-2004 American National Standard Specification for Audiometers, © 2004 with the permission of the Acoustical Society of America, 35 Pinelawn Road, Suite 114E, Melville, NY 11747.

set to a given intensity level is producing the appropriate amount of sound pressure at the eardrum, we compare the sound pressure produced at this specific HL value with the standard. For example, if the audiometer is set at 1,000 Hz at 70 dB HL (standard intensity used for calibration) and TDH-49 earphones are being used, based on Table 4.1 the resulting sound pressure should be 77.5 dB SPL. If the audiometer is set to 4,000 Hz at 70 dB HL, the sound pressure reading should be 80.5 dB. If the actual sound pressure produced by a given audiometer at a given frequency is not exactly the same as the expected value, is the audiometer out of calibration? Not necessarily. ANSI S3.6-2004 allows a range of acceptable values based on frequency (i.e., ±3 dB up to 5,000 Hz and ±5 dB at 6,000 Hz and beyond). Returning to our previous examples, if my audiometer produces 80 dB SPL when it is set to 70 dB HL at 1,000 Hz, it is in calibration because it is within the ±3-dB standard.

What if an audiometer produces 85 dB SPL when it is set to 4,000 Hz (at 70 dB HL)? If you said it is out of calibration, you are correct, because the difference between the expected value of 80.5 dB SPL and the actual value of 85 dB SPL is greater than the ±3 dB allowed. When an audiometer is out of calibration, the best course of action is to contact a technician who services this equipment to make the necessary repairs/adjustments to the audiometer. Table 4.1 provides reference values for insert earphones.

Correction Factors

Although use of **correction factors** is less than ideal, there are times when they can serve as a temporary solution when calibration is known to be faulty and an appointment for service is weeks away. If the intensity level is out of calibration such that the audiometer is delivering a more intense stimulus than the dial reading indicates, the clinician must *add* to the threshold before recording it. Conversely, if the audiometer delivers too weak a signal, the clinician will need to *subtract* from the obtained threshold.

What are the consequences of using an audiometer that is out of calibration? Imagine testing a child with an audiometer that routinely produces too much sound pressure. Hearing assessment yields normal thresholds when, in fact, the child has a hearing loss. Conversely, what if the audiometer is producing less sound pressure than it should? An individual with normal hearing is incorrectly identified with a hearing loss.

Let's think about the equipment needed to perform the calibration just described. A sound level meter is used for the type of calibration just described, and it includes a microphone, which converts the acoustic energy from the audiometer to an electrical signal. Also used is a coupler, which is designed to approximate the conditions that occur during testing under earphones (i.e., the acoustic impedance of the human ear under an earphone and cushion). This coupler connects the earphone to the microphone of the sound level meter. See Figure 4.9 for an illustration. This coupler is commonly referred to as an

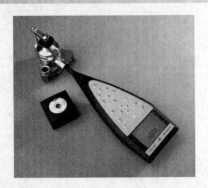

FIGURE **4.9** **2260 Investigator Sound Meter/Analyzer with 4153 Artificial Ear/Coupler.**

Source: Courtesy of Brüel and Kjaer.

TABLE 4.2 **Equivalent Threshold Force Levels for Bone Conduction Output for Mastoid and Forehead Placement at Selected Frequencies**

Frequency in Hz	Placement of Bone Vibrator	
	Mastoid	**Forehead**
250	67.0	79.0
500	58.0	72.0
1,000	42.5	51.0
2,000	31.0	42.5
3,000	30.0	42.0
4,000	35.5	43.5
6,000	40.0	51.0
8,000	40.0	50.0
Speech	55.0	63.5

Source: Excerpted from ANSI S3.6-2004 American National Standard Specification for Audiometers, © 2004 with the permission of the Acoustical Society of America, 35 Pinelawn Road, Suite 114E, Melville, NY 11747.

"artificial ear." Technically correct names for the artificial ear include the NBS-9A and the IEC318. For calibration of the force of bone-conducted signals, very similar procedures are used. Instead of using an artificial ear, an "artificial mastoid" may be used. The technically correct name for an artificial mastoid is mechanical coupler. ANSI standards (S3.6-2004) for the force needed to obtain 0 dB HL are noted in Table 4.2.

Intensity calibration is not the only issue that is of importance in this discussion. Calibration also includes checking the accuracy of frequencies (i.e., does a 1,000-Hz tone actually produce 1,000 cycles per second), checking that each change on the HL dial of the audiometer results in consistent changes in sound pressure (referred to as linearity), and checking for distortion. Frequency and distortion measurements require additional equipment beyond the sound level meter.

Calibration is essential not only for the audiometer but also for the test room in which comprehensive hearing assessment takes place. This acoustically modified room is typically attached to a second separate room where the audiometer is located. Between the two rooms is a window that allows the audiologist to observe the client and vice versa. See Figure 4.10 for a picture of a typical testing room arrangement. It should be noted that the acoustically modified room in which threshold testing is done is a **sound-treated test booth** but not a "soundproof" room. This is a common misconception. Soundproof rooms are also referred to as anechoic chambers, and if we take this word apart we see that the soundproof room allows no echo. Such rooms are very expensive to construct and are typically used by researchers conducting acoustic experiments. Sound-treated rooms are acoustically modified, but not to the degree that anechoic chambers are. Some of the common features of sound-treated test booths include the following:

- Thick metal double doors on the outside of the booth that close tightly
- Incandescent lighting (to avoid the buzz or hum made by other types of lights)

FIGURE **4.10**   **A two-room test suite.**

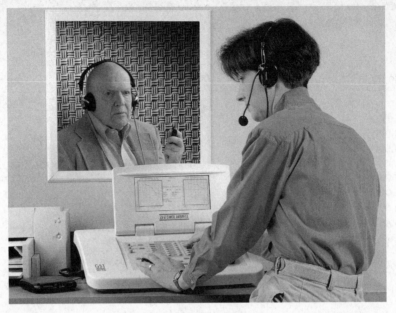

Source: Courtesy of Grason-Stadler, a division of VIASYS Healthcare. Used with permission.

- A ventilation system that includes sound attenuation
- Two layers of thick metal panels (referred to as a double-walled booth) forming the walls of the booth
- Sound-attenuating material inserted between these wall panels (and exposed by small holes in the walls)
- Carpet on the floor
- Multiple windows separating the patient room from the tester room
- The booth raised off the ground to reduce the effects of vibrational noise

In order for a room to be deemed suitable for audiological assessment, noise levels must be sufficiently reduced to allow threshold testing down to 0 dB HL at each of the test frequencies. Remember from earlier discussions that noise can easily mask high-frequency sounds, and if this occurs the client's thresholds for those frequencies will become elevated and unreliable. In addition, the presence of noise in the test environment will result in elevated (poorer) low-frequency thresholds. Values for maximum permissible noise levels for audiological test booths are provided in the ANSI 3.1-1991 standard. The standard includes an "ears covered" requirement, which refers to earphone testing, and an "ears uncovered" requirement, which refers to bone conduction and sound field testing. More noise is permissible in the "ears covered" condition because earphones serve to reduce the amount of background noise perceived by the client.

In addition to a basic understanding of the calibration issues described above, professionals who are using audiometric equipment for diagnostic or screening purposes should also be familiar with the steps in biological (listening) checks of equipment, included in Chapter 11 on screening. Special attention should be paid to calibration when portable audiometers, moved from one location to another, are used, which increases the chance that calibration will be affected.

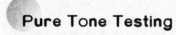

Pure Tone Testing

Before Testing

Before an audiologist begins the pure tone testing of a client, the client is typically greeted and a brief pretest interview is conducted. This pretest interview may be useful in a number of ways. First, audiologists can ask clients questions that will provide insight about their hearing/communication status. For example, a common question is whether the person has concerns about his or her hearing. A good number of the clients who seek out audiologists do so not because they perceive their hearing as a problem, but rather because a family member has complained about the client's hearing. A client who has hearing loss but who reports little to no difficulty hearing may be resistant to later efforts to improve communication through hearing aids.

Information regarding hearing difficulty can also be obtained by asking clients how they perform in specific listening situations. For example, how does the client perform when talking on the telephone or watching TV? Can he understand speech in noisy settings or at distances? Individuals who have sensorineural hearing loss often report understanding speech well in quiet settings but with difficulty in noisier environments. Questions about exposure to noise can be important because noise can be very damaging to the inner ear. Unfortunately, this is a question that should now be asked of teenagers, because of the increased use of headsets that deliver potentially damaging levels of sound to the ear.

Other questions that may be posed during this pretest interview concern potential medical issues that may be affecting hearing. For example, an audiologist may ask if the client has any **tinnitus,** dizziness or balance difficulties, or any pain or drainage from her ears. Also, has the client been seen by an ear, nose, and throat (ENT) physician for medical conditions of the ear or ear surgery? Table 4.3 provides a sample adult case history form with corresponding comments as to the underlying rationale for each question.

In addition to obtaining information about the client's hearing/communication status, the pretest interview also is an opportunity for audiologists to establish rapport with clients so that they will be more relaxed during the testing process. Also, an audiologist can make some preliminary decisions about the possible need to modify the typical test procedures.

Taking the case history provides an opportunity for audiologists to practice audiology that is both humanistic and scientific. During the case history, information is collected that will be important in the diagnostic evaluation process, such as whether there may be a better-hearing ear or if a medical component to the hearing loss is likely to exist. At the same time, the audiologist actively listens and attends to both verbal and nonverbal messages, which are very important to the diagnostic and later case management processes.

Following the pretest interview, an audiologist will perform otoscopy in order to identify any obvious abnormality (e.g., blood in the canal, drainage, wax blockage). **Otoscopy** is visual examination of the ear canal and the eardrum with an **otoscope.**

TABLE 4.3   Sample Adult Case History Form

Case History Question	Rationale
1. What is the reason for your visit here today?	Hearing testing can be done for a variety of purposes (to identify communication difficulties, to rule out medical pathology, to monitor medication effects, etc.), and the answer to this question gives direction to the rest of the case history interview and possibly to the rest of the evaluation.
2. Do you believe that you have a hearing loss? (If yes, discuss time of onset.)	Interestingly, many patients who have hearing loss respond no to this question. This can be important later if recommendations are made for the client to initiate a trial period of amplification. Such clients may be disinclined to pursue such assistance.
3. Do you believe that one ear is better than the other?	In the normal course of events, hearing should be the same in each ear. For example, age-related hearing loss is typically symmetrical. Unilateral or asymmetrical hearing losses can signal some type of medical issues (e.g., an inner ear fistula, an acoustic schwannoma, Meniere's disease). Remember also that the answer to this question directs the audiologist to begin (pure tone) testing with the better ear.
4. Do you believe that your hearing loss is gradual, or have you noted any sudden changes in it?	Sudden changes in hearing could signal some type of medical issue. In the typical course of events, changes in hearing are gradual.
5. How would you describe your ability to understand conversational speech when on the telephone? Watching TV? In noisy environments? At distances?	These questions are more related to the rehabilitation aspect of hearing assessment and will be helpful if the client decides to pursue some type of amplification. Addressing the client's specific listening needs is important to their achieving satisfaction. The question about hearing in noisy backgrounds can be diagnostically significant because the ability to understand speech is related to brainstem function and the central auditory system.
6. Do you experience a sensation of ringing, buzzing, or other noises in your head or ears? If so, do these sounds keep you awake at night?	Tinnitus is a common sign of hearing loss but also can be triggered by medical conditions (middle ear effusion, acoustic schwannoma, etc.) or environmental agents (e.g., medication, excessive caffeine). Asking if the client's sleep is disrupted gives the audiologist an idea of the severity of the tinnitus and could make tinnitus management a primary objective of intervention.
7. Do you experience any pain or drainage from your ears? Do you have a plugged or fullness sensation in one or both of your ears? Have you ever been seen by an ENT physician?	Obviously these questions are medically related to ascertain the degree to which middle ear pathology could be a factor. A sensation of fullness, especially in only one ear, can be associated with an acoustic schwannoma or Meniere's disease.

TABLE 4.3 (*continued*)

Case History Question	Rationale
8. Have you experienced dizziness or a sensation that the room is spinning (vertigo)?	These symptoms can be associated with a number of conditions, including benign paroxysmal vertigo, acoustic schwannoma, labyrinthitis, and inner ear fistula. Remember that hearing assessments are commonly part of the physician's medial workup for individuals who have vestibular symptoms. In these cases, the audiologist is more likely to carry out specific tests to rule out retrocochlear pathology, including masking level difference (MLD), acoustic reflex decay, and auditory brainstem response (ABR).
9. Do you have a history of or are you currently exposed to loud sounds, either through your work or at home or through hobbies/leisure activities?	Because noise exposure can have a devastating effect on high-frequency hearing, it is important to inquire about it. Some clients are not aware of the extent of their noise exposure until this question is asked. If the client answers this question affirmatively, counseling is important to decrease exposure and promote the use of ear protection. Remember to ask this question to teenagers; they tend to listen to music at loud levels.
10. Do you currently wear hearing aids, and are the aids helping you to your satisfaction?	Some patients have come to the audiologist because they need to have their hearing rechecked and their hearing aids adjusted. For those who do not have hearing aids, this question often gives the audiologist some insight into the client's view of hearing aids. For example, some clients comment that they do not wear aids but believe that they are ready to do so, and other clients comment that they will not wear hearing aids.
11. Is there a family history of hearing loss?	Provides insight regarding potential etiology of hearing loss.
12. What do you think may have caused your hearing loss?	Provides the client with an opportunity to reveal information about etiology that was not elicited by the previous questions.

This is a familiar instrument because it is frequently used by physicians to examine patients' ears during physical exams. Audiologists can perform otoscopy in their office or in the sound-treated booth. Otoscopy, as performed by the audiologist, is not performed for purposes of making a diagnosis and is therefore commonly referred to as "nondiagnostic otoscopy." Otoscopy is also important because comprehensive audiological assessment may involve placement of something into the ear canal of the client (e.g., insert earphones, probe for immittance testing). It is not good practice to perform these procedures without first examining the client's ears. In cases where supra-aural earphones are being used, otoscopy should be used to assess the possibility of **collapsing ear canals.** In some clients, the force of the headband connected to the earphones causes the ear canal to close up. If this happens, the hearing test results will be inaccurate because sound will be blocked from traveling through the ear canal. Solutions for this problem are discussed later in this chapter.

A reliable procedure for otoscopy includes first gently pulling the pinna up and back (for adults) or down and back (for children). This opens the ear canal for easier observation of the eardrum. The speculum of the otoscope is then placed into the ear canal and the examiner looks through the otoscope's lens. If the eardrum is not seen, the examiner redirects the beam of light by carefully changing the angle of the otoscope; the otoscope can be moved to the left or right, or up or down, until the eardrum is visualized.

Under normal conditions, the examiner will note some wax in the ear canal, but not enough to occlude (block) the canal. This wax is often orange or brown in color. Also, many individuals have hair in their ear canal, which is noted during this process. The eardrum itself is typically pearly gray in color, and is translucent. This means that it allows light to pass through, but not to the degree that structures behind it can be clearly seen. The manubrium of the malleus may be seen during otoscopy.

The Test Process

The client should now be seated comfortably in the chair located in the sound booth. In some cases, it is advisable to have the client face the audiologist. For example, for those clients who require more reassurance and reinforcement, making eye contact can be very important. If the client is facing the audiologist, every effort should be made not to inadvertently provide the client with any cues regarding when pure tones are being presented. Some clients may pick up on subtle cues that the audiologist is unaware are being provided. For example, the audiologist's head movements, arm movements, eye movements, and/or facial expressions may provide unintended cues to the client. Some audiologists choose to situate the client so that he or she is seated at an angle, facing slightly away from the audiologist. This allows some interaction between the client and audiologist but reduces the opportunity for the client to detect cues.

Instructions for Obtaining Pure Tone Thresholds

The first part of obtaining accurate pure tone thresholds is to provide the client with specific instructions regarding his or her role in the testing. These instructions should include a clear indication that the client must respond to the tones even if the tones are very faint. Remember that most clients, because they are cooperative and honest people, will want to provide reliable responses to the audiologist. In some cases, this desire "not to make any mistakes" causes clients to delay responding until they are sure they have heard the tone. Rather than providing threshold data, this results in suprathreshold findings, which make the client's hearing appear to be worse than it actually is. Therefore, when giving instructions to clients for pure tone testing, it is important to emphasize the necessity of responding to the very faint tones.

Another important part of the instructions to clients involves the response mode. What will clients do to indicate that they have heard the tone? Will they raise their hand? Will they say "yes" or "I hear it?" Will they depress a response button? The choice of response is best made by the audiologist, who has assessed the client's capabilities during the case history interview and who has some knowledge of potential difficulties with various response techniques. For example, hand raising can be problematic if a client fails to raise his hand fully when he hears the tone and then lower it fully. Some clients who are uncertain about their perception of very faint tones will raise their hand halfway, making interpretation of the response difficult for the audiologist. The advantage of requiring a verbal response from clients to indicate that they have heard the sound may be to reduce the need to look at clients for visual confirmation of every response, thereby reducing the potential for "cueing" clients.

Similarly, when using a response button, some individuals, especially older clients, have a tendency to continue depressing the response button long after the tone has been terminated. This requires that the audiologist repeatedly remind the client to remove her finger from the button. Because older people sometimes lose some of their touch sensitivity, it may be difficult for them to know that their finger is still on the button. Sometimes, instructing clients to "tap" the response button is effective in communicating that they should not hold the button down. Special modifications of response techniques for clients can be found in Chapters 8 and 9.

Earphone Placement

When placing conventional earphones on clients, care should be taken to ensure that the diaphragm of the earphone is directly over the client's ear canal. Otherwise, the signal will be reduced in intensity and the person's air conduction hearing levels will appear poorer than they really are. Similarly, when placing the bone vibrator on the client's head (mastoid process or forehead), be sure that the bone vibrator is in firm contact with the skull. If this is not the case, a weaker signal than intended will reach the cochlea, and the client's hearing levels will again appear worse than they truly are.

Threshold Search

Regarding the actual presentation of pure tones to clients, the American Speech-Language-Hearing Association (ASHA) guidelines for manual pure tone audiometry (2005) suggest that tones be 1 to 2 sec in duration, and that the interval between tones be varied but not shorter than the test tone. In addition, audiologists should begin the testing by familiarizing clients with the testing process by delivering a tone that is intense enough to elicit a clear response. Consistent with ASHA guidelines, many audiologists do this by presenting a tone of 30 dB, and if no response occurs, increasing the intensity to 50 dB. If no response results, the tone is increased in 10-dB steps until a response is noted.

Once the client has responded to the initial tone, the clinician decreases its intensity by 10 dB and presents that signal. If the client responds to this less intense signal, the tone is decreased in intensity, again by 10 dB, and is presented. Every time the client responds to a signal, the intensity is decreased by 10 dB; if the client does not respond, the signal is increased by 5 dB. This "down 10, up 5" process (**ascending–descending approach**) continues until the client's **threshold** is identified, which is defined as "the lowest decibel hearing level at which responses occur in at least one half of a series of ascending trials. The minimum number of responses needed to determine the threshold of hearing is two responses out of three presentations at a single level" (ASHA, 2005, p. 4).

In a departure from previous ASHA guidelines, pure tone diagnostic threshold testing now routinely includes 3,000 and 6,000 Hz (ASHA, 2005). This means that threshold measures should be made at 250, 500, 1,000, 2,000, 3,000, 4,000, 6,000, and 8,000 Hz. In cases of low-frequency hearing loss, 125 Hz should also be measured. These frequencies represent a portion of the total range of frequencies (20 to 20,000 Hz) that are audible to the normal human ear. This restricted range used in audiometric testing represents those frequencies that are most important to our understanding of speech. ASHA (2005) also recommends that interoctave measurements be made in cases in which a difference of 20 dB or more exists between the thresholds at any two adjacent octave frequencies between 500 and 2,000 Hz. Testing typically begins at 1,000 Hz in the better ear (if case study information suggests that one ear is better than the other).

The choice of 1,000 Hz as a starting frequency is based on the fact that this is a relatively easy signal to perceive and that many clients have normal hearing at this frequency. If there is no knowledge or suspicion that one ear is better, many audiologists begin testing in the right ear. Testing typically proceeds to the higher frequencies (2,000, 3,000, 4,000, 6,000, 8,000 Hz), back to 1,000 Hz for a reliability check, and then to 250 and 500 Hz. In the event that the client does not readily respond to the 1,000-Hz signal, two basic strategies may be used. First, audiologists can increase the intensity of the signal by 20 dB and see if a response is elicited. If so, proceed with testing (down 10, up 5 procedure). If not, the second strategy would be to switch to 500 Hz at the same intensity level. This may be effective if the client has better hearing sensitivity at 500 Hz.

Now that we have examined the process of obtaining pure tone thresholds, let's examine Case 1 in Figure 4.11. What have been plotted on this audiogram are two air conduction thresholds in the right ear. At 1,000 Hz a threshold of 10 dB is noted, and at

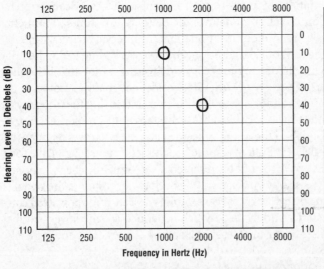
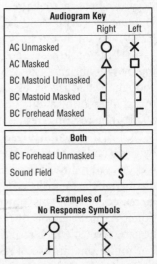

FIGURE **4.11** **Air conduction thresholds at 1,000 and 2,000 Hz in the right ear.**

2,000 Hz a threshold of 40 dB is noted. Let's review how the audiologist obtained these thresholds. First, the tone was presented at 1,000 Hz at 30 dB. Using one of the response modes described previously, the client responded. Because the audiologist is attempting to assess the client's threshold, the intensity of the tone was decreased to 20 dB (down 10) and the tone was presented again. The client again responded and the intensity was further decreased to 10 dB. Because this 10-dB tone was also heard, the audiologist decreased the tone to 0 dB; this did not elicit a response from the client. The audiologist then increased the intensity of the tone to 5 dB (up 5). This 5-dB tone also did not elicit a response from the client, so the intensity was increased again to 10 dB (up 5 again). Once again, the 10-dB tone was heard by the client.

At this point the client has responded twice at 10 dB HL. The audiologist keeps this in mind as the search for the client's right ear air conduction threshold continues. Decreasing to 0 dB, the audiologist presents the tone, but no response is elicited. Increasing in 5-dB steps, no response is noted at 5 dB but a response is noted at 10 dB. We can conclude that 10 dB represents this client's air conduction threshold in the right ear, so a circle is recorded on the audiogram at 1,000 Hz at 10 dB HL.

The process of threshold testing for 1,000 and 2,000 Hz in Case 1 is summarized in Table 4.4.

It is important to note that threshold testing is not always as efficient as suggested by these examples. For instance, consider the client who has responded twice to a tone at 10 dB at a given frequency. The audiologist decreases the signal intensity to 0 dB and no response is elicited. The intensity is then increased to 5 dB and the client responds. Why is the client responding at 5 dB now when he did not respond previously at this level? One possible reason is that the client is getting better at the task of listening at threshold. Also, a client's threshold can fluctuate within a 5-dB range and is affected by his or her attention to the task at that given moment. Changes of 5 dB from one test session to another are not considered true changes, but rather reflect test–retest reliability. Human responses to sound reflect the combined factors of auditory sensation (acoustics) and perception (psychology). The combined study of psychology and acoustics is **psychoacoustics.**

TABLE 4.4	Case 1: Threshold Search, 1,000 and 2,000 Hz		
Presentation Level in HL	**Client Response**	**Presentation Level in HL**	**Client Response**
1,000 Hz		**2,000 Hz**	
30 dB	Response	30	No response
20 dB	Response	50	Response
10 dB	Response	40	Response
0 dB	No response	30	No response
5 dB	No response	35	No response
10 dB	Response	40	Response
0 dB	No response	30	No response
5 dB	No response	35	No response
10 dB	Response	40	Response

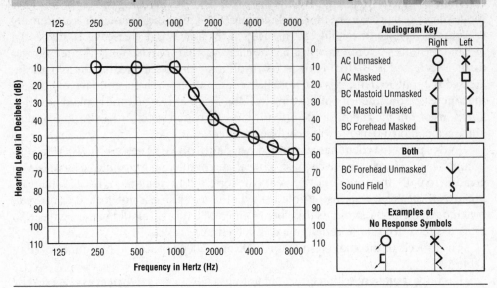

FIGURE **4.12** **Frequencies 250 to 8,000 Hz tested in the right ear.**

Resuming the search for this client's threshold, the audiologist now makes a mental note that the client has responded twice at 10 dB and once at 5 dB. Beginning at minus 5 dB (a decrease of 10 dB from the previous response level of 5 dB), the audiologist increases the intensity of the tone in 5-dB steps. If the client fails to respond at 5 dB but does respond at 10 dB, the threshold is 10 dB because the client has provided two responses out of three presentations at the same level.

Depicted in Figure 4.12 is an audiogram of the right ear pure tone air conduction thresholds as tested at all of the standard test frequencies and the interoctave frequency of 1,500 Hz. This interoctave frequency is tested because the difference noted in the threshold at 1,000 Hz and the threshold at 2,000 Hz is more than 20 dB (i.e., $40 - 10 = 30$ dB).

Pure Tone Average

One common calculation made after pure tone audiometry has been completed is the **pure tone average.** This is the average of the air conduction thresholds for a given ear at 500, 1,000, and 2,000 Hz. Like most averages, the pure tone average is calculated to provide a summary of information regarding the client's hearing loss. Additionally, the calculated value may not accurately reflect/summarize the overall data. For example, in Figure 4.12, the pure tone average is 20 dB ($10 + 10 + 40 \div 3$), which falls within the normal range of hearing for adults. Examination of the pure tone audiogram, however, indicates that although this client does have normal hearing sensitivity in the low to middle frequencies (i.e., 250 to 1,000 Hz), she also has hearing impairment in the important high-frequency range. In fact, adults who have a hearing loss with this degree and slope regularly report difficulty understanding conversational speech when the room acoustics are poor or if background noise is present. Further, children with this hearing loss often have a range of articulation/phonological and language difficulties. The mathematical average, which included two normal frequencies and one abnormal frequency, has resulted in a value that underestimates the difficulty that this client will experience. In the next chapter we will discuss how the pure tone average can be valuable to the audiologist in determining whether internal consistency exists among the tests. It is important to remember that the pure tone average should not be used to describe the degree of hearing loss a client has.

It is permissible to use variations of the traditional three-frequency pure tone average described above, depending on the configuration of the hearing loss and the purpose of the calculation. For example, in the case just discussed, use of a two-frequency average (eliminating the abnormal frequency) would further underestimate the client's hearing levels. Use of a four-frequency average (500, 1,000, 2,000, 4,000 Hz divided by 4) would provide a more accurate reflection of the potential impact of the hearing loss on speech understanding and communication. The specific pure tone average used can depend on the configuration of the hearing loss or other factors such as requirements of a specific state or organization (e.g., public funding agency or workers' compensation board).

As noted earlier, there are currently two primary options for directing pure tones by phone: supra-aural earphones, which are the standard phones that are placed over the client's ears; and insert earphones, which are inserted directly into the ear canals of the client. Disadvantages of insert earphones include their expense (the foam plugs are disposable) and their lack of popularity with some children (who may object to them because they are somewhat invasive). Also, insert earphones may not be appropriate for clients who have a discharge or infection in the ear canal. Advantages of insert earphones include the considerable reduction in the need to use masking (discussed in detail in the Appendix to this chapter), because sound is less likely to cross over to the non-test ear.

Also, unlike supra-aural earphones, inserts do not cause collapsing ear canals. Photos of supra-aural and insert earphones are shown in Figure 4.13 and 4.14. One last type of earphones that clinicians may encounter is *circumaural earphones,* which resemble earmuffs and fit around the external ear. These are the least commonly encountered type of earphone. Whatever type of earphone is used should be compatible with the particular audiometer and calibrated appropriately.

Pure Tone Bone Conduction Testing

The process of assessing pure tone bone conduction thresholds is essentially the same as that described for air conduction thresholds. The main difference is that the transducer selected on the audiometer is now bone rather than phone. Also, the right and left selections are not relevant because when the bone vibrator is placed on the client's skull, the better cochlea picks up the sound. Even if the bone vibrator is placed on

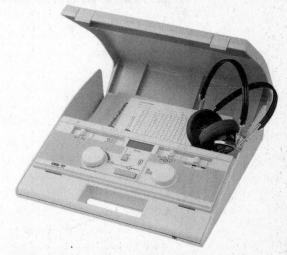

FIGURE **4.13** **Supra-aural earphones.**

Source: Courtesy of Grason-Stadler, a division of VIASYS Healthcare. Used with permission.

FIGURE **4.14**   **Insert earphones.**

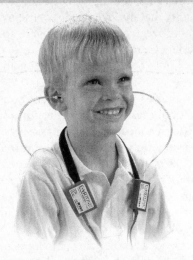

FIGURE **4.14**   **Insert earphones.**

Source: E-ARTONE® Insert Earphone photo courtesy of Aearo Technologies.

the right mastoid, the sound can be picked up by the left cochlea with little to no loss of intensity (attenuation). ASHA (2005) recommends that bone conduction thresholds be obtained at octave intervals from 250 to 4,000 Hz and at 3,000 Hz. In addition, higher frequencies can be tested if the bone oscillator and equipment being used are adequate for this purpose. Because unmasked bone conduction testing is done with the ears uncovered, individuals with normal or near normal low-frequency hearing levels must be tested in an appropriately sound-treated environment. Also, because sending sound vibrations to the cochlea by way of the skull requires more intensity, the maximum output intensity levels the audiometer can produce at different frequencies for bone conduction are less than those for air-conducted tones. Figure 4.15 provides a case example to illustrate.

One decision that an audiologist makes when performing bone conduction testing is whether to place the vibrator on the part of the mastoid bone located behind the pinna or on the forehead. Although not commonly used, one advantage of forehead placement is that the bone vibrator is generally held in place by a band that fits around the client's skull. With mastoid placement,

FIGURE **4.15**   **Use of no response (⌡) symbol to indicate no response at the limits of the audiometer for bone conduction testing.**

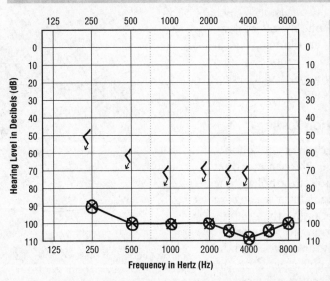

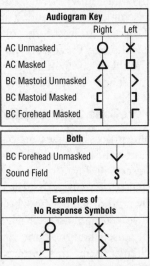

the bone vibrator itself, which is enclosed in a plastic case, must press directly against the skin of the mastoid area. Even though the vibrator is attached to a tension headband for purposes of securing it in place, it can move or even suddenly fall off the client's head.

In addition to the advantage of a more secure fit, some audiologists prefer forehead placement because it is more convenient when introducing masking. As will be discussed, there are times when noise must be directed into one ear (by air conduction) while simultaneously assessing tones by bone conduction. Forehead bone conduction placement allows for easy introduction of masking. In fact, some audiologists prefer to place earphones on the patient along with the forehead bone vibrator before bone conduction testing begins, so that they do not have to go back into the sound room to add earphones for masking.

Placing the bone vibrator on the mastoid of the test ear is a common approach. An important advantage of mastoid placement for bone conduction testing is the fact that placing the bone vibrator directly on the mastoid allows thresholds to be obtained with less vibration. This is important because, as noted previously, bone-conducted signals require more intensity than air-conducted signals, which consequently limits the range of intensities for which bone conduction can be tested. Use of forehead placement may limit this even further. For clients who have significant hearing loss, this can mean the difference between being able to measure a bone conduction threshold or not.

Masking

Masking is a subject of considerable discussion in the field of audiology. In fact, in the fifth edition of Katz's *Handbook of Clinical Audiology* (2002) there are sixty subheadings in the subject index under the word *masking*. Nicolosi, Harriman, and Kresheck (1989) define masking as: (1) noise of any kind that interferes with the audibility of another sound; (2) in audiology, noise used in an attempt to eliminate the participation of one ear while the opposite ear is being tested. Similarly, the American National Standards Institute (ANSI S3.6-2004, pp. 6–7) defines masking in this way:

1. The process by which the threshold of hearing for one sound is raised by the presence of another (masking) sound
2. The amount by which the threshold of hearing for one sound is raised by the presence of another (masking) sound, expressed in decibels

While our primary interest is the use of masking in the clinical setting, there are many times throughout the day when sounds we are trying to hear are "masked" by other sounds, as discussed in Chapter 2 regarding environmental acoustics. In effect, our hearing thresholds become "poorer" due to the presence of the secondary (masking) noise. In the clinic, this phenomenon is useful when we are trying to eliminate the participation of the non-test ear.

In clinical work, we intentionally use masking to eliminate the participation of the non-test ear. Goldstein and Newman (1994) state that clinical masking involves two main concepts: a second signal is introduced that interferes with the primary (test) signal and a shift in threshold generally occurs.

Why would it be necessary to eliminate the non-test ear during audiological assessment? Recall that cases of **asymmetrical hearing loss,** in which the air conduction responses from each ear are not the same, were discussed in Chapter 2. If one ear has a severe hearing loss and the other ear is within normal limits, as indicated at 1,000 Hz in Figure 4.16, it is possible for the signal being presented to the poorer (in this case, left) ear to be so intense that it is heard by the better (in this case, right) ear. We often say that the more intense signal has "crossed over" to the other ear. If this occurs, the left-ear thresholds may be inaccurate because they have been obtained with some participation from the non-test ear. Elimination of the non-test ear through masking is done in order to obtain reliable thresholds in the poorer ear. Masking is not necessary when a **symmetrical hearing loss** exists, in which air conduction thresholds are the same in both ears.

Review the diagram of the audiometer in Figure 4.8. Note that the audiometer has two channels. One of the purposes of a two-channel audiometer is that the audiologist can deliver a tone to one ear while at the same time sending masking noise into the other ear. Based on the case in Figure 4.16, the tone would be directed from channel 1 to the left ear because this is the test ear. At the same time, noise would be directed from channel 2 to the right ear.

Note also that on this audiometer there are three different types of noise from which to choose. Which one is most effective for masking pure tones? Research suggests that all maskers are not created equal. A masker should be efficient, which means the masker uses the least amount of sound pressure needed to complete the task. The work of Fletcher (1940) and Fletcher and Munson (1937) showed that the use of a narrow band of noise centered around the test frequency provided masking of the test tone. Use of

FIGURE 4.16 Discrepancy between right and left air conduction thresholds illustrates the need for masking of the right ear.

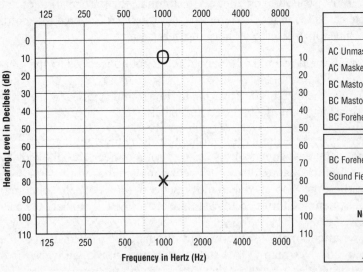
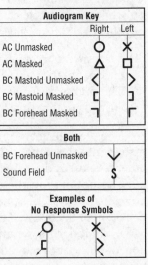

additional bands of noise did not increase the masking effect, but served to add to the overall loudness of the masker. This phenomenon is related to the "critical band" concept, which says that the only parts of the noise that have a masking effect on the test tone lie within a restricted band with the test tone at its center. When masking is needed during pure tone testing, narrow-band noise, centered around the frequency of interest (i.e., the test frequency), is used. During speech audiometry, speech noise is used for masking.

Effective Masking

Effective masking (EM) is defined by ANSI as the dB HL to which threshold is shifted by a given level of noise (Yacullo, 1996). If we have 40 dB EM, then the threshold of a pure tone air conduction signal will be shifted to 40 dB HL. In the presence of 40 dB EM, a 40-dB HL pure tone will be just audible. Yacullo has explained that this definition is used by most authorities on clinical masking and is consistent with the critical band concept discussed earlier.

A goal of audiological evaluation is to assess the hearing sensitivity of each ear. In cases where a difference in hearing exists of sufficient magnitude between the two ears, masking has to be used to keep the non-test ear occupied. In these cases, without the use of masking, we would not be able to isolate the test ear from the non-test ear, and the test results would be inaccurate. The use of contralateral masking accomplishes the goal of separating the test ear from the non-test ear. With this conceptual framework, when to mask will be discussed. For the interested student, a discussion on how to mask is included in Appendix A. Appendix A also includes information about undermasking, overmasking, the occlusion effect, and the plateau method for masking.

When to Mask

Air Conduction Threshold Testing

Remember that interaural attenuation is defined as a reduction in the energy of the signal as it is transmitted (for the most part by bone conduction) from one side of the skull to the other. This transmission is possible because signals presented to one ear that are sufficiently intense reach the cochlea on the opposite side. If the opposite cochlea is sensitive enough to detect the portion of the signal that has crossed over, this will interfere with audiological testing. The generally recommended minimum interaural attenuation for air conduction is 40 dB HL (Martin, 1974; Martin & Clark, 2003). This value assumes that supra-aural earphones are used. If insert earphones are employed, the interaural attenuation is greater, and can range from approximately 75 dB in the lower frequencies to 50 dB in the higher frequencies. A conservative minimum interaural attenuation value is 50 dB. Clinically, this means that the use of insert earphones affords greater "protection" from cross-hearing (sound traveling from one side of the skull to the other via bone conduction), and a more intense signal may be presented before masking is necessary to isolate the test ear.

The first step in masking is to recognize that cross-hearing can possibly occur in a given set of circumstances. These circumstances generally involve different hearing between the client's ears. Minimum interaural attenuation of 40 dB HL means that the presence of the head between the two ears prevents cross-hearing of up to 40 dB HL. In cases where the difference in hearing between the two ears exceeds 40 dB HL, the clinician must consider whether masking is needed. Although it is tempting to base masking decisions on the difference between the two ears' responses to air-conducted signals, the truth is that the bone conduction threshold of the non-test ear is the critical variable to consider when determining the need for masking during air conduction testing.

This can also be stated in a "formula" that can be applied to threshold data to determine the need for masking during air conduction testing. The formula reads as follows:

$$ACT\ (TE) - IA \geq BCT\ (NTE)$$

where

IA (AC) = 40 dB for supra-aural earphones

IA (AC) = 50 dB for insert earphones

Translation: if the air conduction threshold (ACT) of the test ear minus the minimum interaural attenuation (40 dB HL) is greater than or equal to the bone conduction threshold (BCT) of the non-test ear, then masking is needed to occupy (in effect, to "raise the threshold") of the non-test ear, to eliminate its participation in the test.

Consider the audiological data and decide whether masking is necessary for air conduction testing of the poorer ear in the following four sample masking cases. Answers appear at the end of this chapter, starting on page 122.

Sample Case 1: Unmasked Results

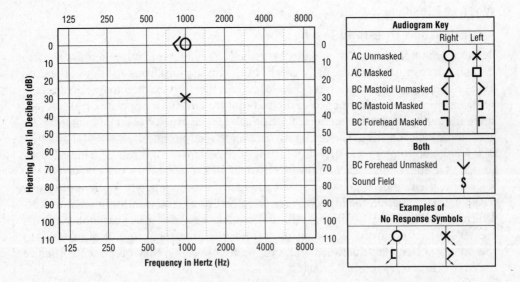

Q: Is masking needed for AC testing of the left ear?

Sample Case 2: Unmasked Results

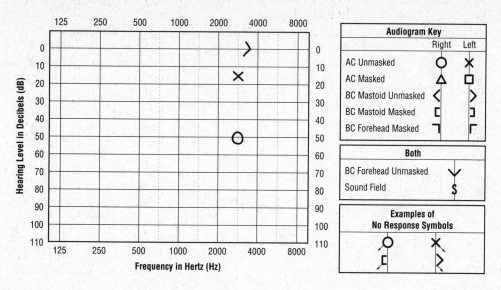

Q: Is masking needed for AC testing of the right ear?

Sample Case 3: Unmasked Results

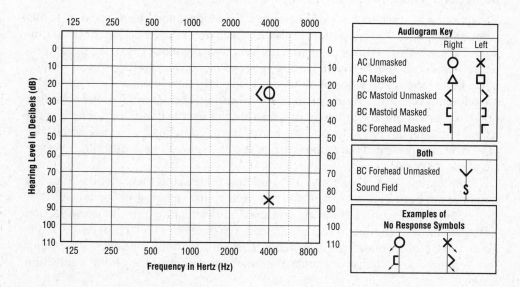

Q: Is masking needed for AC testing of the left ear?

Sample Case 4: Unmasked Results

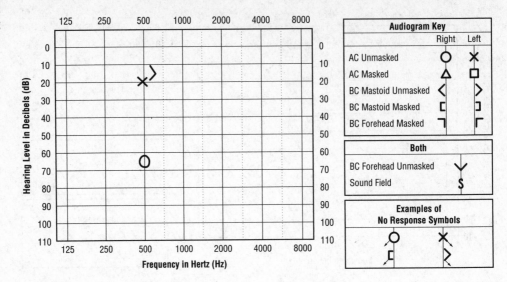

Q: Is masking needed for AC testing of the right ear?

Bone Conduction Threshold Testing

The question of when to mask during bone conduction could be answered by saying "most of the time." The reason for this is that the interaural attenuation for bone conducted signals is 0 dB HL, meaning that the head does not block any of the signal from reaching one cochlea or the other. During bone conduction testing, the physical location of the **bone conduction vibrator** (sometimes called the bone oscillator) on the skull is not relevant, because the more sensitive (better-hearing) cochlea will respond regardless of the placement of the vibrator. In other words, placing the bone vibrator behind the left ear pinna, on the mastoid process, in no way assures the clinician that the left cochlea is receiving the presented pure tone signal or that the patient's response reflects the status of the left cochlea.

Considering these concepts, you should now understand that any time there is a potential air–bone gap *in the test ear,* you need to use masking in the non-test ear during bone conduction testing. This means that, during pure tone bone conduction testing, if the bone conduction results are better than the air conduction results at any point in the process, masking will be needed to determine bone conduction thresholds for the poorer ear. Stated as a formula, the "rule" for masking during bone conduction testing is

$$\text{ABG} > 10 \text{ dB in the TE}$$

Translation: any time there is an air–bone gap (ABG) greater than 10 dB in the test ear (TE), use masking in the non-test ear during bone conduction testing. Practically speaking, when a difference between the two ears exists, the clinician usually bases the masking for bone conduction decision on the "best bone" responses. If the best bone responses suggest the potential for air–bone gaps in the test ear, masking will be needed to determine the type of hearing loss in the test ear.

On the other hand, there are many cases of symmetrical sensorineural hearing loss that do not require masking during bone conduction testing. Why not? If the "best" *unmasked* bone conduction thresholds are the same as (or within 5 dB of) the thresholds obtained by air conduction, no additional information would be gained by using masking because there is no air–bone gap to begin with. The thresholds by bone conduction would remain essentially the same if masking were used, and the clinical picture would be unchanged. Based on this information, in most cases of bilateral symmetrical sensorineural hearing loss, most clinicians opt to test unmasked bone conduction thresholds. Because the interaural attenuation by bone conduction is 0 dB, it does not matter where on the skull the bone vibrator is placed (it could be on either the mastoid process or the forehead, for example).

Consider whether masking is needed to determine bone conduction thresholds for the following cases. Remember that accurate bone conduction information is necessary to determine the type of hearing loss present. Refer to the end of this chapter for answers.

Sample Case 1: Unmasked Results

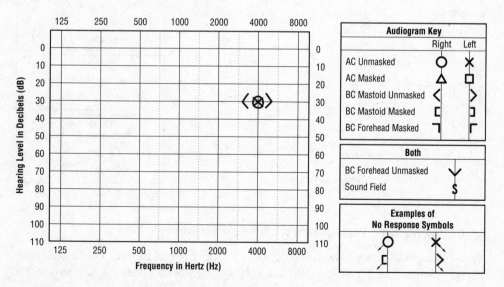

Q: Is masking needed during bone conduction (BC) testing?

Sample Case 2: Unmasked Results

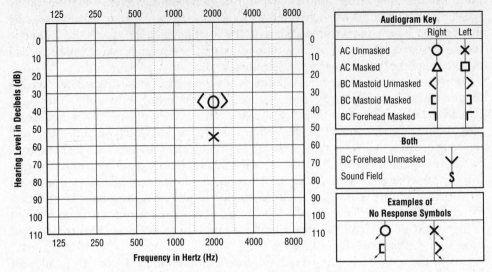

Q: Is masking needed to determine the BC threshold for the left ear at 2,000 Hz?

Sample Case 3: Unmasked Results

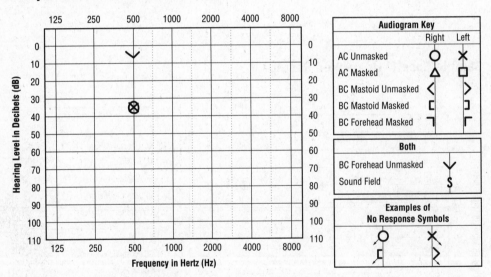

Q: Where is masking needed?

Recording Masked Test Results for Air Conduction

As discussed in Chapter 2, the symbol for the test ear changes from its unmasked counterpart when masking has been used to establish a threshold. For example, consider the following data:

AC RE 4,000 Hz: 25 dB HL; BC: 25 dB HL

AC LE 4,000 Hz: 85 dB HL

In this case, masking would be delivered to the non-test (right) ear to establish the AC threshold of 85 dB HL in the left ear. The left ear threshold at 4,000 Hz would be recorded as a □ rather than a cross (✕). This would alert anyone reading the audiogram that masking noise was delivered to the non-test ear when the threshold at 4,000 Hz for the left ear was being established. In the case where the right ear is the poorer ear, and masking was used in the left (non-test) ear, the right ear threshold would be recorded using a Δ rather than a O. Again, this would tell the reader that the non-test ear was isolated from the test ear during testing.

Recording Masked Test Results for Bone Conduction

Instead of using the < and > symbols used during unmasked bone conduction testing for the right and left ear, respectively, when masking is delivered to the non-test ear during bone conduction testing, the symbols change to [for the right ear and] for the left ear. So, in the case where the symbol [is encountered, the reader should conclude that this represents a masked bone conduction threshold for the right ear, and that masking noise was delivered to the left ear in the process of establishing that (right ear) bone conduction result.

Can Bone Conduction Thresholds Be Worse Than Air Conduction Thresholds?

This is a question that has been asked by students and clinicians alike. Some argue that since air conduction measures the entire auditory pathway (outer, middle, and inner ears) and bone conduction measures primarily the inner ear, bone conduction thresholds could not possibly be worse than air conduction. However, Barry (1994) says that the answer to this question is yes, bone conduction thresholds can be worse than air conduction thresholds, for a number of reasons. Reasons that bone conduction results may be poorer than air conduction thresholds include:

- The mechanism by which we hear through bone conduction is not perfectly understood; we do know that there are both ossicular (bones of the middle ear) and meatal (external ear) contributions to bone conduction sensitivity that can influence test outcomes, which means that, although bone conduction does measure inner ear function, other parts of the auditory system may be contributing to the final result.
- Both within and across individuals there are differences in the efficiency of signal transmission through AC and BC pathways.
- Threshold measurement involves a behavioral task, subject to variability inherent in a measure of this type.
- Small discrepancies between thresholds obtained by air versus bone conduction should be expected due to measurement error; large discrepancies (greater than 10 dB HL) may be due to calibration problems or may be because the client is not responding reliably.

In short, from a statistical point of view, we should expect that occasionally bone conduction thresholds will be poorer than air conduction thresholds. Knowing this, you should record the result that is obtained, particularly when it is in the 5- to 10-dB "negative air–bone gap" range. The best practice is to record the results that were obtained in the test session. Discrepancies of greater than a 15-dB negative air–bone gap warrant investigation of equipment calibration.

Some Thoughts on Traditional Test Protocols

The landscape in clinical audiology is ever changing. Air and bone conduction testing have been with us for over 50 years. Other techniques, including immittance testing, otoacoustic emissions, and auditory brainstem response testing will be covered in Chapter 6. Immittance testing (tympanometry), which assesses middle ear function, was not widely available for clinical use until the 1970s. Auditory brainstem response testing has been used since the late 1970s to measure auditory system function. Otoacoustic emissions, a measure of cochlear function, were discovered in 1978 by David Kemp, and became available as a clinical tool in the 1990s. Students in audiology courses are taught both traditional test techniques and new techniques for assessing the auditory system.

James Hall III (2001) has challenged clinicians' thinking about traditional audiometric techniques and practices, ranging from the use of insert earphones versus supraaural earphones to whether bone conduction testing is necessary in all cases. He makes the case that, in some cases, middle ear dysfunction can be effectively ruled out by using immittance audiometry and other objective techniques that rely on normal middle ear function. In other cases, bone conduction is needed to quantify the degree of conductive hearing loss when middle ear involvement is either known or suspected. Once clinicians are well versed about the types of information the various clinical techniques yield, they are in a position to discern what battery of tests will most effectively answer the individual clinical questions that confront them. It is important that testing be done in a manner that answers the questions at hand accurately and efficiently. Rethinking traditional clinical protocols based on proven technology should be a regular part of clinical practice and discussion among colleagues.

Potential Pitfalls in Pure Tone Testing

False Positive and False Negative Responses

Clearly, an audiologist's goal during threshold testing is to obtain reliable data. Because threshold testing is designed to determine the softest level at which the client is just barely able to detect the tone, it requires considerable attention to the task on the client's part; if this attention is inconsistent, errors can result. This is true whenever you engage in behavioral test techniques. As noted previously, the client may fail to respond even though he or she heard the tone. This is referred to as a *false negative response.* Such responses lead to suprathreshold data, meaning that the client is responding when the tone is more intense than his threshold. These data, of course, can suggest a hearing loss even though no loss exists. Conversely, if a client responds when no tone has been presented, a *false positive response* has occurred, which could result in data that are better than the true thresholds. In this case, a person may appear to have normal hearing even though she does have a hearing impairment.

Collapsing Ear Canals

This condition typically affects older individuals and very young individuals and results from reduced elasticity in the cartilage of the external ear. The force of the headband of the supra-aural earphones can cause the ear canals to collapse during audiological testing,

FIGURE **4.17** **Collapsing ear canal resulting in false conductive hearing loss.**

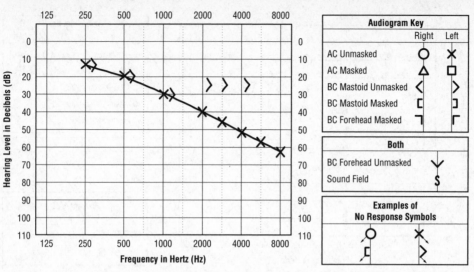

resulting in air conduction results that are poorer than they should be. However, bone conduction results are not affected. Unless the audiologist takes steps to avoid collapsing ear canals in those clients who may have them, invalid air–bone gaps will result, creating a false (usually high-frequency) conductive hearing loss, as illustrated in Figure 4.17. Some audiologists test the client in the sound field (with the non-test ear masked) to determine whether collapsing ear canals have interfered with test results. Other solutions to this problem include repositioning the earphones, using material such as foam to relieve the force imposed by the headband of the earphones, or using insert earphones.

Standing Waves

Recall from Chapter 2 that wavelength can be determined by dividing the speed of sound in air by frequency ($w = v/f$). Coincidentally, the wavelength of an 8,000-Hz pure tone (approximately 4.2 cm) is very similar to the distance between the eardrum and the diaphragm of the earphone. If these two values are very close, a **standing wave** can develop in the ear canal and, due to phase differences, can cancel out the 8,000-Hz tone being presented. The audiologist should monitor this potential problem by noting thresholds at 8,000 Hz that are very discrepant from thresholds at 4,000 Hz. Repositioning of the supra-aural earphones or use of insert earphones can be helpful in these cases. A sample audiogram is found in Figure 4.18.

Tactile Responses

Tactile responses refer to responses made by the client, usually during bone conduction testing, because vibrations of the bone oscillator are felt (rather than heard). This is common in individuals who have severe hearing loss and is more common with low-frequency

FIGURE **4.18** **Standing-wave interference suggested by the discrepant threshold at 8,000 Hz in the right ear.**

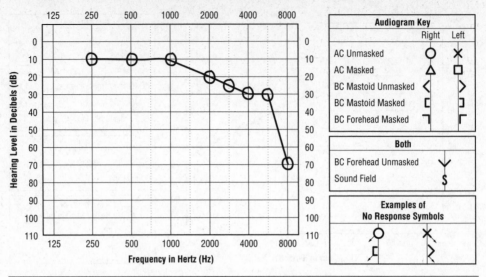

tones (250 and 500 Hz). Illustrated in Figure 4.19 is an example of tactile responses. Note that because the tactile responses occur for bone conduction and not typically for air conduction, a false conductive hearing loss is exhibited at 250 and 500 Hz. Knowing that such responses can occur when the hearing loss is severe, audiologists should verify that the client is feeling the vibration rather than hearing it, and denote this on the audiogram.

FIGURE **4.19** **Vibrotactile response at 250 and 500 Hz in a client with a severe sensorineural hearing loss.**

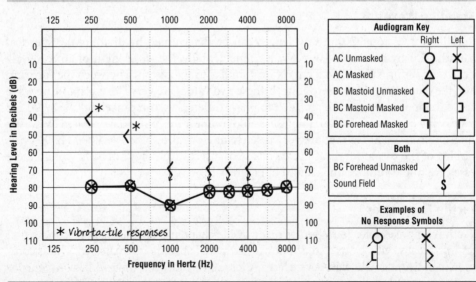

CHAPTER SUMMARY

Pure tone testing was presented in this chapter, including the value of pure tones, the use of the audiometer, and calibration issues. The reasons for using pure tone stimuli were discussed, and the relationship between pure tone findings and speech understanding was emphasized. The case history was discussed as an important component of the overall test battery, and illustrated some of the humanistic aspects of gathering audio-logical data.

Techniques for obtaining air conduction and bone conduction thresholds were covered, as was the use of masking to isolate the non-test ear when necessary. Sample cases were provided. Potential pitfalls to avoid in pure tone testing were also addressed.

QUESTIONS FOR DISCUSSION

Discuss the following questions when considering the sample audiograms that appear below:

1. What is the type (nature) and degree of hearing loss in each ear?
2. For each ear identified with hearing loss, what is the affected part or parts of the auditory system?
3. Identify when masking was used. In cases where masking was used, discuss why masking was needed.
4. Considering the entire audiogram, describe the potential effects of the hearing loss on the client's ability to understand conversational speech.
5. For each of the case examples, speculate what information might have been obtained during the case history discussion with the client.

Sample 1

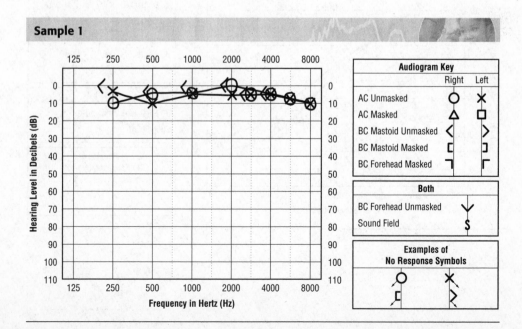

Sample 2

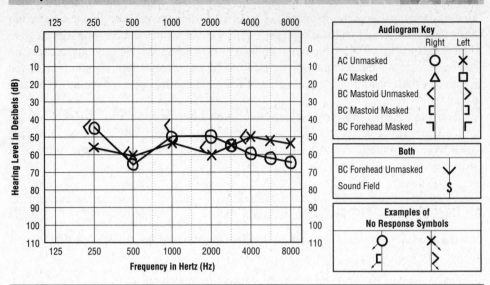

Sample 3

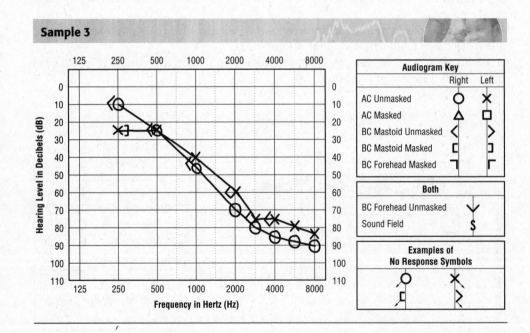

Sample 4

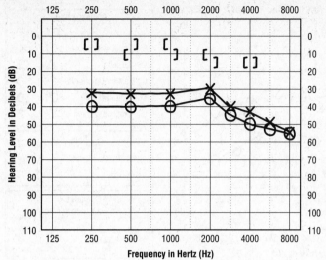

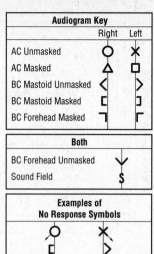

Sample 5

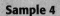

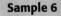

Sample 6

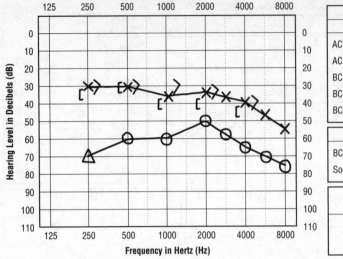

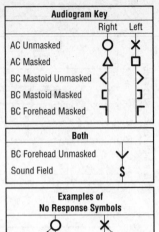

RECOMMENDED READING

American Speech-Language-Hearing Association. (2005). *Guidelines for manual pure-tone threshold audiometry.* Rockville, MD: Author. Available from http://www.asha.org /members/deskref-journals/deskref/default

Staab, W. (1992). *Basic masking: An explanation and procedure* (2nd ed.). Dammeron Valley, UT: Author.

REFERENCES

American National Standards Institute (ANSI). (2004). Specifications for audiometers. ANSI S3.6-2004. New York: Author.

American Speech-Language-Hearing Association. (2005). *Guidelines for manual pure tone threshold audiometry.* Rockville, MD: Author.

Barry, S. Joseph. (1994). Can bone conduction thresholds really be poorer than air? *American Journal of Audiology, 3*(3), 21–22.

Fletcher, H. (1940). Auditory patterns. *Review of Modern Physics, 12,* 47–65.

Fletcher, H., & Munson, W. A. (1937). Relation between loudness and masking. *Journal of the Acoustical Society of America, 9,* 1–10.

Gelfand, S. (2001). *Essentials of audiology* (2nd ed.). New York: Thieme.

Goldstein, B. A., & Newman, C. W. (1994). Clinical masking: A decision-making process. In

Katz, J., Ed., *Handbook of clinical audiology* (pp. 109–131). Baltimore: Williams & Wilkins.

Hall, J. III. (2001). Page ten: Rethinking some traditional procedures. *The Hearing Journal, 54*(4), 10–17.

Katz, J. (2002). *Handbook of clinical audiology* (5th ed.). New York: Lippincott, Williams & Wilkins.

Martin, F., & Clark, J. (2003). *Introduction to audiology* (8th ed.). Boston: Allyn & Bacon.

Martin, F. N. (1974). Minimum effective masking levels in threshold audiometry. *Journal of Speech and Hearing Disorders, 39,* 280–285.

Mueller, G., & Killion, M. (1990). An easy method for calculating the articulation index. *The Hearing Journal, 45*(9), 14–17.

Nicolosi, L., Harryman, E., & Kresheck, J. (1989). *Terminology of communication disorders* (3rd ed.). Baltimore: Williams & Wilkins.

Olsen, W., Hawkins, D., & Van Tasell, D. (1997). Representations of the long-term spectra of speech. *Ear and Hearing, 8*(45), 1003–1085.

Staab, W. (1992). *Basic masking: An explanation and procedure* (2nd ed.). Dammeron Valley, UT: Author.

Yacullo, W. S. (1996). *Clinical masking procedures.* Boston: Allyn & Bacon.

Appendix A
How to Mask during Pure Tone Testing

Air Conduction

Sample Case 1

Unmasked results:

> AC right ear 4,000 Hz: 25 dB HL; BC 25 dB HL
>
> AC left ear 4,000 Hz: 85 dB HL

Is masking needed for air conduction (AC) testing of the left ear? Yes, because the difference between the air conduction "threshold" on the left and the bone conduction threshold on the right is 60 dB; the potential for cross-hearing exists because 60 is greater than the minimum interaural attenuation (40 dB HL) afforded by the presence of the head between the two ears.

When masking must be delivered to the non-test ear during air conduction testing, the masking noise is simply delivered to the non-test ear through the earphone that has been in use during the test procedure. In Sample Case 1, you would be delivering the masking noise to the right (non-test) ear to find out the true threshold in the left (test) ear.

The next question is how much noise you need to deliver to the non-test ear. You are seeking an amount of masking noise that will provide "effective masking" and will not undermask or overmask. If you **undermask,** you have not raised the threshold in the non-test ear enough, so it is still contributing to the response we are attributing to the test ear. If you **overmask,** you have used so much masking noise in the non-test ear that the masking is crossing over to the test ear and contaminating the response. There are formulas to help you decide how much masking noise to begin with. First, consider ways to arrive at initial masking and effective masking, and then a procedure to use to arrive at a masked threshold will be discussed.

Initial Masking Level

Initial Masking (IM) during Air Conduction Testing

According to Yacullo (1996), Martin (1974) has recommended that the initial amount of masking to use in the non-test ear is equal to the threshold in the non-test ear plus a safety factor. Yacullo (1996) recommends using Martin's formula for the initial minimum masking level for air conduction, which is

> ACnte + 10 dB safety factor

In Sample Case 1, how much masking would you start with in the right ear? The initial masking amount would be 25 dB HL (the threshold in the non-test ear) plus a safety factor of 10 dB HL, or 35 dB HL in this case.

Yacullo (1996) also provides a formula for minimum masking, which can be used to derive a starting point, and is as follows:

$$\text{M min} = \text{ACte} - \text{IA} + \text{AB Gapnte}$$

Translation: Minimum masking equals the (unmasked) air conduction threshold of the test ear minus interaural attenuation (estimated at 40 dB) plus the air–bone gap in the non-test ear.

If we apply this formula to masking for air conduction in Sample Case 1, minimum masking would equal 85 (the unmasked threshold of the test ear) minus 40 dB (minimum interaural attenuation for air conduction) plus 0 (there is no air–bone gap in the non-test ear in this case) or 45 dB HL.

Either of these formulas can be applied when decisions about initial masking levels (or "where to start") are needed. Using the air conduction threshold in the non-test ear as a starting point has the advantage of requiring less calculation and may therefore appeal to beginning clinicians.

Initial Masking (IM) during Bone Conduction Testing

Martin's (1974) formula for initial masking for bone conduction is

$$\text{ACnte} + \text{OE} + 10 \text{ dB safety factor}$$

To accomplish masked bone conduction testing, the bone vibrator is usually placed behind the "test ear" on the mastoid process. The earphone that will deliver the masking noise to the non-test ear is placed over the non-test ear. The "extra" (unused) earphone is usually placed on the head as illustrated in Figure 4.20.

Before going further, an explanation of OE is needed. OE stands for the **occlusion effect,** which is defined as an improvement (decrease) in the bone conduction threshold of tones of 1,000 Hz and below when the ears are tightly covered with an earphone during bone conduction testing; this effect is seen in normal hearers and in patients with sensorineural hearing losses. The occlusion effect is negligible in patients with conductive hearing losses. During masked bone conduction testing, the masking signal is delivered to the non-test ear via air conduction (through an earphone), making it necessary to consider the occlusion effect. If the occlusion effect is not considered, the low-frequency bone conduction thresholds will appear better than they actually are, incorrectly resulting in air–bone gaps. From this definition, it can be concluded that consideration must be given to the occlusion effect during bone conduction testing of lower frequencies in individuals with normal hearing or sensorineural hearing losses. Because the OE is less problematic in bone conduction testing for individuals with conductive hearing losses, one might assume that it would not be factored into masking calculations for this group. However, because we often do not know if conductive hearing loss exists until masking has been performed, this is not the case.

The occlusion effect varies by frequency, with the greatest effect in the lower test frequencies and a negligible effect in the higher test frequencies. It is possible to derive the occlusion effect for individual frequencies for each client by comparing bone conduction

FIGURE **4.20** **Typical arrangement of (a) the bone vibrator and (b) earphones during masking for bone conduction.**

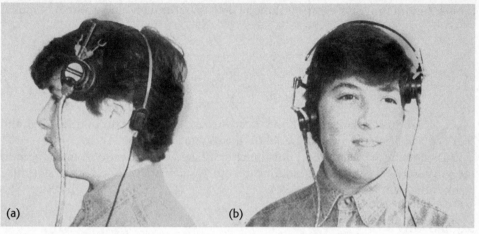

(a)   (b)

Source: From S. A. Gelfand, *Essentials of Audiology.* New York: Thieme Medical Publishers, 2001: p. 312. Reprinted by permission.

---

thresholds *without* an earphone over the non-test ear to bone conduction thresholds obtained *with* an earphone over the non-test ear. Because this is time-consuming, many audiologists make use of standard values to account for the OE. A summary of the occlusion effect by frequency, assuming the use of supra-aural earphones, follows:

250 Hz	30 dB
500 Hz	20 dB
1,000 Hz	10 dB
2,000 Hz	0 dB
4,000 Hz	0 dB

Returning to the formula, ACnte + OE + 10 dB safety factor, we would calculate the amount of initial masking for bone conduction testing of the left ear at 4,000 Hz as follows: 25 dB + 0 + 10 dB = 35 dB HL initial masking amount. If we had the same information except that we were interested in the bone conduction threshold at 1,000 Hz, it would be necessary to add in 10 dB to account for the occlusion effect at that frequency. At 1,000 Hz, applying the formula to arrive at the initial amount of masking for bone conduction testing of the left ear, we would have: 25 dB HL + 10 dB + 10 dB = 45 dB initial masking amount.

Maximum Masking (Overmasking)

Just as it is possible to use too little masking, it is also possible to use too much. **Overmasking** occurs when the amount of masking delivered to the non-test ear crosses over to the test ear and influences (raises) its response. Overmasking will lead to overestimating the degree of hearing loss in the test ear. There are formulas to calculate the level at which overmasking can occur for air and bone conduction testing. The formula for maximum masking is the same for both air and bone conduction testing, because in both cases masking is delivered through an earphone (Yacullo, 1996):

$$M \max = BCte + IA - 5\,dB$$

or

$$OM = EML(nte) - IA(ac) > BCT(te)$$

where OM is overmasking, EML is the effective masking level (of the non-test ear), and BCT is the bone conduction threshold (of the test ear).

Considering Sample Case 1, how much masking would have to be introduced to the non-test (right) ear for overmasking to occur? You may wish to plot these data on a blank audiogram to facilitate analysis.

Sample Case 1

Unmasked results:

AC right ear 4,000 Hz: 25 dB HL; BC 25 dB HL

AC left ear 4,000 Hz: 85 dB HL

Using the first formula above, during air conduction testing we have 25 + 40 − 5, or 60 dB as the point at which overmasking could begin to occur. Why was 25 used as the bone conduction threshold of the test ear? Because at this point in testing, you have only unmasked bone conduction results available, and it is possible that the bone conduction result for the left ear could be as good as 25 dB HL when testing is completed. Of course, it is also possible that the bone conduction result for the left ear will approach the air conduction threshold of 85 dB, indicating a sensorineural loss; or that it will fall somewhere in between and the conclusion will be that a mixed loss exists in the left ear at the test frequency in question.

If we find that the left-ear hearing loss is actually sensorineural, adding a new piece of information to Sample Case 1, what happens to the maximum masking level?

Unmasked results:

AC right ear 4,000 Hz: 25 dB HL; BC 25 dB HL

AC left ear 4,000 Hz: 85 dB HL

New information: Masked BC results for the left ear: 80 dB HL

The formula remains the same, so

$$80 + 40 - 5 = 115\,dB\,HL\,(maximum\,masking)$$

What happens is that the level at which overmasking may occur is really considerably higher than was first thought. Usually, the potential for overmasking is overestimated in cases of sensorineural hearing loss. In cases of conductive hearing loss, overmasking is more problematic during testing. Consider Sample Case 2.

Sample Case 2

Unmasked results:

> AC left ear 500 Hz: 35 dB HL
>
> AC right ear 500 Hz: 35 dB HL
>
> BC left ear 500 Hz: 5 dB HL
>
> BC right ear 500 Hz: 5 dB HL

Using the formula M max = BCte + IA − 5 dB with the right ear as the test ear, we can calculate maximum masking as 5 + 40 − 5 or 40 dB HL. If both ears in fact have a conductive hearing loss, we run the risk of overmasking when only moderate levels of masking are introduced to the non-test ear.

Masking Dilemmas

There are times when it becomes impossible to mask effectively for air or bone conduction testing, a situation referred to as a "masking dilemma." Consider the following information and, using the previously discussed formulas, calculate a minimum masking level and an overmasking level for air conduction and for bone conduction testing, using the right ear as the test ear.

Sample Case 3

Unmasked results:

> AC left ear 500 Hz: 60 dB HL
>
> AC right ear 500 Hz: 65 dB HL
>
> BC left ear 500 Hz: 5 dB HL
>
> BC right ear 500 Hz: 5 dB HL

For air conduction testing, if M min = ACte − IA + AB Gapnte, we have 65 − 40 + 60 or 85 dB HL as our minimum masking level. Using the formula for overmasking, we have M max = BCte + IA − 5 dB, or 5 + 40 − 5 = 40 dB as the point where the potential for overmasking exists.

For bone conduction testing, minimum masking can be derived as follows: ACnte + OE + 10 dB safety factor, or 60 dB + 10 dB = 70 dB HL (since you know the non-test ear has a conductive hearing loss, you do not need to account for the occlusion effect in this case).

In the case of a bilateral conductive hearing loss, in which each ear has air conduction thresholds over 40 dB, the problem of a masking dilemma occurs, wherein the level needed for minimum masking exceeds the level at which overmasking can be expected. As we have seen, this problem can occur for both air and bone conduction testing in the case of a significant bilateral conductive hearing loss. In some cases, use of insert earphones can reduce the problems imposed by a masking dilemma because greater amounts of masking can be delivered to the non-test ear before crossover occurs.

Plateau Method (The Hood Technique)

Once the initial masking level is identified, that amount of masking is introduced to the non-test ear. The patient is instructed beforehand to ignore the masking noise in the left or right (non-test) ear and to respond when the tone is heard. The pure tone threshold in the test ear is then reestablished with the masking noise present in the opposite ear. No change in the pure tone threshold in the test ear means that the original threshold reflects the truth about the test ear. If, however, there is a shift of more than 5 dB in the threshold in the test ear, it become necessary to search for the true threshold in the test ear. This is done by raising the level of the masking noise by 10 dB and reestablishing the threshold. The masking noise is then raised another 10 dB. If the threshold "holds," this is the true threshold. If the threshold shifts by more than 5 dB, the procedure is repeated: raise the masker by 10 dB, and reestablish the threshold in the test ear. Once the masked threshold is established, it is important to promptly remove the masking noise from the client's non-test ear. In order for the threshold in the test ear to be considered "true," it must remain stable over approximately a 20-dB range when the masking noise level is raised (this is the "plateau" shown in Figure 4.21).

Undermasking, the plateau, and overmasking are represented in Figure 4.21, which summarizes the Hood, or plateau, method of masking. Basically, the plateau is the point at which the threshold in the test ear *does not change* with increases in the masking level. This is represented by the portion of the masking function between B and C. This is the point we are seeking: the masking noise is sufficient to occupy the non-test ear, but not intense enough to interfere with the test ear.

The section of the masking function between A and B represents undermasking. At this point, the threshold in the test ear is shifting each time the masking level is raised. This means that the non-test ear is still responding to the test signal, and we have not yet isolated the non-test ear from the test ear.

Overmasking is the portion of the masking function between C and D. At this point, the masking is so intense that it crosses over to the test ear, and interferes with obtaining a true threshold from the test ear. If overmasking is occurring, for each 10-dB increase in the masking noise there will be a corresponding 10-dB increase in the threshold of the test ear.

It should also be noted here that the same considerations about when masking should be used apply to speech audiometry. A sufficient difference in the sensitivity between the two ears will necessitate the use of masking during both threshold speech audiometry procedures (assessing speech recognition thresholds or speech awareness thresholds) and suprathreshold speech audiometry procedures (assessing word recognition scores). This topic will be revisited in Chapter 5.

Answers to Sample Air Conduction Masking Cases

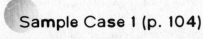

Sample Case 1 (p. 104)

A: No, because the difference between 30 dB HL and 0 dB HL is less than 40 dB HL. This can also be seen using the formula, ACT (TE) – IA $\geq$ BCT (NTE), in which we have 30 minus 40 is not greater than or equal to 0 dB.

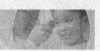

FIGURE **4.21** **The Hood, or plateau, method of masking with representations of undermasking, the plateau, and overmasking.**

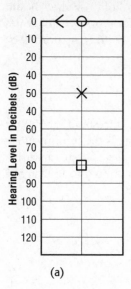

(a)

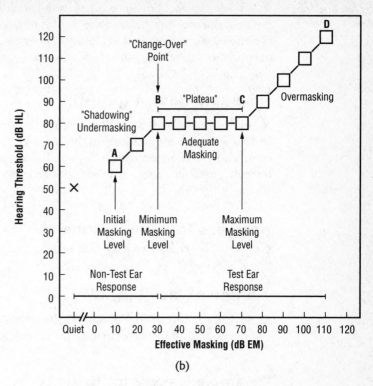

(b)

In this example, there is more than a 40-dB difference between the LE unmasked AC threshold of 50 dB HL and the bone conduction threshold of 0 dB HL in the non-test (right) ear. In this circumstance, it is possible that the LE AC result of 50 dB HL underestimates the true degree of hearing loss in the left ear. Therefore, masking must be delivered to the RE to establish the true LE threshold for this frequency.

Source: William S. Yacullo. *Clinical masking procedures.* Published by Allyn & Bacon, Boston, MA. Copyright © 1996 by Pearson Education. Reprinted by permission of the publisher.

- A is the masking intensity level at which the threshold in the test ear begins to shift; from A to B, undermasking is depicted.
- Effective masking (dB EM) occurs at the plateau between B and C, where the threshold in the test ear *does not change* with increases in the masking level to the non-test ear.
- From C to D, overmasking is occurring.

Note: The starting level for masking will vary with the degree of hearing loss.

Source: Staab, W. (1992). *Basic masking: An explanation and procedure* (2nd ed.). Dammeron Valley, UT: Author. Reprinted by permission.

Sample Case 2 (p. 105)

A: Yes, because the difference between 50 dB HL and 0 dB HL is greater than the minimum interaural attenuation (greater than 40 dB HL) and the potential for cross-hearing exists.

Sample Case 3 (p. 105)

A: Yes, because the difference between the air conduction "threshold" on the left and bone conduction threshold on the right is 60 dB; the potential for cross-hearing exists because 60 is greater than the minimum interaural attenuation (40 dB HL) afforded by the presence of the head between the two ears.

Sample Case 4 (p. 106)

A: Yes, because there is a 50 dB difference between the right ear "threshold" at 500 Hz and the left-ear bone conduction threshold at 500 Hz. This exceeds the minimum interaural attenuation available by air conduction when supra-aural earphones are used; therefore, masking should be used to obtain an accurate air conduction threshold at 500 Hz in the right ear.

Answers to Sample Bone Conduction Masking Cases

Sample Case 1 (p. 107)

A: No, because the air conduction results show symmetrical hearing levels in each ear and the unmasked bone conduction result reveals no air–bone gap for either ear.

Sample Case 2 (p. 108)

A: Yes, because without masking, you obtain the same result as when you tested the right ear by BC (35 dB HL). You should have expected this because you know that the interaural attenuation by BC is 0, meaning that the better cochlea will respond by bone conduction no matter where you place the bone oscillator. The only recourse is to raise the threshold in the non-test (right) ear by adding masking noise to the right ear. By doing this, the type (nature) of the left-ear hearing loss can be determined. There are two possibilities for the type of hearing loss in the left ear at this point. What are they? After masking is used, it is possible that that the BC threshold on the left would remain at 35 dB HL, in which case the nature of the left-ear hearing loss would be mixed. On the other hand, we may find that the BC threshold is really 50 or 55 dB HL, in which case the nature of the loss would be sensorineural.

Sample Case 3 (p. 108)

A: From the available information, you can see that the potential for air–bone gaps exists in both ears. In this case, you need to account for the possibility of an air–bone gap when testing bone conduction for each ear. Since the "best bone" response is in the normal range, there is a good chance that a conductive component exists in at least one ear. It is possible that the other ear has a mixed or sensorineural hearing loss. The only way to find out is to mask the non-test ear during bone conduction testing of the right and left ears.

chapter 5

Speech Audiometry

AFTER COMPLETING THIS CHAPTER, YOU SHOULD BE ABLE TO:

1. Define *speech audiometry* and describe (in general) the usefulness of speech audiometry data for audiologists and speech–language pathologists.
2. List commonly used speech audiometric tests. For each test, describe test administration procedures and the specific value of these data in hearing assessment.
3. Choose three speech audiometry tests and for each explain its relationship to pure tone data.
4. Determine when to use masking during speech audiometry for air and bone conducted signals for specific audiometric profiles.
5. Understand the potential impact of manipulating various test parameters (e.g., use of live voice versus recorded materials, length of word list) on test outcomes.

In Chapter 4 you learned about the value of obtaining pure tone thresholds by air and bone conduction at different frequencies. Some of the relationships between pure tones and the ability to understand speech were described. You also learned that pure tone testing, unlike speech audiometric testing, provides information about the client's hearing sensitivity at specific frequencies.

Despite the valuable information obtained from pure tone threshold testing, there are a number of benefits to be obtained by using speech audiometry as part of comprehensive audiological assessments. The term **speech audiometry** refers to the assessment of a client's hearing using speech stimuli.

Contributions of Speech Audiometry

A client's performance on speech audiometric tasks, especially those that are suprathreshold, can provide an audiologist with a more accurate view of the client's communication performance in the real world. Responses to speech presented at an average conversational level could reveal good speech understanding for individuals with normal or near-normal hearing sensitivity, or could expose reduced ability to understand average conversational speech for individuals with hearing loss. Responses to speech presented at levels greater than an average conversational level may reveal improved speech understanding, which provides useful information for case management purposes. The pure tone audiogram provides information regarding the degree of hearing loss; speech audiometry provides information regarding the degree of hearing communication handicap. It is not uncommon, for example, to find a person with a relatively mild pure tone hearing loss who demonstrates considerable difficulty when tested with speech in a background of noise.

Another contribution of speech audiometry is that it can be sensitive to auditory problems that pure tone testing might miss. *Sensitivity* is a term that is discussed in detail in Chapter 11 on screening and in Chapter 10 on auditory processing disorders. Sensitivity refers to the degree to which a measuring tool identifies individuals who have a specific condition. If the audiologist's goal is to identify a sensorineural hearing loss, pure tone testing is a sensitive tool for that purpose. If, however, the goal is to identify a tumor in the central auditory system, pure tone testing is not a particularly sensitive tool. Because speech stimuli are processed at different places in the auditory system compared to pure tones (i.e., usually higher in the auditory system), speech tests are often more sensitive than pure tones to certain auditory disorders. Later in the chapter, the term *site of lesion* testing will be used, referring to an audiologist's goal of determining in which part of the auditory system (e.g., cochlea, auditory nerve, brainstem) the disorder lies.

A third contribution made by speech audiometry is to check the accuracy or reliability of the client's responses. Although speech and pure tones are different stimuli, they are related in certain ways and you can use your understanding of these relationships to establish that you have confidence in your results. If, for example, a client's responses to pure tones suggest a moderate hearing loss in the right ear, and the responses to speech stimuli suggest hearing within normal limits in that ear, the audiologist is alerted to a lack of consistency. Comparison of the decibel levels at which responses to speech and pure tones are obtained provides a cross-check to ensure reliable data.

Finally, for some clients, using speech audiometry is the only reliable way to assess hearing sensitivity. Unlike speech, which we listen to all the time, pure tones are less familiar and more abstract to many clients. For this reason, sometimes children, older clients, or clients with cognitive deficits have difficulty responding reliably to pure tones. In these cases, speech audiometry can be most helpful. These issues are discussed in more detail in the chapters dealing with pediatrics and assessment of special populations.

The Speech–Language Pathologist and Speech Audiometry

The results of speech audiometry have special relevance for speech–language pathologists working with clients of all ages to improve their communicative competence. Understanding the meaning of speech awareness and recognition thresholds as well as word recognition scores provides fundamental information for planning and counseling purposes. Functional audiometric information is essential to planning therapy goals for young children, school-age children, adults, and older adults with hearing loss, as well as to the counseling of these clients and their families. In this context, functional audiometric information provides answers to pivotal questions such as:

- How clear does speech sound to this client?
- At what hearing level (dB HL) must speech be presented to achieve audibility (hearing)?

- At what hearing level (dB HL) and under what conditions must speech be presented to be intelligible (understood)?
- Are some sounds inaudible to this client even when speech is presented at a comfortably loud hearing level?
- When speech is presented at a conversational intensity level (e.g., 45–50 dB HL or 60–65 dB SPL), what speech sounds does the client have access to without amplification?
- What speech sounds are accessible with amplification?

In considering this list of questions, it is important to note that audibility does not guarantee intelligibility. In other words, just being able to hear the signal does not necessarily mean that the signal has been understood by the listener. The classroom teacher who observes a child respond to his or her name may assume that the child is "hearing," when the child may simply be responding to a portion of the presented signal.

In several chapters, the concept of the audibility index (AI; formerly referred to as the articulation index) has been discussed. The AI is based on knowledge about the frequencies that are most important to speech perception. You know that frequencies between 500 and 4,000 Hz are important for speech perception. In addition, for perception of single words, access to information at 1,900 Hz is critical; for sentence perception, information at 750 Hz is essential (Hall & Mueller, 1997). The "count the dots" method for calculating an articulation (audibility) index, discussed in Chapter 4, provides an individual look at clients' AI, and their access to frequency information important for hearing and understanding speech. Greater weight is assigned to frequencies in the 1,000–3,000 Hz range, since these frequencies contribute the most to the ability to understand speech.

Although certain predictions about an individual's ability to hear and understand speech sounds can be made based on the results of pure tone testing, the results of the pure tone audiogram alone do not provide sufficient insight into an individual's speech perception abilities. Because the relationship between pure tone findings and speech understanding ability does not always follow a predictable pattern, speech audiometry test results should be obtained whenever possible. A variety of tests are available for this purpose.

Speech Audiometry Tests

The most commonly used speech audiometry tests are described next. Information about the tests includes the purpose of the test, the type of stimulus used, the directions to the client, administration, and interpretation of the test results. Variables that are considered in selecting these tests include whether the tests are presented to one ear or both ears, through **monitored live voice testing,** or by recorded material (tape or compact disc), and the type of speech material used (e.g., nonsense syllables, monosyllabic words, spondee words, or sentences). Another variable of relevance is whether the material is presented in quiet or in a background of noise.

Speech Recognition Threshold

Recall from Chapter 4 that a pure tone threshold is "the lowest decibel hearing level at which responses occur in at least one half of a series of ascending trials. The minimum number of responses needed to determine the threshold of hearing is two responses out of three presentations at a single level" (ASHA, 2005, p. 4). Similarly, the **speech recognition threshold (SRT),** formerly referred to as the speech reception threshold, is defined as "the minimum hearing level for speech at which an individual can recognize 50% of the speech material" (ASHA, 1988).

There are a number of stated purposes for the SRT, one of which is to assess the reliability of the pure tone findings. Recall from Chapter 4 that the pure tone average, traditionally calculated by finding the average of the thresholds at 500, 1,000, and 2,000 Hz (or the average of the best two thresholds from these three) in a given ear, can provide summary information about the client's hearing loss. This average should be within ±10 dB of the SRT. If it is not, the client's responses may be unreliable.

Assume for a moment that a client has a flat moderate hearing loss in the right ear, with pure tone thresholds ranging from 45 to 50 dB from 250 to 8,000 Hz. This is illustrated in Figure 5.1 Based on the previous discussion, you would expect that the client's SRT would be somewhere between 45 and 50 dB. If, however, the SRT in the right ear was

FIGURE **5.1** **Flat moderate hearing loss in the right ear.**

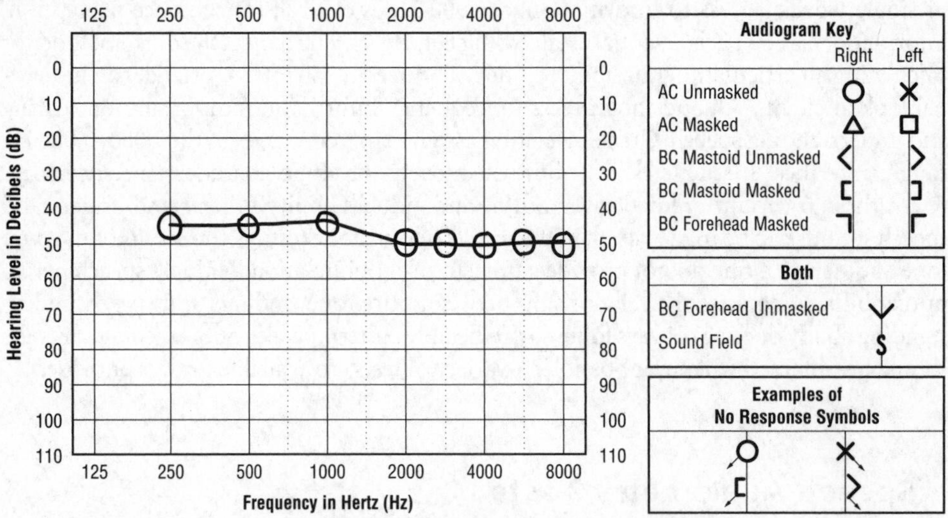

Speech Audiometry

Ear	SRT	SDT	PTA	Test	Word Recognition Level/Percent Correct	MCL	LDL
Right							
Left							
Bone							
Sound Field							
Right Aided							
Left Aided							
Binaural Aided							

found to be 30 dB, suspicion would be raised about the accuracy of the pure tone findings. Such lack of agreement between the pure tone average and SRT may signal a lack of consistency that may require reinstruction of the client and repetition of pure tone testing.

Use of the SRT as an average hearing level can be problematic because it is possible for a client's SRT to reflect only one of the three frequencies often associated with it (e.g., 500, 1,000, 2,000 Hz). Examine the audiograms in Figure 5.2 and you will note that in each case the SRT is consistent not with the average of 500, 1,000, and 2,000 Hz, but rather with only one of these frequencies. For this reason, use of the SRT alone as a general indicator of degree of hearing loss or the degree to which the client's communication ability will be impaired in the real world is not recommended. Speech pathologists

FIGURE **5.2** **Sloping (a) and reverse curve (b) audiograms demonstrating inconsistency between pure tone average and SRT.**

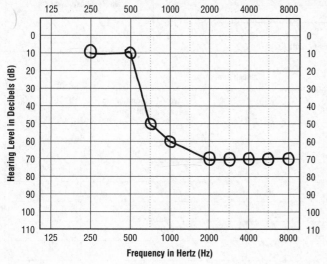

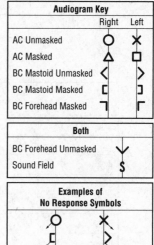

Speech Audiometry

Ear	SRT	SDT	PTA	Test	Word Recognition Level/Percent Correct	MCL	LDL
Right	10						
Left							
Bone							
Sound Field							
Right Aided							
Left Aided							
Binaural Aided							

(a)

(continued)

FIGURE **5.2** *(Continued)*

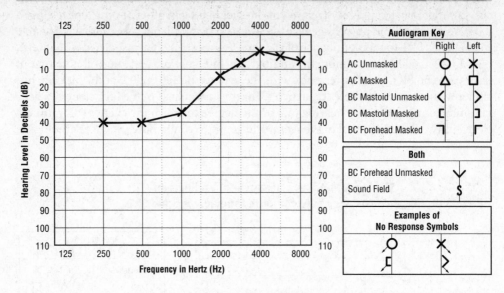

Speech Audiometry

Ear	SRT	SDT	PTA	Test	Word Recognition Level/Percent Correct		MCL	LDL
Right								
Left	*15*							
Bone								
Sound Field								
Right Aided								
Left Aided								
Binaural Aided								

(b)

and other clinicians should note this limitation of the SRT and take care to examine all of the available data about a client's audiological status.

Despite the limitations of the SRT noted above, it can be useful when interpreted carefully (1) as a reference point for presentation of words for suprathreshold speech testing and (2) in testing children and populations requiring special test techniques and/or those who do not respond reliably to pure tones.

Test Setup

Let's now examine the audiometric setup for SRT testing. In Chapter 4 you were introduced to a basic diagram of the audiometer. You also learned that for pure tone testing an audiologist chooses "tone" from the "stimulus" column and then directs that tone to a transducer (e.g., phone, bone, or speaker), based on the particular test being performed. During speech audiometry, the transducer options remain the same and the stimulus selection is microphone or an auxiliary source such as cassette tape or compact disc (CD). As in pure tone testing, the hearing-level dial (also referred to as the attenuator dial) is used to increase or decrease the intensity of the speech stimuli being directed to the transducer. Because speech is complex and, unlike pure tones, does not have a single frequency of vibration, no frequency information appears in the frequency display on the audiometer. For conventional SRT testing, the audiologist chooses microphone and phone, and sets the attenuator dial to an initial hearing level.

Again considering the diagram of the audiometer, find the panel labeled **VU** (volume units) **meter.** This display provides information regarding the intensity of the input signal. Note that the standard scale on the VU meter has a range from −20 to +3 dB. Some audiometers use a VU light bar instead of a meter needle to provide visual feedback about the intensity of the signal being delivered. When the meter or light bar reads 0 dB, the intensity of the input signal is equal to the value on the attenuator dial (in dB HL). If the meter or light bar reads −5 dB as the speech stimulus is delivered, the intensity of the stimulus is 5 dB less than that noted on the attenuator dial.

When audiologists use tape or CD recordings of speech stimuli, a calibration tone that is part of the recorded material is presented first. Adjusting the VU meter to 0 dB in response to the calibration tone ensures that the appropriate intensity level (i.e., that noted on the attenuator dial) is being delivered to the client. When audiologists use live voice presentation of speech stimuli, it is necessary to continuously monitor the VU meter to ensure that the intensity of the stimuli being delivered is not more intense (i.e., VU is greater than 0 dB) or less intense (i.e., VU is less than 0 dB) than intended.

Administering the SRT

To administer the SRT test, the audiologist first gives instructions to the client regarding how to respond to this task. According to ASHA (1988) guidelines, clients should be instructed to repeat back two-syllable words (commonly referred to as **spondee** words), some of which will be very faint. Examples of spondee words include *baseball, hotdog,* and *airplane.* These lists were developed incorporating familiar vocabulary words that are phonetically different from one another. In addition, the nature of spondee words is such that relatively equal stress, resulting in relatively equal audibility, occurs on each syllable. When giving instructions, impress upon clients that they should attempt to respond even if the words are very faint; guessing should also be encouraged.

The following sample instructions may be used as a guide before administering the SRT:

"I am going to review a series of words with you. Please repeat each word that you hear. After this review, I will begin to present these words at softer and softer levels. Please continue to repeat the words that you hear, even if they are quite soft and even if you have to guess."

Test administration begins by familiarizing the client with the list of spondee words. Sample spondee words (ASHA, 1988) used with adults include *sidewalk, woodwork, doormat, eardrum, toothbrush,* and *northwest.* For children, commonly used spondee words include *baseball, hotdog, birthday, toothbrush, ice cream,* and *bathtub.* This is an important part of test administration and allows audiologists to omit words that may not be familiar to the client. After familiarization, the audiologist should remind the client that only the words that were just reviewed will be used in the test. Although ASHA (1988) guidelines suggest use of a descending approach to obtaining the SRT, various approaches (e.g., ascending, descending, or ascending/descending) can yield very similar results when testing in 5-dB steps. The basic idea of all of these approaches is to present a series of spondee words several times, until 50 percent understanding is achieved at one level.

Let's now examine a descending approach, based on the work of Chaiklin and Ventry (1964), that many audiologists find useful. Table 5.1 summarizes the steps that are described.

Referring back to the client described in Figure 5.1 who had pure tone thresholds of 45–50 dB from 250 to 8,000 Hz, assume that a starting level of 50 dB has been established. If at this intensity level the client repeats correctly the first three spondee words presented, additional words are not presented because even if the client misses the next three words (we are dealing with a possible total of six words at each intensity level), the client still has achieved 50 percent correct (i.e., three correct out of six) and the speech recognition threshold is defined as the softest level at which the client can recognize 50 percent of the words. The client's threshold could be at this 50-dB level or at a lower level, so intensity is decreased by 5 dB. If at 45 dB the client once again repeats the first three spondee words presented, he has once again achieved at least 50 percent correct. You now know that 50 dB is not the SRT, but 45 dB may be. The intensity level is

---

TABLE 5.1 **Summary of the Descending Procedure for Obtaining an SRT**

Intensity Level	Patient Response	Interpretation	Decision
50 dB	First three words repeated correctly	Client has achieved at least 50% correct	Decrease intensity by 5 dB
45 dB	First three words repeated correctly	Client has achieved at least 50% correct	Decrease intensity by 5 dB
40 dB	First two words repeated correctly; third word repeated incorrectly	Client has achieved 66% correct for the first three words.	Continue to present words to determine if accuracy remains at at least 50%
	Fourth word repeated correctly	Client has achieved at least 50% correct	Decrease intensity by 5 dB
35 dB	Client repeats back first three words incorrectly	Client has achieved 0% correct for the first three words	Continue to present words to determine if accuracy can reach 50%
	Fourth word is incorrect	Client cannot obtain 50% correct, even if all six words are presented	35 dB is not the SRT; 40 dB is

Source: Chaiklin and Ventry (1964).

decreased again by 5 dB to a level of 40 dB. At 40 dB the client repeats the first two words correctly and the next word incorrectly. Even though the client's performance at this point is 66 percent (two correct out of three), additional words must be presented in order to verify that performance here would remain at at least 50 percent if the entire series of six words were given. So, if the client repeats the next word correctly, 75 percent correct has been achieved (three out of four correct) and, more important, performance would not drop below 50 percent even if the client missed the last two words in the series (three out of six is 50 percent). Decreasing by 5 dB to 35 dB, we find that the client misses the first three words presented. Is it necessary to present more words at this level? Yes, because if the client were to repeat the last three words of the series correctly, he would have achieved 50 percent correct, which would then lead to another decrease in intensity by 5 dB. So, a fourth word is presented and the client misses it. The client has now missed all four words at this level and could not achieve 50 percent correct at this intensity level even if he repeated the final two words correctly. The audiologist has now determined that 35 dB is not the threshold; rather, the threshold is 40 dB.

The above scenario illustrates use of a descending approach to obtaining the SRT. As you have seen, such an approach begins at an intensity level that is above threshold and reduces intensity in the search for threshold. Although descending approaches are more common, there are times when an ascending approach to obtaining the SRT is valuable. One such case is when a client repeats spondee words that are presented at suprathreshold levels but not at threshold levels. In these cases, it can be helpful to begin at a level that is below the client's threshold and systematically increase in intensity until threshold is reached. For additional information regarding special test techniques, refer to the section of Chapter 9 that addresses nonorganic hearing loss.

Although the SRT is considered to be part of the conventional audiometric test battery, it is not always possible to obtain an SRT for a variety of reasons. This is covered in greater detail in the chapters on pediatrics and on special populations. In the event that an SRT cannot be obtained, a speech detection threshold (SDT) may be substituted. Or, the SDT may be obtained in addition to the SRT, depending on the particular case.

Speech Detection Threshold

The **speech detection threshold (SDT),** also referred to as the speech awareness threshold (SAT), is defined as "the minimum hearing level for speech at which an individual can just discern the presence of a speech material 50% of the time" (ASHA, 1988, p. 98). Although the terms SDT and SAT are often used interchangeably, the preferred term to use is SDT.

Note the very important difference between the SDT and the SRT: the SDT requires that the client merely detect the presence of speech; the SRT requires that the client recognize words. Because of these differences, the SRT is typically obtained at hearing levels that are about 10 dB greater in intensity than the SDT. This reflects the fact that it requires more intensity for a client to recognize words than it does to detect them. Therefore, it would not be unusual to find that a client has, for example, an SRT of 25 dB HL and an SDT of 15 dB HL.

Administering the SDT

ASHA guidelines suggest that the methods used for pure tone threshold testing be applied to SDT testing. Stimuli for SDT testing are not standardized. According to ASHA, the exact stimulus used is not critical because the SDT measures detection and not recognition. For purposes of consistency, use of "bup-bup-bup" or "uh-oh" is suggested. Use of the child or client's name should be avoided because it will result in a highly variable stimulus. Other possible speech materials include speech babble, running speech, or familiar words. Regardless of the type of stimuli used, it is important to record the material type on the audiogram for reporting and comparison purposes.

The SDT is not commonly part of routine audiological assessment, probably because it provides less information than other speech measures. In fact, as illustrated in Figure 5.3, a client can have an SDT that is well within the normal range even with significant hearing loss. Note that the SDT of 10 dB reflects the normal hearing sensitivity at 250 and 500 Hz. It is for this reason that students of audiology and speech–language pathology are cautioned not to place great weight on the SDT; it only provides information about a client's hearing for a limited and nonspecific portion of the speech spectrum. This is similar to the caution made earlier regarding use of the SRT.

FIGURE 5.3 Patient with normal SDT and considerable pure tone hearing loss.

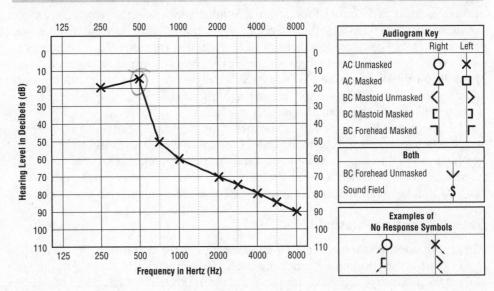

Speech Audiometry

Ear	SRT	SDT	PTA	Test	Word Recognition Level/Percent Correct	MCL	LDL
Right							
Left		10					
Bone							
Sound Field							
Right Aided							
Left Aided							
Binaural Aided							

Finally, it should be noted that the SDT can be helpful in cases where word repetition is impossible or difficult, such as with children or individuals who have special needs.

Word Recognition Testing

Word recognition testing may be defined as a measure of speech audiometry that assesses a client's ability to identify one-syllable words that are presented at hearing levels that are above threshold to arrive at a **word recognition score.** Word recognition testing was previously referred to as word discrimination ability, but that term is no longer current.

Reviewing carefully the above definition of word recognition testing, note that word recognition testing differs from speech recognition threshold testing in several important ways. First, the most common stimuli for word recognition testing are **monosyllabic words** (words of one-syllable), not spondees. In the past, efforts were made to construct word lists that were phonetically balanced. In a **phonetically balanced word list,** the sounds represented in the monosyllabic word lists occur proportionally to their occurrence in spoken English. These lists were developed as part of research to determine how much of the speech signal would have to be transmitted over telephone lines without compromising the listener's understanding. Although phonetic balancing was once viewed as very important in speech audiometry, it is no longer regarded as essential to the construction of word lists used in audiological evaluation. The use of monosyllables for audiological testing is based, in part, on the fact that these words can provide information regarding the client's ability to distinguish subtle acoustic cues in the language. For example, correct perception of the word *take* requires that the client have rather precise perception of the phonemes involved. Otherwise, the client may respond with the word *tape* or *cake.* This same degree of perception is not required to understand spondee words that are perceptually quite distinct from each other (e.g., *hotdog, airplane*).

Another important difference between word recognition testing and the speech recognition threshold is that word recognition is performed at a suprathreshold level. This level is necessary because, as early research showed, understanding of monosyllables requires more intensity than understanding of spondee words. In other words, comparing scores for recognition of monosyllabic versus spondee words presented at reduced intensity levels reveals that more spondee words will be understood.

A variety of lists of monosyllabic words have been developed for use in word recognition testing. Well-known lists of phonetically balanced monosyllabic words include the CID W-22 lists and the PBK-50 lists. The NU-6 list is a commonly used list of consonant–nucleus–consonant (CNC) monosyllabic words that is not phonetically balanced. Clinical experience shows that each of these lists has characteristics that make it applicable in certain clinical situations. For example, the NU-6 lists are generally considered to contain more difficult vocabulary, making them more appropriate for adult clients. The vocabulary words in the W-22 lists are relatively easier, making them more useful for younger age groups or for individuals with special needs. The PBK-50 lists were developed specifically for children of kindergarten age, rendering them useful for children and for individuals with special needs.

Initial audiometric setup for word recognition testing is the same as described for the SRT and SDT. However, there are differences in administering tests of word recognition, and these will be described in a later section. Before addressing test administration, let's examine the various purposes for word recognition testing.

Maximum Word Recognition Score. The primary purpose of word recognition testing is to determine the client's maximum speech understanding for one-syllable words. Ideally, the way to measure this maximum ability is to assess understanding of monosyllables at various intensity levels, in steps beginning near threshold and continuing to intensity levels that are well above threshold. This process is typically referred to as a **performance–intensity (PI)** function. Illustrated in Figure 5.4 (see •) is a typical PI function for an individual who has normal hearing sensitivity. Note that for this client, once the intensity level reaches 40 dB HL, the maximum recognition score (also referred to as PB Max) has been obtained and further increases in intensity do not improve the score. Figure 5.4 also provides an example of a PI function for a client who has a cochlear hearing loss (see △). Although PB max for this client requires greater intensity and is not as high as it was for the client with normal hearing, the PI pattern is the same. Increases in intensity yield increases in word recognition up to a certain intensity. Beyond this level, word recognition ability does not improve.

An important application of the PI function is using it to identify those clients who have retrocochlear pathology, evidenced by "rollover." **Retrocochlear pathology** refers to auditory dysfunction that is beyond the cochlea (e.g., at the auditory nerve or brainstem). **PI rollover** occurs when increasing intensity results in decreasing word recognition. Examine the PI function in Figure 5.4 (see ■) and note that word recognition performance improves until the presentation level reaches 70 dB, at which point an unexpected decrease in the recognition score occurs. This phenomenon is referred to as *rollover*.

FIGURE **5.4** **Performance intensity (PI) functions for individuals with normal hearing, cochlear hearing loss, and retrocochlear involvement.**

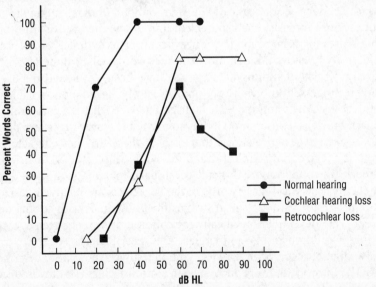

It is important to remember that not all rollover is suggestive of retrocochlear pathology. Formal determination of whether the rollover noted is significant for retrocochlear site of lesion can be made by using the following formula:

$$PB\ Max\ -\ PB\ Min/PB\ Max$$

For this formula, the PB Min used is the minimum score obtained at an intensity level that is above the maximum score. In general, a rollover value of 0.25 to 0.45 is significant, depending on the particular monosyllabic word list used.

Let's now use the above formula to determine whether the PB rollover noted in Figure 5.4 is significant. PB Max (70) minus PB Min (40) divided by PB Max (70) is 30/70, which equals 0.42. This is clearly significant for the NU-6 word list and would likely be significant for other word lists as well.

Surveys of the common practices of audiologists working in clinical settings reveal that most audiologists do not routinely perform PI functions when conducting word recognition testing, in part because doing so is very time-consuming, and also because there are more definitive audiological and medical tests to identify the site of suspected lesions in the auditory system. These other tests include auditory brainstem response (ABR) testing and magnetic resonance imaging (MRI).

Instead, many audiologists attempt to determine the maximum understanding by adding some dB value (e.g., 35 or 40 dB) to the SRT and using this as their level of presentation. For example, in the case described in Figure 5.5, the SRT is 40 dB HL in the right ear. If 35 dB is added to this SRT, the presentation level for word recognition testing is now 75 dB HL. Clients are then asked to repeat a list of words at this single intensity level and a percentage correct is calculated. In the case in Figure 5.5, the client scored 80 percent correct. Some audiologists then interpret this percentage using verbal descriptors, which may be useful in report writing and conveying diagnostic information to clients. Descriptors that may be encountered and corresponding percentage scores are

96–100%	Excellent
88–95%	Very good
80–87%	Good
70–79%	Fair
50–69%	Poor
Less than 50%	Very poor

Caution is advised when using or interpreting these verbal descriptors because they may not be good indicators of the real-world communication abilities of clients. In fact, when word recognition testing is performed in quiet, individuals with various degrees of sensorineural hearing loss perform similarly. This reflects the fact that word recognition tested in quiet is not a very sensitive measure. Later in this chapter we will describe how sensitivity is improved when noise or speech competition is added.

Despite the popularity of testing word recognition at a single intensity level, this time-saving method can result in elimination of helpful diagnostic information. Experts agree that the intensity level required for a client to achieve the maximum understanding of monosyllables varies greatly from client to client. Testing at one intensity level is unlikely to reveal a client's maximum score. Even though adding 35–40 dB to the SRT

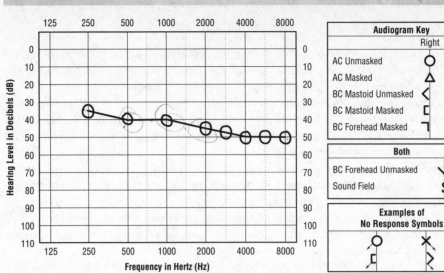

FIGURE **5.5** **Word recognition tested at a level that is 35 dB above the SRT.**

Speech Audiometry

Ear	SRT	SDT	PTA	Test	Word Recognition Level/Percent Correct	MCL	LDL
Right	40			W22	75/80%		
Left							
Bone							
Sound Field							
Right Aided							
Left Aided							
Binaural Aided							

does produce a suprathreshold level, that level will not necessarily yield maximum word recognition ability.

A note once again to the speech–language pathologist. When reading audiological reports, careful attention should be paid to the intensity level at which the word recognition testing was conducted. While the 80 percent score may be termed "good" from a diagnostic point of view, the client's ability to hear average conversational speech may be quite different. In this case, a good word recognition score was achieved at 75 dB HL; however, this does not tell us how the client will perform when speech is presented at a normal conversational intensity level (45–50 dB HL).

Another important factor to consider is that some audiologists record the absolute presentation level used for word recognition testing (e.g., 75 or 50 dB HL) on the audiogram form under the speech audiometry section. Others record the number of decibels they added to the SRT on the audiogram form using a "+" sign for the designation SL (sensation level). For example, if the SRT is 30 dB HL, the audiologist would record "+40 dB" or +40 dB SL to indicate a presentation level of 70 dB HL. You will find speech audiometry reported both ways in this text, to help you develop a critical eye for reviewing audiograms.

Another criticism of the use of the SRT to establish a single level of intensity for deriving the presentation level that will yield maximum recognition ability is illustrated by the audiogram in Figure 5.6. You will note that the client has a sloping hearing loss in the right ear and a flat loss in the left ear. Because the SRT is correlated with low to middle frequencies, and the pure tone hearing loss is the same in each ear at these frequencies, it is not surprising to find that the SRTs are the same for each ear. If you simply add 35 dB to the SRTs and use this as the presentation level, you will not be obtaining information about the maximum recognition ability because the right ear has less access to the high-frequency phonemes than the left ear. Comparing the recognition scores between ears will not be useful in this case.

FIGURE 5.6 **Influence of SRT on word recognition presentation level in cases of asymmetrical hearing loss.**

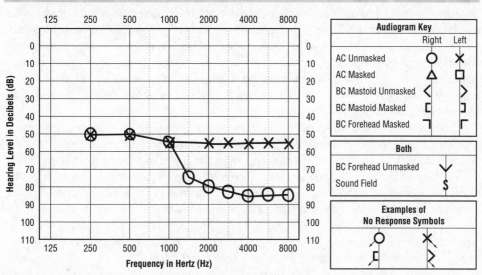

Audiogram Key		
	Right	Left
AC Unmasked	O	X
AC Masked	△	□
BC Mastoid Unmasked	<	>
BC Mastoid Masked	⊏	⊐
BC Forehead Masked	⌐	⌐

Both	
BC Forehead Unmasked	Y
Sound Field	S

Examples of No Response Symbols	

Speech Audiometry

Ear	SRT	SDT	PTA	Test	Word Recognition Level/Percent Correct	MCL	LDL
Right	50			W22	85/68%		
Left	50			W22	85/88%		
Bone							
Sound Field							
Right Aided							
Left Aided							
Binaural Aided							

What should an audiologist do to save time and obtain useful data regarding word recognition ability? One suggestion is to assess recognition ability at one intense level that will likely result in maximum recognition scores and will allow significant rollover to be ruled out (e.g., 80 dB). If the client obtains a score of greater than 80 percent, testing for that ear is complete. If the score is less than 80 percent, a more complete PI function can be obtained.

Most Comfortable Level and Loudness Discomfort Level.   Audiologists perform word recognition testing for purposes other than finding the maximum score. Despite concern that it is not always a reliable measure, some audiologists assess word recognition ability at a level referred to as the client's **most comfortable level** (MCL) and use this to estimate the client's word recognition ability with hearing aids. As you may already have discerned, the client's MCL for speech is the intensity level at which she perceives speech to be most comfortable. The logic of testing word recognition at MCL is that the amount of amplification (often referred to as *gain*) provided by a hearing aid theoretically should amplify incoming speech information to the client's MCL. If, for example, the client's MCL is 70 dB and at that level the client achieves a word recognition score of 88 percent, this suggests that word understanding will be good in the aided condition. If, on the other hand, the recognition ability is 32 percent at MCL, this might suggest limited aided benefit and may lead the audiologist to counsel the client in ways that will keep expectations realistic. Use of the MCL as the presentation level for assessing word recognition is often criticized on the basis that maximum recognition is often not obtained at MCL. However, it is important to remember that finding maximum recognition is not the only goal of word recognition testing.

Let's examine more completely some terms associated with listening comfort levels. The MCL has already been defined above as the intensity level at which the client perceives speech to be most comfortable. Similarly, the **loudness discomfort level** (LDL) for speech, formerly called the uncomfortable level or UCL, is the level at which the client perceives speech to be uncomfortable. It is important to note that when we use the word *uncomfortable,* we are not referring to physical discomfort, which can occur in response to very intense sound. We are referring to a subjective response to sound in which the sound is unpleasant to listen to due to its extreme intensity. The major purposes of word recognition testing are summarized in Table 5.2.

To obtain the MCL and LDL, many clinicians present speech stimuli (words or phrases) to the client at a variety of intensity levels. They ask the client for judgments about each level (e.g., too soft, just right, too loud). Some methods incorporate use of a numeric scale against which loudness judgments are made, and others use pictures (e.g., happy faces or sad faces) for this purpose. The method selected for determining the MCL and LDL should be based on the abilities of the client.

In the following case examples, note that we refer to decibels using the HL reference. This is because we are referring to audiological test results obtained through use of an audiometer calibrated in hearing level (HL). There are times when a different decibel referent is used. For example, when discussing hearing aid specifications, the decibel referent that is typically used is sound pressure level (SPL). In Chapter 4, the conversions from dB SPL to dB HL for specific frequencies and earphones, based on ANSI standards, were given. Speech constitutes a broader signal than pure tones, and is composed of frequencies including, but not limited to, 500–4,000 Hz. Averaging the conversion from HL to SPL for these frequencies results in approximately a 10-dB difference. It is for this reason that conversational speech may be reported as 45–50 dB HL or 55–60 dB SPL. In the ensuing discussion, the HL reference will be used.

Examine the audiogram in Figure 5.7. Note that the SRT is 25 dB HL, the MCL is 65 dB HL, and the LDL is 95 dB HL. These three speech measures represent the client's threshold for speech, most comfortable listening level, and loudness discomfort level, respectively. The difference in dB between the SRT and the LDL is the client's **dynamic range.** In this case it is 70 dB. This means that 70 dB separate the level at which speech is just barely understandable and the level at which it becomes uncomfortable.

TABLE 5.2   Summary of the Major Uses of Word Recognition Scores

Purpose	Procedure	Comment
To assess maximum speech understanding	PI function	This is the traditional purpose of word recognition testing. Use of PI function is the most widely respected method of doing this.
	80-dB presentation level	Use of a very intense level is an accepted short cut. If the client achieves at least 80% correct, the test is terminated.
	Adding 35–40 dB to the SRT to derive the presentation level	Criticized because these levels do not consistently yield PB max. For example, basing presentation levels on the SRT can result in different access to speech sounds in cases of asymmetrical hearing loss.
To rule out retrocochlear pathology	PI-PB rollover	A sensitive measure to retrocochlear pathology. Remember that some rollover is nonsignificant.
To assess speech understanding in noise	Introduce noise under earphones or in the sound field	Can document the effects of noise on speech understanding.
For hearing aid fitting	Test word recognition at conversational levels	This can establish (for the client or family) the need for amplification. Can be repeated with the hearing aids in place to demonstrate improvement.
	Use MCL as the presentation level	If it is assumed that the client will wear hearing aids at their most comfortable listening levels, testing at this level may be useful. MCL is typically a range of numbers and can be an unreliable measure.
	Test word recognition in noise	Can be used to measure the benefits of hearing aids in noise.

FIGURE **5.7** **Normal dynamic range in a right ear with mild to moderate sensorineural hearing loss.**

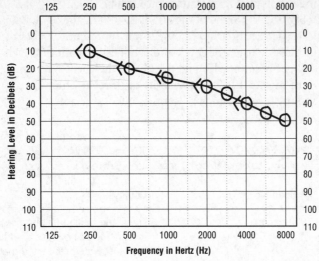

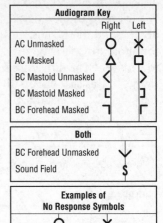

	Audiogram Key	Right	Left
AC Unmasked		○	✕
AC Masked		△	☐
BC Mastoid Unmasked		<	>
BC Mastoid Masked		⊏	⊐
BC Forehead Masked		⊤	⊤

Both	
BC Forehead Unmasked	Y
Sound Field	S

Examples of No Response Symbols

Speech Audiometry

Ear	SRT	SDT	PTA	Test	Word Recognition Level/Percent Correct	MCL	LDL
Right	25					65	95
Left							
Bone							
Sound Field							
Right Aided							
Left Aided							
Binaural Aided							

Now examine the audiogram in Figure 5.8. This client has a sensorineural hearing loss. Note that because of the hearing loss, the SRT of 60 dB HL is much higher than in the first case. Also note that the LDL is 95 dB HL. Now the dynamic range is restricted, at only 35 dB. Complicating this picture is the fact that amplification using hearing aids will be recommended for this client, and the gain provided by these hearing aids will amplify sounds above the SRT but must not amplify them beyond the LDL. The restricted dynamic range noted in this case makes hearing aid fitting challenging. This will be discussed more fully in Chapter 12.

Functional Audiometric Testing. For the final application of word recognition testing, examine the audiogram in Figure 5.9. Note that in this case the audiologist performed word recognition testing in the sound field at a level of 45 dB HL, even though the client's hearing

FIGURE **5.8** **Restricted dynamic range in a right ear with moderately severe sensorineural hearing loss.**

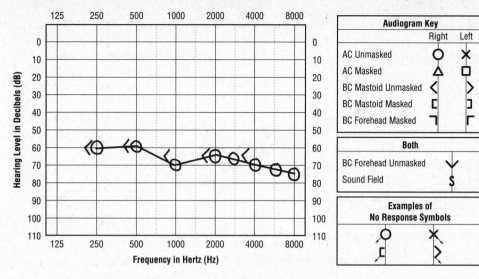

Ear	SRT	SDT	PTA	Test	Word Recognition Level/Percent Correct	MCL	LDL
Right	60						95
Left							
Bone							
Sound Field							
Right Aided							
Left Aided							
Binaural Aided							

Speech Audiometry

loss gives him almost no access to speech sounds at this intensity level. Why would the audiologist do this? First, think about the importance of 45 dB HL. It is the approximate intensity of conversational speech. By testing at this level and documenting that only 20 percent of the words were recognized, the audiologist can counsel the client and the client's family as to the substantial degree to which the hearing loss interferes with speech understanding. Also note for the same case that the audiologist retested word recognition skills at 45 dB, after the client was fitted with hearing aids. Recognition ability is now 76 percent at 45 dB, suggesting that amplification has made speech much more understandable, at least in quiet settings. This information is important to clients' understanding of their communication abilities, to their family members, and to those who work with them. Although testing conducted in a sound-treated room can provide valuable insights about clients' performance, test scores may be different from real-world performance for a variety of reasons.

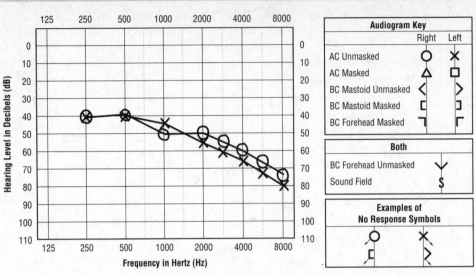

FIGURE **5.9** **Comparison of word recognition scores tested at conversational levels with and without amplification.**

Speech Audiometry

Ear	SRT	SDT	PTA	Test	Word Recognition Level/Percent Correct	MCL	LDL
Right							
Left							
Bone							
Sound Field				*NU6*	*45/20%*		
Right Aided							
Left Aided							
Binaural Aided				*NU6*	*45/76%*		

Because word recognition testing can be done for various purposes and at different presentation levels, it is important that audiologists explain findings in a meaningful way in their report writing so that the client, family members, and other professionals are provided with functional information regarding the client's ability to understand speech in everyday settings. A humanistic approach to audiology requires that the expressed communicative needs of the client be addressed to the greatest extent possible. Providing relevant, understandable information is one aspect of this type of care.

Word Recognition Testing in Noise and Speech Competition

One of the observations made by audiologists regarding word recognition testing is that even clients with considerable hearing loss can perform fairly well in the controlled conditions of the sound-treated booth. As noted, this is due to the limited sensitivity of word recognition testing performed in quiet. In an attempt to make word recognition testing more sensitive to the difficulty clients experience in the real world, many audiologists perform some type of word recognition testing in the presence of noise or speech competition. Although there are no standards for performing speech testing in noise, one method is to introduce **speech noise** (using channel 2 of the audiometer) into the same earphone that is receiving speech (referred to as ipsilateral noise), usually at a level that is slightly less than the level of the speech. For example, if an audiologist wants to assess word recognition in noise and chooses an intensity level of speech of 45 dB HL, the level of the noise may be 35 or 40 dB HL. Recall from our discussion in Chapter 2 that the term *signal-to-noise ratio* is used to describe the intensity relationship between speech and noise. Even though the word *ratio* is used, calculation of the signal-to-noise ratio actually involves subtracting the level of the noise from the level of the speech, because both are decibel values. So, if the speech level is 45 dB and the level of the noise is 35 dB, the signal-to-noise ratio is +10 dB. What would the signal-to-noise ratio be if the level of the noise was 40 dB? You are correct if you said it would be +5 dB.

A method of assessing word recognition with competition is to use recorded multitalker noise (also called multitalker babble) as the competing stimulus. Multitalker babble sounds like the background chatter you hear at a large party. This differs from speech noise in that it has more of a discernable linguistic content and may be more realistic. It may also be a more difficult task for the client's auditory system because it requires listening to the speech being presented (i.e., monosyllabic words) and at the same time squelching the background speech babble.

Although most audiological procedures for speech testing in noise are nonstandard and the data obtained typically have limited reliability, recently standardized tests have been developed that may allow more regular and reliable assessment of the effects of noise on word recognition. One such test is the Hearing in Noise Test (HINT; Nilsson, Soli, & Sullivan, 1994), which is designed to provide a measure of word recognition thresholds for sentences in quiet and in noise. The test consists of twenty-five equivalent lists (ten sentences per list) and speech spectrum noise, making this instrument well suited for measuring the effects of hearing loss on a client's ability to understand speech in noise. After instructing the client to repeat back as much as she can of each sentence presented in a background of noise, the audiologist delivers (via CD) a series of sentences, adjusting the presentation level of the next sentence based on the client's performance on the previous sentence. For example, if a sentence is repeated correctly, the intensity of the next sentence is decreased; if it is repeated incorrectly, the intensity of the next sentence is increased. The intensity level of the speech noise remains constant. Once data have been gathered for several intensity levels, a formula is used to derive the reception threshold for sentences (RTS).

This RTS can be used in a number of different ways. First, it can be compared to normative data provided by the test authors to determine whether the client's performance in noise is consistent with other listeners. Second, the RTS obtained in noise can be compared to the client's RTS in some other noise condition. For example, if the original RTS was obtained with the speech and noise directly in front of the client, the second administration could separate the speech and noise (by 90 degrees) to determine how this affects speech understanding. The test authors state that this provides information about the effects of binaural hearing. Finally, the RTS can be interpreted relative to the resulting changes to the percentage of speech understanding. For example, if a client's RTS is improved by even a few decibels with high-technology hearing aids, research suggests that this will result in a considerable improvement in speech understanding.

Other Tests of Speech Understanding

A number of other tests have been developed to assess clients' ability to understand speech. Given the many factors that can influence speech perception abilities, it is understandable that the conventional test materials developed to assess word recognition thresholds and word recognition scores might not be useful for all clients or for all purposes for which speech audiometry may be used. Although not routinely part of the audiological test battery, these tests are valuable because they can provide insight about word recognition ability for specific clinical questions and for specific client profiles.

Sentence Tests

CID Everyday Sentences

Developed by Davis and Silverman (1970) at the Central Institute for the Deaf (CID), the CID Everyday Sentences consist of ten sets of ten sentences with fifty key words contained within each set of sentences. The number of key words correctly identified out of fifty determines the client's score.

Utley Test of Lipreading

The Utley Test of Lipreading was described in 1946 and was a filmed test of lip-reading ability. The full test consisted of words, sentences, and stories. Many clinics have a list of the sentences used in the Utley Test of Lipreading. The words used by Utley (1946) were taken from lists of commonly used words, and the sentences are commonly used expressions. Although this test was designed to assess lip-reading ability, these sentences, provided with auditory cues only, may be useful during word recognition testing for clients who are unable to repeat monosyllabic words but who have the ability to repeat familiar sentences. The difference in stimulus material may prove helpful since sentence material provides more cues for the listener, including redundancy. In such circumstances, an estimate of the client's speech perceptual skills obtained in a nonstandardized manner may provide useful insight. As with any assessment, the material used to obtain information included in the audiological report should be recorded on the audiogram.

Synthetic Sentence Identification

Speaks and Jerger (1965) developed the Synthetic Sentence Identification (SSI) test. The materials for this test are comprised of nonsense sentences that follow certain syntactic rules but do not "make sense." There are two methods for administering the SSI: ipsilateral competing message tasks (message and competition in the same ear) and contralateral competing message tasks (message and competition in opposite ears). The competition consists of connected discourse, and a closed-set format is used. In a **closed-set** format, the client identifies the presented item from a limited set of items. The rationale for use of this format is to reduce the influence of a listener's knowledge of rules of grammar and syntax on his perception of sentence-length stimuli. An example of an item from the SSI is "Small boat with a picture has become." In administering this test, a verbal response is not required. Rather, the client is provided with a list of the ten sentences in the group and asked to identify the correct sentence from that list. Therefore, the client's ability to read as well as his visual skills must be considered when deciding whether this test is appropriate for a particular individual.

The Speech Perception in Noise Test

The Speech Perception in Noise (SPIN) test was designed by Kalikow, Stevens, and Elliott (1977) to assess a listener's ability to use context cues and linguistic information to perceive auditory information. Two types of sentences are included in the SPIN test, those with high predictability, in which the target word can be "figured out" from the context of the sentence, and those with low predictability, in which the listener cannot discern the target word from the contents of the test sentence. The target word is always the last word in the sentence and is a monosyllabic noun. Comparison of a listener's performance on these two types of test items provides insight regarding whether the listener takes advantage of linguistic/contextual cues or not.

This information can be helpful to clinicians planning aural rehabilitation services. For example, one goal may be to enhance the use of linguistic/contextual cues that are available to the listener. Because even optimal amplification may not provide every acoustic cue to a listener, use of context and other cues to enhance understanding of spoken messages is an important strategy for individuals with hearing loss. Speech–language clinicians have extensive knowledge of "top-down" processing of speech information and can help clients with hearing loss by providing practical applications of this information to their situation.

Sample SPIN test sentences with high predictability are

The watchdog gave a warning *growl.*

She made the bed with clean *sheets.*

The old train was powered by *steam.*

Sample SPIN test sentences with low predictability are

The old man discussed the *dive.*

I should have considered the *map.*

Miss Brown shouldn't discuss the *sand.* (Kalikow et al., 1977)

Additional Test Materials

Depending on the particular assessment purpose, one or more of the following test materials may be useful.

The California Consonant Test

The California Consonant Test (CCT) was described by Owens and Schubert (1977). It is a closed-set test consisting of 100 items with three foils (incorrect choices) for each item and was developed for use with clients with hearing loss. The CCT has a high correlation with the configuration of the hearing loss and is particularly sensitive in cases of high-frequency hearing loss. Owens and Schubert indicated that a potential use of the results of measurement of speech perceptual skills with the CCT is in identifying consonant confusions to assist with planning for aural rehabilitation.

Clinicians may wish to add the CCT to their test battery to provide additional insight into a client's ability to hear consonants when high-frequency hearing loss is present. In some cases, the CCT may reveal difficulty that the standard monosyllabic word lists used for word recognition testing do not. Instructions for the CCT and word lists may be found in Appendix A of this chapter. Potential settings for use of the CCT include the audiometric test suite or face to face with auditory cues, with or without amplification, depending on the clinical question(s) to be addressed.

Word Intelligibility by Picture Identification

Described by Ross and Lerman (1970), the Word Intelligibility by Picture Identification test, or WIPI, is a closed-set test designed to measure speech discrimination (word recognition) ability in young children with hearing loss. The test has twenty-five plates with six pictures on each plate. Children are required to point to the correct picture on each page. Requiring a picture-pointing response has the advantages of (1) limiting the number of vocabulary words used, thereby increasing the chance that the stimuli are within the recognition vocabulary of the child, and (2) eliminating the opportunity for any articulation errors present in the child's speech to interfere with interpretation of responses. In addition to the WIPI's usefulness for children with hearing loss, this closed-set test is also helpful when evaluating individuals with developmental disabilities, expressive aphasia, or motor speech disorders, as well as younger children whose speech is not sufficiently intelligible to permit reliable interpretation of a verbal response. It should be noted that use of a closed-set test can result in scores that are 20 percent higher than if an **open-set** response format were used. In an open-set format, choices are not supplied to the client, requiring him to provide responses that best match the input stimulus, without knowledge of potential alternative responses. This is important when word recognition scores are compared from one year to the next; the type of test stimuli and response should be considered when making such comparisons.

Northwestern University-Children's Perception of Speech

Northwestern University-Children's Perception of Speech (NU-CHIPS) is a standardized, recorded, closed-set word recognition test. It is composed of fifty monosyllabic words with four choices per page. Because this test requires a picture-pointing response, its advantages are similar to those of the WIPI. Developed by Elliott and Katz (1980), the vocabulary used in NU-CHIPS includes words that are familiar to 3-year-old inner-city children.

Minimal Auditory Capabilities Battery

The Minimum Auditory Capabilities (MAC) battery was designed by Owens, Kessler, Raggio, and Schubert (1985) to provide a comprehensive analysis of the auditory skills of individuals with profound postlingual hearing loss. Individuals with this degree of hearing loss typically score at or near zero on conventional tests of word recognition using monosyllabic words, so a need for a different way to evaluate the word recognition skills of these individuals was recognized. The MAC battery consists of thirteen auditory tests and one lip-reading test. The overall goal for the MAC test battery was to provide a consistent method of assessing cochlear implant candidacy. According to the authors, secondary uses of the MAC battery include making comparisons between profoundly deaf individuals who use hearing aids and those who use cochlear implants, assisting in determining whether a profoundly deaf hearing aid user might realize greater benefit from cochlear implant use, and assisting with aural rehabilitation placement. Specific components of the revised (1985) version of the MAC battery are in Appendix B. Beiter and Brimacombe (2000) note that a shortened version of this battery has also been developed for clinical use with adults who are potential cochlear implant candidates.

Ling Six Sound Test

The Ling Six Sound Test (Ling, 1989) consists of the sounds /a/, /u/, /i/, /sh/, /s/, and /m/. Earlier work (Ling, 1976) may refer to the Ling Five Sound test; the /m/ sound was added later. These sounds represent the sounds in the speech frequencies. This informative test is typically used for young clients with amplification, and can also be used to verify and supplement other audiological data. Each of the sounds is presented at a normal conversational intensity level (50 dB) at a distance of 3–5 ft, without visual cues. The child is required to repeat the presented sound, or raise a hand if the sound is heard. Depending on the purpose of the assessment, the sounds may also be presented at increasing distances.

Masking during Speech Audiometry

As we have seen, the fundamental speech audiometric tests are the speech recognition threshold (SRT), a threshold test, and the word recognition score, a suprathreshold test. Recall from Chapter 4 that the use of masking is necessary under certain circumstances to isolate the test ear from the non-test ear during pure tone testing. Masking is also necessary when the possibility of cross-hearing exists during speech audiometric testing. In fact, the possibility of cross-hearing is encountered often during suprathreshold (word recognition) testing. Following is a brief discussion of when to mask during speech audiometry.

Type of Masking Noise Used

As we discussed in Chapter 4, the most efficient masker for use in pure tone testing is a narrow-band noise centered around the test frequency. The use of an efficient masker helps to achieve the goal of raising the threshold in the non-test ear without using any more sound pressure (intensity) than necessary. For speech audiometry, the most efficient masker is speech spectrum noise, which Yacullo (1996) defines as "white noise that has been filtered to simulate the long-term average spectrum of conversational speech" (p. 17). Another masker used during speech audiometry is **white noise,** which is also broad in spectrum but slightly less efficient than speech noise.

When to Mask during Air Conduction Testing

Speech Detection Threshold and Speech Recognition Threshold

The following information can be applied when considering whether masking is needed during assessment of the SDT or SRT:

- The SRT of the test ear should be compared with the *bone conduction thresholds* of the non-test ear, if available, for purposes of determining the need for masking.
- Summed up as a formula (Martin & Clark, 2006, p. 122), there is danger of cross-hearing during SRT testing when:

    $$\text{SRTte} - \text{IA} \geq \text{best BCnte}$$

- If bone conduction has not yet been tested in the non-test ear, assume that the bone conduction threshold in the non-test ear is zero.
- Based on this assumption, once the presentation level for the assessment of the SRT exceeds 40 dB HL, masking should be used in the non-test ear.

In addition, you should note that, in most cases, if unmasked air conduction thresholds do not shift with masking, there is no need to mask when testing the SRT or SDT. However, because speech is a broad-band signal, the clinician should be alert to the possibility of cross-hearing (and the need to use masking) if any frequency in the non-test ear has normal bone conduction sensitivity.

The plateau method described for pure tone testing (Chapter 4, Appendix A) is one method that can be applied when masking is needed to establish the SDT or SRT; the true speech threshold would be ascertained when the masker could be raised or lowered in 5-dB steps at least three times without affecting the threshold (Martin & Clark, 2006). In other words, the size of the plateau we are seeking is 15 dB HL.

Word Recognition Testing

Now that you have learned about masking for the SRT and SDT, let's examine masking for word recognition testing. Remember that word recognition, unlike the SRT and SDT, is a suprathreshold measure, making potential crossover of the signal to the non-test ear even more likely. The following information can be applied when considering whether masking is needed during assessment of word recognition ability:

- Factors influencing the need to mask during word recognition testing include the presentation level to the test ear, interaural attenuation for air-conducted signals, and the presence of air–bone gaps in the non-test ear.
- Expressed as a formula (Martin & Clark, 2006), masking is needed for word recognition testing when

$$PBHLte - IA \geq best\ BCnte$$

where PBHL refers to the hearing level of the stimulus words.
- Conservatively, assuming two ears with symmetrical hearing loss and a presentation level during word recognition testing of 40 dB SL (or 40 dB above the client's speech recognition threshold), masking will be needed.
- In cases where asymmetrical hearing exists between the two ears, masking will be needed during suprathreshold word recognition testing of the poorer ear.

Other Issues in Speech Audiometry

Additional factors to consider when conducting and interpreting speech audiometry are summarized in Table 5.3. Selected factors are discussed in greater detail.

Recorded Material versus Live Voice Testing

One of the most common concerns expressed about word recognition testing by authorities in the field is the persistent tendency among audiologists to present speech stimuli to clients using monitored live voice, rather than by tape or compact disc. Recall from our earlier discussion that monitored live voice refers to presentation of speech by talking directly into the audiometer microphone and monitoring the VU meter to ensure that the intended amount of gain is being delivered. Survey results reported by Martin, Champlin, and Chambers (1998) showed that most audiologists use monitored live voice testing despite evidence that recordings of word lists are more reliable.

TABLE 5.3   Factors Involved in Conducting and Interpreting Speech Audiometric Tests

Test Variables	Client Variables
Recorded material versus live-voice testing	Linguistic background of client
Number of stimulus items	Familiarity with the vocabulary/words
Intensity level	Fatigue
Interpretation of scores and meaningful differences in scores	Attention
	Presence of other disabilities (e.g., apraxia, aphasia, traumatic brain injury, motor disability, vision impairment)

There are probably two major reasons why monitored live voice is so popular with audiologists: it is quicker than use of recorded materials and it is more flexible. Imagine a very cooperative client who has normal hearing and is able to easily repeat the words presented. The audiologist can present words at a fairly rapid pace and complete the word recognition testing with efficiency. Recorded materials, on the other hand, tend to take more time because typically a fixed time interval exists between words. Similarly, when using live voice, the audiologist is able to repeat words that are missed without having to rewind a tape or locate the correct place on the compact disc.

Despite these conveniences, use of monitored live voice in speech audiometry is not recommended because of the great variability in presentation, not only among different audiologists who test the same client but also on the part of the same audiologist on different test sessions. Let's discuss these briefly.

If Mrs. Smith comes in for a hearing test and the evaluation is performed by audiologist #1, that audiologist has a specific fundamental frequency and unique articulation and dialect patterns. When she is seen the following year by audiologist #2 for a reevaluation, the acoustic features of the speaker are now different, which will influence the recognition scores obtained. This makes reliable comparison of the recognition scores obtained in the first visit with those obtained on the second visit difficult.

In addition, because live-voice testing does not allow standardization, some audiologists tend to present words in a very formal manner and overarticulate the words as they are spoken to the client. These audiologists may be motivated by their view that the primary purpose of word recognition testing is to assess the client's maximum understanding of the words. Other audiologists present the words in a very natural, conversational, manner, based on the idea that this will yield scores that are more realistic. Once again, these differences in philosophy and methodology add to the variability of the test results and reduce the consistency of the data. Remember that the variability problems described here do not apply only to different speakers. Even if a client regularly sees the same audiologist, research has shown that live-voice presentation of words is very different between test sessions. Use of recorded materials removes such variability from the testing process.

Testing Non-English Speakers

A common occurrence in audiology and speech–language pathology is the need to provide reliable diagnostic (and rehabilitative) services to individuals who are non-English speakers. Although this issue is challenging in numerous fields, it can be critical in our field because our focus is on the client's communication abilities. Special care must be taken to ensure that the client's language status does not interfere with our ability to obtain credible data regarding communication skills.

In this effort, a growing number of speech–language pathologists and audiologists have become bilingual, learning a second language so that they can better serve their clients. Undergraduate programs in communication disorders also regularly encourage students to minor in a foreign language. In addition, some companies now produce recorded speech audiometry materials in languages other than English. For example, compact discs are available in Spanish for use during speech audiometry. These developments are positive trends and are likely to continue. To further support this, clinicians who encounter the need for speech audiometry materials in other languages should make this known to manufacturers of recorded speech materials.

When non-English speakers are scheduled for audiological assessments, it is important to arrange with the referent for the client to be accompanied by someone who has the ability to provide at least informal interpretation for the purposes of the evaluation. In addition to serving as an informal interpreter, this person can also provide to the audiologist words that might be used for speech audiometry. These words can be spoken by the audiologist or preferably can be spoken by the informal interpreter. The audiologist would monitor the VU meter, as discussed previously, and would adjust the attenuator dial. The audiogram should contain documentation of the test technique used, and any word list generated for test purposes should be kept in the client's file.

Number of Words to Present

When word recognition lists were originally developed, the intention was for the audiologist to present a list of 100 words to each ear in order to determine the percentage correct. Over the years, it has become very common for audiologists to use shorter and shorter lists of fifty words, then twenty-five words, as a means of saving time. Some audiologists use twenty-five words only if the client's performance on those words is very good; others use twenty-five words routinely, regardless of the client's test performance.

The length of the word list used for word recognition testing is important because if affects the reliability of the test scores. Reliability, as you will recall, refers to the consistency or stability of the test results. If word recognition testing is performed on a client on one day and then performed again on the same client one week later, the two scores should be consistent (presuming that there has been no change in the client's auditory status). If the testing on the second day reveals a different score, a lack of test stability is suspected. Because obtaining a greater number of samples better assesses the skill in question (in this case, word recognition ability), longer word lists tend to yield more reliable results. For this reason, use of shortened word lists can be problematic.

Recently, authorities in audiology have proposed protocols that might represent reasonable compromises between audiologists' desire to save time and the need to obtain reliable data. For example, Hall and Mueller (1997) suggest that audiologists present the ten most difficult monosyllabic words via tape or compact disc. If the client scores between 90 and 100 percent, the test is terminated in that ear. As noted previously, if the client obtains such high scores at a level of 80 dB, the audiologist has also ruled out rollover. Runge and Hosford-Dunn (1985) also suggest beginning with the ten most difficult words. The audiologist uses twenty-five words only if the client scores less than 100 percent on these first ten. If the client scores less than 84 percent (four errors) on this list of twenty-five words, the complete fifty-word list is used. This recommendation is reinforced by the work of Hurley and Sells (2003), who analyzed Nu-6 word lists to determine the most difficult words and recommended beginning testing with these.

What Constitutes a Significant Difference in Performance?

Comparison of new audiological results with previous findings is usually of interest, both to the client and to family members, and to clinicians, therapists, and educators who may work with the client. Changes in pure tone thresholds and changes in word recognition scores are of particular interest. Because a decrease in word recognition ability can have a significant impact on communication skills, and could signal other changes in the client's overall auditory system function, serious attention is generally given to reductions in these scores.

Recognizing that numerous factors can affect word recognition scores, clinicians need to consider how to interpret differences in scores from one test to another. Thornton and Raffin (1978) used a mathematical model to study differences in speech discrimination scores (word recognition scores). This is important because clinicians need to know whether a change in word recognition scores from one test to the next is significant. A significant change represents a true change in performance, whereas a nonsignificant change in scores may be due to performance variability caused by factors that are unrelated to word recognition ability. Using Thornton and Raffin's critical differences data, given in Table 5.4, someone with a speech discrimination (word recognition) score of 96 percent on a fifty-word list has a 95 percent probability of obtaining a score between 86 and 100 percent on another fifty-word list. Someone with a word recognition score of 48 percent on a fifty-word list has a 95 percent probability of obtaining a score between 30 and 66 percent on another fifty-word list. From this table, it can be seen that there is little variability at the extreme ends of the distribution of scores. In other words, if scores are near 100 percent (or near 0 percent), a small difference in two subsequent scores suggests a true difference in performance, since the expected range of scores is smaller (a 14 percent range in the 96 percent example versus a 36 percent range in the 48 percent example). Therefore, a larger difference in word recognition scores in the middle of the range is not as significant as a smaller difference in scores at either end of the range. For this reason, it is not possible to offer a specific percentage that constitutes a significant difference between word recognition scores for the entire range of possible scores.

The researchers also examined factors such as the use of half or full word lists. The size of the list changes the variability of the resultant scores. The smaller the word list, the greater is the variability. Use of a longer word list is justified based on the fact that reduced variability is desirable in audiological assessment, particularly when word recognition scores fall in the mid-range. In other words, use of a half-list may be a relatively minor factor when word recognition scores fall at the extreme ends of the range,

TABLE 5.4 Lower and Upper Limits of the 95 Percent Critical Differences for Percentage Scores. Values within the range shown are not significantly different from the value shown in the percentage score columns ($p > 0.05$).

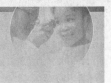

% Score	n = 50	n = 25	n = 10	% Score	n = 100*
0	0–4	0–8	0–20	50	37–63
2	0–10			51	38–64
4	0–14	0–20		52	39–65
6	2–18			53	40–66
8	2–22	0–28		54	41–67
10	2–24		0–50	55	42–68
12	4–26	4–32		56	43–69
14	4–30			57	44–70
16	6–32	4–40		58	45–71
18	6–34			59	46–72
20	8–36	4–44	0–60	60	47–73
22	8–40			61	48–74
24	10–42	8–48		62	49–74
26	12–44			63	50–75
28	14–46	8–52		64	51–76
30	14–48		10–70	65	52–77
32	16–50	12–56		66	53–78
34	18–52			67	54–79
36	20–54	16–60		68	55–80
38	22–56			69	56–81
40	22–58	16–64	10–80	70	57–81
42	24–60			71	58–82
44	26–62	20–68		72	59–83
46	28–64			73	60–84
48	30–66	24–72		74	61–85
50	32–68		10–90	75	63–86

near 100 percent or near 0 percent. For scores in the middle, it may be prudent to use a full list to increase score reliability and validity.

Given this inherent potential variability in word recognition test scores, caution should be exercised in determining whether a significant difference in scores exists from one test to the next. The number of variables that can have an impact on word recognition scores, including the word list used, the number of words presented, and the client's state during testing, argues against applying a single percentage as constituting a clinically significant difference in all cases. One important strategy to assist in making comparisons of test scores from one test to the next is to be exact in recording the type of test material (word list) used, the number of items given, and the presentation level. When as many factors as possible are the same from one test to the next, differences approaching 20 percent can be considered clinically significant for the mid-range of scores, while somewhat smaller differences may be meaningful at the upper limits (90–100 percent) and lower limits (0–10 percent) of the range of scores.

TABLE **5.4** (*continued*)

% Score	n = 50	n = 25	n = 10	% Score	n = 100*
52	34–70	28–76		76	64–86
54	36–72			77	65–87
56	38–74	32–80		78	66–88
58	40–76			79	67–89
60	42–78	36–84	20–90	80	68–89
62	44–78			81	69–90
64	46–80	40–84		82	71–91
66	48–82			83	72–92
68	50–84	44–88		84	73–92
70	52–86		30–90	85	74–93
72	54–86	48–92		86	75–94
74	56–88			87	77–94
76	58–90	52–92		88	78–95
78	60–92			89	79–96
80	64–92	56–96	40–100	90	81–96
82	66–94			91	82–97
84	68–94	60–96		92	83–98
86	70–96			93	85–98
88	74–96	68–96		94	86–99
90	76–98		50–100	95	88–99
92	78–98	72–100		96	89–99
94	82–98			97	91–100
96	86–100	80–100		98	92–100
98	90–100			99	94–100
100	96–100	92–100	80–100	100	97–100

*If score is less than 50%, find % Source = 100-observed score and subtract each critical difference limit from 100.

Source: Thornton, A., & Raffin, M. (1978). Speech-discrimination scores modeled as a binomial variable. *Journal of Speech and Hearing Research, 21,* 515. Used with permission.

CHAPTER SUMMARY

There are a number of benefits to be obtained by using speech audiometry as part of a comprehensive audiological assessment. This chapter described the various threshold and suprathreshold speech audiometric tests that are routinely part of the comprehensive audiological battery, as well as a number of tests that are used to answer specific questions about particular cases. In addition to providing information regarding the purposes of the tests, discussion of test administration and interpretation were noted, with special application to the role of the speech–language pathologist.

The information in this chapter is critical to both audiologists and speech–language pathologists because it serves as the foundation for understanding a client's hearing loss and allows for an understanding of modifications in test procedures that will be described later in the chapters on pediatrics and special populations.

QUESTIONS FOR DISCUSSION

1. List reasons why an audiologist might substitute an SDT for an SRT.
2. Describe the importance of speech audiometry results to the speech–language pathologist.
3. Describe the importance of speech audiometry results to the audiologist.
4. Discuss three broad purposes of word recognition testing. How is test administration influenced by these various purposes?
5. Discuss the contributions of other speech audiometric tests (e.g., sentence materials, speech-in-noise tests) to the diagnostic process? What additional information can be obtained from these tests?
6. Six sample audiograms were included for review in Chapter 4. Speech audiometric information has now been added. Consider the following as you review these cases:
   - Is the speech audiometric data consistent with pure tone findings?
   - Describe the information gained from the word recognition scores about the person's functional communication ability. Consider the presentation level and percent correct.

Sample 1

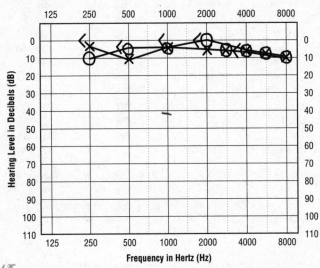

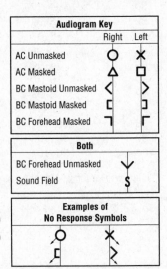

+40

Speech Audiometry

Ear	SRT	SDT	PTA 5 – 2	Test	Word Recognition Level/Percent Correct	MCL	LDL
Right	5		3	NU6	+40/ 100%		
Left	5		7	NU6	+40/96%		
Bone							
Sound Field							
Right Aided							
Left Aided							
Binaural Aided							

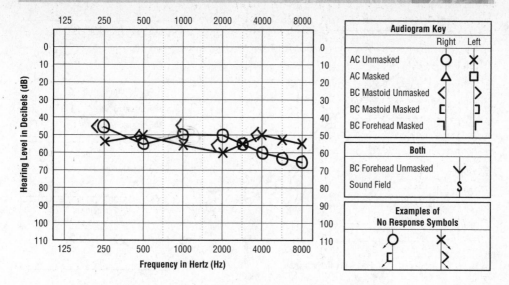

Speech Audiometry

Ear	SRT	SDT	PTA 5 - 2	Test	Word Recognition Level/Percent Correct	MCL	LDL
Right	50		52	NU6	+30/84 %		
Left	55		55	NU6	+30/80 %		
Bone							
Sound Field							
Right Aided							
Left Aided							
Binaural Aided							

RECOMMENDED READING

American Speech-Language-Hearing Association (ASHA). (1988, March). Guidelines for determining threshold level for speech. *ASHA,* pp. 85–89.

Auditec of St. Louis, www.auditec.com

Elliott, L. L., & Katz, D. R. (1980). *Northwestern University Children's Perception of Speech Test (NU-CHIPS).* St. Louis, MO: Auditec.

Ling, D. (1976). *Speech and the hearing impaired child: Theory and practice.* Washington, DC: Alexander Graham Bell Association for the Deaf.

Nilsson, M., Soli, S., & Sullivan, J. (1994). Development of the Hearing in Noise Test for the measurement of speech reception thresholds in quiet and in noise. *Journal of the Acoustical Society of America, 95,* 1085–1099.

Owens, E., Kessler, D. K., Raggio, M. W., & Schubert, E. D. (1985). Analysis and revision of the Minimal Auditory Capabilities (MAC) battery. *Ear and Hearing, 6,* 280–290.

Owens, E., & Schubert, E. D. (1977). Development of the California Consonant Test. *Journal of Speech and Hearing Research, 20,* 463–474.

Sample 3

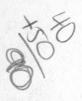

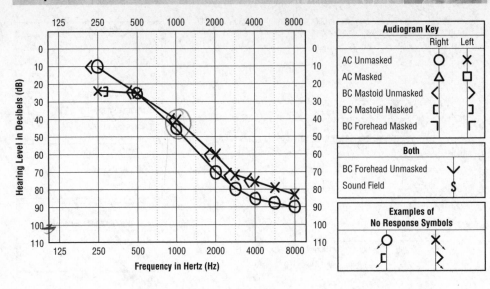

Speech Audiometry

Ear	SRT	SDT	PTA 5 - 1	Test	Word Recognition Level/Percent Correct	MCL	LDL
Right	30		35	NU6	+50/72%		
Left	30		33	NU6	+50/68%		
Bone							
Sound Field							
Right Aided							
Left Aided							
Binaural Aided							

REFERENCES

American Speech-Language-Hearing Association (ASHA). (1988, March). Guidelines for determining threshold level for speech. *ASHA,* 85–89.

American Speech-Language-Hearing Association. (2005). *Guidelines for manual pure tone threshold audiometry.* Rockville, MD: Author. Available from http://www.asha.org/members/deskref-journals/deskref/default

Beiter, A., & Brimacombe, J. (2000). Cochlear implants. In J. Alpiner and P. McCarthy, Eds.,

Rehabilitative audiology: Children and adults (3rd ed. pp. 473–500). Philadelphia: Lippincott Williams & Wilkins.

Chaiklin, J. B., & Ventry, I. M. (1964). Spondee threshold measurement: A comparison of 2- and 5-dB methods. *Journal of Speech and Hearing Disorders, 29,* 47–59.

Davis, H., & Silverman, S. (1970). *Hearing and deafness.* New York: Holt, Rinehart & Winston.

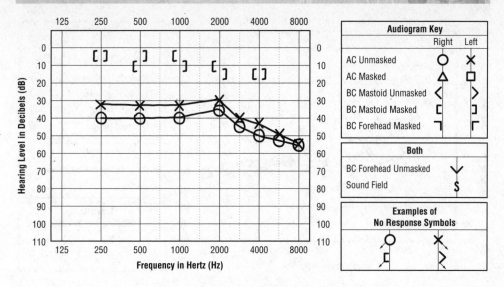

Speech Audiometry

Ear	SRT	SDT	PTA 5 - 2	Test	Word Recognition Level/Percent Correct	MCL	LDL
Right	40		42	NU6	+30/92%		
Left	30		35	NU6	+35/96%		
Bone							
Sound Field							
Right Aided							
Left Aided							
Binaural Aided							

Elliott, L. L., & Katz, D. R. (1980). *Northwestern University Children's Perception of Speech test (NU-CHIPS)*. St. Louis, MO: Auditec.

Hall, J., & Mueller, H. (1997). *Audiologist's desk reference: Volume 1: Diagnostic audiology principles, procedures, and practices*. San Diego: Singular.

Hurley, R., & Sells, J. (2003). An abbreviated word recognition protocol based on item difficulty. *Ear & Hearing, 24*(2), 111–118.

Kalikow, D. N., Stevens, K. N., & Eliott, L. L. (1977). Development of a test of speech intelligibility in noise using sentence materials with controlled predictability. *Journal of the Acoustical Society of America, 61*, 1337–1351.

Ling, D. (1976). *Speech and the hearing impaired child: Theory and practice*. Washington, DC: Alexander Graham Bell Association for the Deaf.

Ling, D. (1989). *Foundations of spoken language for hearing impaired children*. Washington, DC: Alexander Graham Bell Association for the Deaf.

Martin, F. (1997). *Introduction to audiology* (6th ed.). Boston: Allyn & Bacon.

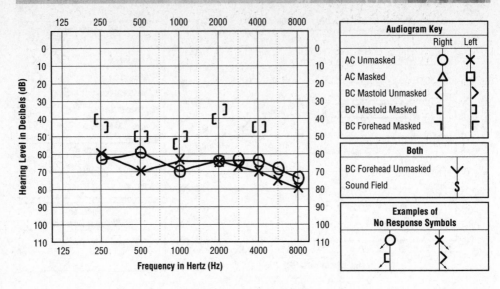

Speech Audiometry

Ear	SRT	SDT	PTA 5-2	Test	Word Recognition Level/Percent Correct	MCL	LDL
Right	65		65	NU6	+25/56%		
Left	65		67	NU6	+25/52%		
Bone							
Sound Field							
Right Aided							
Left Aided							
Binaural Aided							

Martin, F., Champlin, C., & Chambers, J. (1998). Seventh survey of audiometric practices in the United States. *Journal of the American Academy of Audiology, 9,* 95–104.

Martin, F., & Clark, J. G. (2006). *Introduction to audiology* (9th ed.). Boston: Allyn & Bacon.

Nilsson, M., Soli, S., & Sullivan, J. (1994). Development of the Hearing in Noise Test for the measurement of speech reception thresholds in quiet and in noise. *Journal of the Acoustical Society of America, 95,* 1085–1099.

Owens, E., Kessler, D. K., Raggio, M. W., & Schubert, E. D. (1985). Analysis and revision of the Minimal Auditory Capabilities (MAC) battery. *Ear and Hearing, 6,* 280–290.

Owens, E., & Schubert, E. D. (1977). Development of the California Consonant Test. *Journal of Speech and Hearing Research, 20,* 463–474.

Ross, M., & Lerman, J. (1970). A picture identification test for hearing-impaired children. *Journal of Speech and Hearing Research, 13,* 44–53.

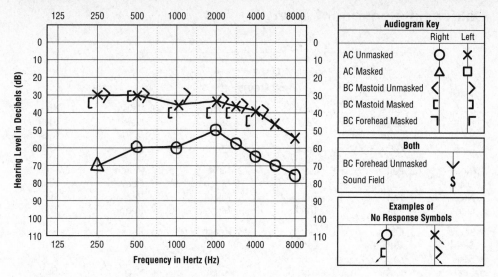

Speech Audiometry

Ear	SRT	SDT	PTA 5-2	Test	Word Recognition Level/Percent Correct	MCL	LDL
Right	50		57	NU6	+25/88%		
Left	30		33	NU6	+30/92%		
Bone							
Sound Field							
Right Aided							
Left Aided							
Binaural Aided							

Runge, C., & Hosford-Dunn, H. (1985). Word recognition performance with modified CID W-22 word lists. *Journal of Speech and Hearing Research, 28,* 355–362.

Speaks, C., & Jerger, J. (1965). Method for measurement of speech identification. *Journal of Speech and Hearing Research, 8,* 185–194.

Thornton, A., & Raffin, M. (1978). Speech-discrimination scores modeled as a binomial variable. *Journal of Speech and Hearing Research, 21,* 507–518.

Utley, J. (1946). A test of lipreading ability. *Journal of Speech and Hearing Disorders, 11,* 109–116.

Yacullo, W. (1996). *Clinical masking procedures.* Boston: Allyn & Bacon.

Appendix A
California Consonant Test

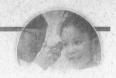

Name _____   Date _____

List 1
Test Items

1. Back	1. Gave	11. Page	21. Shin	31. Vale	41. Kit
Bag	Game	Paid	Sin	Dale	Kick
Batch	Gaze	Pays	Thin	Jail	Kiss
Bath	Gage	Pave	Chin	Bale	Kid
2. Rice	2. Pail	12. Kick	22. Muff	32. Peach	42. Pin
Dice	Sail	Pick	Much	Peat	Kin
Nice	Fail	Tick	Mush	Peak	Tin
Lice	Tail	Thick	Muss	Peep	Thin
3. Seen	3. Cuff	13. Laugh	23. Reach	33. Rack	43. Bus
Seed	Cup	Lash	Reap	Rash	But
Seal	Cuss	Lass	Reef	Rat	Buck
Seat	Cut	Lap	Reek	Rap	Buff
4. Bail	4. Muss	14. Sheep	24. Back	34. Hag	44. Gate
Tale	Much	Seep	Bat	Had	Bait
Sail	Mush	Cheap	Batch	Have	Date
Dale	Muff	Heap	Bath	Has	Wait
5. Leave	5. Fake	15. Gave	25. Tame	35. Tick	45. Laugh
Leash	Fate	Game	Shame	Sick	Lass
Lean	Face	Gage	Fame	Thick	Lash
League	Faith	Gaze	Same	Pick	Lap
6. Rail	6. Till	16. Beach	26. Core	36. Chair	46. Hip
Jail	Chill	Beep	Pore	Care	Hit
Tail	Pill	Beak	Tore	Share	Hiss
Bale	Kill	Beet	Sore	Fair	Hitch
	7. Lease	17. Mass	27. Rage	37. Beach	47. Hick
	Leash	Map	Raise	Beak	Sick
	Leaf	Mat	Rave	Beet	Thick
	Leap	Math	Raid	Beep	Chick
	8. Seep	18. Path	28. Fill	38. Beak	48. Leaf
	Cheap	Patch	Pill	Beep	Lease
	Sheep	Pack	Kill	Beat	Leash
	Heap	Pat	Till	Beef	Leak
	9. Face	19. Gaze	29. Chop	39. Cheek	49. Cheek
	Faith	Gage	Pop	Chief	Cheap
	Fate	Gave	Top	Cheat	Cheat
	Fake	Game	Shop	Cheap	Chief
	10. Bays	20. Sick	30. Muck	40. Cup	50. Rid
	Babe	Chick	Mutt	Cut	Rib
	Bale	Thick	Muss	Cuss	Ridge
	Bathe	Tick	Muff	Cuff	Rig

Source: Used with permission from California Consonant Test, 2515 S. Big Bend, St. Louis, MO 63143.

Appendix B
Selected Tests of the MAC Battery

The following is a description of the 13 auditory tests and one lipreading test of the MAC as used in the present study, in their order of appearance on the battery.

I. **Question/Statement Test:** A 20-item test of prosody in which patients are required to determine if a phrase has a rising or falling inflection. Subjects are instructed to listen only for pitch and to state if a phrase is a "question" or a "statement." All phrases are constructed so that they may be spoken as either a question or a statement. In order to avoid the search for understanding, patients are provided with the printed phrases.

SAMPLE: They're not home? or They're not home.

II. **Vowel Test:** 15 vowels and dipthongs are represented in a four-alternative multiple-choice (closed-set) format. Each phoneme occurs 4 times in CVC context, resulting in a total of 60 items. The patient is instructed to read the four choices, listen as the stimulus word is spoken, and to both say and mark his selection.

SAMPLE: fool-full-fall-foul

III. **Spondee Recognition Test:** A 25-item open-response spondee test in which patients are required to listen and repeat the spoken word. One-half point credit is allowed if one syllable of the word is correctly repeated.

SAMPLE: doorbell (door/bell)

IV. **Noise/Voice Test:** This 40-item, two-choice test attempts to determine if the patient can discriminate between a voice and a noise. The test contains sentences spoken by 5 different voices, both male and female, and 4 different noise spectra in temporal-intensity envelopes derived from the same spoken sentences. The patient is instructed to listen and state whether the stimulus is a "voice" or a "noise."

V. **Accent Test:** A 20-item prosody test consisting of short phrases, each of which contains one accented or stressed word. The patient is required to indicate the stressed word. Since any one of four words in the phrase can reasonably be accented, this is viewed as a four-alternative closed response test. In order to avoid the search for meaning, the patient is provided with the printed phrases.

SAMPLE: Can you **fix** it? Can **you** fix it?

VI. **Everyday Sentences (CID):** Four lists (Nos. 1, 2, 6, 8) of the CID (CHABA) Everyday Sentences are combined, resulting in a test of 40 sentences with 200 key words. The patient is instructed to listen and to repeat as much of the sentence as possible. Scoring is based on the number of key words correct.

SAMPLE: **Do** you **want** an **egg** for **breakfast?**

VII. **Initial Consonant Test:** A 64-item, four-alternative multiple choice test, identical in format to the Vowel Test (II). Instructions to the patients are the same as for the Vowel Test.

SAMPLE: din-bin-fin-gin

VIII. **Spondee Same/Different Test:** A 20-item, two-choice test in which four spondee words are used in contrasting pairs. The patient is instructed to determine and state only whether the two words of a pair are the "same" or "different."

SAMPLE: mailman–playground   mailman–mailman

IX. **Words in Context Test:** This test consists of 50 sentences from the revised high context items of the Speech Perception in Noise (SPIN) Test (Bilger et al., 1979; Kalikow et al., 1977). The last word of a sentence is highly predictable from the words preceding it. The patient is instructed to listen to the whole sentence and to repeat only the final word. Scoring is based on the number of final words correctly repeated.

SAMPLE: The cow gave birth to a calf.

X. **Everyday Sounds Test:** 15 familiar sounds are presented in an open response format. Patients are asked to describe or identify the sounds they hear.

XI. **Monosyllabic Words (NU 6) Test:** The Northwestern University Auditory Test No. 6 (list 1B) was used for a test of one-syllable open response word recognition. Patients are asked to repeat the word they hear.

XII. **Four-Choice Spondee Test:** This test, consisting of 20 times, is a four-alternative choice closed response test, similar in format to the Vowel (II) and Initial Consonant (VII). The stimuli and foils were randomly selected from a pool of 48 spondees. The patient is required to listen to the word and make a selection from a set of four words.

SAMPLE: downtown-streetcar-pancake-doorstep

XIII. **Final Consonant Test:** Identical in format to the Vowel and Initial Consonant Tests, this is a 52-item test in a four-alternative closed-set format.

SAMPLE: rid-rip-rib-ridge

XIV. **Visual Enhancement:** The lipreading test materials consist of 40 CID Everyday Sentences. In order to determine whether amplified sound enhances lipreading ability, testing is done in both the aided and unaided conditions. Lists 9 and 10 are used for unaided lipreading, while lists 5 and 7 are used for aided lipreading. The subject is instructed to repeat as much as possible of each sentence. Scoring is based on the number of key words correct—50 key words per list, or 100 possible key words in each condition. Sentences are presented live.

Source: Owens, E., Kessler, D., Raggio, M., & Schubert, E. (1985). Analysis and revision of the minimal auditory capabilities (MAC) battery. *Ear and Hearing (6),* 280–290. Reprinted by permission.

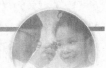

Appendix C
How to Mask during Speech Audiometry

Speech Recognition Threshold Testing

There are basically two options available to the audiologist in masking during SRT testing. Martin (1997) describes a method for determining whether cross-hearing may have occurred during testing to obtain SRTs. If masking is presented to the non-test ear at a level equal to the SRT in that ear and the SRT in the test ear remains the same, or shifts by only 5 dB (central masking), then the SRT in the test ear is true and no further masking is needed. If, however, the SRT in the test ear shifts more than 5 dB with the introduction of masking to the non-test ear, further testing with masking is needed to determine the true SRT in the test ear. In this case, the plateau method may be used, starting with an initial masking level. To use the plateau method, starting with an initial masking level, the following information applies:

- The starting point for masking can be derived using a formula. To find the minimum (initial) masking level for SRT or SDT testing, Yacullo (1996) provides the following formula:

$$M \min = PLt - IA + Max \, ABgapnt$$

where PL is the presentation level in the test ear, IA is interaural attenuation for air conduction (40 dB HL), and Max ABgapnt is the maximum air–bone gap in the non-test ear, considering frequencies from 250 to 4,000 Hz.

A second option during masking for the SRT is to calculate a mid-masking level for use during speech audiometry (Yacullo, 1996). If this alternative is chosen, the following information applies:

- A mid-masking level may be calculated to arrive at a masking level above the minimum and below the point of overmasking. The formula for calculating a mid-masking level is as follows:

$$M \min = \frac{M \max + M \min}{2}$$

The maximum masking level formula is

$$M \max = Best \, BCt^* + IA - 5 \, dB$$

*bone conduction thresholds in the frequency range from 250 to 4,000 Hz (Yacullo, 1996, p. 95).

To illustrate these two approaches, minimum (initial) and mid-masking levels will be derived for the following test in progress:

SRT (RE) = 20 dB HL

The largest air–bone gap, RE, considering 250–4,000 Hz, is 10 dB HL; the best BC threshold for the same frequency region is 10 dB HL.

SRT (LE) = 75 dB HL

The best bone in the test (L) ear is 30 dB HL.

First, is masking needed to determine the true LE SRT? Considering the formula for when to mask,

$$SRTte - IA \geq best \, BCnte$$

is $75 - 40 \geq 10$ dB HL?
Because 35 is greater than 10, masking is needed.

If you choose to use the plateau method and begin masking with an initial masking level, the calculation is as follows:

$$M \min = PLt - IA + Max \, ABgapnt$$

$$= 75 \, dB - 40 \, dB + 10 \, dB$$

$$= 45 \, dB \, HL$$

If you choose to arrive at a mid-masking level, you need to find the maximum masking level using this formula:

$$M\ max = Best\ BCt + IA - 5\ dB$$

$$= 30\ dB\ HL + 40 - 5\ dB$$

Since

$$M\ mid = \frac{M\ max + M\ min}{2}$$

then

$$M\ mid = \frac{75\ dB\ HL + 45\ dB\ HL}{2}$$

$$= 60\ dB\ HL$$

Either of these methods may be used for purposes of masking during speech audiometry. Since the goal of masking during assessment of the SRT is to use masking in the mid-range of the plateau, the calculation of a mid-masking level may be the most desirable and time-efficient method in most instances. According to Yacullo (1996), the advantage of the plateau method is that appropriate masking levels can be selected without having the bone conduction sensitivity of each ear available.

Word Recognition Testing

Martin's (2006) formula for masking during word recognition testing (p. 133) is

$$EM = PBHLte - IA + ABGnte$$

where PBHLte is the level at which monosyllable words are presented to the test ear, IA is the interaural attenuation for air conducted signals (40 dB HL), and ABGnte is the largest air–bone gap in the non-test ear.

Example

SRT in RE: 40 dB HL

SRT in LE: 20 dB HL

No air–bone gap in NTE

Is masking needed for word recognition testing of the RE if a presentation level of +30 dB SL (or 70 dB HL) is used?

Is PBHLte − IA ≥ best Bcnte?

Is 70 dB − 40 dB ≥ 20 dB?

Since 30 is greater than 20, you will need to use masking in the left ear during word recognition testing of the right ear.

Example

SRT in RE: 30 dB HL

SRT in LE: 50 dB HL

Best bone RE = 20 dB HL

Is masking needed for word recognition testing of the LE if a presentation level of +30 dB SL (or 80 dB HL) is used?

Is PBHLte − IA ≥ best BCnte?

Is 80 dB − 40 dB ≥ 20 dB?

Since 40 is greater than 20, you will need to use masking in the right ear during word recognition testing of the left ear.

Example

SRT in RE: 30 dB HL

SRT in LE: 30 dB HL

No air–bone gaps, either ear

Is masking needed for word recognition testing of either ear if a presentation level of +35 dB HL is used?

Is PBHLte − IA ≥ best BCnte?

Is 65 dB HL − 40 dB HL ≥ 30?

Since 25 is less than 30, masking is not needed during word recognition testing for either ear in this case. If increased sensation levels are used, however, the need for masking will have to be reevaluated.

Although typically presented via air conduction (through the earphones), speech stimuli can also be presented via bone conduction (through the bone vibrator). Since speech is a more salient stimulus than pure tones, it may be useful to use speech as the stimulus to establish whether an air–bone gap is present, particularly for pediatric or difficult-to-test clients. If speech stimuli are presented via bone conduction, the same masking rules apply as if pure tone stimuli were used.

As discussed in Chapter 4, if the bone conduction results are better than the air conduction results at any point during testing, masking will be needed. If air-conducted SRTs or SDTs are obtained and an unmasked SRT or SDT is established, revealing an air–bone gap, masking is required to determine the air–bone relationship for each ear. To reiterate the formula for masking during bone conduction testing,

ABG > 10 dB in the TE

Or, whenever you obtain an air–bone gap (ABG) greater than 10 dB in the test ear (TE), masking is needed in the non-test ear during bone conduction testing. Said differently, when you are attempting to obtain a bone conduction score in the poorer ear (TE), you need to deliver masking noise to the better ear (NTE) to raise the threshold in the NTE.

If it becomes necessary to determine the type (nature) of the hearing loss using speech stimuli, masking may be needed, as the following example shows.

Example

SDT (RE, AC) = 40

SDT (LE, AC) = 45

Unmasked SDT (BC) = 10

From our limited air conduction results and unmasked bone conduction result, we know that a moderate hearing loss is present in each ear and that, in at least one ear, a significant conductive component exists. Since the potential for an air–bone gap greater than 10 dB exists, masking must be used to determine the nature of the hearing loss for each ear.

If you use Martin and Clark's (2006) formula for initial masking for bone conduction,

A/Cnte + OE* + 10 dB safety factor

*N/A for conductive hearing loss

then intial masking for B/C testing of the left ear is calculated as follows:

IM = 40 + 10 dB = 50 dB HL

Initial masking of 50 dB HL should be introduced to the right ear and the bone-conducted SDT or SRT reestablished for the left ear using the plateau method. This process should be repeated to establish a bone-conducted SDT or SRT for the right ear.

chapter 6

Physiological Assessment of the Auditory System

AFTER COMPLETING THIS CHAPTER, YOU SHOULD BE ABLE TO:

1. Define *immittance testing.*
2. Describe the relevant features of tympanograms commonly encountered in audiology practice. For each tympanometric configuration (shape), describe an associated middle ear condition.
3. Define *acoustic reflex threshold* and describe guidelines for determining when the reflexes should be present or absent.
4. Define *otoacoustic emissions* and describe two types of them.
5. Explain the contributions of otoacoustic emission testing to the practice of audiology.
6. Define *auditory evoked potentials.*
7. Compare and contrast the use of brainstem auditory evoked potentials for site-of-lesion testing and for estimation of hearing thresholds.
8. Describe other auditory evoked potentials, including electrocochleography, middle potentials, and late potentials, in terms of their relative latencies and the information they provide about the auditory system.
9. Describe the clinical value of stacked ABR.

In the previous chapters on pure tone and speech audiometry you learned about a series of tests that are used in assessing the hearing of clients. These tests are referred to as behavioral tests because they require a response on the part of the client. In other words, we gain information regarding a client's hearing by examining some aspect of his or her behavior in response to sound. For example, when a client raises her hand in response to a tone, this behavior signals the examiner that the stimulus has been heard. Similarly, when a person correctly repeats a word presented through earphones, this behavioral response informs an audiologist about the client's ability to understand speech.

The 1960s saw a proliferation of various behavioral **site-of-lesion tests,** designed to assist in pinpointing the anatomic site of dysfunction in the auditory system. Examples of these tests include: (1) Alternate Binaural Loudness Balance (ABLB); (2) Short Increment Sensitivity Index (SISI); (3) Bekesy; (4) Tone Decay; and (5) Brief Tone Audiometry.

During the 1970s, the **immittance battery** became an integral part of clinical audiological work. Because it is an objective measure of middle ear function, immittance testing adds considerably to an audiologist's ability to identify the specific site(s) of dysfunction in the auditory system during routine evaluations. In the 1980s, audiologists' ability to discern the site of lesion in the auditory system advanced with the increasing use of **brainstem auditory evoked response testing,** an objective measure that provides insight about higher-frequency hearing (1,000–4,000 Hz). **Otoacoustic emissions (OAEs),** discovered by David Kemp (1978), became the test of the 1990s. Applications of OAEs include enhancing our understanding of the biomechanics of the inner ear, assessment of cochlear pathology, and the early identification of hearing loss through infant hearing screening.

Although behavioral responses are very useful to the audiologist, for a variety of reasons, it is not always practical to use them in hearing assessment. Consider the newborn whose hearing will be screened prior to leaving the hospital. Although at this age some behavioral responses to sound can be observed, subjective interpretation of these responses is difficult. Consider the individual diagnosed with severe developmental disabilities who is brought to the clinic for a hearing evaluation. This individual may also not be able to provide reliable behavioral responses. In cases such as these, an audiologist should include more objective measures in the audiological assessment battery. The tests we have selected for this chapter are relatively more objective than their behavioral predecessors (such as the SISI and the Tone Decay test) and have greater sensitivity and specificity in identifying the site of lesion within the auditory system. Therefore, physiological (objective) measures, which rely on recorded changes in the body's response to sound, are the primary subject of this chapter. The objective measures covered include immittance testing, electrocochleography, auditory evoked potentials, and otoacoustic emissions.

Physiological assessment measures are also valuable because they can add information about aspects of the client's auditory system that behavioral measures cannot provide. For example, in the next section of this chapter you will learn about immittance testing, which assesses the functioning of the middle ear. Immittance testing has been shown to be much more sensitive to middle ear disorders than any of the behavioral tests (e.g., pure tones and speech audiometry) that audiologists use. You will also learn about auditory evoked potential testing, which can assist in ruling out **retrocochlear** (beyond the cochlea, i.e., at the auditory nerve or brainstem) **pathology** in ways that the conventional audiometric test battery cannot.

Acoustic Admittance Testing

Acoustic immittance is a term that can be used to refer to acoustic **impedance,** acoustic **admittance,** or both. Think for a moment about your understanding of the words *impedance* and *admittance.* If something is *impeded,* it is blocked, or opposition to it is great. Conversely, if we *admit* something, we allow it to pass through. These terms are reciprocal; if one is high, the other is low. It follows then that if we know the value of one of these components, we can easily determine the other.

Now think about these terms with respect to energy in the middle ear. If impedance in the middle ear is excessively high (and admittance is low), energy is opposed, as might be the case when a child has fluid in the middle ear. Audiologists are obviously concerned about the middle ear's status because reduced admittance of sound energy as it flows into the middle ear system can result in hearing loss.

Because immittance devices used clinically today measure admittance rather than impedance, in this chapter we will use the term *acoustic admittance* when referring to the middle ear test battery. The unit of measure for admittance is the **millimho (mmho).**

It is important to note that acoustic admittance consists of two primary acoustic components: acoustic susceptance and acoustic conductance. Because various structures in the middle ear (e.g., ligaments, muscles, bones) have susceptance and conductance characteristics, pathology of the middle ear alters these components and therefore alters the resulting data.

Information in this chapter regarding test administration will have most relevance to the audiologist because use of acoustic admittance testing for diagnostic purposes is part of the scope of practice of the audiologist. Test interpretation, however, is relevant to the audiologist, the speech–language pathologist, and related professionals. Chapter 11 addresses the use of tympanometry for screening purposes, which is included in the scope of practice for both audiologists and speech–language pathologists. Tympanometry has an important role, for example, in conducting screenings of preschoolers because of the frequency of middle ear pathology in this age group.

The acoustic admittance battery consists basically of tympanometry and acoustic stapedius reflex thresholds. After briefly reviewing the equipment used, we will describe each of these tests and provide case examples.

Equipment for Acoustic Admittance Testing

Note in Figure 6.1 that the probe assembly of the immittance equipment, which is positioned in the ear canal of the client during testing via a probe tip, involves the following:

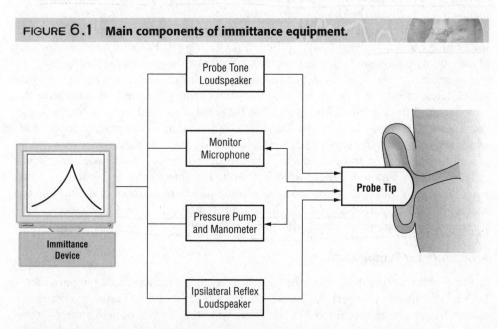

FIGURE 6.1   **Main components of immittance equipment.**

Source: Bess, F. H., & Humes, L. E. (1995). *Audiology: The fundamentals* (2nd ed.). Baltimore: Lippincott, Williams & Wilkins. Reprinted by permission.

- A transducer to produce the probe tone
- An air pump and manometer to vary the air pressure in the ear canal
- A microphone to measure the sound that is reflected from the eardrum

Keep these instrument features in mind as we discuss the first of the two tests in the admittance battery, which is tympanometry.

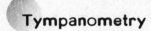

Tympanometry

Tympanometry is the measurement of acoustic admittance of the middle ear as a function of variations of air pressure in the external auditory canal. Variations in pressure, which are delivered automatically by the test equipment, include: (a) delivering positive pressure into the ear canal so that pressure in the canal is greater than atmospheric pressure, or (b) pumping air out of the ear canal so that pressure in the canal is less than atmospheric pressure (referred to as *negative pressure*).

One purpose of tympanometry is to determine the point (measured in pressure in daPa) at which the pressure in the ear canal is equal to the middle ear pressure. In order to understand the significance of this measure, it is important to understand that the acoustic admittance of the middle ear system is maximized when the ear canal pressure is equal to the middle ear pressure.

Remember that pressure on the outside of the eardrum is the result of atmospheric pressure, which is directed against our bodies at all times. Pressure also exists in the middle ear space. In a normal condition, the outside pressure (i.e., atmospheric pressure) and the middle ear pressure are the same because the Eustachian tube opens and closes regularly throughout the day to keep them equal. When the Eustachian tube is not working properly, a difference in pressures develops, often with less pressure noted in the middle ear space. By identifying the point (in pressure) at which the admittance of the middle ear system is maximized, we can estimate the middle ear pressure.

Specifically, how does the acoustic admittance device detect low or high admittance? These measurements are made by assessing changes in sound pressure being directed toward the eardrum. The probe that is placed in the entrance of the ear canal delivers a tone toward the eardrum. This is referred to as the **probe tone.** As this sound, which typically has a frequency of 226 Hz, is directed to the ear canal, some of it will be passed through to the middle ear space and some will be reflected back into the ear canal. Think for a moment about what factor might influence the degree to which this sound energy is reflected. If you said the admittance characteristics of the middle ear space, you are correct. Specifically, reduced admittance will result in considerable reflection of sound energy; normal admittance will result in little reflected energy.

Procedure for Tympanometry

It is important to note that, whenever feasible, otoscopy should precede tympanometry because it is unsafe to insert the probe (or any other instrument) into the client's ear canal without first examining the canal. There will be times when, in the tester's judgment, beginning with the otoscopic exam could compromise the ability to collect any audiological information. An example of this might be a young child who is overtly fearful of the test situation or a child with a diagnosed condition such as a pervasive developmental disorder. In these cases, the more effective course is to collect as much audiological data as possible prior to introducing the otoscope. If an audiologist observed any sign of infection, drainage, blood, or foreign object, a decision may be made to defer tympanometry until medical guidance is sought.

The first step in obtaining a reliable tympanogram is getting an airtight seal. This refers to sealing off the ear canal with the probe tip, which is necessary in order to build up pressure toward the eardrum. In some cases, the plastic probe tips are color-coded or numbered based on size to assist audiologists in choosing one that will seal off the canal efficiently. Often, choosing a probe tip that is slightly larger than the outside diameter of the ear canal is an effective strategy. Also, pulling up and back on the pinna when the probe is being inserted opens up the canal, which can be helpful. As the probe tip is being put into the ear canal, a twisting motion is often helpful to seat the probe tip tightly into the canal.

In the event that an audiologist is unable to obtain an adequate seal, it is important to ask clients if they have a **perforated eardrum** (an eardrum that has a hole or opening in it) or **pressure equalization (PE) tubes.** In some acoustic admittance devices, no seal will be obtained in these clients. Also, audiologists should remember to check for any equipment malfunction that could account for the difficulty in obtaining a seal. An easy way to verify that the problem involves the equipment is to place your finger over the probe tip and attempt to build up pressure. If this is not possible, an equipment problem exists. Some of these problems can be avoided by conducting equipment checks at the beginning of each day, using the cavities supplied by the manufacturer, or by performing a self-tympanogram to ensure proper equipment functioning.

Figure 6.2 illustrates a graph for recording a tympanogram. Note that ear canal pressure (in daPa) is displayed on the *x* axis and admittance (in mmhos) is on the *y* axis. When tympanometry was first becoming common in clinical work, the devices used did not automatically change the air pressure and record the resulting graph, as is routine today. Instead, these earlier acoustic admittance devices required that the audiologist change the air pressure manually and record the resulting admittance values at multiple pressure points. Today's devices are far more convenient than the devices of the past but because they perform the steps so automatically, some students do not develop an understanding of the principles behind the procedure.

With this in mind, let's go through the various steps typically involved in obtaining a tympanogram on an individual with normal middle ear function.

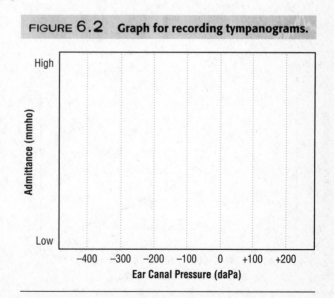

FIGURE 6.2   **Graph for recording tympanograms.**

FIGURE 6.3 Graph of normal middle ear pressure and admittance.

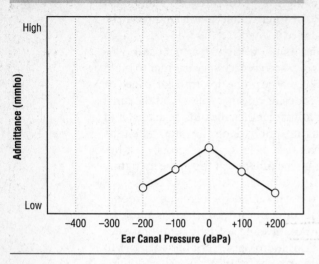

A normal tympanogram is illustrated in Figure 6.3.

First, +200 daPa of pressure is introduced into the ear canal. Because this client has normal middle ear function, this amount of pressure will decrease the acoustic admittance of the middle ear system. In fact, at +200 daPa, the eardrum becomes so tense that middle ear admittance is likely not being measured; only outer ear admittance is. Note the location of the circle at +200 daPa, indicating very low acoustic admittance at this pressure point. Pressure is now decreased slightly from +200 daPa to +100 daPa. What effect will this have on the acoustic admittance of the middle ear system? If you said that the acoustic admittance will improve somewhat, you are correct. Note the circle at the +100 pressure point indicating this change. The middle ear system is less tense than it was at the +200 daPa point so assessment of the middle ear admittance is now in process. When the audiologist introduces 0 daPa into the ear canal this client is likely to exhibit the best acoustic admittance because this means that the atmospheric pressure and the middle ear pressure are equal and that the Eustachian tube is working efficiently. Note on the tympanogram this improvement in acoustic admittance and that 0 daPa is the point at which acoustic admittance is maximized. This is also an estimate of the middle ear pressure, commonly referred to as the **tympanometric peak pressure.** Note also that just as was the case with positive pressure, when negative pressure (e.g., −100 daPa, −200 daPa) is introduced into the ear canal of a client who has a normal middle ear system, acoustic admittance will again decrease.

FIGURE 6.4 Graph of negative middle ear pressure.

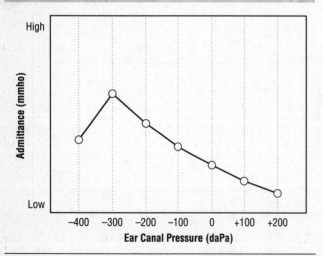

Remember from our earlier discussion that one of the purposes of tympanometry is to estimate the middle ear pressure, which provides information regarding Eustachian tube function. What can be determined about the middle ear pressure of the client whose tympanogram is illustrated in Figure 6.4? Note that the tympanometric peak pressure is at −300 daPa. If maximum acoustic admittance occurs when pressure on each side of the eardrum is equal and maximum acoustic admittance has occurred when −300 daPa is directed toward the eardrum, there must be a similar

174

amount of pressure in the middle ear space. This is referred to as *negative middle ear pressure* and suggests that this client's Eustachian tube is not working as efficiently as it should.

Although tympanometric peak pressure is routinely obtained, its clinical value is limited. This is due in part to the fact that it can be affected by a number of variables, including coughing, sneezing, and the specific manner by which the admittance equipment changes the ear canal pressure. As will be noted in the chapter on screening, tympanometric peak pressure is not included in ASHA's screening criteria.

Peak Compensated Static Acoustic Admittance

In order to understand peak compensated static acoustic admittance, it is first necessary to briefly address the difference between measurement plane tympanograms and compensated measures.

When **measurement plane tympanometry** is being performed, the measures are obtained at the probe tip. Because of this, the resulting admittance values include the acoustic admittance of both the volume of air between the probe tip and the eardrum, as well as the admittance of the middle ear system. Because clinically we may not be interested in the acoustic admittance of the volume of air between the probe tip and the eardrum, it is possible to remove the ear canal contributions (by subtracting them out). This is done automatically by some acoustic admittance devices. When this takes place, the resulting measures are an estimate of the acoustic admittance at the lateral surface of the eardrum and are referred to as **compensated measures. Peak compensated static acoustic admittance,** then, describes the amplitude (height) of the tympanogram measured at the plane of the tympanic membrane.

Interpretation of static admittance involves use of norms that are summarized in Table 6.1 from various research studies. Most authorities believe that low static admittance values support disorders of the middle ear involving increased stiffness (e.g., otosclerosis) and that values which are too high support disorders involving too little stiffness (e.g., a hypercompliant eardrum or ossicular discontinuity). However, authorities also note that these values should be interpreted with caution because static admittance values obtained for individuals with and without middle ear pathology often overlap. For this reason, audiologists should rely on the full acoustic admittance test battery when interpreting results of middle ear analysis. In fact, the results of acoustic admittance testing should be combined with audiometric findings, case history, and other medical/diagnostic information so that a complete picture of the client's status is obtained. The ability to incorporate multiple pieces of data in case interpretation is an important skill for the student of audiology to develop. Also, greater use of higher frequency probe tones would add to the sensitivity of the admittance battery for various middle ear pathologies. This is discussed in more detail later in the chapter.

Initial Interpretation of Tympanometry Using Peak Pressure and Static Acoustic Admittance

At this point we are ready to apply some basic interpretation skills to the information that has been covered. As noted in the beginning of this chapter, understanding how to interpret tympanograms is important not only for audiologists but also for speech–language pathologists and other professionals who receive audiological reports and use this information to make decisions about individuals who are in their care. One of the most useful

TABLE 6.1 **Sample Norms for Interpretation of Acoustic Admittance Data**

Parameter	Normal Values	Interpretation of Abnormal Values
Tympanometric peak pressure	−100 to +50 daPa	Negative pressures greater than −100 are generally associated with Eustachian tube dysfunction; positive pressures greater than +50 may be due to crying or nose blowing.
Equivalent ear canal volume	0.3 to 0.9 cc (young children) 0.6 to 1.5 cc (older children) 0.6 to 2.0 cc (adults)	Small values may be due to wax or a probe that is against the canal wall; large values support a perforation or open PE tube.
Peak compensated static acoustic admittance	*Range of Values* 0.25 to 0.92 mmho (infants) 0.25 to 1.5 mmho (children) 0.3 to 1.7 mmho (adults)	Low values may support too much stiffness; high values, too little stiffness.
Gradient	greater than 0.3	Small values are associated with middle ear fluid; other measures of middle ear function are more sensitive and specific.
Tympanometric width	275 daPa or less	Large values (i.e., wider tympanograms) are associated with middle ear fluid.
Acoustic reflexes	70 to 100 dB HL	Influenced by middle ear status, hearing sensitivity, and neurological integrity.

Note: Normal values provided are general guidelines. Specific values can vary based on differences in the method of measurement, the particular equipment used, and clients tested.

Source: Based on Margolis and Hunter (2000), Nozza et al. (1994), and Silman et al. (1992).

methods of interpreting tympanograms is to describe their pressure and admittance characteristics. As we have discussed, pressure has to do with the location of the peak of the tympanogram; acoustic admittance is related to the height of the peak above the baseline.

Pressure and Acoustic Admittance Characteristics

Audiologists who routinely interpret tympanograms based on a description of the pressure and static acoustic admittance characteristics may do so based on published norms or based on visual observation. Of the two approaches, the normative-based approach is more reliable because decisions are made about pressure and acoustic admittance based on research data.

To facilitate data interpretation and client counseling, some manufacturers of acoustic admittance devices include a box or shaded area on the tympanogram form that illustrates the normative range of values. As noted in Figure 6.5, this particular manufacturer has defined normal middle ear pressure as ranging from +100 to −100 daPa and normal static acoustic admittance values as ranging from 0.3 to 1.5 mmho.

Tympanometric Types

Another method of interpreting tympanograms that have been obtained using a 226-Hz probe tone uses tympanometric types. Developed by Jerger (1970), some audiologists simply refer to tympanograms by their type, rather than providing a verbal description of the pressure and acoustic admittance characteristics. Table 6.2 summarizes the various tympanometric types. Although this method of interpretation is both quick and popular, its disadvantage is that it is only helpful to those who are knowledgeable about this classification system. The speech–language pathologist or school nurse who must review an audiological report will likely make better use of that report if specific descriptions of pressure and acoustic admittance are included.

It is important to emphasize that Jerger's classification system is based on tympanograms measured with a 226-Hz probe tone and that additional patterns may be noted when higher frequency tones are used. For example, Linden and colleagues in the 1970s used an 800-Hz probe tone and noted additional tympanometric shapes. These included a **notched tympanogram** pattern and a pattern of wavelike peaks. Why did this higher frequency tone reveal patterns not identified by the 226-Hz tone? The 226-Hz probe tone is sensitive to stiffness-related conditions (e.g., middle ear effusion) and the higher-frequency probe tone is more sensitive to mass-related conditions such as those that would affect the eardrum or ossicles. Research suggests that clear relationships exist between the acoustic admittance of the middle ear system and changes in probe tone frequency. Even though these relationships could provide valuable diagnostic information, the use of single frequency 226-Hz tympanometry remains the most popular method of tympanometry. It is interesting to note that for infant acoustic admittance testing, research

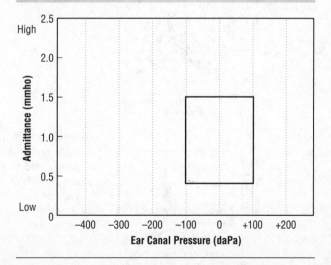

FIGURE 6.5 **Box denoting norms for specific admittance device.**

TABLE 6.2 Tympanometric Types and Descriptions

Type	Description
Type A 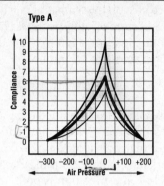	Normal middle pressure and admittance, consistent with normal middle ear function. Normative data: Pressure +50 to −100 daPa Admittance: range of 0.3 to 1.7
Type As 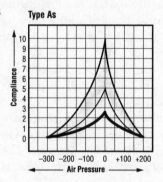	Normal middle ear pressure with reduced admittance, associated with a stiffness-dominated middle ear system, as may occur with tympanosclerosis or otosclerosis.
Type Ad 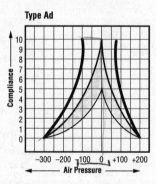	Normal middle ear pressure with markedly increased admittance, associated with a flaccid or hypermobile middle ear system, as may occur with ossicular discontinuity.
Type B 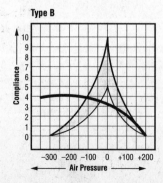	No identifiable point of maximum admittance, consistent with extreme stiffness of the outer and/or middle ear systems, as may occur with otitis media or other middle ear effusion, or impacted cerumen (wax).

TABLE 6.2 *(continued)*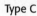

Type	Description
Type C 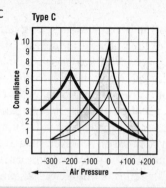	Abnormally negative ear pressure with normal or near normal admittance, as may occur with Eustachian tube dysfunction with or without middle ear fluid present.

Source: Based on Jerger, J. (1970). Clinical experience with impedance audiometry. *Archives of Otolaryngology, 92,* 311–324. Adapted from Northern, J., & Downs, M. (2002). *Hearing in children* (5th ed.). New York: Lippincott, Williams & Wilkins. Used by permission.

studies are inconclusive as to whether a 226-Hz probe tone or a higher-frequency probe tone is optimal.

Additional Important Tympanometric Measures

Equivalent Ear Canal Volume

In addition to pressure and acoustic admittance, equivalent ear canal volume is an important consideration in tympanometric interpretation. It was noted earlier that when the audiologist directs +200 daPa pressure toward the eardrum, the drum becomes so tense that the admittance of the middle ear is essentially not being measured. This allows measurement of the outer ear admittance alone. In addition, if the eardrum is intact, the audiologist can obtain an acoustic admittance estimate of the volume between the probe tip and the eardrum. This measure is referred to as **equivalent** (because it is not a direct measure) **ear canal volume** and should fall within some normative range of values.

A review of the various norms cited in the research literature (see additional readings at the end of this chapter) suggests that normal equivalent ear canal volume measurements are smaller in children than adults and are smaller in females than males. In children up to about 6 years of age, a reading of 1.0 cubic centimeters (cc or cm^3) typically constitutes a large equivalent volume. Wiley and colleagues (1996) report an average value for adult females of 1.28 cc and an average value for adult males of 1.5 cc.

In a client who has an opening in the eardrum, such as would be created by an eardrum **perforation** or a patent (open) pressure equalization (PE) tube, the equivalent ear canal volume becomes an estimate of the acoustic admittance of the volume of the ear canal and the middle ear space. This resulting volume measure will be greater than that found in the average person. When there is some doubt as to how to interpret a borderline equivalent ear canal volume reading, a comparison between ears can be useful. Unless a client had ear surgery on one ear (which can increase the volume), a large difference in the equivalent ear canal volume measures between ears in the same client would not be expected.

You may have noted that although equivalent ear canal volume measures are based on assessment of acoustic admittance (measured in mmho), the units of measure for equivalent ear canal volume values are cubic centimeters. This is based on information from Shanks and Lilly (1981) who noted that when a 226-Hz probe tone is used, a 1-cc volume of air at sea level has an acoustic admittance of approximately 1 acoustic mmho.

Equivalent Volume and Flat Tympanograms

Flat tympanograms present a challenge in interpretation because a flat tracing can be obtained from sources that are unrelated to the status of the outer or middle ear. For example, if one of the openings in the probe assembly is clogged with wax or debris, or if a wire or tube from the probe assembly is disconnected, this can result in a flat tracing. Also, in cases in which the client's ear canals are very small or narrow, the ear canal wall can interfere with the application of pressure to the eardrum, resulting in a false flat tympanogram.

The presence of a perforated eardrum or a pressure equalization (PE) tube in the eardrum can also result in a flat tympanogram. In such cases, however, the flat tracing will be accompanied by a large volume reading. Rather than reflecting abnormally low admittance, flat tracings with large volumes typically reflect a middle ear system that is open. What do you suspect would happen to the equivalent ear canal volume reading if the probe were up against the canal wall or if the ear canal was occluded with significant cerumen (wax)? In such cases, the volume reading might be excessively small. Use of acoustic admittance to gain information regarding equivalent ear canal volume is sometimes referred to as the *physical volume test*.

What might occur in a client who has an eardrum perforation combined with excessive middle ear fluid? It is possible that the equivalent ear canal volume might be within the norms due to the inflamed nature of the middle ear tissues. This could also be the case if the client had both an eardrum perforation combined with a cholesteatoma.

Refer to Figure 6.6, Figure 6.7, and Figure 6.8 for illustrations of these concepts. For the purpose of this discussion, these are results obtained on adults. Figure 6.6 shows a

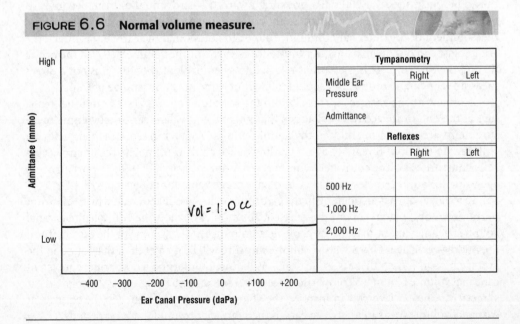

FIGURE 6.6   **Normal volume measure.**

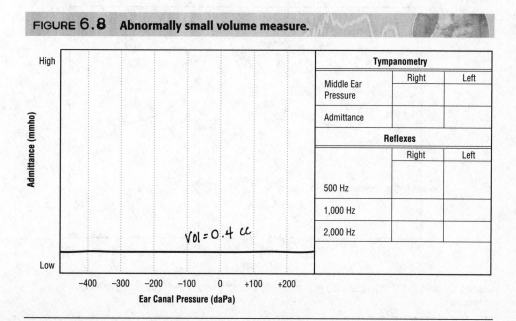

FIGURE **6.7** **Abnormally large volume measure.**

Tympanometry		
Middle Ear Pressure	Right	Left
Admittance		
Reflexes		
	Right	Left
500 Hz		
1,000 Hz		
2,000 Hz		

Vol = 4.6 cc

flat tracing. Because the volume reading is normal, this result is consistent with an intact tympanic membrane. This overall profile is consistent with middle ear dysfunction. Figure 6.7 also shows a flat tracing. In this case, however, the volume measure is abnormally large, consistent with an opening in the tympanic membrane. This overall profile is suggestive of either a perforated tympanic membrane or a patent (open) pressure

FIGURE **6.8** **Abnormally small volume measure.**

Tympanometry		
Middle Ear Pressure	Right	Left
Admittance		
Reflexes		
	Right	Left
500 Hz		
1,000 Hz		
2,000 Hz		

Vol = 0.4 cc

equalization tube. Figure 6.8 shows a flat tracing with an abnormally small volume measure. Possible causes of this finding include excess wax in the ear canal or placement of the probe against the ear canal wall.

Interpreting Tympanograms Using Pressure, Admittance, and Volume

Now let's interpret some tympanograms obtained from a Grason-Stadler acoustic admittance device. Using the norms provided in Table 6.1 and assuming that the clients are adults, refer to the following data and interpret:

Case 1: Pressure = −80 daPa; volume = 1.2 cc; admittance = 1.0 mmho

Case 2: Pressure = −220 daPa; volume = 1.6 cc; admittance = 0.2 mmho

Case 3: Pressure = −60 daPa; volume = 0.9 cc; admittance = 0.1 mmho

Case 4: Pressure = no peak (flat); volume = 5.0 cc

Refer to Appendix A of this chapter for answers.

Tympanometric Width and Gradient

Tympanometric width is a sensitive measure recommended by ASHA in their *Guidelines for Screening Infants and Children for Outer and Middle Ear Disorders, Birth Through 18 Years* (1997). **Tympanometric width** is defined as "the interval in daPa between the sides of the tympanogram at one half [admittance]" (Nozza et al., 1994, p. 312).

Gelfand (2001) also provides a useful example of the method for calculating tympanometric width. Figure 6.9 shows determination of static admittance, which is the

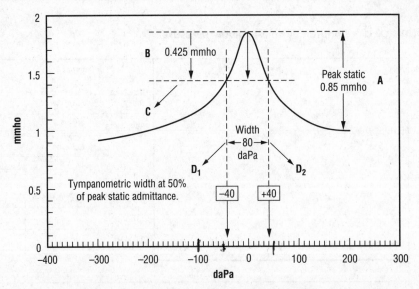

FIGURE 6.9   **Measurement of tympanometric width.**

Source: Gelfand, S. (2001). *Essentials of audiology* (2nd ed.). New York: Thieme. Adapted with permission.

first step in this calculation. In Figure 6.9, A depicts static admittance, which is the difference between the admittance value at +200 daPa and the admittance value at the point of maximum acoustic admittance, which in this case is 0 daPa. Half of the static admittance value is then used to measure down from the peak of the tympanogram. B represents this part of the measurement. Next, a horizontal line is drawn (C) to connect both sides of the tympanogram. Lines are drawn from the two intersection points to the x axis on the graph (lines labeled D1 and D2). Tympanometric width is the total distance, in daPa, between D1 and D2. In this case, the distance between D1 (− 40 daPa) and D2 (+40 daPa) is 80 daPa, a normal value.

As you might expect, the greater the resulting value (in daPa), the wider the tympanogram and the greater the likelihood that middle ear fluid is present. Research by Nozza and colleagues (1992, 1994) suggests that values greater than 200 daPa are consistent with the presence of middle ear fluid; this is the value that ASHA recommends be used in making a recommendation of a rescreening for children ages 1 year to school-age.

A related measure is **gradient.** This measure, which is related to the flatness of the tympanogram, often involves a ratio comparing the mean admittance values at two designated pressure points on the tympanogram with the overall admittance value. An excellent example of the method for calculating gradient is given by Gelfand (2001) and is included in Figure 6.10. Note first that A on the figure shows a horizontal line drawn at the point where the width of the tympanogram is 100 daPa (or mm H_2O depending on the equipment used). The height of the peak above this horizontal line is labeled B in the figure. The total height of the tympanogram is measured from the highest point to the lowest point and is labeled C. Gradient is calculated by dividing B (the height of

---

FIGURE 6.10 Measurement of tympanometric gradient.

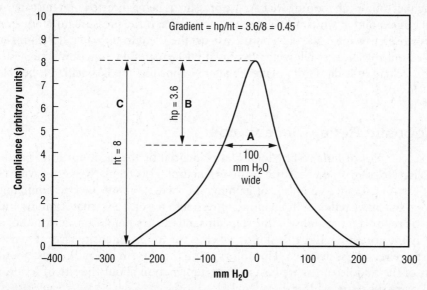

Source: Gelfand, S. (2001). *Essentials of audiology* (2nd ed.). New York: Thieme. Adapted with permission.

the peak) by C (the total height of the tympanogram). In this case, B divided by C (3.6 divided by 8) is 0.45, a normal value.

Gradient values typically range from 0 to 1 in intervals of 0.1. Although research by Nozza and colleagues (1992, 1994) suggests that gradient values that are small (i.e., 0.2 or less) are associated with the presence of middle ear fluid, other tympanometric measures have been found to be both more sensitive and more specific, making gradient measures of limited clinical value.

Eustachian Tube Testing

Although not routinely used by audiologists, specific tests of Eustachian tube function can be carried out with acoustic admittance equipment. The purpose of Eustachian tube testing is to assess the Eustachian tube's ability to equalize air pressure. These tests can be divided into those performed on clients whose eardrums are intact and those who have "open" systems (e.g., perforation, patent PE tube). Hall and Mueller (1997) provide procedures that can be used for intact and open middle ear systems.

On an intact middle ear system, first obtain a tympanogram and save it for future reference. Then, direct +400 daPa into the ear canal and instruct the client to swallow by sipping water. Perform a second tympanogram and note if the pressure peak is slightly negative compared to the initial tympanogram. A change in pressure supports good Eustachian tube function. Next, introduce −400 daPa into the ear canal and instruct the patient to swallow. Perform a third tympanogram and note if the pressure peak is slightly positive compared to the initial tympanogram. Once again, this finding supports good Eustachian tube function.

On an open system, in which the eardrum has either a perforation or a patent PE tube, attempts to build up pressure in the ear canal will often be unsuccessful if the Eustachian tube is functioning well. As the pressure is being directed into the canal, note the pressure point at which it releases back to 0 daPa. If the pressure does not spontaneously release by the +200 daPa point, instruct the client to sip water. If the pressure is released only by client swallowing, decreased Eustachian tube function is suggested. If the Eustachian tube does not open even after swallowing, the Eustachian tube is likely to be closed.

Acoustic Reflex Thresholds

Reflexes are part of human physiology, as evidenced by the flexion of the leg when a physician taps sharply on the knee. Similarly, neurologists regularly assess a wide range of reflexes in patients as a means of gaining information about the functioning of the nervous system. A **reflex** is an involuntary response to some external stimulus and the **acoustic reflex** is the response of the stapedius muscle to sound. Clinically, audiologists identify the **acoustic reflex threshold,** which is the lowest intensity level at which the acoustic reflex can be detected. This information can inform the audiologist about the status of the middle ear, as well as provide information about the site of lesion (i.e., cochlear versus retrocochlear disorder).

It is important to note the underlying mechanism by which the acoustic admittance device measures reflexes. Basically, when an acoustic reflex occurs, the acoustic admittance

FIGURE 6.11 **Depiction of ipsilateral acoustic reflex deflection.**

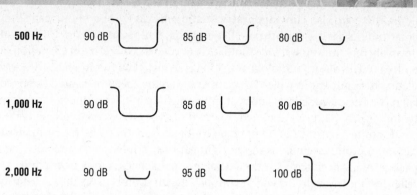

device detects a temporary increase in the impedance or decrease in the admittance of the middle ear. An acoustic reflex is detected by the admittance device as a decrease in the flow of energy through the middle ear.

Acoustic reflexes are typically noted by a decrease in admittance as illustrated in Figure 6.11. Most audiologists look for a certain minimum change in admittance in order to deem the response an acoustic reflex. For example, at 500 Hz at 80 dB some change is noted in response to the sound but it is so minimal that it is not likely to be accepted as a reflex. The change noted at 85 dB, however, is clear. Visual detection of the presence of acoustic reflexes can lead to errors and increased variability in test interpretation. Some admittance equipment uses computerized measurements with specific criteria for the amount of change needed to determine the presence of a reflex (e.g., 0.02 mmho for 226-Hz probe; 0.06 mmho for the 678-Hz probe). These objective measures decrease variability and add objectivity for improved test interpretation. Audiologists may provide results in hard copies or may report acoustic reflex data (hearing levels at which the reflexes occurred) on a form included with their written test summary.

Recording Acoustic Reflexes

Here you will learn how to record **ipsilateral** (probe and stimulus in same ear) **acoustic reflexes.** Using the data noted in Figure 6.11, you would record the following information:

Frequency	Ipsilateral Acoustic Reflex Thresholds
500 Hz	85 dB HL
1,000 Hz	85 dB HL
2,000 Hz	95 dB HL

Note that when recording acoustic reflex thresholds, the convention is to record data for the ear receiving the stimulus. When recording ipsilateral reflexes this is very straightforward because the probe assembly that measures both the response (reflex) and provides the stimulus is in the same (ipsilateral) ear. In addition to ipsilateral acoustic reflexes, there are also **contralateral acoustic reflexes** (probe in one ear, stimulus in the other ear). In fact, the acoustic reflex is a bilateral phenomenon. This means that in a normally functioning system, stimulation of one ear will result in elicitation of a reflex in both ears. This allows audiologists to obtain acoustic reflexes in one of two ways: by stimulating the same ear in which the tympanogram has been measured (referred to as ipsilateral or uncrossed reflexes) or by stimulating the ear that is opposite the ear in which the tympanogram has been obtained (referred to as contralateral or crossed reflexes).

Examine Figure 6.12 and note the configuration for acoustic admittance testing. Because the probe assembly is in the right ear of the client, we know that the right tympanogram has been tested. If the audiologist then chooses to perform ipsilateral acoustic reflex testing, the right ear will be stimulated with sound (using the same probe assembly that allowed assessment of tympanometry) to assess acoustic reflex thresholds. If the audiologist wants to obtain contralateral acoustic reflexes, stimulation of the left ear will be required. Note in the figure that the left ear is covered with an earphone for this purpose.

Recording contralateral acoustic reflexes is more complicated. Remember, the convention, based on the ANSI Standard (S3.39-1987), is to record the data for the stimulus ear. This means that if the probe is in the left ear and you stimulate the right ear, you are obtaining *right* contralateral reflexes. Conversely, if the probe is in the right ear and you stimulate the left ear, you are obtaining *left* contralateral reflexes. Figure 6.13 demonstrates this recording process.

General Procedure for Obtaining Acoustic Reflex Thresholds

Acoustic reflex thresholds are obtained using the same equipment that is used during tympanometry. In fact, the standard procedure for measuring acoustic reflex thresholds is to first obtain a tympanogram. Once this is completed, the equipment automatically returns to the tympanometric peak pressure, which is the point at which the acoustic admittance of the middle ear is maximized. The test frequency is selected (500, 1,000, and 2,000 Hz are commonly measured) and the starting intensity level is chosen. Because acoustic reflexes are typically noted at levels of 70 to 100 dB HL in the normal population, a starting level of 90 dB is reasonable. The audiologist then monitors the acoustic admittance device for an indication that the reflex has occurred in response to the sound. If a reflex is noted, intensity of the tone is decreased by 5 dB and the softer signal is presented. If there is no reflex, an increase in tone intensity is required. This process is continued at the frequencies noted until testing is completed.

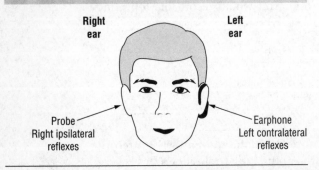

FIGURE 6.12 **Location of probe and earphone in assessing right ipsilateral/left contralateral acoustic reflexes.**

Right ear

Left ear

Probe
Right ipsilateral
reflexes

Earphone
Left contralateral
reflexes

Interpretation of Acoustic Reflex Thresholds

Interpretation of acoustic reflex thresholds is made easier when you understand the

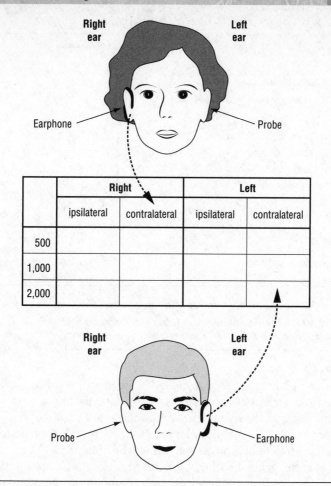

	Right		Left	
	ipsilateral	contralateral	ipsilateral	contralateral
500				
1,000				
2,000				

anatomy and physiology of the acoustic reflex, commonly referred to as the acoustic reflex arc. For a more detailed description of the acoustic reflex arc, refer to Chapter 3. Remember that the acoustic reflex arc has three components: a sensory component, a motor component, and a central pathway component.

In general, as illustrated in Figure 6.14, for ipsilateral reflexes, sound stimulation is directed through the ear canal to the middle ear, cochlea, eighth nerve, and lower brainstem structures, which comprise the sensory or *afferent* portion of the reflex arc. If the afferent portion of the reflex arc is intact, the ipsilateral acoustic reflexes will be present.

Impulses then travel to cranial nerve (cn) VIII and then to two parts of the brainstem, referred to as the ventral cochlear nucleus and the superior olivary complex. From here, impulses travel to the motor nucleus of the facial nerve and then to the facial nerve itself (cranial nerve VII). Finally, impulses stimulate the stapedius muscle, which contracts.

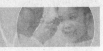

FIGURE **6.14** **Diagram of ipsilateral and contralateral acoustic reflex pathways.**

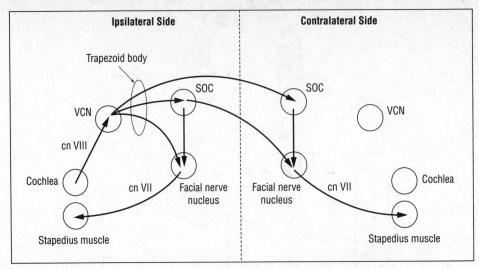

Note: SOC refers to the superior olivary complex. VCN refers to the ventral cochlear nucleus.

Source: Gelfand, S. (2002). The acoustic reflex. In J. Katz (Ed.), *Handbook of clinical audiology.* Baltimore: Lippincott, Williams & Wilkins, p. 206. Reprinted by permission.

The motor component of the acoustic reflex arc, which is composed of nerve cells in or near the motor nucleus of the facial nerve, the stapedial branch of the facial nerve, the stapedius muscle, and the middle ear components in the "probe" ear, is also known as the *efferent* portion of the acoustic reflex arc. If the efferent portion of the acoustic reflex arc is intact, contralateral acoustic reflexes will be obtained.

Note now that the general pathway for the contralateral acoustic reflex involves a crossing over of impulses from the superior olivary complex on one side of the brainstem to the facial nerve on the other side. In this way, stimulation of one ear creates an acoustic reflex in both ears. This is because impulses from the cochlear nucleus go to both superior olivary complexes (SOCs). Nerve cells and fibers in the superior olivery complex are part of the central component of the acoustic reflex arc for contralateral acoustic reflexes.

At first glance, students sometimes believe that as the stimulating sound enters the middle ear, it causes the stapedius muscle to contract. This, of course, is not possible because in order for any muscle to move, some part of the neurological system (in this case the brainstem) must be involved in the process. Now that you have a basic familiarity with the acoustic reflex arc, let's use this knowledge to address issues of acoustic reflex interpretation. We might begin this discussion by noting three broad principles regarding absence of acoustic reflexes.

The first principle is that acoustic reflexes will likely be absent in clients when even a small conductive component exists in the probe ear. This means that in cases where even minimal air–bone gaps exist, acoustic reflexes are likely to be absent because the conductive component interferes with our ability to measure the change in admittance of the middle ear on the affected side. Even if air–bone gaps are not measured, if a tympanogram supports some abnormality, this can create absent acoustic reflexes in the affected ear. Middle ear disorders, such as middle ear effusion, are a common efferent abnormality that causes the acoustic reflex to be absent in the probe ear. Figure 6.15 illustrates this.

The second principle is that acoustic reflexes will likely be absent when the degree of hearing loss in the ear being stimulated is so great as to prevent adequate intensity to elicit a reflex. For example, an abnormality of the afferent system in one ear, such as a severe or profound unilateral sensorineural hearing loss, will cause the ipsilateral acoustic reflexes to be absent. Remember that the ear being stimulated could be the same as the probe ear (ipsilateral reflex) or could be the ear opposite the probe ear (contralateral reflex).

FIGURE 6.15 **Conductive pathology in the right ear and absent ipsilateral acoustic reflexes.**

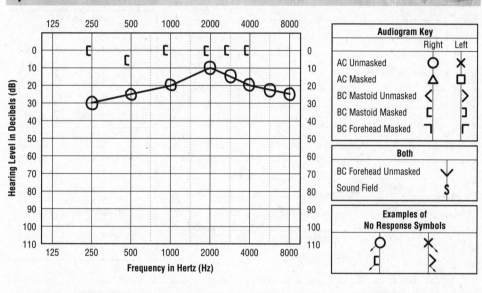

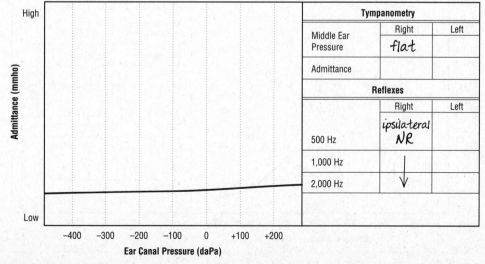

Related to this second point is that if we assume that the maximum intensity level that will be delivered to the client's ear in attempting to obtain an acoustic reflex is 125 dB HL, the acoustic reflex will likely be absent if the ear being stimulated has a cochlear loss greater than 80 dB. The reason for this, as noted previously, is that even for individuals with normal hearing, elicitation of the acoustic reflex requires considerable intensity. When the cochlear hearing loss exceeds 80 dB, there is typically not enough intensity to stimulate the auditory system to create the reflex response. This is shown in Figure 6.16.

FIGURE 6.16 **Severe to profound sensorineural hearing loss in the right ear and absent ipsilateral acoustic reflexes.**

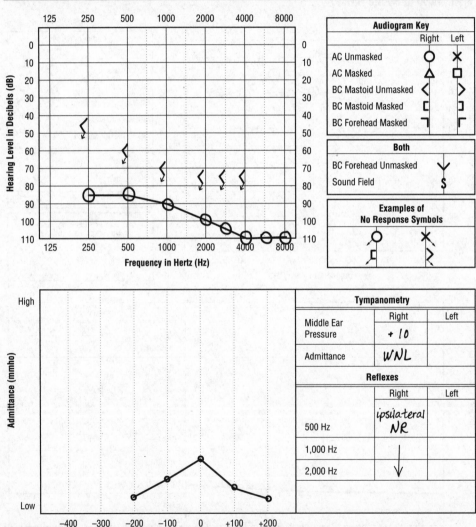

What about a case in which we are attempting to obtain an acoustic reflex with contralateral stimulation in an ear with a conductive hearing loss? Generally, a conductive hearing loss that is more than mild in degree, as shown in Figure 6.17, will likely result in absent reflexes because the stimulating intensity has to be great enough not only to elicit the reflex but also to overcome the conductive component. Note that when the conductive hearing loss is mild in degree, as in Figure 6.18, *stimulating* the ear does elicit

FIGURE 6.17 **Moderate unilateral conductive hearing loss (in the right ear) and resulting ipsilateral and contralateral acoustic reflex pattern.**

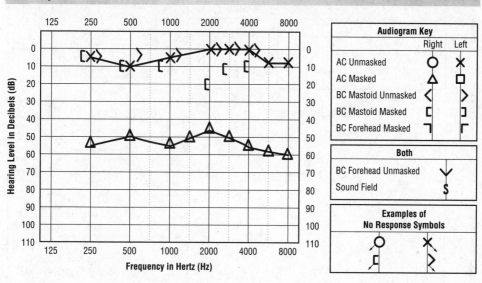

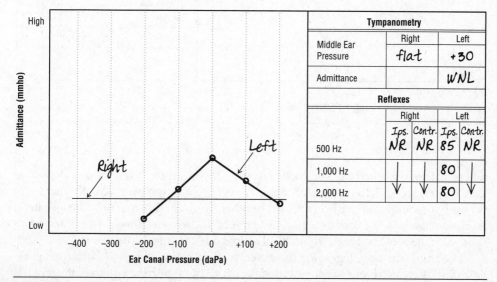

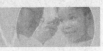

FIGURE 6.18 **Unilateral conductive pathology (in the right ear) and resulting ipsilateral and contralateral acoustic reflex pattern.**

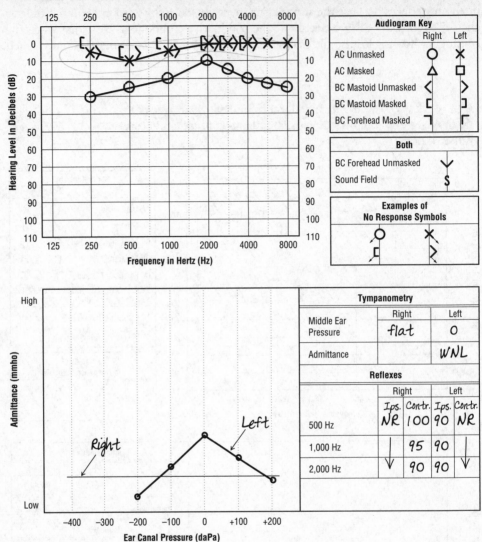

reflexes. However, when the conductive hearing loss is greater than mild in degree, as shown in Figure 6.17, the reflexes are absent in every condition involving stimulation of the ear with the conductive hearing loss. In other words, in this case only the ipsilateral acoustic reflexes in the unaffected ear are present. If there was conductive hearing loss bilaterally, the acoustic reflex would be obscured (absent) in all conditions.

The third principle regarding the absence of acoustic reflexes is that acoustic reflexes will likely be absent when pathology exists to those portions of cranial nerve VII and VIII and the brainstem that are involved in the acoustic reflex arc. This is an example of a combined efferent (cranial nerve VII or facial nerve) and afferent (cranial nerve VIII or auditory nerve) disorder. Figure 6.19 shows that both ipsilateral and contralateral acoustic reflex results are affected for an individual with such involvement on the right. Audiometric profiles and the acoustic reflex (AR) patterns associated with each are summarized in Table 6.3 (pp. 194–195).

FIGURE 6.19 **Eighth cranial nerve hearing loss in the right ear and the resulting ipsilateral and contralateral acoustic reflex pattern.**

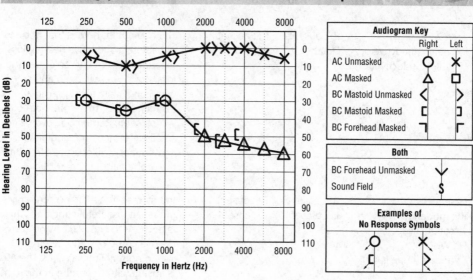

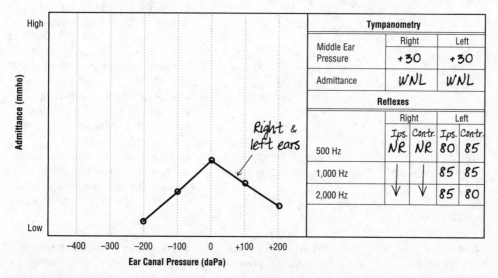

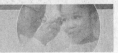

TABLE 6.3   Audiometric Profiles and Associated Acoustic
Reflex (AR) Patterns

Audiometric Profile	Ipsilateral AR	Contralateral AR	Comment
Case 1 RE: mild conductive LE: hearing WNL (no air–bone gaps)	RE: absent LE: present	RE: present LE: absent	You would expect the AR to be absent whenever the probe is in the ear with conductive pathology. Because the degree of conductive hearing loss is mild, it is possible to elicit the AR when stimulating the RE in this case.
Case 2 RE: mild conductive LE: mild conductive	RE: absent LE: absent	RE: absent LE: absent	The main point here is that in cases of bilateral conductive hearing loss, regardless of the degree of hearing loss, the probe will be in an ear with conductive pathology in all test conditions; therefore, no AR will be seen. Remember, even a small air–bone gap (conductive component) will obscure the AR in the probe ear.

Case 3
RE: moderate
    conductive
LE: WNL
    (no air–bone gaps)
	RE: absent
	LE: present
		RE: absent
		LE: absent
			In this case, the AR is present only in the left ipsilateral condition. This is because the left ear has no conductive pathology and hearing within normal limits (WNL). The AR is absent with the probe in the right ear (ipsilateral right and contralateral left conditions) because of the conductive pathology in the right ear. The AR is absent in the contralateral right (probe left) condition because the degree of conductive hearing loss cannot be overcome by the sound pressure level of the stimulus.

Case 4
RE: mild cochlear*
    loss
LE: WNL
    (no air–bone gaps)
	RE: present
	LE: present
		RE: present
		LE: present
			Because there is no conductive pathology, no auditory nerve involvement, and a mild degree of cochlear loss, AR are present in all conditions.

Case 5 RE: moderate cochlear* loss	RE: present LE: present	RE: present LE: present	Because there is no conductive pathology, no auditory nerve involvement, and a moderate degree of

TABLE 6.3 *(continued)*

LE: WNL (no air–bone gaps)			cochlear loss, AR are present in all conditions.

Case 6
RE: severe cochlear*
   loss
LE: WNL
   (no air–bone gaps)
	RE: absent
	LE: present
		RE: absent
		LE: present
			Each time the RE is stimulated with sound, the AR are absent due to the degree of cochlear hearing loss. Acoustic reflexes are present upon LE stimulation because the left ear has hearing WNL and there is no conductive involvement in either ear.

Case 7 RE: mild neural loss LE: WNL (no air–bone gaps)	RE: absent LE: present	RE: absent LE: present	Note that when the RE is stimulated, the AR are absent. When the LE is stimulated, the AR are present. Absence of the AR for ipsilateral and contralateral stimulation of the RE in the presence of a mild hearing loss with no conductive pathology is an important diagnostic clue and points toward neural involvement on the right.

Case 8
RE: hearing WNL
   (no air–bone gaps)
LE: hearing WNL
   (no air–bone gaps)
Client reports right
   facial numbness
   and weakness of
   recent onset.
	RE: absent
	LE: present
		RE: present
		LE: absent
			In this case, the acoustic reflex is absent with the probe in the affected (right) ear. This is because the seventh (facial) nerve is abnormal on the right side, and is not capable of transmitting the stimulation from the ventral cochlear nucleus and/or superior olivary complex to the stapedius muscle. Therefore, the acoustic reflex is absent on ipsilateral right and contralateral left stimulation (i.e., when the probe is in the right ear).

Cochlear is used here rather than the term *sensorineural* to denote a specific problem with the cochlea. Sensorineural is a nonspecific term referring to hearing loss arising from the cochlea and/or auditory nerve (cranial nerve VIII).

Acoustic Reflex Decay

There are cases of retrocochlear pathology in which all of the acoustic reflexes are present but they do not behave as expected when stimulated. The acoustic reflex decay test involves stimulating the ear contralaterally for 10 seconds at an intensity level that is 10 dB above the reflex threshold. In the normal condition (i.e., no acoustic reflex decay), the amplitude of the reflex remains essentially the same for the 10-second period. This is illustrated in Figure 6.20. In cases of acoustic reflex decay, a reduction of more than 50 percent

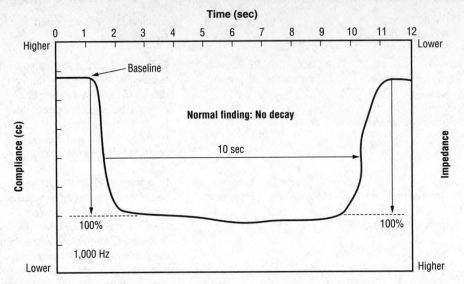

FIGURE 6.20 **Negative acoustic reflex decay test results.**

Source: *Audiologists' Desk Reference, Volume I, Diagnostic Audiology Principles, Procedures and Practices,* 1st edition, by Hall. 1997. Reprinted with permission of Delmar Learning, a division of Thomson Learning: www.thomsonrights.com. Fax 800-730-2215.

of initial amplitude is noted within the 10-second stimulation period. This is considered an abnormal finding and is illustrated in Figure 6.21, in which the amplitude has decreased by more than half its initial magnitude. What might account for acoustic reflex decay? Decay typically results when a mass (e.g., a **vestibular schwannoma**) compromises the auditory nerve, resulting in an inability for the nerve to maintain activity over time.

Otoacoustic Emissions

We know from earlier discussions about the anatomy, physiology, and pathways of the auditory system in Chapter 3 that sound travels through the auditory system beginning with the outer, then middle, then inner ear, to the brainstem with a destination of the auditory cortex and auditory association areas in the brain. With the discovery of otoacoustic emissions, it can be seen that this "one-way" transmission route does not tell the entire story. In fact, dynamic processes that take place in the cochlea produce sound that can be measured through the use of recording equipment in the external auditory canal.

Otoacoustic emissions (OAEs) are defined as sound generated in the cochlea that can be measured in the ear canal. OAEs were described by David Kemp (1978) as an "acoustic impulse response waveform" that was elicited in response to stimuli presented to healthy ears but was absent in ears with cochlear hearing loss of moderate or greater degree.

In the same article, Kemp (1978) discusses possible physiological reasons for OAEs. He concludes that these emissions arise from a cochlear source related to the activity of sensory cells in the cochlea, and speculates that the outer hair cells (OHCs) of the cochlea may be responsible for generation of the mechanical energy we know as OAEs.

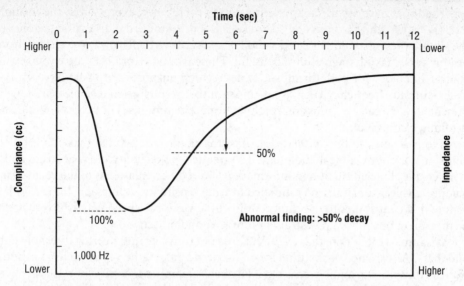

Source: *Audiologists' Desk Reference, Volume I, Diagnostic Audiology Principles, Procedures and Practices,* 1st edition, by Hall. 1997. Reprinted with permission of Delmar Learning, a division of Thomson Learning: www.thomsonrights.com. Fax 800-730-2215.

Although early descriptions of OAEs referred to them as "echoes," this analogy is over-simplified because more recent information has revealed that they result from dynamic processes taking place in the inner ear. In summary, Burch-Sims and Ochs (1992) report that OAEs arise from movement of OHCs in a normally functioning cochlea. Additional information about outer and inner hair cells is found in Chapter 3. As a preneural event, the presence of OAEs does not provide information about the function of cranial nerve VIII or beyond, but allows us to conclude that the auditory system has a normal response to stimulation through the outer, middle, and inner (cochlear) portions of the ear.

Types of OAEs

There are two major types of otoacoustic emissions: spontaneous and evoked. **Spontaneous otoacoustic emissions** are sounds generated by the cochlea and recorded in the ear canal in the absence of sound stimulation. Spontaneous OAEs are found in about half of individuals with normal hearing. Since spontaneous OAEs are not uni-versally present in individuals with healthy cochleas, their clinical usefulness is limited.

Evoked otoacoustic emissions are sounds generated by the cochlea and recorded in the ear canal that follow presentation of a stimulus. The particular type of stimulus de-termines the emission. The three types of evoked otoacoustic emissions are

1. Transient evoked otoacoustic emissions (TEOAEs)
2. Distortion product otoacoustic emissions (DPOAEs)
3. Stimulus frequency otoacoustic emissions (SFOAEs)

Transient evoked OAEs are elicited using presentation of a brief stimulus, such as a click. **Distortion product OAEs** are the result of presenting two different tones to the ear. The tones have a particular relationship to each other, expressed in the formula $2 \times (f1 - f2)$, and the emission that results is a third tone, the distortion product of the stimuli presented. Both TEOAEs and DPOAEs can virtually always be elicited from healthy ears, making them clinically useful. These two types of OAEs are employed in clinical audiology for both diagnostic and screening purposes. A third type of evoked OAE, **stimulus frequency OAE,** is an emission that results when a single pure tone is presented to the ear. The emission resulting from this stimulus is difficult to obtain and has limited clinical utility.

Kemp, Ryan, and Bray (1990) described the characteristics that make otoacoustic emissions useful in clinical audiology. The frequency specificity of otoacoustic emissions enable clinicians to obtain information about different aspects of the cochlea, including cochlear function and estimated hearing sensitivity, at the same time. Another feature that contributes to the clinical utility of OAEs is the speed with which they can be measured. In addition, OAES are noninvasive and objective.

It is important to note that OAE data does not translate into hearing threshold data and that OAEs are not a substitute for audiometric data, rather, they are used in addition to conventional audiometric data. Further, remember that for TEOAEs, ears with cochlear pathology will yield "no response," whether the associated hearing loss is in the 40-dB HL range or in the 95-dB HL range. This means that a test battery approach will be needed with OAEs comprising a useful part of the clinical picture, but not the only part.

Equipment for OAE Testing

Since Kemp's description of OAEs, the equipment used to obtain them has undergone an evolutionary process, incorporating features to increase ease of use in clinical settings. Features that were a part of the first commercially available instrumentation for obtaining OAEs are also applicable to the current generation of equipment. These features include noise artifact rejection, attention to the design and fit of the otoacoustic probe, calibration, standardization, and consistency across instruments. The first generation of OAE equipment included TEOAE, DPOAE, and SOAE testing capability. In 1992, Lonsbury-Martin et al. suggested that future instruments might incorporate additional features, such as combined OAE and ABR instruments for use in **neonatal hearing screening.** In fact, such equipment is now available in the marketplace. The main components of equipment used for OAE testing are shown in Figure 6.22.

OAE Measurement Techniques, Protocols, and Pitfalls

Because OAEs are weak sounds, noise artifact rejection is a necessary component of OAE instrumentation. Rejection of artifacts is combined with signal enhancement techniques such as averaging to ensure that reproducible and reliable OAEs can be obtained. The design and fit of the otoacoustic probe are critical components of successful OAE measurement. In addition to the actual manufacturing design of probes used in measuring otoacoustic emissions, the tester must have a good seal, similar to the technique used in tympanometry, to obtain OAEs. The difference in OAEs obtained with good and poor seals is illustrated in Figure 6.23. With a good fit/seal, the typical adult ear yields a

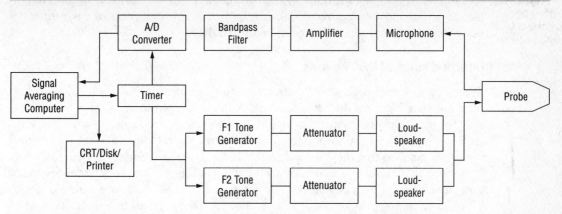

FIGURE 6.22 **Diagram of main components of equipment used to measure otoacoustic emissions.**

Source: Clinical Audiology: An Introduction, 1st edition, by Stach. 1998. Reprinted with permission of Delmar Learning, a division of Thomson Learning: www.thomsonrights.com. Fax 800-730-2215.

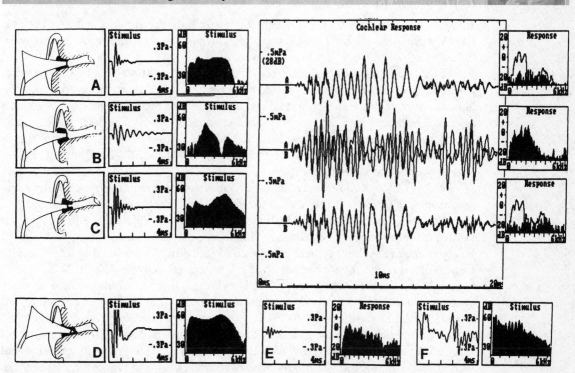

FIGURE 6.23 **OAEs with good and poor seals.**

Source: Kemp, D., Ryan, S., & Bray, P. (1990). A guide to the effective use of otoacoustic emissions. *Ear and Hearing, 11*(2), 93–105. Reprinted by permission.

good stimulus waveform (short transient) and a good cochlear emission waveform with noise levels well below the emission level (see Figure 6.23, example A). A poor seal will result in a long, ringing stimulus waveform (due to oscillation or ringing produced in the ear canal) and an obscured cochlear response (due to the effect of environmental noise) with poor reproducibility, as in Figure 6.23B.

Interpretation of OAE Results

According to Kemp et al. (1990), "the primary value of otoacoustic emissions is that their presence indicates that the preneural cochlear receptor mechanism (and necessarily the middle ear mechanism as well) is able to respond to sound in a normal way" (p. 94). There are several important points to remember. First, OAEs are a preneural response, meaning that they provide information about the auditory system including the outer, middle, and inner ears up to, but not including, the auditory nerve. Second, if outer and/or middle ear function is compromised, the OAE response will be affected. Third, OAE testing provides information about auditory system functions that underlie hearing, but is not a direct measure of hearing.

As noted previously, the various types of OAEs are named for the stimuli that are used to elicit them, most commonly a brief (transient) stimulus or a combination of two frequencies that results in the emission of a third frequency (distortion product).

Relationship between Audiometric and OAE Data

TEOAEs provide binary (yes/no) information about the function of the cochlea. DPOAEs provide additional insight regarding threshold and suprathreshold function in the cochlea.

TEOAEs are characterized as a fixed-frequency (not multiple-frequency) response, which does not allow them to be used to test a particular frequency range. Although the binary nature of this auditory system response does not provide information about a discrete frequency region, its applicability to neonatal hearing screening is well established; for additional information, refer to Chapter 11 on screening. The typical presentation levels for diagnostic OAE testing using TEOAEs are 82–83 dB peSPL. Figure 6.24 shows normal TEOAE results.

DPOAEs allow audiologists to assess various frequency regions in the auditory system, from 1,000 to 8,000 Hz, and to assess hair cell function at both threshold and suprathreshold levels. Lonsbury-Martin and Martin (1990) indicated that DPOAEs can be used to look at outer hair cell function in individuals with hearing loss up to 45–55 dB HL, whereas TEOAEs are typically not seen in individuals with hearing losses greater than 30 dB HL. DPOAEs are elicited using two tones, referred to as f1 and f2. The resulting third tone, the DPOAE, is usually 60 dB less intense than the stimulus tones, and may be expressed as $2(f1-f2)$. For clinical purposes, the stimulus is often presented at two levels (L1 and L2) that differ by 10–15 dB. For purposes of identifying hearing loss, stimulation of the cochlea is most effective at moderate intensity levels (Stover et al., 1996). An example of DPOAE stimulus levels is 65/50 dB SPL. A DP-gram for an individual with normal hearing, using stimulus levels of 65/55, is shown in Figure 6.25. Figure 6.26 illustrates a comparison of DP-grams for an individual with normal hearing through 4,000 Hz and for an individual with a high-frequency sensorineural hearing loss.

FIGURE 6.24 **Normal TEOAE results.**

201

Otoacoustic
Emissions

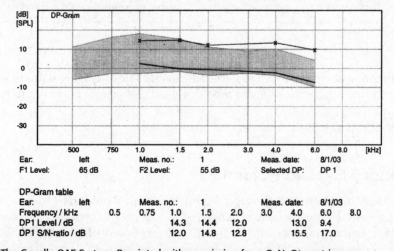

TEOAE band analysis						
Ear:	left				Meas. date:	8/1/03
Frequency / kHz	0.75-1.25	1.25-1.75	1.75-2.50	2.50-3.50	3.50-4.50	Overall:
Correlation / %:	90	98	92	92	0	90
Emis. strength / dB:	8.1	16.0	10.1	11.5	-1.0	18.8
S/N-ratio / dB:	10.5	20.7	13.6	14.0	0.1	13.0

Source: The Capella OAE System. Used with permission from G. N. Otometrics.

In summary, OAEs add the following information to the practice of clinical audiology:

- An ability to distinguish between cochlear (sensory) and neural involvement
- An objective screening of auditory system function, particularly in the 1,000–4,000-Hz range, useful in infant hearing screening

FIGURE 6.25 **Normal DPOAE.**

DP-Gram table								
Ear:	left			Meas. no.:	1		Meas. date:	8/1/03	
Frequency / kHz	0.5	0.75	1.0	1.5	2.0	3.0	4.0	6.0	8.0
DP1 Level / dB			14.3	14.4	12.0		13.0	9.4	
DP1 S/N-ratio / dB			12.0	14.8	12.8		15.5	17.0	

Source: The Capella OAE System. Reprinted with permission from G. N. Otometrics.

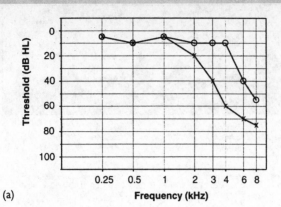

(a)

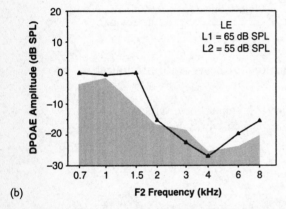

(b)

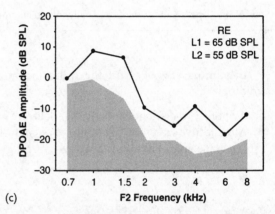

(c)

Source: Musiek, Frank E., and Jane A. Baran, *The Auditory System: Anatomy, Physiology, and Clinical Correlates.* Published by Allyn and Bacon, Boston, MA. Copyright © 2007 by Pearson Education. Reprinted by permission of the publisher.

- Information about the cochlear status and an estimate of hearing status of individuals who are unable/unwilling to provide reliable behavioral responses to auditory stimuli
- An ability to monitor changes in cochlear function

Auditory Evoked Potentials

It is perhaps best to introduce the topic of **auditory evoked potentials** by first defining the word *potential*. A **potential** is a change in nerve or muscle activity. One example of the measurement of brain potentials is found in **electroencephalography (EEG).** In this testing, scalp electrodes are placed on the client and the ongoing electrical brain potentials are measured and recorded on a graph, referred to as an electroencephalogram.

EEG involves measurement of ongoing electrical brain activity that is the result of the brain's processing of incoming information. Think for a moment what would occur if, during this measurement of ongoing electrical brain activity, an intense sensory signal (e.g., a flash of light, an intense sound) was presented to the client. Presuming that the client's sensory system was intact, this stimulation would cause some change in the ongoing brain activity because the stimulus would be processed by the brain. This is the underlying premise of evoked potential testing, which assesses the change in ongoing electrical activity that results from some sensory stimulation.

Historically, one of the challenges in performing evoked potential testing was that the change in electrical activity created by the introduction of the stimulus was very small, and therefore difficult to pick out from the ongoing brain activity, which was large. This challenge is addressed by special computerized equipment that has the capability of amplifying the activity that is of interest and averaging out the unnecessary background activity.

Thus far, we have used the broad term *evoked potentials testing.* Now examine the term *auditory evoked potential testing.* This term refers to a group of tests, all of which "evoke" brain activity by the introduction of auditory stimuli. The various tests that are included under the heading of "auditory evoked potentials" differ in the time window in which the potentials appear. By time window, also referred to as *latency,* we mean the time at which the evoked potential appears following stimulation. Examine Figure 6.27 and you will note that potentials observed very early reflect activity that is at a relatively lower level in the system, such as the cochlear hair cells and the auditory nerve. Potentials that are noted later provide information at "higher" centers. This is logical because auditory evoked potential tests are basically time-conduction tests and it requires more time to record information about auditory sites that are more central and less time to record information about auditory sites that are more peripheral.

In this next section of the chapter, we examine the various auditory evoked potential tests, moving from the earliest to the latest measures. One of the important distinctions that should be understood is the difference between endogenous and exogenous components of evoked potentials. Briefly:

- *Exogenous* components are controlled by external events.
- *Endogenous* components are regulated by internal aspects of brain activity.

In general, the early evoked potentials are considered exogenous and arise from identifiable sites within the auditory system. They are more dependent on the stimulus used than the later potentials, and are relatively less affected by the client's state of arousal or use of sedation. Generator sites for the later auditory evoked potentials, which are considered endogenous, have been more difficult to identify, and the probability is that these responses arise from multiple sites in the auditory system. These potentials are less contingent on the stimulus used per se and are significantly influenced by the client's state of arousal.

Auditory Brainstem Response

ASHA (1990) states that audiologists who perform auditory brainstem response (ABR) testing should demonstrate four competencies. These include knowing:

FIGURE 6.27 **Auditory evoked potentials.**

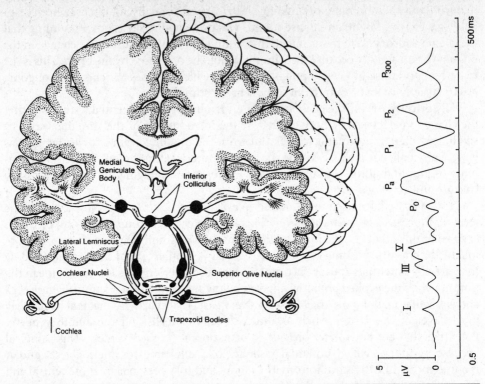

Time Frame	Evoked Potential	Probable Site of Neural Generation
First (0–2 msec) (not shown)	EcochG (EcoG)	Cochlear microphonic, summating potential and acoustic nerve response
Early or fast (2–10 msec)	ABR (BSER, BAER)	Acoustic nerve and auditory brainstem response
Middle (8–50 msec)	AMLR (MLR)	Thalamus and auditory cortex
Late (50–300 msec)	Late potential or slow vertex potential (SVP)	Primary and secondary areas of areas of cerebral cortex
Auditory P-300 (300+ msec)	P-300 (cognitive potential)	Primary and association areas of cerebral cortex

Sources: American Speech-Language-Hearing Association. (1987*). Short latency auditory evoked potentials, a relevant paper by the audiological evaluation working group on auditory evoked potential measurements.* Rockville, MD: Author. Copyright by the American Speech-Language-Hearing Association. Reprinted by permission. Jerry L. Northern. *Hearing Disorders*, 3e. Published by Allyn and Bacon, Boston, MA. Copyright © 1996 by Pearson Education. Reprinted by permission of the publisher.

1. Who should be referred for the test
2. What test protocols are most appropriate for each particular client
3. Interpretation of the results
4. Making appropriate recommendations

It should also be noted that there are a number of different terms that all refer to ABR testing. For example, brainstem auditory evoked response (BAER) testing and brainstem auditory evoked potentials (BAEP) are also commonly used. Another term that you will see is brainstem evoked response (BSER) testing. Finally, sometimes ABR testing is simply referred to as the "early response."

There are two broad purposes of ABR testing: to rule out retrocochlear site of lesion and to estimate hearing thresholds. Historically, it was more common to use ABR testing for the purpose of ruling out retrocochlear involvement. ABR is also used for identifying auditory neuropathy/dys-synchrony as well as for intraoperative monitoring purposes. In addition, with the proliferation of universal newborn hearing screening programs, use of ABR for purposes of threshold estimation has increased. This section begins with the use of ABR as a site-of-lesion test. The information described in that context (e.g., absolute and interpeak latencies and stimulus type) provides a foundation for the subsequent information on ABR and threshold estimation.

Recall from our earlier discussion of acoustic reflexes and acoustic reflex decay that there are cases in which an audiologist suspects that a client has a retrocochlear site of lesion. Although in these cases the physician may refer the client directly for a CT scan or an MRI, it is common for physicians to request that ABR testing be done first. This testing is typically performed by an audiologist.

Test Protocol

The equipment used and physical setup for ABR testing that is described in this section is the same for either application of the testing (i.e., to rule out retrocochlear site of lesion or to estimate hearing thresholds). Figure 6.28 shows the various equipment

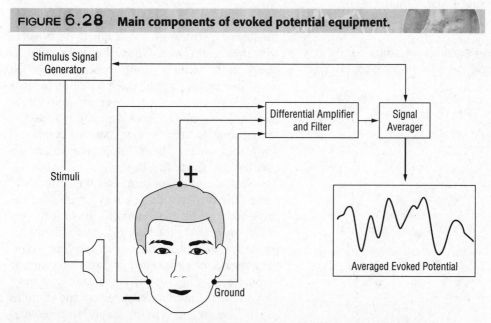

FIGURE 6.28   Main components of evoked potential equipment.

Source: Gelfand, S. (2001). Essentials of audiology (2nd ed.). New York: Thieme. Reprinted by permission.

components used for ABR testing. Clients are seated in a comfortable chair, often a recliner, so that they will become relaxed and have adequate body support. Instructions about the purpose of the test and about the reasons for electrode placement should be provided, because these can be useful in relieving any anxiety that the client may be experiencing about the procedure.

Depending on the particular type of equipment that is being used, several areas of the client's head are cleaned thoroughly with a slightly abrasive solution so that when the scalp electrodes are in place, they will make good contact and will efficiently pick up the electrical activity from the brain. If those areas where the electrodes are to be placed are not cleaned sufficiently, oil, dirt, or skin can decrease the quality of the measured response by increasing the impedance. Remember from our discussion earlier in this chapter that impedance refers to opposition to the flow of energy. In the current test situation, we are attempting to keep impedance as small as possible so that the electrodes can effectively measure changes in electrical activity. In general, electrode impedance should not exceed 5,000 ohms (or 5 kohms). More important than the absolute impedance value for each electrode is that the variation among the impedance values for each of the electrodes should be kept to a minimum. A common electrode montage (configuration) used in ABR testing is shown in Figure 6.29. Typically, for adults, when two-channel equipment is used, the electrodes are secured in the following locations: Cz (the top of the head, at midline); FpZ (the middle of the forehead); and the right and left earlobes. The exact placement of the electrodes may vary depending on the particular equipment used.

Although we are measuring brain activity, we are placing electrodes on the skull. This is referred to as **far-field testing** and is one of the advantages of most types of auditory evoked testing. In other words, even though we are obtaining information about auditory sites that are part of the brainstem, we can do so with noninvasive surface electrodes placed on the skull.

FIGURE 6.29 **Common locations for electrodes for auditory evoked potential testing.**

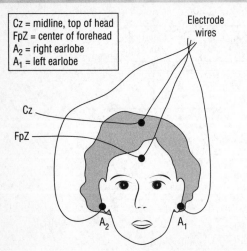

Cz = midline, top of head
FpZ = center of forehead
A_2 = right earlobe
A_1 = left earlobe

Electrode wires

Cz

FpZ

A_2 A_1

After the scalp electrodes are securely in place, clients are instructed to sit as quietly as possible with their eyes closed. Often, the client's chair is placed in the reclining position. Some clients fall asleep during the testing, which is helpful because controlling unnecessary movement allows for more efficient collection of data and reduces the testing time. Either insert or standard earphones are placed on the client, impedance values are checked, and the testing begins.

Next, the audiologist directs the stimulus to one of the two ears. A click is typically used because its acoustic characteristics allow it to very effectively activate the auditory nerve fibers that produce the auditory brainstem response. Typically, the better ear is tested first, just as is routine in pure tone audiometry. The audiologist must also decide the number of sweeps of the stimulus that will be presented to the ear and the presentation rate. For example, the audiologist may present 2,000 sweeps or 4,000 sweeps of the click stimulus at a rate of 11 clicks per second. The greater the number of sweeps used, the better the waveform morphology (shape and definition of the waves). A slower rate of presentation may also result in improved waveform morphology; however, it takes a longer time to obtain. Often 2,000 sweeps are presented at a in a range of 11 to 33 per sec. Similar to pure tone and speech audiometry, masking is employed if the possibility of stimulating the non-test ear exists during ABR testing.

Another decision that must be made is the intensity of the stimulus. The choice of click intensity level that will be used is often made based on the available norms. For example, if the audiologist has normative data for the specific piece of equipment being used based on an intensity level of 85 dB, this is the intensity level that the audiologist should use. When ABR testing is done for purposes of ruling out a retrocochlear site of lesion, levels of 80 to 90 dB are typically recommended. Intensity levels greater than 95 dB are not recommended because of the increased possibility of elicitation of an acoustic reflex, which can reduce the intensity of the signal to the cochlea.

At this point, brief mention should be made about denoting intensity in ABR testing. A process by which intensity in dB SPL is converted to dB HL was described earlier. You will recall that for each frequency, the smallest average amount of sound pressure required to create threshold was renamed as 0 dB HL. Similarly, a common method of denoting the intensity level of clicks used in ABR testing is to determine the average softest intensity level (from a group of individuals who have normal hearing) where the click can be heard. This mean click threshold is referred to as 0 **dB nHL.** For this reason, when referring to intensity levels in ABR, dB nHL is used rather than dB HL.

ABR Data Interpretation

Once both ears have been tested, the audiologist interprets the data. There are several different parameters on which to judge the ABR results, and three of the four that will be discussed involve a comparison of the client data with normative data. Although general normative data is available and can be used for interpretation of ABR results, it is recommend that audiologists collect their own normative data using their own equipment. When doing this, it is important to collect separate norms for males and females, because females tend to have shorter absolute and interpeak latencies than males. Also, some audiologists divide their norms by age, using categories that include adults under 40 years, adults over 40 years, and elderly. Let's now examine some of the main parameters on which ABR findings are judged.

Absolute Wave Latency.   **Absolute wave latency** refers to the time at which each of the individual waves appears. Remember that for the ABR response, the total time window is only about 10 msec. Although adult latency values will vary with equipment, age, and gender, in general, wave I is noted at latencies between 1.5 and 2.0 msec, wave III between 3.5 and 4.3 msec, and wave V between 5.0 and 6.1 msec. Based on the normative data, audiologists determine if any of the waves occur outside of (i.e., later than) the norms.

Illustrated in Figure 6.30 is a normal ABR in an adult male. Examine the peaks for waves I, III, and V and note that the absolute latencies all fall within these norms.

FIGURE 6.30   **Absolute and interpeak latencies of an ABR on a normal adult male.**

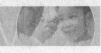

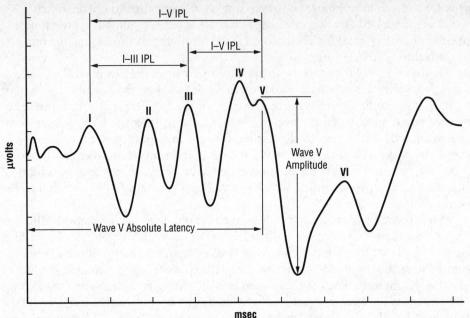

Source: Jacobson, John T. *Principles and Applications in Auditory Evoked Potentials.* Published by Allyn and Bacon, Boston, MA. Copyright © 1994 by Pearson Education. Reprinted by permission of the publisher.

Interpeak Latencies.   In addition to the absolute latencies, audiologists also calculate the time differences between the following waves: I and III, III and V, and I and V, which are referred to as the **interpeak latencies.** Once again, audiologists refer to norms to determine if any of the times noted from the client data exceed the norm values. In general, the interpeak difference should not exceed 2.2 msec for the I–III and III–V interval and should not exceed 4.2 msec for the I–V interval. Figure 6.30 also demonstrates calculation of interpeak latencies. Perform these calculations and be sure that the obtained values fall within these norms.

Interaural Latency Difference.   The **interaural latency difference (ILD)** refers to the difference in time (latency) between the absolute latency of wave V in each ear. Most authorities agree that this difference should not exceed 0.4 msec. Examine the ABR data in Figure 6.31 and note that the wave V latency in the right ear is 5.3 msec and the latency in the left ear for wave V is 5.5 msec. The difference between these two latencies is 0.2 msec, which is less than 0.4 msec and therefore not consistent with retrocochlear pathology.

Morphology.   The word *morphology* in this context refers to the shape or definition of the waves. This is important for two reasons. First, retrocochlear disorders can result in

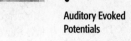
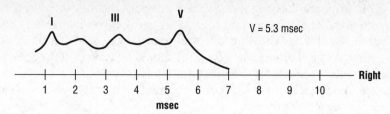

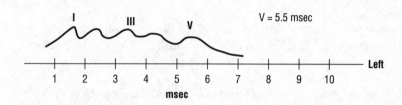

poor **wave morphology,** as illustrated in the left-ear tracing in Figure 6.32. Second, although ABR is commonly described as an objective measure, its interpretation requires that the audiologist make subjective judgments about the location of the peaks of the waves. If morphology is poor, these judgments become more difficult, which increases the chance of error in interpretation of ABR data.

Using these parameters of the ABR data, an audiologist determines whether abnormality of the auditory brainstem response can be ruled out. This process can be

FIGURE 6.32 **Abnormal wave morphology in left ABR tracing.**

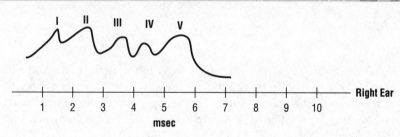

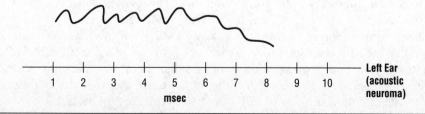

complicated by the presence of hearing loss, which can interfere with the intensity of the sound used to "evoke" the brainstem response. Audiologists must be able to distinguish the effects of peripheral hearing loss on the wave pattern from the effects of retro-cochlear pathology. This is important because in many cases clients who have retro-cochlear pathology also have hearing loss. It is important to note that the ABR should not be interpreted in isolation; rather, the ABR should be viewed in the context of au-diometric and other available test information.

There are some general rules that guide interpretation of the waveform pattern in cases where hearing loss is present:

- In cases of conductive hearing loss, wave I is commonly quite delayed, reflecting the considerable influence hearing loss has on wave I. The interpeak intervals are typically normal.
- In cases of sensorineural hearing loss, wave I is commonly delayed, once again due to the hearing loss. Wave I is also commonly difficult to identify. Interpeak intervals are often within normal limits, and sometimes the I–V interval is shortened because wave I is late and wave V is on time.
- In cases of retrocochlear site of lesion, wave I is typically noted at a normal latency (reflecting normal cochlear function), but later waves such as III and V may be delayed. Interpeak latencies may also be abnormal (i.e., greater than the norm).

It should also be noted that correction factors, which were once used in an attempt to compensate for the effects of high-frequency hearing loss on the latency of wave V, are no longer recommended. Also, in cases of asymmetrical hearing loss, the ear with the greater loss can be stimulated at a more intense level than the less-impaired ear. As is true in behavioral pure tone audiometry, bone conduction ABR testing can be used to assist in determining the type (nature) of hearing loss. If results of ABR testing do not allow retrocochlear pathology to be ruled out, the physician will most likely order addi-tional tests, such as an MRI or CT scan, to gain more information regarding the client's status.

Stacked ABR

Definition

Dr. Manuel Don, in a 2005 interview in *Audiology Online,* defined **stacked ABR** as an attempt to record the sum of the neural activity across the entire frequency region of the cochlea in response to click stimulation. This section will discuss the use of stacked ABRs and how they are obtained. For a discussion of the mechanisms underlying stacked ABRs, refer to Don et al. (2005) and Hall (2007).

As you now know, ABR is used as a site-of-lesion test, and has been shown to be sen-sitive to acoustic tumors (vestibular schwannomas). However, as Hall (2007) points out, early studies that suggested ABR was highly sensitive to retrocochlear pathology were conducted before magnetic resonance imaging (MRI) was available. We have since learned that the ABR is sensitive to larger tumors; however, one limitation of ABR test-ing is its relatively poor sensitivity for small (less than 1 cm) acoustic tumors. Dr. Don and his colleagues at the House Ear Institute have studied the stacked ABR measure as a way to enhance the sensitivity of ABR in detecting smaller tumors.

With the existence of imaging techniques that can detect small tumors, why would it be beneficial to have an ABR measure that is sensitive to small tumors? Don (2005) points out that MRI equipment is not available in all localities or geographic regions. In addition, greater costs are associated with MRI than with ABR testing and, for some clients, claustrophobia makes MRI difficult.

Don (2005) has hypothesized that the reason standard ABR measures do not detect small tumors is that they rely on latency changes of wave V of the ABR. Don (2005) further points out that the wave V latency measure is influenced primarily by high-frequency fibers. If the tumor size is small, it is possible that the high-frequency nerve fibers are not affected, and ABR results will miss the presence of a tumor.

How Are Stacked ABR Measures Obtained?

The stacked ABR measure is done using click stimulation and high-pass pink noise masking. Stacked ABR is the composite of activity from *all* frequency regions of the cochlea (versus only the high-frequency region). Obtaining a stacked ABR involves (1) obtaining ABR responses to clicks and high-pass masking noise; (2) obtaining "derived-band" ABRs; and (3) shifting and aligning the wave V peaks of the derived-band responses (i.e., "stacking" the waveforms with the waves V lined up); and (4) adding the waveforms together.

Derived-band ABRs are obtained by subtracting each of the ABRs obtained for a sequence of frequencies (8,000, 4,000, 2,000, 1,000, and 500 Hz) from the one before it. By doing this subtraction technique, you obtain five derived-band ABRs that reflect the neural contributions from five different octave-wide frequency regions in the cochlea (Don, 2005). The amplitude of the stacked ABR is then compared with the amplitude of the click-evoked ABR from the same ear. Don (2005) explains that in a normal ear, the sum of the stacked ABR will have the same amplitude as the click-evoked ABR. The presence of even a small tumor would result in a *reduction* in the amplitude of the stacked ABR, compared with the click-evoked ABR (see Table 6.4).

Clinical Utility

The primary purpose for using stacked ABR measures is to help screen for and detect the presence of small (less than or equal to 1 cm) acoustic tumors (vestibular schwannomas). Don et al. (2005) reported that this technique demonstrated 95 percent sensitivity and 88 percent specificity in identifying small acoustic tumors in a study of fifty-four individuals with small acoustic tumors that had been identified through MRI. Stacked ABR was far more sensitive than conventional ABR in this population. However, Hall (2007) notes that Don and colleagues have reported preliminary evidence that patterns of abnormalities occur when the stacked ABR measure is applied to individuals with Meniere's disease.

Threshold Estimation

Another major use of ABR testing is for estimation of thresholds for hearing. As we have already discussed, there are clients for whom behavioral testing is impossible or unreliable. Specifically, very young children, individuals with developmental disabilities, and individuals with nonorganic hearing loss are candidates for ABR testing for purposes of threshold estimation. ABR measures are not tests of hearing (they are measures of neural synchrony), but because there are some predictable relationships between stimulation

TABLE 6.4   **Obtaining a Stacked ABR**

Step	Rationale	Result
An ABR is obtained using clicks with high-pass masking noise.	Use of ipsilateral masking with pink noise masks the ABR evoked by the click stimulus.	ABR response to conventional click stimulus.
High-pass masking noise with five different low-frequency cutoffs (8,000, 4,000, 2,000, 1,000, and 500 Hz) is used to generate additional ABR responses.	Each ABR in the series is generated by activity in a particular frequency region (versus the broad neural involvement resulting from a click stimulus).	Five ABR waveforms, each resulting from a defined set of nerve fibers.
Each ABR waveform is digitally subtracted from the one generated before it (the "derived-band" ABRs).	Because these ABRs resulted from a specific frequency region, these "derived bands" reflect frequency-specific activity. The characteristic frequencies seen in the derived bands are: 11,300 Hz, 5,700 Hz, 2,800 Hz, 1,400 Hz, and 700 Hz. These represent the center frequency for the particular region in the cochlea responsible for generating the ABR response for each of the derived bands.	Hall (2007) indicates that the derived bands behave in a predictable manner: those with the higher characteristic frequencies have the shorter latencies.
All of the wave Vs from the derived-band ABRs are lined up, one on top of the other, resulting in the stacked ABR.	If all of the frequency bands in the cochlea are represented normally, the resulting stacked ABR should have the same latency as the click-evoked ABR; however, a tumor affecting any of the frequency regions would be expected to affect the ABR derived from that frequency region.	Comparing the stacked ABR with the click-evoked ABR helps to determine whether retrocochlear pathology is present.

Sources: Don (2005) and Hall (2007).

levels, hearing status, and wave patterns, ABR testing can be used to estimate hearing sensitivity.

Use of ABR testing for threshold estimation is important to both audiologists and speech–language pathologists. Audiologists need to know how to perform ABR testing,

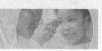
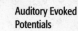
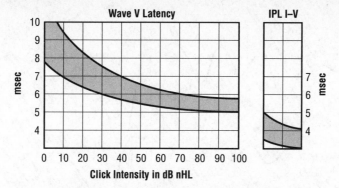

Source: *Audiologists' Desk Reference, Volume I, Diagnostic Audiology Principles, Procedures and Practices,* 1st edition, by Hall. 1998. Reprinted with permission of Delmar Learning, a division of Thomson Learning: www.thomsonrights.com. Fax 800-730-2215.

how to interpret the data, and how to incorporate the data to plan meaningful aural rehabilitation. Knowledge of the specific purposes of ABR testing and the information such testing can provide will enable the speech–language pathologist to make appropriate referrals.

Let's begin this discussion of hearing estimation by stating that for adults, test preparation and instructions are the same as those described previously. Use of ABR with children will be discussed shortly. One of the major differences between ABR testing to rule out retrocochlear pathology and testing to estimate hearing is that for hearing estimation the intensity of the signal will not remain at its original (rather intense) level. In order to observe the effects of intensity on the wave patterns, it is necessary to decrease the intensity of the stimulation level in a series of steps. Because the procedure involves examination of wave V latency associated with changes in intensity, the term **latency–intensity function** is used to describe the resulting graph. This graph is shown in Figure 6.33. The shaded area represents the normative latency values for wave V as click intensity is decreased.

Before specifically examining the latency–intensity function for this client, let's examine Figure 6.34, which represents the overall auditory brainstem wave pattern for a client who has normal hearing. Stimulation began at 80 dB, just as it would when testing to rule out retrocochlear site of lesion. Note that at this intensity level the wave morphology is very good; it is very easy to identify not only the major waves (I, III, and V) but also waves II and IV. Although for this client the ABR is being used to estimate hearing and not to assess retrocochlear status, the fact that at 80 dB the absolute and interpeak latencies are within the norms that we have discussed previously does support a normal brainstem response and rules out retrocochlear pathology.

At this point, note what happens to both the morphology and wave latency as the intensity is decreased from 80 to 60 dB. The morphology becomes slightly poorer and the latency of the waves increases, as noted by the pattern shifting to the right. As the

FIGURE 6.34 **Effects of decreasing intensity on latency and morphology of wave V in individual with normal hearing sensitivity.**

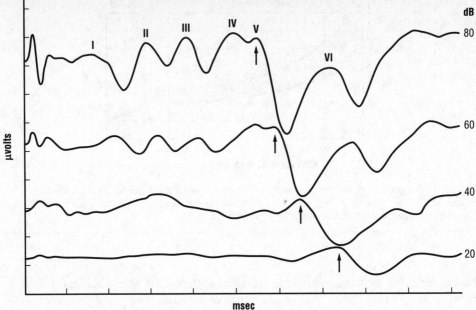

Source: Jacobson, John T. *Principles and Applications in Auditory Evoked Potentials.* Published by Allyn and Bacon, Boston, MA. Copyright © 1994 by Pearson Education. Reprinted by permission of the publisher.

intensity is decreased again to 40 dB, morphology further worsens, with wave I barely identifiable. Once again, latency increases.

Now, addressing the latency–intensity function specifically, note that all of the wave V latencies fall within the normative data graphed in Figure 6.35. An important additional observation is that at the very reduced intensity level of 20 dB, wave V is still observable. Wave V is often referred to as "robust" for this reason. The presence of wave V at an intensity level of 20 dB is correlated with normal hearing in the 1,000–4,000-Hz region.

What would happen to the latency–intensity function if a client had a conductive hearing loss like the one in Figure 6.36? Note that air–bone gaps of 20 dB on the average exist in the right ear and this results in a shift in wave V latencies of about 20 dB, reflecting the attenuation of the sound intensity. Note also that the shift in latency is most pronounced as the intensity of the stimulus decreases.

For sensorineural hearing loss that is essentially moderate, note in Figure 6.37 that at the more intense levels wave V is within the "norms" area on the graph. For softer levels, however, there is not enough intensity to stimulate the brainstem adequately; therefore wave V latency values fall outside of the normal range.

Now that we have examined some of the issues related to threshold estimation using ABR with adults, let's examine the same testing with children. First, the brainstem

FIGURE 6.35 Latency–intensity function in case of normal hearing.

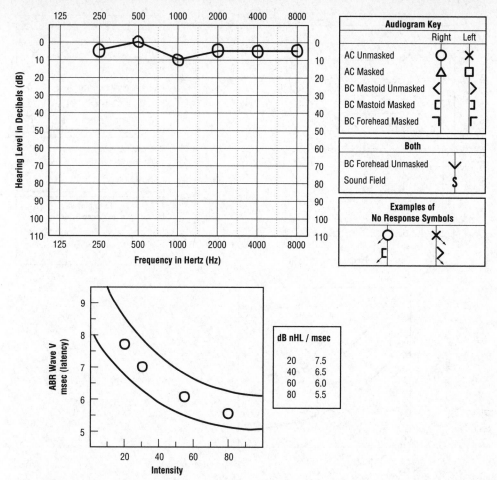

response of children younger than about 18 months of age is different than that of the more mature child and adult. For example, the brainstem response of the very young child is characterized by waves I and V and the absence of other waves. Also, overall morphology is reduced at very young ages. Finally and very importantly, absolute and interpeak wave latencies decrease as the child matures. In view of this information, it is not surprising that audiologists who perform ABR testing on newborns and very young children use separate normative data collected specifically on children in these age ranges.

As noted earlier, client comfort is important in order to limit the degree of movement the client will make during the testing. For infants up to approximately 3 to 4 months of age, this may be accomplished by feeding the baby and having a parent rock him to sleep before beginning the testing. As children become older and less cooperative,

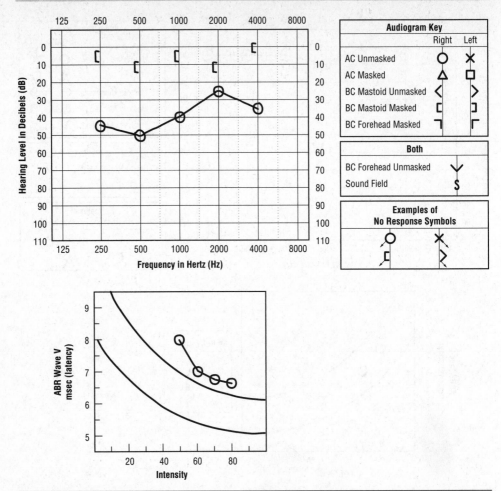

FIGURE 6.36 **Latency–intensity function in case of conductive hearing loss.**

it is often necessary to use sedation so they will remain still during testing. Each institution conducting ABR testing on clients requiring sedation will have developed a policy and procedures for the use of conscious sedation. For additional guidelines, refer to ASHA's (1992) technical report concerning sedation and topical anesthetics.

One of the most commonly used sedatives for this purpose is chloral hydrate in liquid form. In some settings, the parent fills the prescription for the medication prior to the appointment and brings it with her to the appointment. Before the audiologist is ready to begin the testing, the medication is given so that the child will remain sleeping for the entire test session. Sedation does not influence the auditory brainstem response.

Finally, it is important for audiologists, speech–language pathologists, and related professionals to understand that although auditory brainstem testing can be used to estimate hearing thresholds, ABR testing is not a direct test of hearing. Consider the

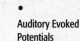
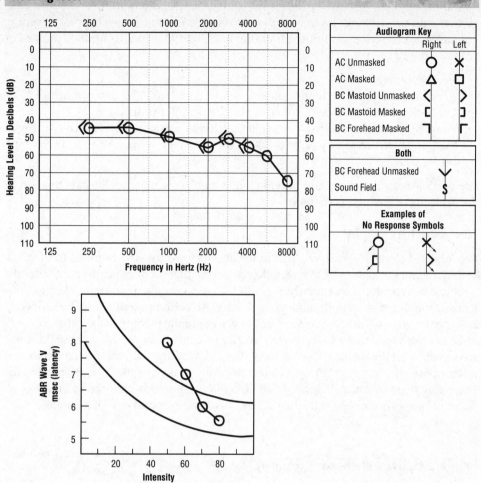

anatomy involved in the auditory brainstem response. Although the test is certainly assessing the integrity of structures that are critical to the process of hearing, it does not tap auditory areas that go beyond the rostral brainstem. This means that the very important areas of auditory reception located in the temporal lobe are not included in this assessment. In addition, because most ABR testing uses only click stimuli, low-frequency hearing is not assessed. Therefore, when testing infants, ABRs should also include low-frequency tonal stimuli (e.g., 500 Hz) and responses should be compared with established norms. In addition, despite some established correlations between performance on the ABR and responses to pure tones, there is little information regarding relationships between ABR performance and a client's understanding of speech. Because the response of interest is generated from the brainstem, it can be absent or abnormal in clients who have brainstem pathology. For example, a client with multiple sclerosis can have normal hearing bilaterally based on comprehensive audiological assessment and also yield absent or abnormal auditory brainstem responses.

Sininger (2005) discusses an electrophysiological test battery for use with infants in need of a diagnostic audiological assessment referred from newborn hearing screening programs. She describes an initial minimum test battery for infants under 6 months of age as including:

- Tympanometry
- Acoustic reflexes with a high-frequency probe tone (1,000 Hz is recommended)
- Otoacoustic emissions (either transient or distortion products)
- Frequency-specific electrophysiologic threshold measures (such as ABR) using at least one high-frequency (2,000–4,000 Hz) and one low-frequency (500 Hz) tone bursts.

Use of such a test battery would provide important frequency-specific data to assist in the planning of any necessary follow-up.

Electrocochleography

Recording of electrical potentials within the auditory system is not limited to the well-known auditory brainstem response. Other responses that occur either before or after the ABR can be recorded. **Electrocochleography** is the recording of compound action potentials from the cochlea and eighth cranial nerve. An **action potential** may be defined as a change in nerve or muscle activity. Electrocochleography is abbreviated either ECochG or ECoG, with the former being preferred. The ECochG response is composed of three waves, which are the cochlear microphonic (CM), the action potential (AP), and the summating potential (SP). According to Hall (2007), the AP is also called N1, referring to the first negative peak, and ABR wave I. The ECochG response is pictured in Figure 6.38. These responses occur within the first 1.5 to 2 msec following an abrupt stimulus.

FIGURE 6.38 Electrocochleography.

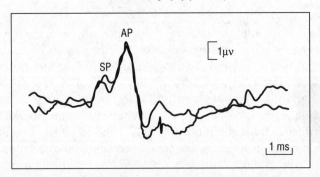

Electrocochleography (ECochG)

Source: Hall, James W., III. *Handbook of Auditory Evoked Responses,* 1e. Published by Allyn and Bacon, Boston, MA. Copyright © 1992 by Pearson Education. Adapted by permission of the publisher.

The anatomic sites responsible for generation of the components of the ECochG are as follows:

CM: outer hair cells

SP: hair cells

AP: distal eighth nerve (Hall, 2007)

There are two methods for recording evoked responses: near field and far field. In near-field recording the electrode is placed in close proximity to or on the site of interest, whereas in far-field recording, the electrode placement is relatively distant from the anatomic site that generates the response. The CM and SP are the result of near-field recording of the hair cell response from the cochlea. The AP response of the ECochG, which can be recorded using either near-field or far-field techniques, is the response from the auditory nerve (N1, N2), reflecting the firing of eighth nerve fibers.

The most effective recordings of the ECochG response are obtained using a near-field recording technique, meaning that the electrode placement is near the cochlea. If the eardrum is intact, this involves placing a needle electrode through the tympanic membrane and positioning it on the promontory of the cochlea. Placement of the electrode can be accomplished during ear surgery when the middle ear is exposed. Many studies of ECochG were done on patients undergoing middle ear surgery for this reason. Noninvasive electrodes have also been designed for ECochG recording, making it possible to utilize electrocochleography in a wider variety of clinical settings.

Clinical Utility of ECochG

The ECochG response is dependent on hearing sensitivity in the 1,000–4,000-Hz region. The major purposes of measuring ECochG include monitoring of cochlear and auditory nerve function during surgery, which could result in compromise of these functions, and improving the ease with which wave I is identified during ABR testing (Hall, 2007). Another area of clinical interest and application of the ECochG response is in the differential diagnosis of Meniere's disease. **Meniere's disease** is a disease of the inner ear, characterized by fluctuating hearing loss, vertigo, and tinnitus.

Middle Components of the Auditory Evoked Response

Auditory middle latency responses (AMLR) are relatively less well known than their earlier (auditory brainstem response) counterparts. These responses occur from 8 to 50 msec poststimulus. Early controversy regarding whether the middle components of the auditory evoked response originated from nerve or muscle activity (neurogenic versus myogenic) prevented them from being widely used clinically.

The actual components of the middle response are labeled as follows: No, Po, Na, Pa, and Nb. Pa is generally the most robust of the waves. As noted in Figure 6.39, approximate latencies for the middle components are as follows:

No: 8–10 msec   Pa: 30–45 msec

Po: 10–13 msec   Nb: 40–60 msec

Na: 16–30 msec   Pb: 55–80 msec

FIGURE **6.39** **Auditory middle response.**

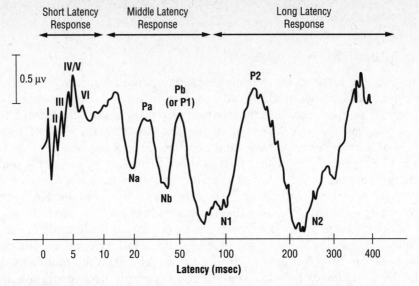

Sources: Gelfand, S. (2001). *Essentials of audiology* (2nd ed.). New York: Thieme. Reprinted by permission. American Speech-Language-Hearing Association Audiologic Evaluation Working Group on Auditory Evoked Potentials. (1987). *Short latency auditory evoked potentials.* Copyright by the American Speech-Language-Hearing Association. Reprinted by permission.

Actual latencies are relative and depend on the filter settings selected by the audiologist.

Recording the middle components requires a technique similar to that used in recording the ABR. Specifically, computer averaging is used to amplify the activity of interest and average out unnecessary background activity, such as biological activity. Similar to the ABR, the middle components reflect a potential difference between two electrodes. Summating these responses enables them to be used for diagnostic purposes. The electrode configuration used in recording the ABR and the AMLR is the same. Differences in recording the AMLR compared to ABR recording include:

	ABR	*AMLR*
Recording window	10–20 msec	50–100 msec
Rate of signal presentation	11–33/sec	8–10/sec
Filter settings	100–3,000 Hz	25–175 Hz

Note that, compared to recording the ABR, the AMLR involves a longer recording window, a slower stimulus repetition rate, and a lower frequency filter setting. The recording window for the AMLR is shown in Figure 6.39.

Effects of Subject State on the AMLR

Kraus et al. (1987) have shown that various factors affect recording of AMLRs, including:

- Sleep
- Sedation
- Age-related changes
- Filtering parameters
- Rate of stimulation
- Electrode placement

According to Hall (2007), the AMLR can be reliably recorded during light sleep, after mild sedation, and in different states of subject attention in adults. Studies have shown variable findings on the effects of sleep, sedation, and attention in the AMLR response of infants and children. This variability warrants and has resulted in further investigation to enhance the clinical usefulness of the AMLR.

Clinical Utility of the AMLR

One method of determining the usefulness of an evoked response involves manipulating factors such as those listed above to determine their effects on the AMLR. For example, a variety of filter settings might be used to determine the effect of a change in filter setting on the AMLR in a given population. Or researchers investigating the AMLR might look at this evoked response in individuals with various types of lesions to determine possible anatomic generator site(s) responsible for this evoked response. From work of this nature involving individuals with various defined cortical lesions, as well as studies that looked at the subject's state during recording of the AMLR (e.g., sleeping, sedated), the following general points were derived:

- Multiple generator sites appear to contribute to the AMLR, from the auditory pathway central to the brainstem. From their work with individuals with cortical lesions, Kraus, Ozdamar, Hier, and Stein (1982) suggested that the auditory cortex and thalamic projections are implicated as generator sites of Pa of the AMLR and, like the acoustic reflex, monaural stimulation produces Pa bilaterally. In other words, the generation of Pa appears to be bilateral for monaural stimulation.
- The most robust of the AMLR waves are Na and Pa (Kraus et al., 1982).
- Amplitude of Pa increases with age up to a certain age (Kraus et al., 1987).
- Recording of the AMLR is affected by filter settings; Kraus et al. (1987) found that use of high-pass filter settings ranging from 10 to 15 Hz resulted in a larger AMLR amplitude.
- The AMLR has been shown to mature over the first decade of life. There is a systematic increase in the detectability of wave Pa from birth through adolescence (Kraus et al., 1985).
- AMLRs are useful in the estimation of low-frequency hearing sensitivity (500–1,000 Hz); however, variability is greater in children than in adults.
- Kraus et al. (1985) concluded that the strong age effect that they saw in the AMLR made it difficult to draw conclusions about children's hearing from the presence or absence of an AMLR. In other words, an absent AMLR in a child does not necessarily correlate with hearing loss or auditory pathway dysfunction.
- Presence of the AMLR is unpredictable in children. This clinical limitation makes it necessary to use a test battery approach including the ABR for children. Simultaneous recording of the ABR and AMLR is possible.

The Auditory Steady-State Response

The **auditory steady-state response (ASSR)** has also been called the 40-Hz response and/or the **steady-state evoked potential (SSEP)**. This evoked potential differs from the previously described ABR and AMLR in that it is considered an "event-related potential." Unlike the previously discussed evoked potentials, which are elicited with brief duration clicks or tones, steady-state evoked potentials are elicited using steady-state tones.

In general, event-related potentials (ERPs) such as the auditory steady-state response are more influenced by the subject state of arousal and involve processing of the stimulus to some extent (Hall, 1992). ERPs are those evoked responses that are elicited with stimuli other than a sequence of brief duration clicks or tones (examples include the ASSR, the 40-Hz SSEP, and the P-300 response).

In the past, authors referred to the 40-Hz response as the 40-Hz event-related potential or 40-Hz ERP, while others referred to this response as a steady-state evoked potential (SSEP). Hall (2007) differentiates between the traditional 40-Hz response and more current auditory steady-state response (ASSR) research, which uses faster rates of amplitude and frequency modulation. The ASSR is a relative newcomer to electrophysiologic testing that has potential clinical use in supplementing the information available through ABR testing.

Recording Equipment and Techniques

ASSR responses are recorded in the same way as the ABR—the stimulus is delivered through earphones and the response is recorded via electrodes that have been placed on the client. The two main manufacturers of ASSR equipment are Bio-Logic System Corporation, Inc., which makes a device called the MASTER (for multiple auditory steady-state response), and GSI/VIASYS, which produces the Audera device. The MASTER can produce multiple independent amplitude and frequency modulation (IAFM) stimuli, allowing for simultaneous presentation and evaluation of multiple stimuli. The Audera device also does "traditional" auditory evoked response testing (e.g., ABR, electrocochleography, and AMLR testing). When obtaining ASSR measurements, the waveform takes place over a time span of 1,024 msec (or approximately 1 sec). Each time span is equal to an "epoch" and 16 epochs strung together equal 1 "sweep."

Stimulus Parameters

Audiologists are interested in ASSR as a way to help predict behavioral thresholds in individuals who cannot provide a behavioral response. Researchers are learning the types of stimuli that will provide this information. As you now know, ASSRs are obtained using a steady-state (versus brief or transient) stimulus. The steady-state stimulus (pure tone carrier frequency) can be modulated in amplitude or frequency or both, according to Venema (2005). Thus, the types of stimuli used in obtaining ASSR are pure tones that are either amplitude modulated (AM), frequency modulated (FM), or both (mixed modulation or MM).

Effect of Subject State and Physical Characteristics

The steady-state evoked potential, or 40-Hz response, is affected by the client's state of arousal, which limited its clinical use. For auditory steady-state responses elicited with faster stimulus rates, Hall (2007) and Dimitrijevic et al. (2004) note that sleep has a minimal effect. Hall further notes that there are no formal studies of the possible effects of attention and state of arousal on the ASSR. Dimitrijevic et al. also noted that the ASSR response amplitudes for IAFM stimuli are affected by physical characteristics including head size and skull thickness. Small and Stapells (2006) found that infant bone-conducted ASSR thresholds are very different from those of adults, and indicated that the differences are probably due to skull maturation. They also found differences in bone conduction ASSRs comparing preterm and older infants in this initial study of bone-conducted ASSRs in infants.

Clinical Utility of the ASSR

Wong and Stapells (2004) point out that ASSR is a promising method for prediction of hearing thresholds for both normal-hearing individuals and for listeners with hearing loss. They further note that an advantage of ASSR, compared to brainstem auditory evoked responses, is that analysis of ASSR is generated automatically. Thus, unlike ABR interpretation, ASSR analysis does not require subjective judgment about the presence or absence of certain waveforms.

John and colleagues (2004) studied the use of ASSRs in young infants, and recommended that ASSRs be used *after* the neonatal period to maximize accuracy. In addition to finding that a larger ASSR response is evoked when combined modulations of AM and FM stimuli are used (versus AM or FM tones alone), John et al. (2004) found that responses were easier to detect in relatively older infants (3–15 weeks of age) than in newborns. They further noted the need for more normative and clinical data on ASSRs.

Tests such as the ASSR help audiologists estimate hearing thresholds in individuals who cannot provide behavioral responses to sound, such as young children or people with developmental disabilities. Hall (2007) describes the main clinical advantage of the ASSR as its ability to define severe to profound hearing loss, specifically estimating hearing thresholds in the 80 to 120 dB range, something that is not possible with ABR. He advocates the use of ABR and ASSR in conjunction to assess the auditory abilities of children. The ability to estimate thresholds in this range would improve clinicians' ability to fit appropriate amplification, and enhance aural habilitation efforts for young children with hearing loss.

The study of ASSR has generated questions that require further research. While numerous studies have been conducted on adults, less information is known about ASSR in children. More information is needed to

- Establish the relationship between ASSR thresholds and behavioral thresholds in children
- Establish normative data for ASSR thresholds for various clinical devices for air-conducted and bone-conducted stimuli, particularly for infants and very young children
- Determine the optimal ASSR stimuli so that the response will be detected quickly and test time can be reduced

Results of a survey reported by Tannenbaum (2005) indicate that ASSR is gaining acceptance as a clinical tool that complements ABR. Current constraints reported by Tannenbaum included contending with noise, which increases the test time necessary to obtain accurate results. Clinicians also noted that future use of wireless communication would allow for the elimination of the wires and cables currently needed for ASSR testing, and allow for greater mobility for clients and audiologists.

Late Evoked Potentials

The **late auditory evoked potentials** occur from 50 to 250 msec after presentation of an auditory stimulus. They differ from their earlier counterparts in that the client's state plays a much greater role in the response obtained. In addition, the stimulus itself is presented at a slower rate. According to Hall (2007), the major waveforms that comprise the late auditory evoked potentials are illustrated in Figure 6.40 and include:

P1 (occurs in the range of 50–80 msec)

N1 (occurs in the range of 100–150 msec)

P2 (occurs in the range of 150–200 msec)

N2 (occurs in the range of 180–250 msec)

Stimulus Parameters

Hyde (1994) refers to the late evoked responses as the slow vertex potential (SVP) and indicates that a wide variety of stimuli may be used to elicit these responses, including clicks, tonebursts, syllables, as well as gaps in a tone or noise, with the most common stimulus being the toneburst. Typically, the toneburst is over 5 msec in duration, delivered at a rate of 2 per sec or less.

Clinical Utility of the Late Evoked Potentials

The late evoked potentials can be used to estimate auditory thresholds; however, the time required to estimate each threshold is approximately 5 to 10 minutes, making threshold estimation a lengthy procedure. In addition, unlike the earlier evoked responses, the late potentials are affected by the subject's state of arousal and cannot be obtained from a sedated individual. The clinical utility of these responses is further limited by a high degree of variability in the response, both within a single subject and between subjects.

Auditory P-300 Response

The **P-300 auditory evoked response** is an event-related potential that is affected by subject state and activity. The presentation rate used is relatively slow compared with the stimulus rates used to evoke the earlier potentials. The P-300 is typically recorded using an "oddball" paradigm. This means that the subject is presented with two or more different auditory stimuli, which are presented in a random sequence. One of the stimuli (e.g., tones or syllables) occurs less frequently (oddball stimulus). The subject is required to count the rare stimulus (the one occurring less frequently, typically 15 to 20 percent of the time). The resulting P-300 response is pictured in Figure 6.41 and is a arge vertex positive wave that occurs approximately 300 msec after the oddball stimulus. Because obtaining the P-300 response involves the subject's participation and attention to the task, this evoked potential is referred to as an endogenous response.

FIGURE 6.40 **Auditory late response.**

Auditory Late Response (ALR)

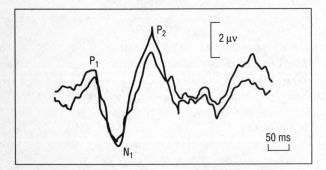

Source: Hall, James W., III. *Handbook of Auditory Evoked Responses,* 1e. Published by Allyn and Bacon, Boston, MA. Copyright © 1992 by Pearson Education. Adapted by permission of the publisher.

FIGURE 6.41 **Auditory P-300 response.**

225

•

Auditory Evoked
Potentials

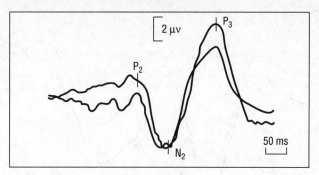

Auditory P-300 Response

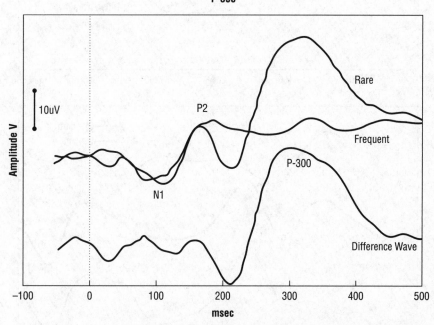

P-300

Source: Hall, James W., III. *Handbook of Auditory Evoked Responses,* 1e. Published by Allyn and Bacon, Boston, MA. Copyright © 1992 by Pearson Education. Adapted by permission of the publisher.

Clinical Utility. The same factors that play a role in obtaining the P-300 response (e.g., attention to the task, ability to discriminate stimuli from one another) are those that are of interest in studying higher-level auditory functions, such as those involved in auditory processing. Research regarding the relationships between the P-300 response and auditory perceptual tasks (e.g., understanding speech in noise) in various populations may result in more widespread application of this event-related potential to clinical investigation of auditory processing abilities.

FIGURE 6.42   **Mismatched negativity response.**

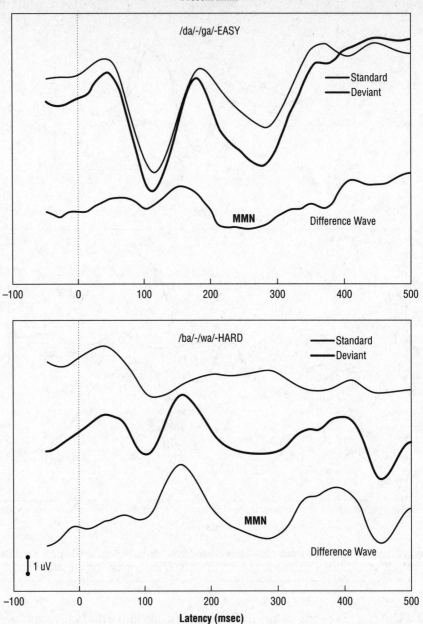

Source: Kraus, N., McGee, T., Ferre, J., Hoeppner, J., Carrell, T., Sharma, A., & Nicol, T. (1993). Mismatch negativity in the neurophysiologic/behavioral evaluation of auditory processing deficits: A case study. *Ear and Hearing, 14*(4), 223–234. Reprinted by permission.

Mismatched Negativity

Mismatched negativity (MMN) is a cortical event-related potential. Kraus et al. (1993) characterize the mismatched negativity (MMN) evoked potential as a recording of sensory processing within auditory cortex. Additional features of the MMN response described by Kraus et al. include the following:

- MMN is a passively elicited, objective measure.
- MMN does not require a behavioral response.
- MMN is a neuronal response to minimal changes in acoustic parameters such as frequency, intensity, location, and duration.
- MMN can be elicited by speech stimuli such as syllables, including relatively easier versus more difficult minimal contrast pairs.

MMN is reportedly more variable and difficult to record than the other evoked potentials reviewed. Kraus et al. (1993) indicate that a statistical analysis procedure is used to verify the presence of the MMN. Presence of the response is illustrated in Figure 6.42 and an absent response is shown in Figure 6.43. The general characteristics of the MMN response described above make it appealing to researchers in the investigation of the relative contribution of peripheral and central aspects of the auditory pathway to the processing of auditory information.

FIGURE 6.43   Absence of mismatched negativity response.

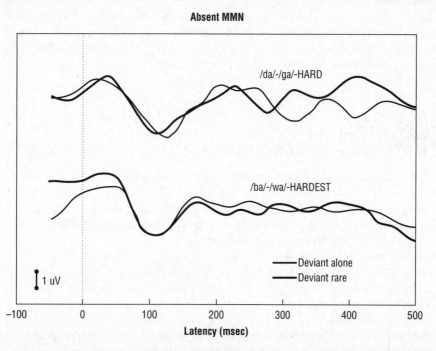

Source: Kraus, N., McGee, T., Ferre, J., Hoeppner, J., Carrell, T., Sharma, A., & Nicol, T. (1993). Mismatch negativity in the neurophysiologic/behavioral evaluation of auditory processing deficits: A case study. *Ear and Hearing, 14*(4), 223–234. Reprinted by permission.

CHAPTER SUMMARY

This chapter presented a number of objective ways to measure auditory system function. Middle ear function can be assessed using the immittance test battery, which includes tympanometry and acoustic reflex testing. Otoacoustic emissions were defined and discussed. Early, middle, late, and cortical auditory evoked potentials were introduced and their clinical uses were discussed. Stacked auditory brainstem response and the auditory steady-state response were also defined and described.

At this point, we have seen that there are behavioral and objective ways to measure auditory system function. Often, a combination of these assessment methods is necessary to obtain a complete picture of a client's auditory system. It is important that clinicians understand the questions they are attempting to answer about an individual's auditory system function and select the test(s) that will provide the information in the most efficient manner. In addition, clinicians must understand the potential interactions among different tests. For example, absent ABR responses may be related to a severe hearing loss or to an auditory nerve/brainstem disorder.

In addition, the order in which the tests are given can be altered to make the test battery serve the client's needs. For example, starting the test session with tympanometry makes sense if ruling out middle ear involvement is a primary concern. Establishing the status of the middle ear can eliminate the need for bone conduction testing (when middle ear function is normal) or clue the clinician that bone conduction testing with masking is likely to be required during the session (when middle ear function is abnormal).

In closing, it is incumbent on clinicians to make use of a variety of information and to tailor audiological assessment to the individual needs of each client. This is consistent with ASHA standards for service provision, which require that clinicians strive to use all available tools to meet the needs of people in their care.

QUESTIONS FOR DISCUSSION

1. Discuss advantages and disadvantages of objective versus behavioral tests of the auditory system.
2. Name and describe the components of the immittance test battery.
3. Discuss the two main purposes of auditory brainstem response (ABR) testing. Include differences in test administration and interpretation.
4. Describe the clinical utility of middle, late, and cognitive evoked potentials.
5. Discuss the clinical information that otoacoustic emissions provide. Include the specific aspects of the auditory system that are assessed using this technique.
6. What types of stimuli are used to generate the auditory steady-state response?
7. What is the main advantage of the ASSR compared with the ABR?
8. How would this advantage be helpful in early hearing detection and intervention programs?
9. Briefly describe the steps involved in obtaining stacked ABRs.
10. What are some advantages of using ABR versus MRI in the detection of acoustic tumors?

RECOMMENDED READING

American Speech-Language-Hearing Association (ASHA). (1997). *Guidelines for screening infants and children for outer and middle ear disorder, birth through 18 years.* Volume IV-74k-74r.

American Speech-Language-Hearing Association (ASHA). (2002). Guidelines for competencies in auditory evoked potential measurement and clinical applications. *ASHA* (Suppl. 23), pp. 35–40.

American Speech-Language-Hearing Association (ASHA). (2003). Guidelines for competencies in auditory evoked potential measurement and clinical applications. *ASHA* (Suppl. 23), in press.

Cone-Wesson, B., Dowell, R., Tomlin, D., Rance, G., & Ming, W. (2002).The auditory steady-state response: Comparisons with the auditory brainstem response. *Journal of the American Academy of Audiology, 13*(4), 173–187.

Hall, J. (2000). *Handbook of otoacoustic emissions.* New York: Delmar Thomson Learning.

Hall, J. W. III. (2007). *The new handbook of auditory evoked responses.* Boston: Allyn & Bacon.

Kei, J., Allison-Levick, J., Dockray, J., Harrays, R., Kirkegard, C., Wong, J., Maurer, M., Hegarty, J., Young, J., & Tudehope, D. (2003). High-frequency (1000 Hz) tympanometry in normal neonates. *Journal of the American Academy of Audiology, 14*(1), 20–28.

Rance, G., & Rickards, F. (2002). Prediction of hearing thresholds in infants using steady-state evoked potentials. *Journal of the American Academy of Audiology, 13*(5), 236–245.

Roeser, R. J. (1996). *Roeser's audiology desk reference.* New York: Thieme.

Wiley, T., & Stoppenbach, D. (2002). Basic principles of acoustic immittance measures. In J. Katz (Ed.), *Handbook of clinical audiology* (5th ed.). New York: Lippincott, Williams & Wilkins.

REFERENCES

American National Standards Institute (ANSI). (1987). Specifications for instruments to measure aural acoustic impedance and admittance (aural acoustic immittance). ANSI S3.39-1987. New York: Author.

American Speech-Language-Hearing Association (ASHA). (1990). Competencies in auditory evoked potential measurement and clinical applications. *ASHA, 32*(Suppl. 2), 13–16.

American Speech-Language-Hearing Association (ASHA). (1992). Sedation and topical anesthetics in audiology and speech-language pathology. *ASHA, 34*(Suppl. 7), 41–42.

American Speech-Language-Hearing Association (ASHA). (1997). *Guidelines for screening infants and children for outer and middle ear disorder, birth through 18 years.* Volume IV-74k-74r.

Bess, F. H., & Humes, L. E. (1995). *Audiology: The fundamentals* (2nd ed.). Baltimore: Lippincott, Williams & Wilkins.

Burch-Sims, P., & Ochs, M. T. (1992). The anatomic and physiologic bases of otoacoustic emissions. *The Hearing Journal, 45*(11), 9–10.

Dimitrijevic, A., John, M. S., & Picton, T. W. (2004). Auditory steady-state responses and word recognition scores in normal-hearing and hearing-impaired adults. *Ear & Hearing, 25*(1), 68–84.

Don, M. (2005). The stacked ABR: An alternative screening tool for small acoustic tumors. *The Hearing Review,* 30–32.

Don, M. A., Kwong, B. A., Tanaka, C. B., Brackmann, D. C., & Nelson, R. C. (2005). The stacked ABR: A sensitive and specific screening tool for detecting small acoustic tumors. *Audiology & Neuro-Otology, 10*(5), 274–290.

El-Kashlan, H. K., Eisenmann, D., & Kileny, P. R. (2000). Auditory brainstem response in small acoustic neuromas. *Ear and Hearing, 21*(3), 257–262.

Gelfand, S. (2001). *Essentials of audiology* (2nd ed.). New York: Thieme.

Gelfand, S. (2001). The acoustic reflex. In J. Katz (Ed.), *Handbook of clinical audiology* (p. 206). Baltimore: Lippincott, Williams & Wilkins.

Hall, J., & Mueller, H. G. (1997). *Audiologist's desk reference volume 1: Diagnostic audiology principles, procedures and practices.* San Diego: Singular.

Hall, J. W. III. (1992). *Handbook of auditory evoked responses.* Boston: Allyn & Bacon.

Hall, J. W. III. (2004). ABRs or ASSRs? The application of tone-burst ABRs in the era of ASSRs. *The Hearing Review, 11*(9), 22–30, 60–62.

Hall, J. W. III. (2007). *The new handbook of auditory evoked responses.* Boston: Allyn & Bacon.

Hyde, M. L. (1994). The slow vertex potential: Properties and clinical applications. In J. T. Jacobson (Ed.), *Principles and applications in auditory evoked potentials* (pp. 179–218). Boston: Allyn & Bacon.

Interview with Manuel Don, Ph.D., Electrophysiology Department Head, House Ear Institute, Los Angeles, California. (2005, April 11). *Audiology Online Interview.* Available from http://www.audiologyonline.com/interview/interview_detail.asp?interview_id=336

Jerger, J. (1970). Clinical experience with impedance audiometry. *Archives of Otolaryngology, 92,* 311–324.

Jerger, J. F., & Hayes, D. (1976). The cross-check principle in pediatric audiometry. *Archives of Otolaryngology, 102,* 614–620.

John, M. S., Brown, D. K., Muir, P. J., & Picton, T. W. (2004). Recording auditory steady-state responses in young infants. *Ear & Hearing, 25*(6), 539–553.

Kemp, D. (1978). Stimulated acoustic emission from the human auditory system. *Journal of the Acoustical Society of America, 64,* 1386–1391.

Kemp, D. T., Ryan, S., & Bray, P. (1990). A guide to the effective use of otoacoustic emissions. *Ear and Hearing, 11*(2), 93–105.

Kraus, N., McGee, T., Ferre, J., Hoeppner, J., Carrell, T., Sharma, A., & Nicol, T. (1993). Mismatch negativity in the neurophysiologic/behavioral evaluation of auditory processing deficits: A case study. *Ear and Hearing, 14*(4), 223–234.

Kraus, N., Ozdamar, O., Hier, D., & Stein, L. (1982). Auditory middle latency responses (MLRs) in patients with cortical lesions. *Electroencephalography and Clinical Neurophysiology, 54,* 275–287.

Kraus, N., Reed, N., Smith, D. I., Stein, L., & Cartee, C. (1987). High-pass filter settings affect the detectability of MLRs in humans. *Electroencephalography and Clinical Neurophysiology, 68,* 234–236.

Kraus, N., Smith, D., Reed, N. L., Stein, L. K., & Cartee, C. (1985). Auditory middle latency responses in children: Effects of age and diagnostic category. *Electroencephalography and Clinical Neurophysiology, 62,* 343–351.

Lonsbury-Martin, B. L., & Martin, G. K. (1990). The clinical utility of distortion-product emissions. *Ear and Hearing, 11,* 144–154.

Lonsbury-Martin, B. L., McCoy, M. J., Whitehead, M. L., & Martin, G. K. (1992). Otoacoustic emissions: Future directions for research and clinical applications. *The Hearing Journal, 45*(11), 47–52.

Margolis, R. H., & Hunter, L. L. (2000). Acoustic immittance measurements. In R. J. Roeser, M. Valente, & H. Hosford-Dunn (Eds.), *Audiology diagnosis* (pp. 381–423). New York: Thieme.

Nozza, R., Bluestone, C., Kardatzke, D., & Bachman, R. (1992). Towards the validation of aural acoustic immittance measures for diagnosis of middle ear effusion in children. *Ear and Hearing, 13,* 442–453.

Nozza, R., Bluestone, C., Kardatzke, D., & Bachman, R. (1994). Identification of middle ear effusion by aural acoustic admittance and otoscopy. *Ear and Hearing, 15,* 310–323.

Shanks, J. E., & Lilly, D. J. (1981). An evaluation of tympanometric estimates of ear canal volume. *Journal of Speech and Hearing Research, 24,* 557–566.

Silman, S., Silverman, C. A., & Arick, D. S. (1992). Acoustic-immittance screening detection of middle-ear effusion in children. *Journal of the American Academy of Audiology, 3,* 262–268.

Sininger, Y. S. (2005). Following up on newborn hearing screening, or why are all my patients such babies? *The Hearing Journal, 58*(5), 10–15.

Small, S. A., & Stapells, D. R. (2004). Artifactual responses when recording auditory steady-state responses. *Ear & Hearing, 25*(6), 611–623.

Small, S. A., & Stepells, D. R. (2006). Multiple auditory steady-state response thresholds to bone-conduction stimuli in young infants with normal hearing. *Ear & Hearing, 27*(3), 219–228.

Stach, B. (1998). *Clinical audiology: An introduction* (p. 314). San Diego: Singular.

Stover, L., Gorga, M., Neely, S., & Montoya, D. (1996). Toward optimizing the clinical utility of distortion product otoacoustic emission measurements. *Journal of the Acoustical Society of America, 100,* 956–967.

Tannenbaum, S. (2005). Clinician survey: ABRs & ASSRs in post-newborn screening applications. *The Hearing Review,* 50–51, 94.

Venema, T. (2005, June). The ASSR revisited: A clinical comparison of two stimuli. *The Hearing Review,* 54–59, 70–71.

Wiley, T., Cruickshanks, K., Nondahl, D., Tweed, T., Klein, R., & Klein, B. (1996). Tympanometric measures in older adults. *Journal of the American Academy of Audiology, 7,* 260–268.

Wong, W. Y. S., & Stapells, D. R. (2004). Brain stem and cortical mechanisms underlying the binaural masking level difference in humans: An auditory steady-state response study. *Ear & Hearing, 25*(1), 57–67.

Appendix A
Answers to Tympanogram Cases 1–4

Case 1. Normal middle ear pressure, normal tympanic membrane admittance, and normal ear canal volume. This is consistent with normal middle ear mobility and Eustachian tube function.

Case 2. Negative middle ear pressure, reduced admittance, and normal ear canal volume. The finding of negative middle ear pressure is consistent with Eustachian tube dysfunction. Reduced compliance suggests some middle ear stiffness.

Case 3. Normal middle ear pressure, reduced admittance, and normal ear canal volume. The finding of reduced compliance may be consistent with a stiffness-dominated middle ear system. A typical cause of this tympanometric pattern is otosclerosis, a condition discussed in Chapter 7.

Case 4. Large ear canal volume. A large ear canal volume is consistent with an open middle ear system, meaning that we are measuring the volume from the end of the probe up to and including the middle ear cavity. The most likely causes for this result include a perforated tympanic membrane, a patent (open) pressure equalization (PE) tube; less commonly, a surgically altered ear. Remember, ideally, tympanometric results would be interpreted along with other parts of the immittance and audiological test battery and other medical/diagnostic information.

chapter 7

Disorders of the Auditory System

AFTER COMPLETING THIS CHAPTER, YOU SHOULD BE ABLE TO:

1. Describe disorders that can affect the outer ear and their effects on audiological assessment and test results.
2. Describe conditions that can affect the middle ear, including effects on hearing and on development of speech and language skills.
3. Describe disorders that can affect the inner ear, including effects on hearing.
4. Understand the effects of vestibular schwannomas in earlier versus later stages.
5. List three disorders of the central auditory system and their potential effects on a person's communication function.
6. Name and identify the relevant inner ear structures involved in balance.
7. Briefly describe the three systems that provide input for balance.
8. Define *nystagmus* and describe its role in balance testing.
9. Describe the major tests that make up comprehensive balance testing.
10. Distinguish between stable and unstable lesions and discuss how they affect vestibular rehabilitation.

The clinical work of audiologists and speech–language pathologists relies on a solid foundation in normal anatomy and physiology of the auditory system and the pathological conditions that may affect the auditory system. In addition, practicing clinicians typically have established relationships with primary health care providers so that when issues requiring medical attention are identified, appropriate referrals can be made. According to the American Speech-Language-Hearing Association (2003) Code of Ethics, one rule of ethics provides that "individuals shall use every resource, including referral when appropriate, to ensure that high-quality service is provided" (p. 1). This is consistent with a humanistic approach to provision of audiological care.

In this section you will learn about some pathological conditions of the outer, middle, and inner ears. Generally speaking, conditions that affect the outer and middle ear systems should be assessed by health care providers and may be remediated through medical assessment and intervention. For example, individuals with clinical test results including a reddened tympanic membrane and middle ear analysis results indicating a

TABLE 7.1 Selected Conditions of the Outer, Middle, and Inner Ears

Outer Ear	Middle Ear	Inner Ear
(Acute) external otitis	Tympanic membrane perforation	Vestibular schwannoma
Infection	Discontinuity of ossicular chain	Diabetes
Injuries	Otosclerosis	Facial nerve disorders
Carcinoma of external ear	Malleus fixation	Meniere's disease
Cysts	Eustachian tube dysfunction	Noise-induced hearing loss/noise trauma
Tumors	Otitis media	
Collapsing ear canal	Barotrauma	Ototoxicity
Cerumen (wax)	Glomus jugulare tumor	Presbycusis
Stenosis		Head trauma (concussion, temporal bone fracture)
Atresia/microtia		
Otalgia		

fluid-filled middle ear (commonly referred to as an "ear infection") would be referred first to their primary health care provider for assessment and medical management as appropriate. Conversely, an individual with a sensorineural hearing loss due to aging (for whom there is no medical or surgical treatment) may have a brief consultation with the primary physician and receive a referral directly to the audiologist, who will diagnose the hearing loss and may recommend a trial period with hearing aids.

Table 7.1 summarizes selected conditions that may affect the outer, middle, and inner ears that practicing clinicians may encounter.

Selected Conditions That May Affect the Outer Ear

External Otitis

Acute **external otitis** is an infection of the external ear characterized by thickened skin on the external ear and external auditory canal. External otitis is also called "swimmer's ear." In this condition, fluid collects in the tissues along with red blood cells and the ear becomes very tender. As the condition worsens, "weeping" of the skin may be observed. Following the symptoms of pain and drainage, the individual commonly experiences hearing loss, as the lumen (opening) of the external auditory meatus closes off. Treatment for external otitis typically involves prescription of eardrops by a health care provider.

Infection: Cellulitis and Perichondritis

Other types of infections that may affect the outer ear include cellulitis and perichondritis. **Cellulitis** is defined as an infection of the skin, not involving the perichondrium, (nutritive connective tissue). If this condition continues untreated, an abscess may occur.

An **abscess** is a collection of living and dead bacteria. **Perichondritis,** named because it does affect the perichondrium, is the next level of external ear infection, and is characterized by edema (swelling), redness, and tenderness. If untreated, this condition progresses to involve the cartilage of the external ear and can lead to serious complications.

Injuries

Injury to the external ear can occur due to sunburn, frostbite, chemical injuries, and radiation. In addition, trauma to the ear canal may be caused by aggressive use of cotton swabs or insertion of a foreign object (common in children).

Carcinoma of the External Ear

Tumors may be benign (noncancerous) or malignant (cancerous) in nature. Three types of malignant tumors affecting the ear are (1) basal cell carcinoma, (2) squamous cell carcinoma, and (3) melanoma.

In **basal cell carcinoma,** the basal skin layer grows "out of control" but does not metastasize; it may spread locally and is malignant. This condition is usually related to sun exposure and may occur anywhere on the pinna (external ear).

Squamous cell carcinoma is the most common malignant tumor of the pinna; it is more invasive because it can travel via blood vessels and the lymph stream/system. Presentation is generally on the pinna in males and near the concha in females.

Melanoma is a malignancy of the pigment cells that spreads through the bloodstream; a high mortality rate is associated with this condition.

In addition to cancerous changes of the outer ear, a number of types of benign cysts (growths that are liquid and contain spaces) and tumors (abnormal growth of tissue) may affect the ear. A sample of the various types of cysts and tumors are summarized in Table 7.2.

Collapsing Ear Canal

Although not necessarily a pathological condition, **collapsing ear canal** deserves to be mentioned because it can affect the outcomes of both audiological testing and rehabilitation efforts. This condition typically affects older individuals and young infants and results from a loss of elasticity in the cartilage of the external ear. The force of the headband connected to the supra-aural earphones can cause the ear canals to collapse during audiological testing. Recall our earlier discussion of air and bone conduction testing. You should be able to appreciate how this would interfere with reliable hearing assessment. The collapsed canals cause air conduction results to be poorer than they should be, but bone conduction results are not affected. A false (usually high-frequency) conductive hearing loss is often recorded. This problem can sometimes be alleviated by repositioning the earphones or using a handheld earphone. Another option is the use of insert earphones, which direct sound to a tube that is inserted into the ear canal. Use of insert earphones has other advantages over supra-aural earphones, which were discussed in Chapter 4.

Cerumen

Cerumen, or earwax, is formed from a combination of secretions from ceruminous and sebacious glands that line the outer third of the external auditory canal. Cerumen is a

TABLE **7.2**   **Cysts and Tumors of the Pinna and External Auditory Canal**

Cyst	Definition/Characteristics
Pseudocyst	Has no lining; no secretory function. A collection of fluid in a tissue space without an epithelial lining; may be due to trauma (e.g., a hematoma) or infection (e.g., perichondritis).
Sebacious cyst	Comprised of a wall around fluid; results from blockage of sebaceous glands.
Preauricular cyst and fistula	Congenital abnormalities resulting from faulty developmental closure of the first and second branchial arches; may be unilateral or bilateral. These present as a pitlike depression just in front of the helix and above the tragus, or the depression may lead to a cyst or epidermis-lined fistulous tract with intermittent or continuous foul discharge (in scant amounts).
Dermoid cyst	A congenital cyst; composed of skin containing hair follicles, sweat glands, and sebaceous glands, found below the skin surface, typically behind the pinna; appendages have secretory function.

Tumor	Definition/Characteristics
Osteoma	Rare condition, usually unilateral; consists of skin covered by bone growth; may cause pain with increase in size; may obstruct normal migration of squamous epithelium outward. Four characteristics: (1) round, (2) narrow base, (3) usually unilateral, (4) skin covered.
Exostosis	All bone; attached to osseous portion of ear canal; "classic" history involves cold water exposure (e.g., swimming in the ocean). Five characteristics: (1) very wide base, (2) usually bilateral, (3) history of exposure to cold, (4) can occlude the ear canal, (5) not round.
Lipoma	A fatty tumor, primarily poses a cosmetic problem.
Keloid	Usually related to ear trauma; involves an overabundance of collagen; associated with ear piercing.

waxlike substance that has a protective function, trapping substances that might enter the ear canal. Although in the normal condition cerumen moves on its own to the outer part of the ear canal, in some cases it accumulates and the external auditory canal becomes closed off (occluded). This causes a conductive hearing loss. Possible causes of wax accumulation include overly aggressive use of cotton swabs, narrow ear canals, and use of hearing aids. Treatment typically involves removal of the wax, either by irrigation or by use of a curette, which is a special instrument with a loop at the end designed for this purpose. Because wax can sometimes become hard and adhere to the wall of the ear canal, use of a softening agent (applied as drops) for several days prior to actual removal is often helpful. Some audiologists pursue specialized training to enable them to perform cerumen management for their clients. Figure 7.1 compares a normal external auditory canal (EAC) with a wax-filled EAC.

FIGURE **7.1** **Normal and wax-filled external auditory canal.**

237

•

Selected
Conditions That
May Affect the
Outer Ear

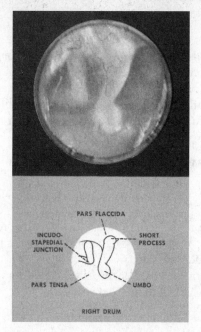

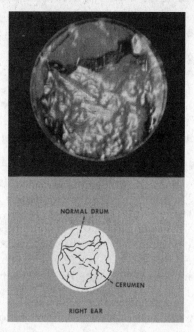

Source: Reprinted by permission of Abbott Laboratories.

Stenosis

Stenosis is the formal term for narrowing of an opening; in this case it refers to narrowing of the external auditory canal. Stenosis may occur for a variety of reasons, including trauma, inflammation due to infection, and genetics. Also, aging can cause stenosis, as the muscles supporting the walls of the ear canals become weak.

Atresia and Microtia

Atresia is a disease of the external auditory canal involving absence of the normal opening to the canal. Atresia may be congenital (present at birth) or acquired (e.g., by trauma). As was discussed previously, the first one-third of the ear canal courses through cartilage (referred to as the membranous portion) and the remaining two-thirds courses through bone (referred to as the osseous portion). Atresia may be membranous or bony. If it is membranous, a dense soft tissue plug will be present between the external auditory canal and the middle ear space. Bony atresia involves a wall of bone that separates the ear canal from the middle ear space. In either case, there will be associated conductive hearing loss. Surgical construction is the typical intervention, presuming cochlear function is good. **Microtia** may be defined as an abnormally small pinna and typically occurs with atresia. The term *microtia* is also sometimes used to refer to a broader range of abnormalities of the pinna. In some cases the external ear affected by microtia has the normal landmarks of the pinna but is smaller in size; in other cases the pinna is composed of tissue that does not resemble the shape of a normal external ear.

Otalgia

Although it is technically not a condition of the ear, *otalgia* is a term students and clinicians should be familiar with. **Otalgia** is the term used for ear pain, and although it may seem logical to think that the presence of ear pain means some pathology of the ear, the fact is that more than half of the time ear pain is the result of pathology in a different part of the body. When this occurs, the term *referred pain* is used. Four main nerves innervate the ear and can be sources of referred pain:

1. Cranial nerve V (trigeminal): innervates the tympanic membrane (eardrum), jaw, and temporomandibular joint (TMJ)
2. Cranial nerve VII (facial): drives the muscles of the face and has a branch in the ear canal
3. Cranial nerve IX (glossopharyngeal): provides the main sensory input for the throat, back of the mouth, tonsil area, and part of the tongue; also innervates the inside of the tympanic membrane and middle ear cavity
4. Cranial nerve X (vagus): provides sensation to part of the external auditory canal and collateral innervation with cranial nerve IX to the back of the throat

After reviewing the innervation sites, it should be clear why common sources of referred pain are the teeth, tongue, tonsils, and throat.

Selected Conditions That May Affect the Middle Ear

Table 7.3 includes conditions that are known to affect the middle ear.

Tympanic Membrane Perforation

A **tympanic membrane perforation** may be defined as an abnormal opening in a structure of the membrane. There are three types of perforations: (1) central perforations, (2) marginal perforations, and (3) retraction pockets (not true perforations). Hearing loss due to perforation of the tympanic membrane may range from 0 to 40 dB, depending on the size and location of the perforation and the presence or absence of purulent (infected) or other drainage from the middle ear. The condition of the mucous membrane lining the middle ear is also a factor. A large equivalent ear canal volume, as

---

TABLE **7.3** **Selected Conditions Affecting the Middle Ear**

Tympanic membrane perforation	Eustachian tube dysfunction
Cholesteatoma	Otitis media
Discontinuity of ossicular chain	Barotrauma
Otosclerosis	Glomus jugulare tumor
Malleus fixation	

discussed in Chapter 6, is a key measure in the diagnosis of tympanic membrane perforation. Before discussing these specific types of perforations, it should be noted that causes of perforations include trauma, thermal burns, foreign bodies in the ear canal, skull fractures, and ear infections. Trauma, the most common cause of perforations, involves a quick buildup of air pressure, causing changes in the hydraulic system of the tympanic membrane and ear. Thermal burns are more likely than other types of injury to lead to a permanent perforation. A thermal burn could occur, for example, as a result of a welding accident or mishandling of fireworks. Foreign bodies in the ear canal may cause perforations to occur either on entry or when removal is attempted. Perforations resulting from middle ear infections result from the pressure of fluid from the middle ear space pressing against the eardrum. These generally heal once the infection is cleared.

Central perforations are perforations in the pars tensa of the tympanic membrane in which the rim of the perforation does not make contact with the annulus. Common causes of central perforations are trauma and infection.

Marginal perforations are perforations involving the annulus in which skin can migrate into the middle ear space. The opportunity for skin to migrate into the middle ear space differentiates marginal perforations from central perforations and makes marginal perforations more dangerous. Why? Because migration of skin into the middle ear space can result in a tumorlike mass referred to as a **cholesteatoma**. Chronic otitis media can also be a cause of this growth. Symptoms of cholesteatoma can include otorrhea, hearing loss, vertigo, tinnitus, pain, headaches, facial nerve paralysis, and Eustachian tube dysfunction. Management generally involves surgical removal of the cholesteatoma. Objectives of management are threefold: elimination of the disease, restoration of hearing through rehabilitation, and prevention of further complications, including bone erosions and intracranial complications. Figure 7.2A shows a small perforation on a right tympanic membrane (TM). Figure 7.2B shows a large marginal perforation on a right TM.

Depending on the size and exact location of the perforation, spontaneous healing sometimes occurs. In other cases, surgical repair, referred to as **myringoplasty**, is performed. A broader term associated with reconstructive surgery performed on the middle ear is **tympanoplasty**.

Retraction "perforations" are also referred to as "attic retraction pockets" and occur when negative middle ear pressure causes the eardrum to retract (pull in) and a pocket forms in the area of the pars flaccida. The pocket then fills with squamous debris that can further develop into an attic cholesteatoma.

Figure 7.3 (page 241) shows an audiogram of a unilateral right conductive hearing loss on a child. Note that the ear canal volume on the right side exceeds the normative values, a finding consistent with an open middle ear system, caused in this case by a perforated right TM.

Important Things to Remember in Cases Such as This

1. In reporting the results to the physician, it is important for the audiologist to point out the pattern of test results and to include information about a potential cause(s). Although audiologists do not make medical diagnoses, their results are important to the confirmation of a diagnosis by an otolaryngologist or pediatrician. It is important to pay attention to the ear canal volume when reporting immitance

FIGURE **7.2**   **Small and large tympanic membrane perforations.**
Small tympanic membrane perforation (a) and large marginal
perforation (b).

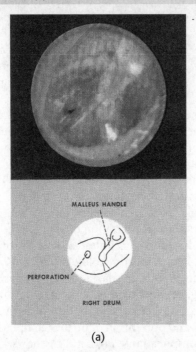

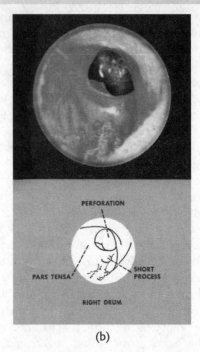

(a)   (b)

Source: Reprinted by permission of Abbott Laboratories.

results. An ear canal volume that significantly exceeds the normative values is most
commonly associated with a perforated tympanic membrane.

2. Next steps following diagnosis of conductive hearing loss should include management of the condition by a physician. Next, if the hearing loss persists despite medical
management, an assessment of the degree to which the hearing loss interferes with
the client's communication ability is needed. In cases of young children with conductive hearing loss, attention must be given to their speech and language development.
For school-age children, classroom performance should be monitored closely. For
some individuals, medical management does not alleviate the hearing loss associated
with conductive involvement, and amplification, with otologic clearance, is needed.

Discontinuity of the Ossicular Chain

Damage to the ossicular chain can involve one or all of the ossicles. A break or fracture
can occur in the manubrium (handle of the malleus), the long process of the incus, or
in the stapes. The incus can become dislocated. Discontinuity of the ossicular chain can
result from head trauma with or without a skull fracture, or from direct trauma to the
tympanic membrane (e.g., resulting from insertion of a cotton swab or other object too
far into the ear canal). Audiometric findings typically include a large unilateral conductive hearing loss; elevated admittance is noted on tympanometry. For clients with

FIGURE **7.3** **Unilateral right conductive hearing loss.**

241

Selected
Conditions That
May Affect the
Middle Ear

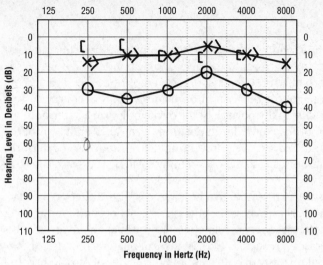

Audiogram Key

	Right	Left
AC Unmasked	○	×
AC Masked	△	☐
BC Mastoid Unmasked	<	>
BC Mastoid Masked	⌐	⌐
BC Forehead Masked	⌐	⌐

Both

BC Forehead Unmasked   ⋎
Sound Field   S

**Examples of
No Response Symbols**

Speech Audiometry

Ear	SRT	SDT	PTA 5-2	Test	Word Recognition Level/Percent Correct	MCL	LDL
Right	25		28	W22	+40/96%		
Left	10		8	W22	+40/100%		
Bone							
Sound Field							
Right Aided							
Left Aided							
Binaural Aided							

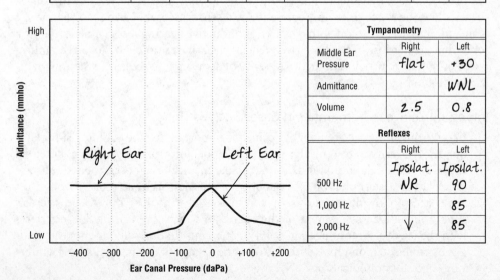

Tympanometry

	Right	Left
Middle Ear Pressure	flat	+30
Admittance		WNL
Volume	2.5	0.8

Reflexes

	Right	Left
500 Hz	Ipsilat. NR	Ipsilat. 90
1,000 Hz	↓	85
2,000 Hz	↓	85

ossicular discontinuity, surgical techniques are often possible to repair the bones involved or to replace an ossicle with wire or teflon.

Otosclerosis

Otosclerosis may be defined as a lesion of the osseous or bony portion of the inner ear and of the stapedial footplate. In this condition, a layer of new bone is laid down at the same time older bone is resorbed, producing a spongy type of bone. For this reason, perhaps a more appropriate name for this condition is *otospongiosis*. This abnormal bone growth most typically occurs in the portion of the oval window just anterior to the stapes footplate, causing the footplate to wedge in position (also called **ankylosis** of the stapes in the oval window) and fixing it (i.e., preventing it from moving) posteriorly. Nearly half of the clients with otosclerosis report a family history of disease, and it is twice as common in females.

Otosclerosis typically results in a conductive hearing loss in the affected ear. The degree of hearing loss generally progresses as the stapes footplate becomes more fixed. Otosclerosis usually affects both ears (occurs bilaterally), but unilateral involvement is reported in 10–15 percent of cases (Derlacki, 1996). In cases of bilateral otosclerosis, the condition may not occur simultaneously in both ears, and the degree of otosclerosis and associated hearing loss may not be the same. When otosclerosis occurs, the tympanic membrane (eardrum) is almost always normal, so diagnosticians must depend on the client's history and audiometric findings, which will have characteristic features (including audiometric air–bone gaps signifying conductive involvement in the hearing loss and middle ear testing supporting "stiffness" in the middle ear system).

In addition, in the initial stages of the disease, the shape (configuration) of the audiogram is upward-rising, meaning that hearing is less impaired in the higher frequencies. As the disease progresses, the shape becomes flatter. Also, a unique feature of otosclerosis is the presence of Carhart's notch on the audiogram. This refers to what appears as bone conduction loss of approximately 15 dB at 2,000 Hz. Actually, it is an artifact related to impairment of bone conduction that is caused by fixation of the stapes footplate. The fact that this notch disappears following surgery to remove the stapes suggests that the notch does not represent a real sensorineural hearing loss. Figure 7.4 is an audiogram of a person with a bilateral conductive hearing loss characterized by a somewhat greater loss in the lower frequencies, a Carhart's notch at 2,000 Hz, and reduced admittance by tympanometry. Absence of acoustic reflexes is consistent with bilateral air–bone gaps.

Important Things to Remember in Cases Such as This

1. In reporting the results to the physician, it is important for the audiologist to point out the pattern of test results and to include information about a potential cause(s). Although audiologists do not make medical diagnoses, their results are critical to the determination of a diagnosis of otosclerosis by an otolaryngologist.
2. Next steps following diagnosis of conductive hearing loss due to otosclerosis should include an assessment of the degree to which the hearing loss interferes with the client's communication ability. After consultation with an otolaryngologist or otologist, individuals with this condition may opt for medical/surgical intervention or for amplification.

FIGURE **7.4** **Bilateral conductive hearing loss.**

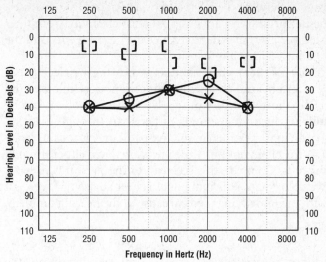

Audiogram Key		
	Right	Left
AC Unmasked	○	✕
AC Masked	△	☐
BC Mastoid Unmasked	＜	＞
BC Mastoid Masked	⊏	⊐
BC Forehead Masked	⌐	⌐

Both	
BC Forehead Unmasked	Ⅴ
Sound Field	S

Examples of No Response Symbols	
○	✕

Speech Audiometry

Ear	SRT	SDT	PTA 5-2	Test	Word Recognition Level/Percent Correct	MCL	LDL
Right	30		30	W22	+30/96%		
Left	40		35	W22	+30/92%		
Bone							
Sound Field							
Right Aided							
Left Aided							
Binaural Aided							

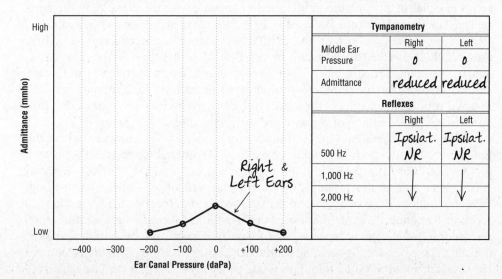

Tympanometry		
	Right	Left
Middle Ear Pressure	0	0
Admittance	reduced	reduced

Reflexes		
	Right	Left
500 Hz	Ipsilat. NR	Ipsilat. NR
1,000 Hz	↓	↓
2,000 Hz	↓	↓

Treatment options may include surgery to restore middle ear function through a **stapedectomy**, which is a surgical procedure in which the stapes is removed and is replaced with a synthetic prosthesis between the incus and oval window. In some cases, individuals choose not to pursue surgery and are given medical clearance from their physician to obtain a hearing aid (or aids) in order to reduce the negative effects of the hearing loss on their understanding of speech information.

Think about a scenario in which a client with a conductive hearing loss decides not to pursue medical management and instead chooses amplification. Certain outer and middle ear conditions, especially those that do not involve active pathology, can be effectively managed by amplifying incoming sounds rather than through medical/surgical treatment. In other words, in some cases conductive pathology is causing hearing loss and the physician offers the client options to deal with that loss either through surgery or by wearing hearing aids. Compare this scenario to the person who has a cholesteatoma or a painful wax blockage. This individual is best advised to seek out medical treatment and deal with the underlying medical cause of the hearing problem.

Malleus Fixation

Malleus fixation is an uncommon middle ear disorder that involves fixation of the malleus head. This condition may be total or partial and may result from infection, tympanosclerosis, otosclerosis, or a fracture of the attic wall, according to Jaffe (1977). In addition to acquired malleus fixation, congenital malleus fixation can occur. Audiometric results will include a significant conductive hearing loss in cases of total malleus fixation, due to poor mechanical transmission of mechanical energy from the tympanic membrane to the incus. Management will include otological evaluation (evaluation by a physician who specializes in disorders of the ear) to establish the diagnosis and to explore treatment options, one of which is surgery to free the fixed bone.

Eustachian Tube Dysfunction

As noted earlier, the **Eustachian tube** provides ventilation of the middle ear space and serves to equalize the pressure in the middle ear space with the pressure in the atmosphere. The Eustachian tube is closed in its resting state, and opens when individuals yawn, chew, sneeze, swallow, or phonate. Possible causes of Eustachian tube dysfunction include (1) swelling due to allergy or infection, (2) obstruction due to enlarged adenoids or a tumor, (3) neurological disorders that interfere with the opening of the tube, and (4) craniofacial anomalies. Compromise of Eustachian tube function typically involves insufficient opening of the tube, which disrupts this pressure equalization function, resulting in a buildup of negative pressure in the middle ear space.

According to Bernstein (1977), complications arising from faulty Eustachian tube function may be divided into two main categories: (1) retraction pocket of the posterior pars tensa and/or (2) accumulation of serous or mucoid fluid in the middle ear space. Persistent Eustachian tube dysfunction is associated with otitis media, discussed in the following section. The goal of medical management is to restore normal Eustachian tube function. Sometimes this can be achieved through the use of medicine, including antibiotics and/or decongestants. In some cases, however, Eustachian tube dysfunction is very difficult to treat, resulting in ongoing conductive hearing loss. Young children commonly have Eustachian tube dysfunction. This is due partly to the fact that the Eustachian tube position in young children tends to be more horizontal than in older children and adults. Treatment for Eustachian tube dysfunction depends on the cause. Allergy mediation, antihistamines, decongestants, and antibiotics may be used in cases of allergies, sinusitis, and infection. In other cases, surgery to remove the obstruction is required.

Patulous Eustachian tube is a condition in which the Eustachian tube is abnormally open. This may be associated with rapid weight loss over a short period of time or with neuromuscular disorders involving the muscles of the nasopharynx. Symptoms reported by an individual with a patulous Eustachian tube may include aural fullness, autophony (hearing one's own voice louder than normal), and hearing respiratory sounds.

Otitis Media

Possibly the most well-known condition affecting the middle ear and resulting in numerous visits to both primary health care providers and audiologists is **otitis media (OM)** which is defined as inflammation of the middle ear. Howie (1977) defines OM as any condition that results in the accumulation of middle ear fluid. There are many types of otitis media, classified based on the particular effusion present and the duration of the condition. **Effusion** is defined as escape of a fluid into a body space; middle ear effusion is the fluid resulting from otitis media.

Regarding the nature of the effusion present in the middle ear space, *serous* otitis media refers to middle ear inflammation accompanied by a thin, watery liquid. *Mucoid* otitis media is OM with a thicker effusion. *Suppurative* otitis media is a condition in which the middle ear is inflamed and contains infected fluid with pus. *Adhesive* otitis media includes a thickening of the fibrous tissue of the tympanic membrane that may be accompanied by severe retraction of the tympanic membrane and negative pressure in the middle ear space. Progression of this condition may result in the formation of a retraction pocket in the superior portion of the pars tensa of the tympanic membrane, setting the stage for the development of a cholesteatoma. Another potential complication associated with otitis media is **mastoiditis,** which occurs when infection in the middle ear spreads to the mastoid bone via the attic portion of the middle ear. This is a serious complication that is less common since the introduction of antibiotics.

Regarding the duration of otitis media, *acute* otitis media is characterized by sudden presentation of severe ear pain, redness of the tympanic membrane, and fever. *Recurrent* and *chronic* are terms used to differentiate otitis media relative to its frequency of occurrence and duration. *Recurrent* otitis media occurs three or more times in a 6-month period, while *chronic* OM lasts for a period longer than 8 weeks. One additional distinction is *persistent* OM, which is middle ear inflammation with fluid that lasts 6 weeks or longer after the initiation of antibiotics. Figure 7.5 shows an eardrum affected by otitis media.

Treatment options can be similar to those listed for Eustachian tube dysfunction, with use of oral antibiotics being quite common. In chronic cases, the surgical procedure referred to as a myringotomy is performed by an ear, nose, and throat (ENT) physician. This involves an incision in the eardrum to drain middle ear fluid. Following this, a pressure equalization (PE) tube is inserted into the incision to keep it open and to prevent the reoccurrence of negative middle ear pressure. The PE tubes effectively perform the pressure equalization role normally assumed by the Eustachian tubes. Hopefully, once the PE tubes are extruded from the eardrums (a time period that is generally between several months and one year), the Eustachian tubes of the child are working more efficiently and healthy middle ear systems can be maintained.

Many medical experts believe that the widespread use of antibiotics has led to the development of antibiotic-resistant bacteria, and it has been documented by Andalabi et al. (2001) that since the introduction of antibiotics a significant increase in cases of chronic otitis media has occurred. This has led researchers to work toward the development of innovative methods of treating otitis media, based on knowledge of the molecular basis of the disease. In addition, researchers hope to be able to learn how naturally occurring cells in the middle ear can combat bacteria, thus reducing or eliminating the need for antibiotics.

It is worth noting that one of the more controversial topics in audiology is the question of whether early otitis media has long-term effects on a child's development. This question is an important one because if the answer to it is yes, efforts to treat it should be aggressive. If, however, there are no long-term consequences to early otitis media, parents and physicians may be more comfortable with less aggressive treatments. Remember that the question here is not whether there are any consequences of otitis media. There is little doubt that otitis media is commonly associated with conditions including hearing loss, tympanic membrane perforation, and cholesteatoma. The difficult question is whether early otitis media has long-term effects on aspects of development such as language abilities, reading, attending, and general auditory processing.

Figure 7.6 shows typical audiological test results for an individual with bilateral otitis media. Note the presence of audiometric air–bone gaps, flat tympanograms bilaterally, and absent acoustic reflexes. This pattern of immittance results is quite typical and is consistent with middle ear dysfunction, most commonly middle ear effusion.

FIGURE **7.5** **Eardrum affected by otitis media.**

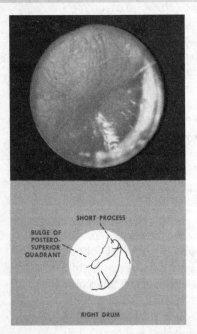

Source: Reprinted by permission of Abbott Laboratories.

Important Things to Remember in Cases Such as This

1. In reporting the results to the physician, it is important for the audiologist to point out the pattern of test results and to include information about a potential cause(s). Although audiologists do not make medical diagnoses, their results are important to the confirmation of a diagnosis by an otolaryngologist or pediatrician. Potential diagnoses include otitis media with effusion, cholesteatoma, or tympanosclerosis.

2. Next steps following diagnosis of conductive hearing loss should include management of the condition by a physician. Next, if the hearing loss persists despite medical management, an assessment of the degree to which the hearing loss interferes with the client's communication ability is needed. In cases of young children with conductive hearing loss, attention must be given to their speech and language development. For school-age children, classroom performance should be monitored closely. For

FIGURE 7.6 **Bilateral conductive hearing loss.**

247

Selected
Conditions That
May Affect the
Middle Ear

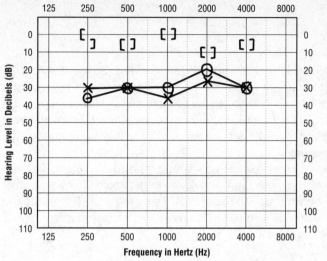

Audiogram Key		
	Right	Left
AC Unmasked	O	X
AC Masked	△	□
BC Mastoid Unmasked	<	>
BC Mastoid Masked	⊏	⊐
BC Forehead Masked	⌐	⌐

Both	
BC Forehead Unmasked	Y
Sound Field	S

Examples of No Response Symbols
O   X

Speech Audiometry

Ear	SRT	SDT	PTA 5-2	Test	Word Recognition Level/Percent Correct	MCL	LDL
Right	25		27	W22	+30/96%		
Left	30		30	W22	+30/92%		
Bone							
Sound Field							
Right Aided							
Left Aided							
Binaural Aided							

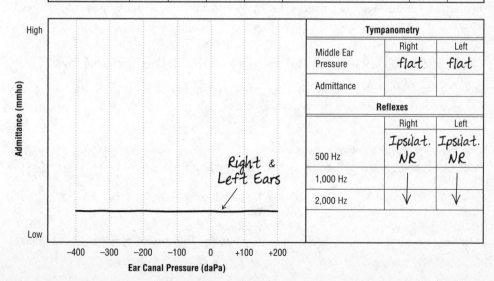

Right & Left Ears

Tympanometry		
	Right	Left
Middle Ear Pressure	flat	flat
Admittance		

Reflexes		
	Right	Left
500 Hz	Ipsilat. NR	Ipsilat. NR
1,000 Hz		
2,000 Hz	↓	↓

some individuals, medical management does not alleviate the hearing loss associated with conductive involvement, and amplification, with otologic clearance, is needed.

Barotrauma

As you have learned, the tympanic membrane and Eustachian tube are designed to accommodate changes in atmospheric pressure. The pars flaccida of the tympanic membrane functions as a type of safety valve, and the Eustachian tube provides pressure equalization for the middle ear to prevent buildup of extremely negative (or positive) pressure values in the middle ear space. Either of these conditions could result in perforation of the tympanic membrane.

Marked changes in atmospheric pressure associated with rapid airplane descents and/or poorly pressurized cabins or with rapid ascents by underwater divers may result in **barotrauma,** leading to perforation of the tympanic membrane. Less dramatic changes in air pressure may also result in perforations of the tympanic membrane if Eustachian tube function is compromised.

Glomus Jugulare Tumor

Glomus tumors are the most common tumor of the middle ear, and are the most common tumors of the temporal bone after acoustic neuromas (covered in the next section). These tumors can occur on the jugular bulb (a protrusion on the floor of the middle ear space), hence the name *glomus jugulare* tumor. Glomus tumors may also form in the middle ear (*glomus tympanicum*) or along the vagus nerve (*glomus vagale*). While the glomus tympanicum tumor generally produces auditory symptoms, including conductive hearing loss and pulsatile tinnitus, the other two types of glomus tumors noted (jugulare and vagale) often involve the labyrinth and cranial nerves. In these cases, other symptoms, such as facial nerve paralysis, may be present. Depending on the type of middle ear tumor and its location, the resulting hearing loss may be sensorineural, conductive, or mixed. The most common treatment option is surgical removal.

Selected Conditions That May Affect the Inner Ear

Table 7.4 lists various conditions that may affect the inner ear. Symptoms and treatment for these conditions are described in this section.

TABLE **7.4** Selected Conditions Affecting the Inner Ear	
Vestibular schwannoma	Noise-induced hearing loss/noise trauma
Diabetes	Ototoxicity
Facial nerve disorders	Presbycusis
Meniere's disease	Head trauma (concussion, temporal bone fracture)

Vestibular Schwannoma

Until proven otherwise, every unilateral sensorineural hearing loss should be considered a potential acoustic tumor or retrocochlear lesion. Asymmetrical sensorineural hearing losses should be viewed with similar suspicion. Acoustic tumors, or tumors affecting the auditory nerve (cranial nerve VIII), typically arise from the vestibular portion of the auditory nerve, specifically affecting the Schwann cells that form the sheath covering the nerve, hence the proper name for these tumors: **vestibular schwannoma.** Most vestibular schwannomas begin inside the internal auditory canal (IAC), although occasionally they begin outside the IAC.

In the initial stage, tumors are very small, with no associated signs or symptoms of their presence. As the tumors grow in size, they begin to compress the superior vestibular nerve, which can result in vestibular symptoms, such as dizziness. This is not always the case, however, because the individual's system may adapt to the changes (called central compensation) if they occur slowly over time.

As a vestibular schwannoma becomes larger, the auditory system will be affected. For example, when the typically smooth, organized neural firing of the auditory nerve is interrupted due to compression, hearing loss occurs. In addition, word recognition (speech discrimination) ability is usually reduced to a degree that is out of proportion to the degree of hearing loss.

Continued growth of the tumor causes pressure on the bone of the internal auditory canal. Tumor growth takes place along the path of least resistance, along the eighth cranial nerve toward the brainstem, and results in progressive sensorineural hearing loss. Because the seventh cranial nerve (facial) is not covered by a sheath, it is not affected by the presence of a vestibular schwannoma until late in its progression.

Intracanalicular vestibular schwannomas are confined to the internal auditory canal. (Take a closer look at the first word in this sentence and you will see that it defines itself. *Hint: intra* means within.) Such tumors may be classified as small (2 cm), intermediate (2–4 cm), and large (greater than 4 cm). At 2 cm, a vestibular schwannoma may affect the fifth (trigeminal) cranial nerve; at this point, the tumor begins affixing itself to the brainstem. Absence of a corneal reflex provides clinical evidence of the compromise of cranial nerve V. At 2–4 cm, a shift may be seen in the brainstem itself. Involvement of the cerebellopontine angle occurs as the tumor increases in size. Larger tumors may extend to involve cranial nerves IX through XII, particularly IX and X.

Typically, the audiologist who suspects that a client may have an acoustic neuroma communicates to the referring physician, who then orders additional diagnostic tests (e.g., auditory brainstem testing, CT scan, MRI) to confirm the presence of the tumor and to determine its location and size. If a tumor is confirmed, surgery is a common form of treatment, although in some cases, depending on the size and growth rate of the tumor, a watch-and-wait approach might be taken. In addition to successful removal of the tumor, surgical success is based on preservation of facial nerve function and hearing on the affected side. While vestibular schwannomas are not malignant tumors, their location can make them life threatening. Figure 7.7 shows a typical audiogram for someone who has a vestibular schwannoma.

Figure 7.7 reveals a markedly asymmetrical sensorineural hearing loss affecting the right ear. Significant findings also include very poor word recognition ability in the right ear at 75 dB HL that worsens at a more intense presentation level. This finding is

FIGURE **7.7** **Unilateral, mid- to high-frequency sensorineural hearing loss with significant asymmetry.**

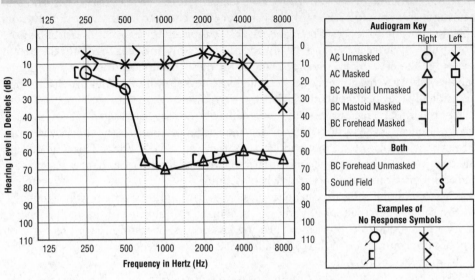

Speech Audiometry

Ear	SRT	SDT	PTA	Test	Word Recognition Level/Percent Correct	MCL	LDL
Right	35		—	W22	+40/44%*		
Left	15		8	W22	+40/92%		
Bone							
Sound Field					*at +50 dB = 32%		
Right Aided							
Left Aided							
Binaural Aided							

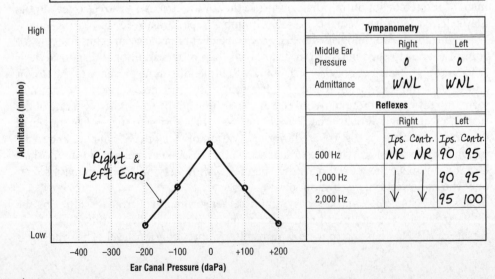

suspicious for retrocochlear pathology. How is this suspicion further supported by the acoustic reflex findings?

Important Things to Remember in Cases Such as This

1. The case history should include information about the onset of the hearing loss (sudden, gradual), feeling of fullness in the ear, tinnitus, and vestibular status (dizziness, vertigo).
2. Because there is a marked difference in thresholds between the two ears, masking is needed for air and bone conduction testing as well as for word recognition testing in the right ear.
3. Next steps following diagnosis of this sensorineural hearing loss should include referral to the client's primary health care provider for consultation to rule out retrocochlear involvement.
4. The most likely cause of a hearing loss with this configuration is retrocochlear involvement (e.g., a vestibular schwannoma) on the right.

Another type of schwannoma is **neurofibromatosis,** the cause of two different diseases: neurofibromatosis 1 (von Recklinghausen's disease) and neurofibromatosis 2. NF-1 results in multiple tumors on the skin and the spinal cord. Acoustic schwannomas are rare in this condition. NF-2 involves bilateral acoustic schwannomas, which unfortunately grow at a faster rate than the unilateral type described above. In addition to the presence of tumors, cranial nerve VIII can also experience inflammation, resulting in a condition referred to as *cochlear neuritis.* When this occurs, the normal functioning of auditory neurons is disrupted and hearing loss can result. As noted earlier, sometimes speech understanding is affected to a greater degree than pure tone sensitivity. If the vestibular portion of cranial nerve VIII is affected, balance problems can also exist.

Diabetes

Diabetes is a metabolic disease affecting the pancreas. Individuals with this disease have a deficiency of insulin and do not utilize glucose normally. Jerger and Jerger (1981) note that the auditory system may be affected by diabetes, either as a result of the direct effect of elevated blood glucose levels on the inner ear or as a result of small blood vessel changes in the body that commonly occur in diabetics. In either case, the most common result is a progressive, bilateral sensorineural hearing loss, with the greatest loss present in the higher test frequencies.

Facial Nerve Disorders

Facial nerve disorders involve the seventh cranial (facial) nerve. A variety of conditions can affect the facial nerve, such as edema (swelling), compression of the nerve, reduced blood flow, or viral infections. Symptoms depend on the location of the pathology. Possible symptoms of facial nerve involvement include impaired tearing (lacrimation), eyelid function, salivation, and taste. Facial muscle weakness is also a common symptom. Bell's palsy is perhaps the most common facial nerve disorder that audiologists encounter. The main audiometric finding relates to the acoustic (stapedial) reflex results. Depending on the exact location of the facial nerve lesion, the acoustic reflexes may be absent. For example, in cases where the pathology is closer to where the stapedius muscle innervation occurs, the acoustic reflex will be absent with the probe in the affected side.

Meniere's Disease

Meniere's disease is a benign (i.e., non-life-threatening) disorder of the inner ear. Although its exact cause is unknown, experts believe that it results from increased endolymphatic fluid pressure, which results in a characteristic group of symptoms including **tinnitus** (the sensation of sound in the head or ears), fullness, and/or pressure in the ear, fluctuating sensorineural hearing loss, and **vertigo** (the sensation of motion or spinning). This condition is characterized by remissions (symptom-free periods) and exacerbations, and individuals may have any combination of the above symptoms. Meniere's disease is one of a number of conditions that can affect a client's hearing and balance systems. This is discussed further in a later section of this chapter.

Noise-Induced Hearing Loss

Think for a moment of the types of individuals who are at risk for hearing loss resulting from noise exposure. Some of these are fairly obvious, such as the factory or construction worker, or the rock musician. But what about the college student who turns his personal stereo up so loud that others can hear it across the room? Or the hairdresser who, over a period of years, experiences loss of hearing from repeated use of a blow dryer? **Noise-induced hearing loss** affects many of us, and its prevention is an important part of an audiologist's work.

In most cases, noise-induced hearing loss occurs gradually over time, the cumulative effect of exposure to sound pressure levels capable of damaging the hair cells in the cochlea. The basal portion of the cochlea (which transmits high-frequency sounds) is the first to show deterioration from noise exposure, resulting in a high-frequency hearing loss with a characteristic pattern exhibiting the greatest hearing loss measured at or near 4,000 Hz. This pattern is sometimes referred to as a "4K notch" or a "noise notch." Noise-induced hearing loss is progressive in nature and depends on a number of factors, including the intensity of the noise, the duration of exposure, individual susceptibility, and the use of personal hearing protection. In some cases, a temporary threshold shift occurs, and serial (repeated) audiograms demonstrate recovery of hearing thresholds following an incident of noise exposure. Repeated exposure results in a permanent threshold shift and involvement of additional frequencies, often accompanied by communicative difficulty, particularly in noisy settings.

Figure 7.8 shows audiological results typical of someone with a history of noise exposure. The results are characterized by a high-frequency sensorineural hearing loss with the greatest loss noted at 4,000 Hz and some recovery by 8,000 Hz. This characteristic shape, also called a *noise notch*, is most often associated with noise exposure. Note also that immittance findings are within normal limits.

Important Things to Remember in Cases Such as This

1. The case history should include information about the client's history of noise exposure, both on and off the job.

FIGURE 7.8   Noise-induced cochlear hearing loss.

253

Selected
Conditions That
May Affect the
Inner Ear

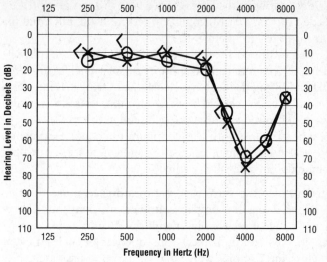

Audiogram Key		
	Right	Left
AC Unmasked	○	✕
AC Masked	△	□
BC Mastoid Unmasked	く	>
BC Mastoid Masked	⊏	⊐
BC Forehead Masked	⌐	⌐

Both	
BC Forehead Unmasked	⋎
Sound Field	S

Examples of No Response Symbols	
○	✕

Speech Audiometry

Ear	SRT	SDT	PTA 5 – 2	Test	Word Recognition Level/Percent Correct	MCL	LDL
Right	15		15	W22	+45/84%		
Left	15		13	W22	+50/84%		
Bone							
Sound Field							
Right Aided							
Left Aided							
Binaural Aided							

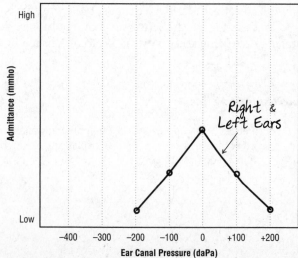

Right & Left Ears

Tympanometry		
	Right	Left
Middle Ear Pressure	0	0
Admittance	WNL	WNL

Reflexes		
	Right	Left
	Ipsilat.	Ipsilat.
500 Hz	85	80
1,000 Hz	85	85
2,000 Hz	90	90

2. Because there is no difference in thresholds between the two ears, and no air–bone gaps on unmasked bone conduction testing, masking is not needed for bone conduction testing. However, depending on the levels chosen for word recognition testing, masking may be needed during word recognition testing if the potential for cross-hearing exists in the lower test frequencies.

3. Next steps following diagnosis of this cochlear hearing loss should include counseling as appropriate regarding the potential effects of noise on hearing. Hearing protection may be indicated. In addition, the degree to which the hearing loss interferes with the client's communication ability should be assessed. Other tests that measure speech understanding in a background of noise may be useful in these cases.

4. The most likely cause of a hearing loss with this configuration is noise exposure. Other factors such as heredity, ototoxic medications, and aging may also contribute to the hearing levels documented in cases such as this.

Hearing loss resulting from noise exposure is sometimes due to noise trauma, which occurs when the ear is exposed to a high-impact sound of sufficient sound pressure level to detach the organ of Corti from the basilar membrane. Examples of this type of noise exposure include explosions and gunshots. Consequences of such an event include sensorineural hearing loss and tinnitus, which may or may not dissipate.

Ototoxicity

Degenerative changes may occur in the inner ear as a result of the use of certain drugs that are **ototoxic**. As the term implies, these drugs are poisonous to some part of the inner ear, and their damaging effects can involve the cochlea and/or vestibular system. Ototoxicity may be congenital, resulting from maternal ingestion of ototoxic drugs during pregnancy, or acquired from an ototoxic drug at any age. Drugs known to be ototoxic include antibiotics in the aminoglycoside family, as well as quinine, salicylates (aspirin), some diuretics, and chemotherapy agents. Table 7.5 contains examples of each of these ototoxic agents. Factors influencing the overall effect of ototoxic drugs on the auditory system include the individual's general health, particularly kidney function, the amount and duration of exposure to the ototoxic agent, and individual susceptibility.

How does ototoxic medication typically affect hearing? The most typical profile is a bilateral sensorineural hearing loss. In cases for which there is no choice but to use a medication that is ototoxic, monitoring of hearing sensitivity can be accomplished by

TABLE **7.5** **Examples of Various Ototoxic Agents**		

Aminoglycoside antibiotics:
   gentamycin
   amikacin
   streptomycin
   kanamycin
   neomycin
   tobramycin
	Diuretics:
	   ethacrynic acid
	   furosimide (lasix)
		Chemotherapy agent:
		   cisplatin

obtaining a baseline (pretreatment) audiogram and periodic repeat audiograms during the course of the drug therapy. When available, ultrahigh-frequency audiometry (testing frequencies above 8,000 through 20,000 Hz) may be useful in monitoring changes in cochlear function because changes in hearing sensitivity due to ototoxicity often occur at ultrahigh frequencies before changes in traditional test frequencies are observed. In addition to repeat testing, the client is advised to notify medical personnel if changes in hearing or changes in tinnitus are noted.

Presbycusis

As people get older, their bodies change in ways that sometimes interfere with their ability to function effectively in the world. One example of this is presbycusis. **Presbycusis** is a progressive loss of hearing resulting from the aging process. The typical result of age-related changes in the inner ear is a bilateral, symmetrical sensorineural hearing loss affecting the higher frequencies, particularly 2,000–8,000 Hz. The onset and degree of presbycusis vary widely. In addition, it is not possible to separate out the other factors, such as noise exposure or disease, which may contribute to the presence of hearing loss in older individuals. Boettcher (2002) summarizes three types of presbycusis that can occur. These are also described by Schuknecht (1964, 1993). It is common to think of loss of cochlear hair cells when considering the changes that occur in the hearing of older individuals. Research suggests, however, that although this does occur, it is not a major factor in presbycusis, and it is typically confined to the very low- and high-frequency regions. This type of presbycusis is referred to as *cochlear* presbycusis.

A second type of presbycusis is *neural* presbycusis. This refers to degeneration of the spiral ganglion, which is made up of the cell bodies of the auditory nerve fibers. Research does support loss of nerve fibers in older humans and animals.

Metabolic presbycusis is a third type of presbycusis. The stria vascularis is a key structure in maintaining the difference in potential between the endolymph of the scala media and surrounding tissue. Animal studies suggest that the area of the stria vascularis suffers reduced blood supply with age. This results in reduced responsiveness of hair cells leading to reduced hearing sensitivity.

In addition to changes in the ear itself, older individuals may experience changes in their auditory processing system. Auditory processing disorders are described in detail in a later chapter, but for now remember that the ability to understand speech and benefit from amplification is not only related to the functioning of the ear but also to those structures that code and relay information to the brain. If this system has undergone major changes with age, reducing the communication difficulties imposed by a hearing loss becomes more challenging. As noted in Chapter 10, changes in auditory processing abilities with age can affect the ability to use binaural listening cues and perception of frequency and time information in speech. As a result, auditory abilities such as localization, understanding speech in adverse listening environments, and perception of the suprasegmental aspects of speech can be compromised.

Figure 7.9 shows typical audiological test results for an individual with hearing loss due to aging. This hearing loss is characterized by a gradual slope with better hearing in the low frequencies, no air–bone gaps (sensorineural loss), and a decline in word recognition ability. As expected, all immittance findings are within normal limits.

FIGURE 7.9 Age-related cochlear hearing loss.

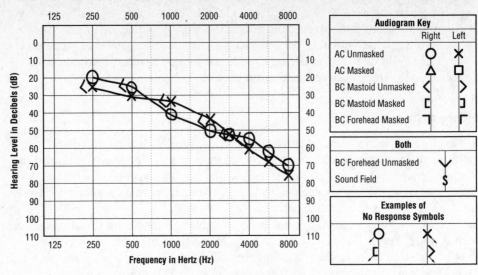

Audiogram Key	Right	Left
AC Unmasked	O	X
AC Masked	△	□
BC Mastoid Unmasked	<	>
BC Mastoid Masked	⊐	⊏
BC Forehead Masked	⌐	⌐

Both	
BC Forehead Unmasked	Y
Sound Field	S

Examples of
No Response Symbols

Speech Audiometry

Ear	SRT	SDT	PTA 5-2	Test	Word Recognition Level/Percent Correct	MCL	LDL
Right	30		38	W22	+40/80%		
Left	30		36	W22	+40/84%		
Bone							
Sound Field							
Right Aided							
Left Aided							
Binaural Aided							

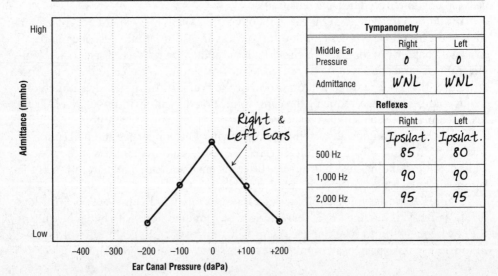

Right & Left Ears

Tympanometry	Right	Left
Middle Ear Pressure	0	0
Admittance	WNL	WNL

Reflexes	Right	Left
	Ipsilat.	Ipsilat.
500 Hz	85	80
1,000 Hz	90	90
2,000 Hz	95	95

Important Things to Remember in Cases Such as This

1. This audiometric pattern is one an audiologist will see over and over again. It is common for cochlear hearing loss to be bilateral and symmetrical.
2. Because there is no difference in thresholds between the two ears, and there are no air–bone gaps on unmasked bone conduction testing, masking is not needed for bone conduction testing. However, masking will be needed during word recognition testing, which is conducted at suprathreshold intensity levels because the potential for cross-hearing exists in the lower test frequencies.
3. Next steps following diagnosis of this cochlear hearing loss should include an assessment of the degree to which the hearing loss interferes with the client's communication ability. Adults with this hearing loss frequently report, "I hear the person's voice, but I don't always understand what they are saying." Children with this hearing loss may be late-diagnosed because their relatively good low-frequency hearing allows them to respond to a variety of sounds in their environment. However, they are missing critical speech sounds carried in the higher frequencies.
4. Possible causes of a bilaterally symmetrical cochlear hearing loss include heredity, ototoxic medications, and aging.

Trauma

Trauma to the head, particularly skull fractures, can cause permanent hearing loss. When motor vehicle accidents involve severe injury to the head, the ear is the most affected sensory structure. Fractures, concussions, and labyrinthine fistulas (an abnormal opening) are potential results of trauma to the head.

Fractures of the temporal bone may be *longitudinal* or *transverse,* and the type of hearing loss that occurs differs according to the type of fracture. In 80 percent of cases, the fracture is longitudinal. In these cases, the fracture extends down the external ear canal (the posterior superior canal wall), tears the tympanic membrane, and causes havoc in the middle ear, with less or no effect on the cochlea. Ossicular damage may include a fracture of the malleus and/or separation of the incudo-malleolar joint. Leakage of cerebrospinal fluid may accompany a longitudinal fracture of the temporal bone. A **hemotympanum** (accumulation of blood in the middle ear) may also occur. The hearing loss resulting from a longitudinal temporal bone fracture will typically be conductive in nature.

Transverse fractures of the temporal bone violate the cochlea, semicircular canals, and/or the internal auditory canal, through which cranial nerves VII and VIII course. This type of fracture is typically the result of a blow to the back of the head and is also associated with a high incidence of facial nerve paralysis. Passage of the fracture lines through the cochlea or vestibule results in significant sensorineural hearing loss or vertigo in the affected individual. Possible consequences of a transverse fracture include perilymph leak and rupture of the oval and/or round windows. Surgical exploration to locate the fistula is common, followed by repair using fatty tissue or vein graft. While most temporal bone fractures are unilateral, both sides require evaluation to rule out involvement. The possibility of a *contracoup* effect (damage to the side of the brain that is opposite the side of the impact) also exists. Of the two types of temporal bone fractures, a higher mortality rate is associated with transverse fractures.

Selected Conditions That May Affect the Central Auditory System

Disorders of the central auditory system include blood flow disruption, tumors, and demyelination and various neuropathies at the level of the brainstem, summarized in Table 7.6. In Chapter 9 you will learn about one of the most significant disorders of the central auditory system: cerebral vascular accidents, also called "strokes." Chapter 10 covers auditory processing disorders. Because of the extensive treatment they receive later in the text, these two disorders are not described in this chapter.

Remember that beyond the cochlear nuclei, there are both ipsilateral and contralateral pathways by which signals can reach the cerebral cortex. This is important because thinking about the numerous pathways by which auditory information can reach the brain helps you understand why pathology of the central auditory system does not always result in hearing loss. In some instances, the effects on hearing are related to the type of test that is given. For example, pure tones may be heard normally but the client's ability to understand speech, which often requires greater processing in those brainstem areas where the pathology exists, may be impaired.

Disrupted Blood Supply

Central auditory pathology is often the result of some problem at or near the brainstem. For example, disruption of blood supply at the brainstem or beyond can be a medically serious problem. Whether hearing loss occurs and the extent of the loss depends on the degree to which blood supply is reduced and the location of that disruption.

Multiple Sclerosis

Multiple sclerosis is a disease of the central nervous system characterized by destruction of the myelin sheath of nerve fibers. The term used for this process is *demyelination.* Because this disease results in the formation of sclerotic plaques on the brainstem, hearing may be affected. Changes in portions of cranial nerve VIII are also noted with this disease.

Hereditary Motor Sensory Neuropathies

From our earlier discussion of anatomy, remember that after auditory nerve fibers leave the cochlea, travel through and exit the modiolus, the cell bodies of these neurons form the spiral ganglion. Certain disorders, called *hereditary motor-sensory neuropathies* (HMSN), can affect the spiral ganglia and may produce auditory symptoms and/or abnormal results on tests of auditory function. HMSNs involve degeneration and atrophy of peripheral motor and sensory neurons.

Two such conditions are Friedrich's ataxia and Charcot-Marie-Tooth disease. Work by Satya-Murti, Cacace, and Hanson (1979) showed that in subjects with hereditary

TABLE 7.6 Selected Conditions Affecting the Central Auditory System

Disrupted blood supply
Multiple sclerosis
Hereditary motor-sensory neuropathy
Tumors

259

•

Selected
Conditions That
May Affect the
Central Auditory
System

neuropathies, it was possible to have abnormal results on short-latency brainstem auditory evoked potentials with normal audiograms. Satya-Murti et al. (1979) speculated at the time that the abnormal brainstem auditory evoked potentials were due to abnormalities in the spiral ganglia of the auditory nerve neurons. When you consider the site in the auditory system affected by motor-sensory neuropathy, it becomes clear that if the more peripheral outer, middle, and inner ear structures are unaffected, the result will be normal pure tone findings. If structures beyond the inner ear are compromised, tests that assess the function of those structures, such as brainstem auditory evoked potentials, will likely be affected.

The availability of otoacoustic emissions, which is a test that taps the function of the cochlea and is thought to reflect outer hair cell activity in the cochlea, has increased our knowledge of site-specific auditory dysfunctions. In more recent literature, the term *auditory neuropathy/dys-synchrony* is used to describe individuals whose profiles include normal otoacoustic emissions (reflecting auditory system integrity up to the point of the cochlea/outer hair cells) and abnormal results on brainstem auditory evoked potentials (reflecting an abnormality in the auditory system at the auditory nerve or beyond). Currently there are no agreed-upon treatment protocols for individuals with auditory neuropathy/dys-synchrony.

Finally, tumors can arise in the brainstem or brain from any number of structures, including blood vessels, glands, and nerves. Although different tumors can be named and classified based on the type of cell from which the tumor developed (e.g., schwannoma), the general term *neoplasm* is used to refer to a growth or tumor. As noted previously, it is possible, and even common, for individuals with brainstem or temporal lobe tumors to be free of auditory symptoms. Especially in cases of temporal lobe tumors, symptoms often include nonauditory concerns such as paralysis, memory changes, seizures, visual disruptions, and loss of language function. Because the contralateral fibers of the central auditory system are dominant (over the ipsilateral fibers), when auditory symptoms do exist, they typically appear in the ear opposite the affected side of the brain. As with most tumors, as they grow, they affect adjacent structures, causing the client's symptoms to increase.

Auditory Neuropathy/Dys-Synchrony

Now you know that certain hereditary motor-sensory neuropathies can result in abnormal brainstem auditory evoked potentials with normal audiograms. Now that otoacoustic emission testing is widely available, knowledge of the specific site of auditory dysfunction is increasing. In a very useful article by Hood (1998), **auditory neuropathy** is defined as a condition in which the patient displays auditory characteristics that support normal outer hair cell function and abnormal (i.e., dys-synchronous) responses from the eighth cranial nerve and brainstem. In other words, the site of dysfunction lies somewhere between the outer hair cells and the brainstem. It is important to note that, unlike space-occupying lesions (e.g., tumors), which can be identified by CT scans or MRI testing, auditory neuropathy cannot be identified in this way. The audiometric pattern is typically one in which otoacoustic emission testing is normal and auditory brainstem responses are abnormal or absent. Expected test results for clients with auditory neuropathy are summarized in Table 7.7.

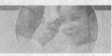

TABLE **7.7**   **Expected Test Results in Clients Who Have Auditory Neuropathy**

Test	Outcome
Pure tone thresholds	Normal to severe/profound hearing loss (any configuration: can be asymmetric)
Speech recognition in quiet	Variable: slightly reduced to greatly reduced
Otoacoustic emissions	Normal
Middle ear muscle reflexes	
Ipsilateral	Absent
Contralateral	Absent
Nonacoustic	Absent
Cochlear microphonic	Present (inverts with stimulus polarity reversal)
ABR	Absent (or severely abnormal)
Masking level difference (MLD)	No MLD (i.e., 0 dB)
Efferent suppression of TEOAEs	No suppression
Speech recognition in noise	Generally poor

Source: Hood, L. (1998). Auditory neuropathy: What is it and what can we do about it? *The Hearing Journal, 51*(8), 10–18. Reprinted by permission.

It is important to address this topic of auditory neuropathy because children who have this condition may be misdiagnosed as having a significant peripheral hearing loss or some type of auditory processing deficit.

Consider the following case. Ashley, age 2 years, is referred for audiological assessment due to significant delays in speech and language development and lack of responsiveness to auditory stimuli. As noted in Figure 7.10, behavioral testing suggests a severe to profound sensorineural hearing loss bilaterally; auditory brainstem response testing is consistent with this finding. Admittance findings are consistent with normal middle ear function and acoustic reflexes are absent, as expected in view of the degree of hearing loss. Aural rehabilitation is initiated with high-powered amplification and speech and language services. After several months the observation is made that Ashley's speech, language, and auditory responsiveness remain unchanged.

Consider for a moment that in the assessment of Ashley it is presumed that the recorded hearing loss and abnormal brainstem finding are the result of abnormality of the cochlea. The decision to use high-powered amplification is consistent with this presumption. Now, consider the possibility that Ashley has auditory neuropathy/dys-synchrony and that her abnormal responses to sound reflect some problem in the area of the inner hair cells, the auditory neurons, or the eighth cranial nerve. This may lead us to question the wisdom of using high-powered amplification and may alter the overall approach to aural rehabilitation. In fact, Berlin and colleagues (2002) advocate early use of sign language and cued speech to provide language in visual form followed by a program of cochlear implantation and auditory-verbal therapy for those families who want their child to be part of the hearing world. Other authorities begin with a trial period of low-gain amplification even though the value of traditional amplification in these cases has been

FIGURE **7.10** **Audiogram of child with auditory neuropathy.**

261
•

Selected
Conditions That
May Affect the
Central Auditory
System

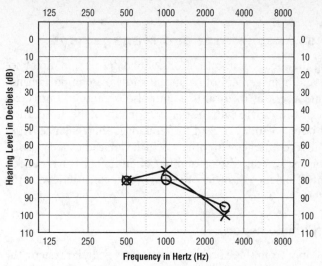

Audiogram Key	Right	Left
AC Unmasked	○	×
AC Masked	△	□
BC Mastoid Unmasked	<	>
BC Mastoid Masked	⊏	⊐
BC Forehead Masked	⌐	⌐

Both	
BC Forehead Unmasked	∨
Sound Field	S

Examples of No Response Symbols

Speech Audiometry

Ear	SRT	SDT	PTA	Test	Word Recognition Level/Percent Correct	MCL	LDL
Right							
Left							
Bone							
Sound Field							
Right Aided							
Left Aided							
Binaural Aided							

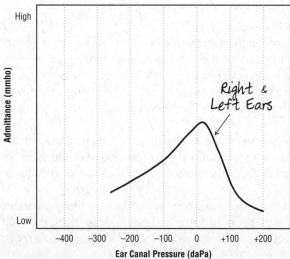

Right & Left Ears

Tympanometry	Right	Left
Middle Ear Pressure	+50	+50
Admittance	WNL	WNL

Reflexes	Right	Left
500 Hz	NR	NR
1,000 Hz	↓	↓
2,000 Hz	↓	↓

questioned. Clearly, auditory neuropathy/dys-synchrony is a topic that will continue to hold a place of importance for audiologists who strive to diagnose hearing loss in children.

Balance Disorders: Assessment and Management

Balance disorders are among the most common reasons why older people might see their physicians. Assessment and management of balance disorders are important not only because they can indicate a serious medical issue but also because, if untreated, balance disorders can significantly interfere with the person's quality of life. In addition to the obvious concern that poor balance can lead to frequent falling, balance issues can also reduce a person's ability to interact with others, which can lead to social isolation and depression. Over the last several years, a number of audiologists have added assessment and management of balance disorders to their work, consistent with the position taken by ASHA (2004).

Balance as a Multisensory Phenomenon

The balance system relies on input from three broad systems: the vestibular system, the visual system, and the somatosensory/proprioceptive system. The systems are described briefly in this section.

The Vestibular System

You will recall from Chapter 3 that the vestibule has two types of sensory receptors: the semicircular canals (horizontal, superior, posterior) and the otolithic organs (utricle and saccule). The hair cells in the vestibule consist of bundles of cilia made up of multiple stereocilia and one kinocilium. **Stereocilia** are rows of hairs at the top of hair cells of the sensory receptors; **kinocilium** is the single long hair cell adjacent to the stereocilium. These are illustrated in Figure 7.11.

You will also recall that in the process of hearing, hair cells make contact with the tectorial membrane and are sheared as endolymph moves. Similarly, for balance, the cilia bundles of the vestibular system make contact with overlying gelatinous structures. This structure is the **otolithic membrane** for the macula (of the urticle and saccule) and the **cupula** for the cristae (of the semicircular canals).

For both types of sensory receptors, displacement of cilia of the hair cells occurs when head movement occurs and is part of the process of maintaining balance. In addition, the otolithic membrane contains crystals of calcium carbonate, **otoconia,** which make these hair cells more sensitive to linear acceleration and changes in gravity when the head is placed in different positions. The semicircular canals respond to angular acceleration of the head.

To take this process one step further, if the stereocilia are displaced toward the kinocilium, an increase in the firing rate (excitation) of the cochleo-vestibular nerve results. If the stereocicilia move away from the kinocilium, a decrease in firing rate (inhibition) occurs.

Consider the person who is turning his head to one side. The resulting movement of fluid will cause increased neural activity on the ipsilateral side (side to which the head is turning) and decreased neural activity on the contralateral side. This asymmetry in

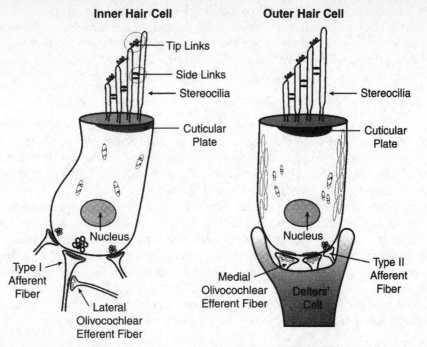

Source: Musiek, Frank E., and Jane Baran. *The Auditory System: Anatomy, Physiology, and Clinical Correlates.* Published by Allyn and Bacon, Boston, MA. Copyright © 2007 by Pearson Education. Reprinted by permission of the publisher.

neural input signals the brain that angular or linear motion is occurring and results in compensatory eye movement, which will be discussed in the next section.

Now, consider the client who is experiencing a vestibular weakness on one side, which prevents the appropriate neural information from being sent by the semicircular canals as the head is turned. Only the input from the contralateral side is received, resulting in a balance problem.

With this background information in mind, describe what is happening regarding neural firing and input to the central nervous system when a person's head is still.

The Visual System

We mentioned in our previous discussion that when the brain receives information that head movement is occurring, compensatory eye movement occurs. Specifically, the **vestibulo-ocular reflex (VOR)** causes the eyes to move in the opposite direction as the head movement and allows the eyes to remain still during head movement. This is possible because of neurons that connect the balance organs with the extraocular muscles, which are located around the eyes.

A second system of the eye movement, called the **saccade system,** is a resetting eye movement, which quickly brings the eyes back in the direction of the head turn. The key feature of the saccade system is to produce a single, rapid eye movement in order to capture a visual image.

A third system of oculo-motor control is the **smooth pursuit system,** which allows a person to track a visual target with smooth, continuous eye movements. This system would likely be used when watching a low-flying airplane travel across the sky.

Finally, the **optokinetic system** combines features of smooth pursuit and saccade movements to support stable visual images during head movement.

Nystagmus

At this point in our discussion it should be clear that changes in head acceleration result in specific input to the vestibular organs, as well as to the ocular system. **Nystagmus** is a particular pattern of eye movement involving a slow component in one direction and a fast component in the other direction (Stach, 2003). Nystagmus results from the neural connections that exist between the vestibular and visual systems.

Because analysis of nystagmus can help determine the nature of a client's balance disorder, clinical recording of nystagmus is a critical component of balance testing and is commonly done using **electro-oculography.** This procedure involves attaching electrodes in specific arrangements around the eyes and then measuring and recording the resulting patterns with a chart recorder. Figure 7.12 is an illustration of a right-beating nystagmus measured as a client turns his head to the right (with compensatory eye movements to the left). Electro-oculography is most commonly used in performing electronystagmography (ENG), which is discussed later in the chapter.

Somatosensory/Proprioceptive System

The third system contributing to balance, the **somatosensory/proprioceptive system,** supports balance during standing and walking and involves tactile cues, pressure sensors, and input to muscles regarding posture, movement, and position in space. In order to maintain balance, a person must make use of these cues; in the case of a weakness in the vestibular system, these cues become even more important. This third system supporting balance is quite broad and involves regulation of muscle force, coordination of limb and trunk movement, and cortical activities that allow a client to use strategies to maintain balance.

Anatomically, as noted in Figure 7.13, fibers of the **cortico-spinal tract,** which extend the full length of the spinal cord, influence fine motor movements of the upper extremities. In addition, brainstem nuclei and basal ganglia influence gross motor movements. Such movements might be noted when a person is walking over an uneven surface and has to quickly shift his or her center of gravity in order to avoid falling.

Assessment

Visit to the ENT Physician

Although the focus of this section is the assessment and management of chronic balance problems, it is important to note that clients who experience an initial acute episode of dizziness or vertigo should be seen by their physician, whose first goal is likely to rule out a life-threatening cause. For example, ruling out a serious neurologic or cardiac condition would be common for these clients. Often a CT scan or MRI is ordered to rule out

FIGURE **7.12** **Right beating nystagmus.**

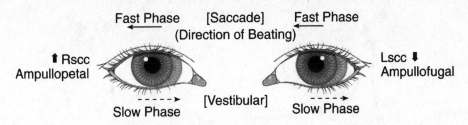

RIGHT BEATING NYSTAGMUS
(Rotating to the Right; RW; LC)

Fast Phase   [Saccade]   Fast Phase
(Direction of Beating)

⬆ Rscc   Lscc ⬇
Ampullopetal   Ampullofugal

Slow Phase   [Vestibular]   Slow Phase

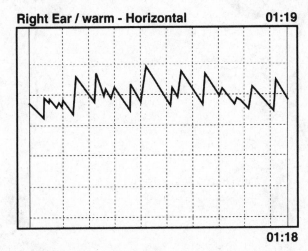

Right Ear / warm - Horizontal   **01:19**

01:18

Source: Koike, K. (2006). *Everyday audiology: A practical guide for health care professionals.* San
Diego, CA: Plural Publishing. Reprinted by permission.

a tumor that is affecting balance. If auditory symptoms exist, a complete audiological
evaluation would also be necessary.

Another important goal is to attempt to determine if the underlying condition is of
a peripheral or central nature. A balance disorder that is peripheral in nature is one that
involves the inner ear itself or the eighth cranial nerve. A central balance disorder
involves some part of the brainstem or brain.

Now consider the patient who has already had an initial exam when balance issues
(caused by labyrinthitis) first developed and who returns to the physician one year later
due to ongoing vertigo brought about by head movement. This client may have incomplete or failed vestibular compensation of their peripheral balance disorder. **Vestibular
compensation** is the process by which the central nervous system recovers spontaneously after injury to the balance organs of the inner ear (Shepard & Telian, 1996). The
physician will investigate why recovery has been limited for this patient, and attempt to

FIGURE **7.13**   **The cortico-spinal tract.**

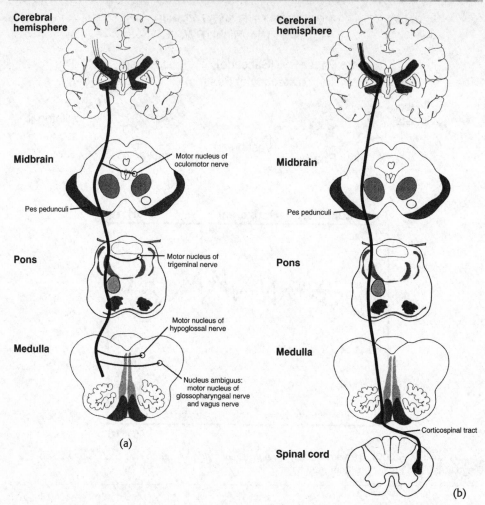

(a)

(b)

Source: Bhatnagar, S., & Andy, O. (1995). *Neuroscience for the study of communicative disorders.*
Baltimore: Lippincott, Williams, and Wilkins. Reprinted by permission.

provide some plan of treatment. Comprehensive balance testing, which will be discussed later in the chapter, will be very important to accomplishing these goals.

Another important aspect of this office visit is the detailed medical interview in which the physician gathers data regarding: (1) what brings on the symptoms, (2) how long a given episode of vertigo lasts, and (3) what other symptoms (e.g., hearing loss, tinnitus) accompany the episode. These questions are designed to help with the differential diagnosis process.

Also, during this exam, the ENT is likely to perform otoscopy to check for middle ear pathology and perform a basic check of cranial nerve function. The physician is also likely to check for abnormal nystagmus by having the client move her head into various positions. For example, by having the client move her eyes back and forth to follow a moving target, **spontaneous** and **gaze-evoked nystagmus** can be assessed. Generally, allowing the client to visually fixate on a target (eyes opened) will result in reduced nystagmus if the condition is peripheral. Because of this, the client is often asked to wear special glasses, which are lighted on the patient's side. These glasses, called **Frenzel lenses,** prevent fixation as the physician examines the eyes for nystagmus.

Comprehensive Balance Testing

The purposes of balance testing include: (1) diagnosing disorders, (2) gaining insight about a client's functional balance abilities, and (3) understanding the extent to which vestibular rehabilitation might be effective. Comprehensive balance testing consists of (1) ENG, (2) oculo-motor testing, (3) rotational chair testing, and (4) postural control assessment.

ENG (Electronystagmography).   The most commonly used test of balance is the ENG. As discussed previously, this test makes use of electro-oculography to measure eye movement and gain information about the vestibular organs and their central vestibulo-ocular pathways. Although these eye movements have traditionally been recorded using electrodes, a newer option is to video record images of eyeball movement and save them on a computer. This is referred to as **videonystagmography (VNG).** The ENG/VNG test primarily assesses functioning of the semicircular canals. According to Shepard and Telian (1996), the recommended order of the tests making up this test battery is as follows: (1) oculo-motor evaluation; (2) Dix-Hallpike maneuver; (3) Positional Tests; and (4) Calorics.

Oculo-Motor Evaluation.   Consistent with our earlier discussion of the visual system's role in balance, **ocular-motor testing** includes assessment of the saccade, smooth pursuit, and optokinetic systems, as well as gaze fixation. In the absence of visual disorders, these measures tend to be sensitive to balance disorders of a central nature.

The saccade testing of rapid eye movement evaluates the client's ability to rapidly move their eyes in the horizontal plane as they visually follow a moving target. Figure 7.14A illustrates an example of a resulting normal pattern and Figure 7.14B illustrates a case of eye movement disorder usually caused by some form of brainstem pathology. Figure 7.15A illustrates an example of the sinusoidal pattern that results during smooth pursuit testing when the client is asked to track a slowly moving target as it moves back and forth. Figure 7.15B demonstrates an abnormal smooth pursuit tracing in a client who is able to follow the visual stimulus to the right, but cannot follow it to the left due to some central nervous system disorder. The optokinetic test employs visual tracking of a repeating pattern that fills the visual field and provokes optokinetic nystagmus. Both normal and abnormal tracings are illustrated in Figures 7.16 A and B. Finally, during gaze fixation, the client is asked to maintain a fixed gaze on a visual target, which is directly in front and then moved to the right, left, up, and down. Figure 7.17 A and B illustrate examples of a normal response and significant spontaneous nystagmus. The presence of significant spontaneous nystagmus may result from either a peripheral or central vestibular lesion.

FIGURE **7.14**   **Normal (a) and abnormal (b) saccade test results.**

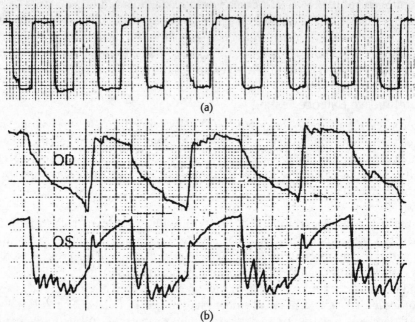

(a)

(b)

Source: Stockwell, C. (2001). Catalog of ENG abnormalities. Schaumburg, IL: G.N. Otometrics. Reprinted by permission.

FIGURE **7.15**   **Normal (a) and abnormal (b) smooth pursuit test results.**

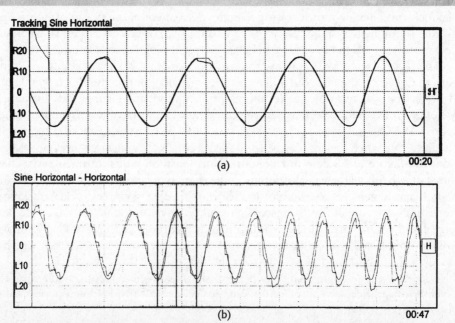

(a)

(b)

Source: Stockwell, C. (2001). Catalog of ENG abnormalities. Schaumburg, IL: G.N. Otometrics. Reprinted by permission.

FIGURE 7.16 Normal (a) and abnormal (b) optokinetic test results.

269
●

Balance Disorders: Assessment and Management

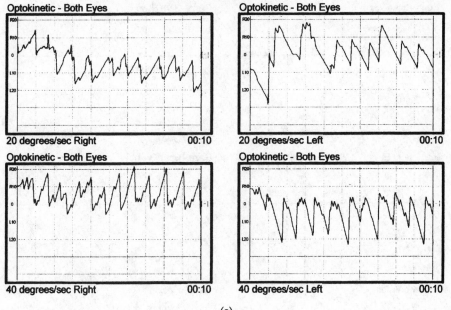

(a)

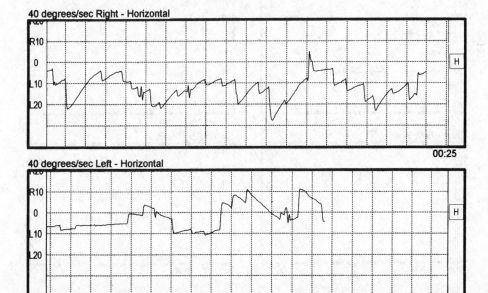

(b)

Source: Koike, K. (2006). *Everyday audiology: A practical guide for health care professionals.* San Diego, CA: Plural Publishing. Reprinted by permission.

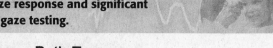

Gaze - Both Eyes

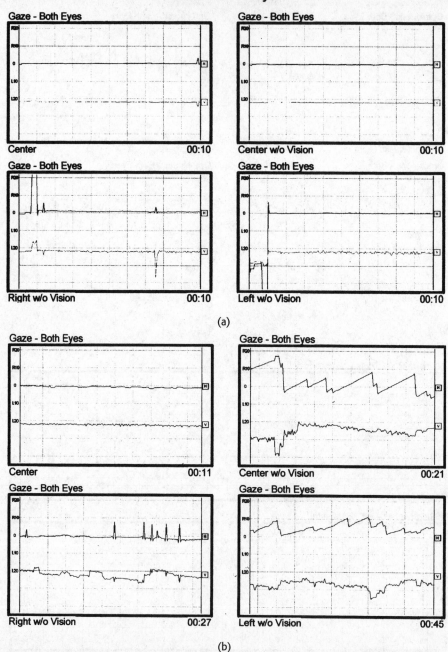

(a)

(b)

Source: Koike, K. (2006). *Everyday audiology: A practical guide for health care professionals.* San Diego, CA: Plural Publishing. Reprinted by permission.

Dix-Hallpike Maneuver. The **Dix-Hallpike maneuver** is illustrated in Figure 7.18 and involves rapidly laying the client back so that his head hangs over one shoulder. As this is done, the examiner directly observes the client's eyes for possible nystagmus or if the equipment is available, records directly the nystagmus with video-recording equipment. The client is then assisted to a sitting position, the eyes are monitored again, and then the procedure is repeated with the head hanging over the opposite shoulder.

FIGURE **7.18**   **The Dix-Hallpike maneuver.**

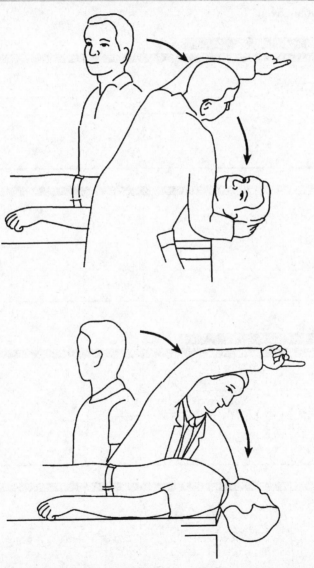

Source: Koike, K. (2006). *Everyday audiology: A practical guide for health care professionals.* San Diego, CA: Plural Publishing. Reprinted by permission.

The Dix-Hallpike maneuver is the only test of the posterior semicircular canals and its primary purpose is to assess for **benign paroxysmal positional vertigo (BPPV)**, a common peripheral vestibular condition. When the test is positive for this condition, a nystagmus that beats toward the underneath ear (and which begins approximately 1 to 10 seconds after the initial maneuver is done) is then noted. If the same maneuver is repeated multiple times, lessening of the nystagmus and associated symptoms is also commonly noted (Shepard & Telian, 1996). Figures 7.19 A and B illustrate normal and abnormal responses.

FIGURE 7.19   Normal (a) and abnormal (b) responses to the Dix-Hallpike maneuver.

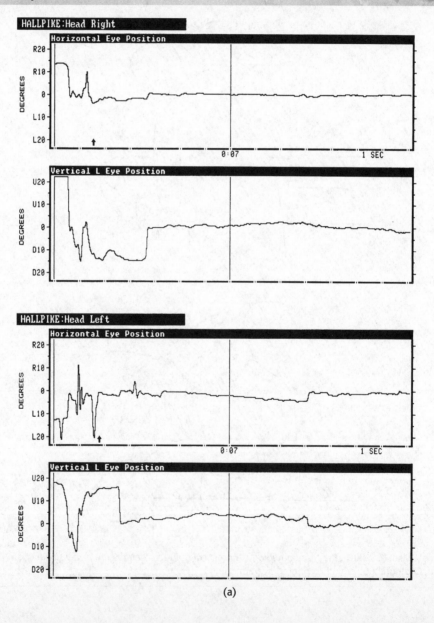

(a)

FIGURE **7.19**   *(continued)*

273
•
Balance Disorders:
Assessment and
Management

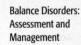

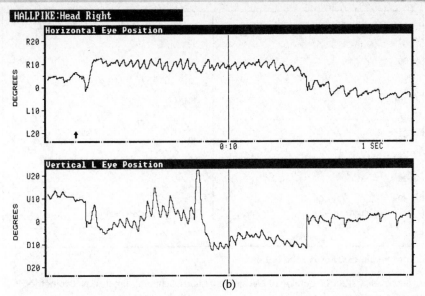

(b)

Source: Koike, K. (2006). *Everyday audiology: A practical guide for health care professionals.* San Diego, CA: Plural Publishing. Reprinted by permission.

Determining which of the semicircular canals are involved in a particular client's BPPV requires careful examination of the nystagmus that is produced by the maneuver. This information is particularly important for planning treatment.

Finally, the Dix-Hallpike maneuver is frequently done by physicians during the initial office visit. Frenzel lenses are not usually necessary because the type of nystagmus produced by this procedure is not easily suppressed by visual fixation. This procedure is typically not performed in cases in which the client has significant back or neck problems.

Positional Tests.   For this part of the ENG battery, the client is slowly moved into stationary positions with her eyes closed to assess the effects of these changes in head position. The positions used typically include: (1) sitting; (2) head turned to the right; (3) head turned to the left; (4) lying on the back (supine); (5) supine and head left; (6) supine and head right; (7) lying on the right side; (8) laying on the left side; and (9) head and shoulders elevated. Although positional nystagmus is commonly peripheral in nature, interpretation is based on the amplitude of the nystagmus and whether the nystagmus beats in only one direction or changes direction.

Calorics.   **Caloric testing** involves heating and cooling the endolymph of the vestibular system by directing temperature-controlled water or air into the ears. The patient is in the supine position with head elevated 30 degrees. Warm water is typically 40 degrees centigrade and cool water is typically 30 degrees centigrade. The purpose of this test is to assess the relative sensitivity of the vestibular organs based on the resulting nystagmus recordings, which is possible because of the effect of changing temperature on endolymph. Heated endolymph becomes less dense, rises, and the cupula moves

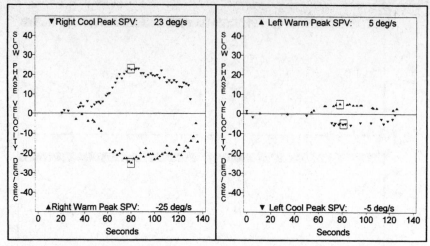

FIGURE 7.20   Left unilateral weakness on caloric testing.

Caloric weakness: 66% in the left ear

Source: Stockwell, C. (2001). Catalog of ENG abnormalities. Schaumburg, IL: G.N. Otometrics.
Reprinted by permission.

---

toward the utricle. Cooled endolymph becomes more dense causing movement away
from the utricle.

The caloric portion of the ENG is the only test in the battery designed to provide
separate right- and left-ear data regarding the horizontal semicircular canals. By comparing the intensity of the nystagmus in each ear, the examiner can assess whether
pathology exists in one of the horizontal semicircular canals or on the vestibular nerve
of the weak ear. This is illustrated in Figure 7.20 where normal caloric responses are
noted for the right ear, with weak responses in the left. These data support a **unilateral
weakness** in the left ear. Although the caloric test is considered to be the least pleasant
of the tests in the ENG battery because it can bring about nausea and vertigo, it is also
one of the more sensitive and useful measures in the battery.

Rotational Chair Testing.   Research and clinical observations strongly suggest that
clients may have negative ENG findings (no abnormalities) but still experience considerable balance difficulties. One reason why this might occur is that the range of head and
body movements to which the vestibular system responds is quite wide and cannot be
fully assessed by ENG. For example, caloric stimulation actually assesses only a limited
part of the horizontal semicircular canals, comparable to a head rotation of .003 Hz
(Hamid, Hughes, & Kinney, 1987).

In view of this information, authorities now recommend that clients who have balance disorders have ENGs and **rotational chair testing** to gain more information
regarding the horizontal semicircular canals. Depicted in Figure 7.21, this testing
involves placing the client in a lightproof booth with her head secured to the chair so
that the head can be moved at various rates of oscillation. Horizontal eye movements are

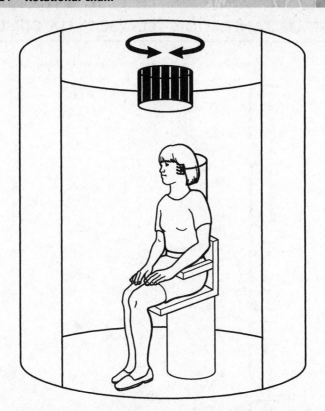

Source: *Practical Management of the Balance Disorder Patient,* 1st edition, by Shepard. 1997.
Reprinted with permission of Delmar Learning, a division of Thomson Learning:
www.thomsonrights.com. Fax 800-730-2215.

recorded. You will recall from our earlier discussion that head movement results in compensatory eye movements. These movements are recorded and analyzed.

Postural Control Evaluation.   ENG and rotational chair testing are performed to assess possible abnormalities of the vestibular and oculo-motor systems. Although some important information can be obtained from these tests, they do not effectively measure the functional balance capacity of the client. **Computerized dynamic posturography (CDP)** is a way to assess a client's ability to maintain balance under conditions similar to what might be encountered in everyday life. CDP consists of two subtests: sensory organization and motor control.

The purpose of the **sensory organization test** is to determine which input cues (vestibular, visual, proprioceptive) are being used to maintain balance. This is done by changing these cues and recording the client's center of mass. As depicted in Figure 7.22, these changes are accomplished by alternating the client's visual input (eyes opened or closed) and/or the orientation of the floor support (fixed or sway). A common pattern of difficulty is decreased

FIGURE **7.22**   **Sensory organization test (SOT).**

SENSORY ORGANIZATION TEST (SOT)-SIX CONDITIONS

	Condition	Sensory Systems
1.	Normal Vision / Fixed Support	
2.	Absent Vision / Fixed Support	
3.	Sway-Referenced Vision / Fixed Support	
4.	Normal Vision / Sway-Referenced Support	
5.	Absent Vision / Sway-Referenced Support	
6.	Sway-Referenced Vision / Sway-Referenced Support	

VISUAL INPUT
RED denotes 'sway-referenced' input. Visual surround follows subject's body sway, providing orientationally inaccurate information.

VESTIBULAR INPUT

SOMATOSENSORY INPUT
RED denotes 'sway-referenced' input. Support surface follows subject's body sway, providing orientationally inaccurate information.

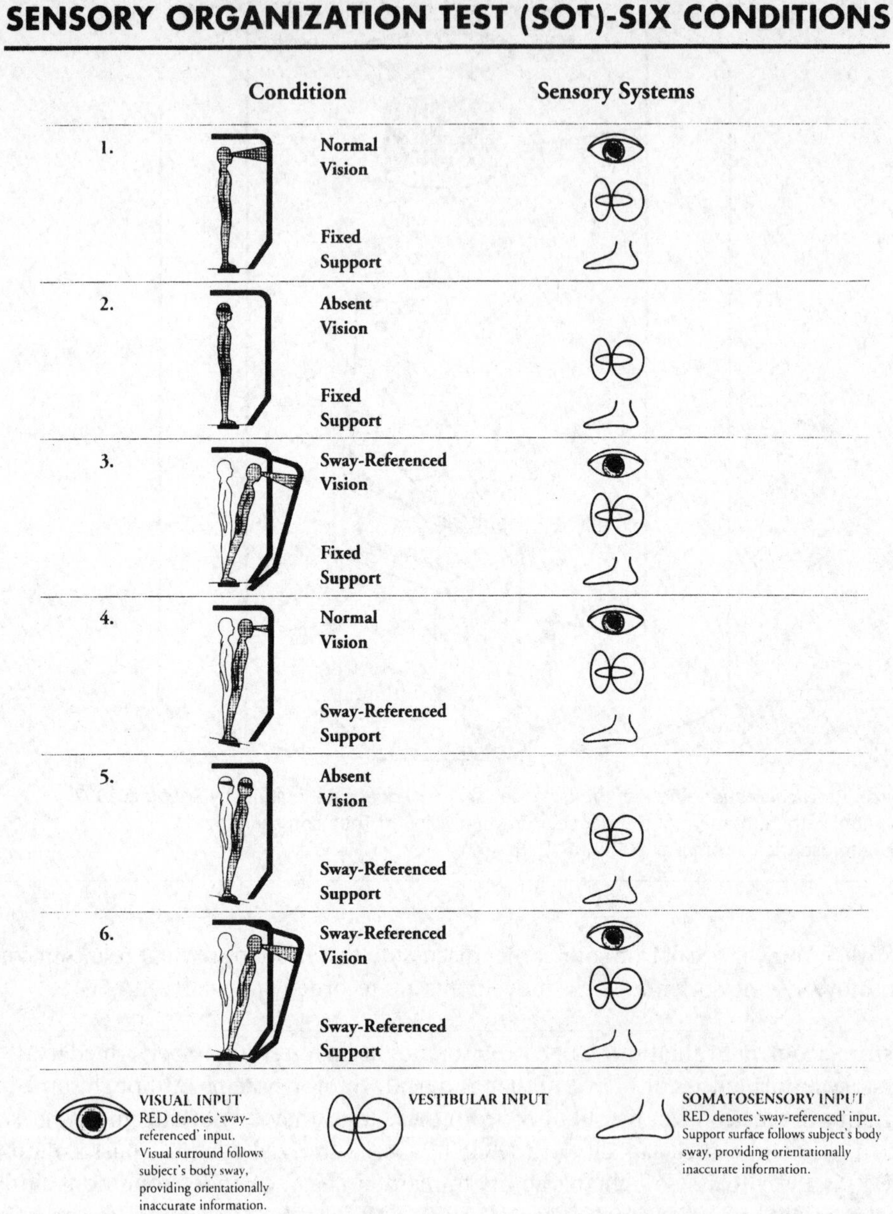

Source: Used courtesy of NeuroCom® International, Inc.

performance on conditions 5 and 6, which suggest that the client needs visual and proprioceptive cues to support balance; vestibular cues alone are insufficient.

The second subset of CDP is the **motor control test,** which focuses on the muscles involved in maintaining posture. This is accomplished by introducing abrupt anterior and posterior changes in the floor support, as well as rotations of the support. Client movement is measured by floor sensors. Reduced performance on this test could be related to incorrect strategies that have developed over the years on the client's part and could provide important information for planning rehabilitation.

Finally, it should be noted that physicians and audiologists who routinely provide services to clients with balance disorders often administer the **Dizziness Handicap Inventory (DHI;** Jacobson & Newman, 1990) in order to assess the physical, functional, and psychological impact of balance issues on clients. Results of the DHI have been shown to correlate with data from the CDP. The DHI can also be used after a period of vestibular rehabilitation as a way to measure improvements.

Management

An important consideration in determining treatment options for individuals who have chronic balance disorders is whether the vestibular disturbance is stable or unstable. The client who reports an initial acute attack of vertigo followed by continuing attacks of lesser severity most likely has a stable disorder. The presence of continuing symptoms also suggests that central vestibular compensation is not complete.

Vestibular rehabilitation programs are designed to help these individuals by facilitating habituation of the system's negative response (e.g., vertigo, nausea) to stimuli that evoke them (e.g., head movement). Such programs therefore require that the client perform those activities repeatedly in order to lessen the resulting symptoms. Vestibular rehabilitation programs also often include work on overall balance and conditioning.

For treating patients who have been diagnosed with BPPV, at-home exercises may be useful. In some cases, however, a specific in-office treatment may be necessary which attempts to reposition the otoconia of the otolithic membrane by moving the client's head into various positions from sitting, to one side, and then rapidly to the opposite side (Brandt & Daroff, 1980; Semont, Freyss, & Vitte, 1980). In many cases a single treatment is sufficient to resolve the problem.

Now consider the client who has been diagnosed with Meniere's disease and whose episodes of vertigo have continued over a period of years following the initial episode. Because this person's vestibular disorder is viewed as unstable, a vestibular rehabilitation plan is not the first course of treatment. Most likely, this client would first be advised to follow a low salt diet and drink plenty of water. Sometimes the antihistamine meclizine is prescribed to help control symptoms. In some cases these clients pursue surgical treatment, which may include total removal of the pathological inner ear (labyrinthectomy) or sectioning of the vestibular nerve. Clients who choose surgery may also undertake a postsurgical vestibular rehabilitation program to facilitate functional balance improvement by promoting central vestibular compensation.

Figure 7.23 illustrates an audiogram for an individual with Meniere's disease. Note that the right ear has a low-frequency sensorineural hearing loss with somewhat reduced word recognition ability. All immittance findings are within normal limits. Audiological findings point toward cochlear (versus retrocochlear) involvement. It is the combination of audiological findings, the case history reported by the client (e.g., fluctuating hearing loss, tinnitus, aural fullness, vertigo), and the results of an overall vestibular workup that help to diagnose this condition.

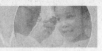

FIGURE **7.23**   **Unilateral low-frequency sensorineural hearing loss in a client with Meniere's disease.**

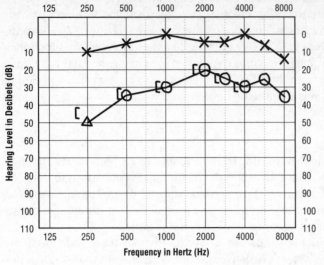

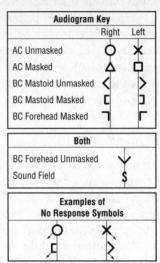

	Audiogram Key	
	Right	**Left**
AC Unmasked	○	X
AC Masked	△	□
BC Mastoid Unmasked	<	>
BC Mastoid Masked	[	]
BC Forehead Masked	⌐	⌐

Both	
BC Forehead Unmasked	Y
Sound Field	S

Examples of No Response Symbols	
○	X

Speech Audiometry

Ear	SRT	SDT	PTA	Test	Word Recognition Level/Percent Correct	MCL	LDL
Right	30		28	W22	+35/84%		
Left	5		3	W22	+35/100%		
Bone							
Sound Field							
Right Aided							
Left Aided							
Binaural Aided							

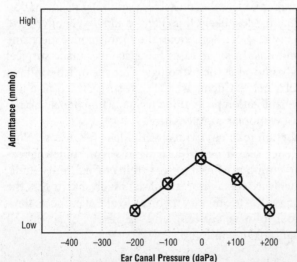

Tympanometry		
	Right	**Left**
Middle Ear Pressure	0	0
Admittance	WNL	WNL

Reflexes				
	Right		**Left**	
	Ips.	cont	Ips.	cont
500 Hz	85	85	80	85
1,000 Hz	85	85	85	85
2,000 Hz	80	85	80	80

CHAPTER SUMMARY

This chapter presented information about disorders that can affect the outer, middle, inner, and central parts of the auditory system. In addition, an overview of the vestibular system was provided, including the complex nature of balance, assessment protocols used by physicians and audiologists, and surgical and nonsurgical management approaches. Disorders and their characteristics were defined for the more commonly encountered conditions. Characteristic audiograms and associated communication and management implications were integrated within the chapter.

The relationships between the anatomic site of lesion in the auditory and vestibular systems, the symptom(s) an individual experiences, and the type of audiologic and vestibular test results that typically occur are important because they assist clinicians in accurately assessing the auditory system so that appropriate intervention can be pursued.

QUESTIONS FOR DISCUSSION

1. Describe three disorders that can affect the outer ear, and their effect on audiological assessment and test results.
2. Describe two conditions that can affect the middle ear, including effects on hearing and on development of speech and language skills.
3. Compare and contrast causes and characteristics of the following inner ear conditions: presbycusis, noise exposure, Meniere's disease, and vestibular schwannoma.
4. Compare and contrast the effects of vestibular schwannomas in earlier versus later stages.
5. List and discuss two disorders of the central auditory system and their potential effects on an individual's communication function.
6. Briefly describe the three systems involved in the balance mechanism.
7. Create a table that summarizes the tests which are part of the ENG battery and how each might be useful in assessing balance disorders.
8. How might management differ for a client whose balance disorder is stable compared with a client with an unstable disorder?
9. Why is additional testing beyond the ENG battery useful for many clients with balance disorders?

RECOMMENDED READING

Martin, F., & Clark, J. G. (1996). *Hearing care for children.* Boston: Allyn & Bacon.

Northern, J., Ed. (1996). *Hearing disorders.* Boston: Allyn & Bacon.

REFERENCES

American Speech-Language-Hearing Association (ASHA). (1994). Code of ethics. *ASHA, 36*(Suppl. 13), 1–2.

American Speech-Language-Hearing Association (ASHA). (2004). Scope of practice in audiology. *ASHA Supplement, 24,* in press.

Andalibi, A., Li, J.-D., Webster, P., & Lim, D. (2001, September). Advances in treating middle ear infections in children: An update on research into treating otitis media. *The Hearing Review,* 32–38.

Berlin, C., Li, L., Hood, L., Rose, K., & Brashears, S. (2002). Auditory Neuropathy/dys-synchrony: After the diagnosis, then what? *Seminars in Hearing, 23*(3), 209–214.

Bernstein, J. (1977). Middle ear effusions. In B. Jaffe (Ed.), *Hearing loss in children.* Baltimore: University Park Press.

Boettcher, F. (2002). Presbycusis and the auditory brainstem response. *Journal of Speech, Language, and Hearing Research, 45,* 1249–1261.

Brandt, T., & Daroff, R. (1980). Physical therapy for benign paroxysmal positional vertigo. *Archives of Otolaryngology, Rhinolaryngology, and Laryngology, 106,* 484–485.

Derlacki, E. (1996). Otosclerosis. In J. Northern (Ed.), *Hearing disorders.* Boston: Allyn & Bacon.

Hamid, M., Hughes, G., & Kinney, S. (1987). Criteria for diagnosing bilateral vestibular dysfunction. In M. Graham & J. Kemink (Eds.), *The vestibular system: Neuropsychological and clinical research* (pp. 115–118). New York: Raven Press.

Hood, L. (1998). Auditory neuropathy: What is it and what can we do about it? *The Hearing Journal, 51*(8), 10–18.

Howie, V. (1977). Acute and recurrent otitis media. In B. Jaffe (Ed.), *Hearing loss in children.* Baltimore: University Park Press.

Jacobson, G., & Newman, C. (1990). The development of the dizziness handicap inventory. *Archives of Otolaryngology—Head and Neck Surgery, 116,* 424–427.

Jaffe, B. (1977). Middle ear isolated anomalies. In B. Jaffe (Ed.), *Hearing loss in children.* Baltimore: University Park Press.

Jerger, S., & Jerger J. (1981). *Auditory disorders: A manual for clinical evaluation.* Boston: Little, Brown.

Musiek, F., & Baran, J. (2007). *The auditory system: Anatomy, physiology, and clinical correlates.* Boston: Allyn & Bacon.

Satya-Murti, S., Cacace, A., & Hanson, P. (1979). Abnormal auditory evoked potentials in hereditary motor-sensory neuropathology. *Annals of Neurology, 5,* 445–448.

Schuknecht, H. (1964). Further observations on the pathology of presbycusis. *Archives of Otolaryngology, 80,* 369–382.

Schuknecht, H. (1993). *Pathology of the ear* (2nd ed.). Philadelphia: Lea & Febiger.

Semont, A., Freyss, G., & Vitte, E. (1988). Curing the BPPV with a liberatory maneuver. *Advanced Otorhinolaryngolgy, 42,* 290–293.

Shepard, N., & Telian, S. (1996). *Practical management of the balance disorder patient.* San Diego: Singular.

Stach, B. (2003). *Comprehensive dictionary of audiology illustrated.* Clifton Park, NY: Thomson Delmar Learning.

chapter 8

Pediatric Audiology

AFTER COMPLETING THIS CHAPTER, YOU SHOULD BE ABLE TO:

1. Describe the importance of audiologists developing skills in behavioral assessment of young children.
2. Understand basic elements of embryological development of the auditory system.
3. Understand essential terms related to genetics of hearing loss.
4. Discuss four key principles that guide the audiologist in carrying out pediatric assessments.
5. Describe the major behavioral test techniques available and then discuss the suitability of each of these for children of various ages.
6. Define client-specific protocols and discuss their value in pediatric assessment.
7. Understand the impact of nonaudiological variables (e.g., temperament, degree of separation anxiety) on pediatric audiological assessment.
8. Understand how to convey information to parents/caregivers after the audiological evaluation.

There was a time when childhood was not considered the unique period of development that it is today and when children were regarded as small adults. This, of course, was prior to the formal study of childhood and the establishment of the body of knowledge that now exists describing how children are qualitatively different from adults in terms of how they think and learn, how they communicate, the control they have over their own actions, and how they interact with others in the world. Because audiologists must be able to diagnose hearing problems in children accurately, it is important that they familiarize themselves with basic information regarding child development and then apply this information to effective pediatric audiological assessment and aural rehabilitation.

Auditory Development and Pediatric Audiology

The term *childhood* is a rather broad one and has been divided into various categories. Before describing detailed audiometric test techniques for children of various ages, let's begin this discussion by describing some general developmental characteristics of three groups of children who may pose special challenges for the audiologist: infants, toddlers, and preschoolers. Specific auditory developmental information for these and other age groups is summarized in Table 8.1 in the Developmental Index of Audition and Listening (DIAL).

Infants

Contrary to popular belief, infants are not helpless little beings who are unaware of what is going on around them. In fact, research on infants has increasingly revealed that they come into the world with a tremendous curiosity about their environment, an ability to learn quickly about it, and perhaps some sophisticated skills that are present at birth.

One area of early skill is speech perception. Research suggests that infants as young as 4 months of age not only can discriminate their mother's voice from a stranger's but also can discriminate vowels and voiced versus voiceless consonant sounds. In addition, infants show a preference for their native language. Although most infants have normal hearing at birth, an infant's ability to demonstrate responses to very faint sounds is limited by the immaturity of the central nervous system. Because of this, infants tend to respond better to louder signals, signals that are more complex in nature, and those that have a longer duration. At approximately 5 months, infants have the neurological development to coordinate a head turn toward a sound that they hear. Prior to this, infants typically respond to sound in more subtle ways, including eye widening, smiling, crying, or a change in breathing pattern. Infants also often exhibit startle responses to sounds around them.

By approximately 7 months the infant has developed strong feelings of attachment to the primary caretaker and often shows anxiety when separated from the caretaker and/or when in the company of a stranger. Separation anxiety typically subsides as the child understands that the parent's absence is temporary.

Toddlers

A toddler is a child who falls in the approximate age range of 1 to 3 years. The normally developing toddler is able to explore the environment by walking without assistance and exhibits increasing motor skill, including walking up stairs and kicking a ball. By about the age of 1½ years, toddlers understand over fifty words and have the cognitive and language skills to be able to comply with requests made by adults. Expressive language typically changes dramatically during the toddler period, growing from the one-word utterance stage to the use of two-word combinations and short sentences.

Preschoolers

The preschool years are marked by increasing independence in all areas, including motor, cognitive, and social development. The preschooler is typically able to perform a variety of motor tasks independently, including running, using a fork, and dressing independently. Language development allows the child to communicate using multiword utterances and to understand even nonliteral language, such as that used in humor. Although preschoolers have the ability to understand adult requests, they often resist attempts by others to exercise control over their behavior.

TABLE 8.1 Developmental Index of Audition and Listening (DIAL)

Age Group	Specific Age	Milestone
Infant	0–28 days	Startle response; attends to music and voice, soothed by parent's voice; some will synchronize body movements to speech pattern; enjoys time in "en face" position; hears caregiver before being picked up
	1–4 months	Looks for sound source; associates sound with movement; enjoys parent's voice; attends to noisemakers; imitates vowel sounds
	4–8 months	Uses toys/objects to make sounds; recognizes words; responds to verbal commands—bye bye; learning to recognize name; plays with noisemakers; enjoys music; enjoys rhythm games
	8–12 months	Attends to TV; localizes to sounds/voices; enjoys rhymes and songs; understands NO; enjoys hiding game; responds to vocal games (e.g., So Big!!)
Toddler	1 year	Dances to music; sees parent answer telephone/doorbell; answers to name call; attends to books
	2 years	Listens on telephone; dances to music; listens to story in group; goes with parent to answer door; awakens to smoke detector; attends to travel activities and communication
Preschool	3 years	Talks and listens on telephone; sings with music; listens to books on tape; smoke detector means danger; enjoys taped books; attends to verbal warnings for safety
	4 years	Telephone play; attends movie theater; dance/swim lessons; watches TV/videos with family; neighborhood play
	5 years	Music lessons; attends to children's service in church; learns to ride bike; plays at playground at a distance from parent
Early school age	6–8 years	Uses telephone meaningfully; enjoys iPod/headphones; uses alarm clock independently; responds to smoke detector independently
Late elementary	8–10 years	Uses television for entertainment & socializing; attends to radio; responds to sirens for street safety; participates in clubs and athletics; enjoys privacy in own room; enjoys computer/audio games; plays team sports
Middle school	10–14 years	Uses telephone as social vehicle; attends movies/plays; develops musical tastes; watches movies/TV with friends
Older adolescent	14–18 years	Goes to dances; begins driving (e.g., needs to hear sirens/turn signal); participates in school groups/clubs; employment/ADA
	18–22 years	Employment/career decisions; travels independently; listens in college lecture halls/classrooms; participates in study groups/extracurricular activities

Source: Elaine Mormer, Communication Science and Disorders, School of Health and Rehabilitation Sciences. University of Pittsburgh, 4033 Forbes Tower, Pittsburgh, PA 15260. Reprinted by permission.

Early Identification and Early Intervention for Hearing Loss

Recent research has reinforced what audiologists, speech–language pathologists, and teachers of the deaf and hard of hearing have been aware of—**early identification** of hearing loss, accompanied by appropriate **early intervention** services, makes a positive difference in the communication and language outcomes for children with hearing loss. The work of Yoshinaga-Itano et al. (1998), comparing language outcomes in children with hearing loss who are identified and served earlier in life with those identified and consequently served later, clearly demonstrates that earlier is better. The advent of universal newborn hearing screening programs, discussed further in Chapter 11, has facilitated earlier identification of infants with potential hearing loss. At the same time, infant hearing screening programs have increased the number of young children who require either rescreening or diagnostic audiological evaluations. These additional procedures are designed to rule out hearing loss or to further define the nature and degree of the hearing loss so that appropriate aural habilitation can be planned and implemented.

This chapter has as its primary focus the provision of audiological evaluations and services to young children for several reasons. First, competent early identification and habilitation for young children with hearing loss is advantageous for communication and language outcomes, as well as for social-emotional development. Second, audiological assessment of this population is challenging, requiring special skills and experience. Third, audiologists and related professionals need to reconsider their roles and responsibilities in the assessment of young clients in light of changes in public policy related to the expansion of newborn hearing screening programs. In other words, a variety of professions are being called on to provide services for younger and younger children. A primary focus of this chapter is on behavioral test techniques for younger clients, children from infancy through age 5. In general, "older" children can participate in hearing tests that use conventional or adult test techniques, with little or no modification required. Test adaptations for clients with special needs are addressed in Chapter 9. The use of an individualized approach aimed at answering the clinical question(s) relevant to children and their families while considering their collective strengths, needs, and abilities is the overarching goal for conducting audiological evaluations for this population.

Components of Auditory System Development

An overview of auditory system development is presented here to introduce relevant terminology and to provide a background against which to consider congenital anomalies that may cause hearing loss in young children. This information relates to considerations about the etiology (cause) of sensorineural hearing loss in infants and young children, which may be extrinsic or intrinsic. **Extrinsic causes of hearing loss** include tumors, infections, injuries, metabolic disorders, prescription or nonprescription drug use, ototoxic drugs, and congenital causes that are nongenetic. Hearing loss is also associated with a number of genetic disorders. **Genetic disorders,** considered **intrinsic causes of hearing loss,** have various patterns of inheritance.

Basic Embryology

Development of the auditory structures that support hearing occurs from approximately the 3rd week of **gestation** through the 37th week. Table 8.2 summarizes the embryologic development of the three parts of the human ear.

TABLE **8.2**   **Embryology Summary of the Ear**

Fetal Week	Inner Ear	Middle Ear	External Ear
3rd	Auditory placode; auditory pit	Tubotympanic recess begins to develop	
4th	Auditory vesicle (otocyst); vestibular-cochlear division		Tissue thickenings begin to form
5th			Primary auditory meatus begins
6th	Utricle and saccule present; semicircular canals begin		Six hillocks evident; cartilage begins to form
7th	One cochlear coil present; sensory cells in utricle and saccule		Auricles move dorsolaterally
8th	Ductus reuniens present: sensory cells in semicircular canals	Incus and malleus present in cartilage; lower half of tympanic cavity formed	Outer cartilaginous third of external canal formed
9th		Three tissue layers at tympanic membrane are present	
11th	Two and one-half cochlear coils present; nerve VIII attaches to cochlear duct		
12th	Sensory cells in cochlea; membranous labyrinth complete; otic capsule begins to ossify		
15th		Cartilaginous stapes formed	
16th		Ossification of malleus and incus begins	
18th		Stapes begins to ossify	
20th	Maturation of inner ear; inner ear adult size		Auricle is adult shape but continues to grow until age 9
21st		Meatal plug disintegrates, exposing tympanic membrane	
30th		Pneumatization of tympanum	External auditory canal continues to mature until age 7
32nd		Malleus and incus complete ossification	
34th		Mastoid air cells develop	
35th		Antrum is pneumatized	
37th		Epitympanum is pneumatized; stapes continues to develop until adulthood; tympanic membrane changes relative position during first 2 years of life	

Source: Northern, J., & Downs, M. (2002). *Hearing in children* (5th ed.). New York: Lippincott, Williams & Wilkins. Reprinted by permission.

According to Northern and Downs (2002), there are three germ layers, the **ectoderm, mesoderm,** and **endoderm,** in embryonic development. These layers become differentiated during fetal development and various anatomic parts arise from each of the layers. Generally, the outer skin layers, the nervous system, and the sense organs are developed from ectoderm. Structures associated with the mesoderm include skeletal, circulatory, and reproductive structures, as well as the kidneys. The digestive canal and respiratory canal originate from the endoderm.

Inner, Middle, and Outer Ear Development

The development of the ear takes place during the embryonic (first 8 weeks of gestation) and fetal (remainder of gestation) phases. The inner ear arises from ectodermal tissue. Some of the landmarks in the development of the inner ear include: the development of the auditory vesicles, or otocysts, at approximately 30 days; the development of vestibular structures (utricle and saccule) at approximately 6 weeks; and, the presence of two and one-half cochlear coils by the 11th week of fetal development, at which time the auditory nerve attaches to the cochlear duct. Additional details are provided in the summary in Table 8.2.

The middle ear, which arises from endodermal tissue, also begins developing at the 3rd fetal week. By the 8th week, two of the three middle ear ossicles, the malleus and incus, are present in cartilage, and by the 9th fetal week the three tissue layers of the tympanic membrane are present. Development of the middle ear continues through the 37th week of gestation, and some structures continue to develop until adulthood.

The external ear, like the inner ear, arises from ectodermal tissue, from the first and second branchial arches. The **branchial arches** begin as paired grooves that are formed at about the 3rd week of fetal development. They come together at the midline to form arches; there are six branchial arches in all. The four visible branchial arches are shown in Figure 8.1. The external ear begins to form at the 4th week of fetal development, and by 6 weeks, six **auricular hillocks** can be seen. The external ear forms from these six hillocks, or growth centers, which appear as thickenings on the first branchial groove. By the 20th week of fetal development, the external ear, or auricle, reaches its adult shape. The external ear continues to grow in size until age 9 years.

Consistent with the development of other major body systems, significant construction of the auditory structures to support hearing also occurs within the first trimester of pregnancy. In addition, the inner and external portions of the ear come from ectodermal tissue, and the middle ear arises from endodermal tissue. Because the internal and external ear structures originate from the same tissue, any observable anomaly of the external ear warrants suspicion about the structural integrity of the inner ear. Some significant external ear abnormalities, such as atresia and microtia, are described in Chapter 7; however, as illustrated in Figure 8.2, more subtle irregularities of the external ear may be present, including preauricular pits and skin tags that should alert clinicians to the possibility of an associated inner ear disorder that could result in hearing loss.

Genetics: Basic Information and Terminology

As students of communication disorders learn, many times one condition, such as hearing loss, is associated with another, such as a congenital malformation or syndrome. There are also instances when hereditary deafness occurs without associated abnormalities.

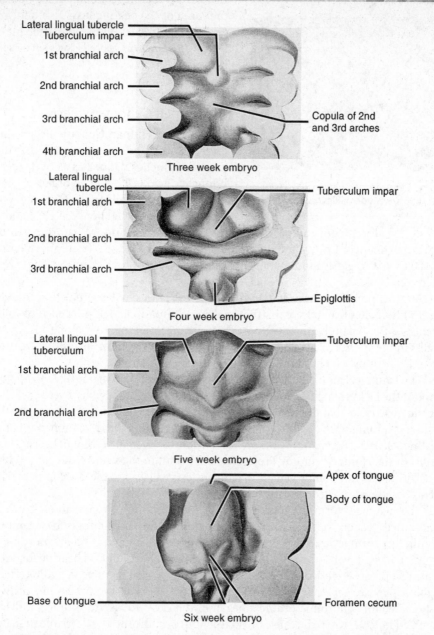

Three week embryo

Four week embryo

Five week embryo

Six week embryo

Source: Zemlin, Willard R. *Speech and Hearing Science: Anatomy and Physiology,* 4e. Published by Allyn and Bacon, Boston, MA. Copyright © 1998 by Pearson Education. Reprinted by permission of the publisher.

FIGURE **8.2**   **Preauricular pits.**

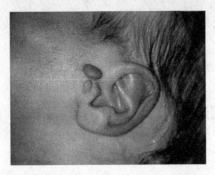

Source: Dermatlas and Christoph U. Lehmann, M.D.; http://www.dermatlas.org.

Often, when childhood hearing loss is identified, family members are interested in learning the cause of the hearing loss. This information can have an impact on the management of the hearing loss and on related issues such as family planning.

The Human Genome Project

Work on the Human Genome Project has increased our understanding of the human genome, which is defined as all of the deoxyribonucleic acid (DNA) in an organism, including its genes. The Human Genome Project, which was conducted between 1990 and 2003, was designed to identify all of the genes in human DNA, and was coordinated by the U.S. Department of Energy and the National Institutes of Health. There are an estimated 30,000 to 40,000 genes in human DNA, which consists of four chemicals that are often referred to as *bases.*

Another purpose of the Human Genome Project was to determine the sequences of the 3 billion chemical base pairs that make up human DNA. Knowledge of these sequences is important because the particular arrangement of bases along a DNA strand results in the specific traits that make one organism different from another (e.g., a bacterium, a fruit fly, or a human).

The Human Genome Project then took this information a step further, to identify regions of the DNA that differ from individual to individual. These discoveries will help to explain differences in individuals' abilities to see or hear. These differences may be the key to understanding the cause of certain diseases and guiding the development of effective treatments. Because genetic factors are responsible for over 50 percent of hearing loss, the results of the Human Genome Project are important to the study of hereditary hearing loss. Ultimately, developing genetic diagnostic tests will lead to the development of treatments based on knowledge of the underlying causes of a disorder.

The two main forms of genetic hearing loss are nonsyndromic and syndromic. In other words, genetic hearing loss can occur alone (nonsyndromic) or be accompanied by other abnormalities, such as in Waardenburg syndrome or Usher syndrome (syndromic). For a list of some genetic conditions related to childhood hearing loss, refer to Table 8.3. Because syndromes have distinguishing clinical features in addition to hearing loss, they are generally more easily recognized. Work to localize and identify genes responsible for syndromic deafness began in the early 1990s. An important discovery occurred in 1992, when the cause of Waardenburg syndrome was determined to be mutations in the PAX3 gene (Tekin, Arnos, & Pandya, 2001). Similarly, information about the specific gene mutations responsible for conditions such as Pendred syndrome, Jervell syndrome, and Usher syndrome has become available (Tekin et al., 2001).

Most hereditary hearing loss is nonsyndromic. Because nonsyndromic hearing loss is very heterogeneous (highly variable), and most families are small in size, identifying the genes that cause this type of hearing loss is more difficult (Tekin et al., 2001).

TABLE 8.3   Genetic Conditions Related to Childhood Hearing Loss

1. Deafness occurring alone
   - Michel's aplasia
   - Mondini's aplasia
   - Scheibe's aplasia
   - Alexander's aplasia

2. Deafness occurring with other syndromes
   - Waardenburg's syndrome (deafness may be delayed)
   - Albinism
   - Hyperpigmentation
   - Onychodystrophy
   - Pendred syndrome
   - Jervell syndrome
   - Usher syndrome

3. Chromosomal abnormalities
   - Trisomy 13–15
   - Trisomy 18

4. Delayed deafness occurring alone
   - Familial progressive sensorineural hearing loss
   - Otosclerosis

5. Delayed deafness occurring with other abnormalities
   - Alport's disease
   - Hurler syndrome
   - Klippel-Feil syndrome
   - Refsum's disease
   - Alstrom's disease
   - Paget's disease
   - Richards-Rundel syndrome
   - Von Recklinghausen's disease
   - Crouzon's disease

Source: Adapted from Paparella, M. (1977). Differential diagnosis of childhood deafness. In F. Bess (Ed.), *Childhood deafness: Causation, assessment, and management* (pp. 3–18). New York: Grune & Stratton.

Nonsyndromic autosomal inherited hearing loss has been distinguished on the basis of audiometric configuration, as described in Table 8.4. By 1997, gene linkage studies had resulted in the identification of twelve different genotypes for autosomal dominant hereditary nonsyndromic forms of hearing loss according to Stinckens and colleagues (1997). Tekin and colleagues (2001) noted that over twenty of seventy mapped nonsyndromic hearing loss genes had been identified, including eleven autosomal dominant, nine autosomal recessive, and two X-linked recessive. Mutations in a particular gene, called *connexin 26,* have been found to be responsible for a significant proportion of childhood genetic deafness in certain populations. Types of hereditary deafness that

TABLE 8.4 Hereditary Hearing Loss with No Associated Abnormalities

Type	Mode of Inheritance	Onset	Progression	Severity	Type	Audiometric Features
Dominant congenital severe hearing loss	Autosomal dominant	Congenital	–	Severe	Neural	
Dominant progressive nerve loss	Autosomal dominant	Childhood	Slow	Mild to severe	Neural	Hearing loss includes high frequencies first, then all frequencies
Dominant unilateral hearing loss	Autosomal dominant	Congenital	–	Severe	Neural	Hearing loss usually unilateral, occasionally bilateral
Dominant low-frequency hearing loss	Autosomal dominant	Childhood	Slow	Mild to severe	Neural	Low frequencies involved first, progressing to all frequencies
Dominant mid-frequency hearing loss	Autosomal dominant	Childhood	Slow	Mild to severe	Neural	Hearing loss generally begins in mid-frequencies, progression to all frequencies
Otosclerosis	Autosomal dominant	Adult	Slow	Mild to moderate	Conductive	
Recessive congenital severe hearing loss	Autosomal recessive	Congenital	–	Severe	Neural	Several different types have been described
Recessive early onset neural hearing loss	Autosomal recessive	Infant or Childhood	Rapid	Severe	Neural	
Recessive congenital moderate hearing loss	Autosomal recessive	Congenital	None	Moderate	Neural	No progression of hearing loss has been found
Sex-linked congenital hearing loss	X-linked recessive	Congenital	–	Severe	Neural	
Sex-linked early onset hearing loss	X-linked recessive	Congenital	Rapid	Moderate to severe	Neural	
Sex-linked moderate hearing loss	X-linked recessive	Childhood	Slow	Mild to moderate	Neural	Hearing loss involving the high frequencies

Note: Vestibular findings are normal in all types described.

Source: Adapted from Holmes, L. (1977). *Medical genetics in hearing loss in children,* B. Jaffe, Ed. Baltimore: University Park Press, 253–265.

occur alone and their characteristic patterns and audiometric features may be found in Table 8.4. Note that the time of onset of hearing loss varies depending on the particular condition. Stinckens and colleagues (1997) speculate that genetic investigation techniques will allow researchers and clinicians to tell types of sensorineural hearing loss apart that were formerly indistinguishable from one another.

The Human Genome Project has led to identification of a small genome, referred to as the *mitochondrial genome.* Mitochondria are the main source of cell energy and possess their own DNA (mtDNA). According to Tekin and colleagues (2001), mutations in the mitochondrial genome can result in numerous conditions, one of which is hearing loss. The hearing loss is maternally inherited (Keats, 2002) and may or may not involve exposure to aminoglycosides (antibiotics). In some cases, the presence of mitochondrial mutation combined with the use of antibiotics resulted in hearing loss; in other cases, the mitochondrial mutation alone was the cause of the hearing loss.

A basic understanding of terms associated with genetics and the common transmission routes can be helpful both in the diagnosis and management of hearing loss in childhood, offering insight about the onset of the loss and whether it may be expected to be stable or progressive. This information is important to clinicians who provide diagnostic and intervention services for children with hearing loss and their families. Table 8.5 provides the essential terminology for understanding the transmission of characteristics, including hearing loss, from one generation to the next.

Dominantly inherited traits are generally characterized by milder presentation of the condition, although a wide range of clinical presentations is possible. They are also **heterozygous,** meaning that affected individuals transmit the condition to their offspring. All individuals with the condition will have one similarly affected parent; not all offspring will have the condition because there is a 50 percent chance of its occurrence. In **autosomal recessive** inheritance, which accounts for the majority of genetic hearing losses, the affected individual must receive the same abnormal gene from each parent. In this case, both parents must be carriers (heterozygous) for transmission to occur. There is a 25 percent chance that each child of two carriers will be affected by the condition, a 50 percent chance that each child of two carriers will be carriers, and a 25 percent chance that each child will not inherit the abnormal gene from either parent. Chances of autosomal recessive genetic inheritance are generally low, but increase when two parents have a common ancestor (i.e., in cases of consanguinity).

For example, a type of hearing loss called *dominant congenital severe hearing loss* is characterized by dominant transmission and congenital onset, as its name implies. The associated degree of hearing loss is severe, and the type of the loss is sensorineural and does not progress. Vestibular findings are normal and there are no other associated abnormalities with this diagnosis. In Pendred's disease, the genetic transmission is recessive and onset is congenital. The associated hearing loss is typically moderate to severe in degree and sensorineural in type. Vestibular findings are depressed. This condition is also characterized by the development of goiter in adolescence. Usher syndrome has been found to have an autosomal recessive inheritance pattern and is a group of six clinically different disorders. One of the forms of Usher syndrome that has been identified involves both hearing and vision impairment, with eventual loss of vision (Keats, 2002). Considering these three examples, it can be seen that early identification of hearing loss coupled with accurate knowledge about the etiology and type of hearing loss is critical for counseling the family and developing the most appropriate management strategies.

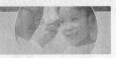

TABLE 8.5 Essential Terms for Understanding Genetic Transmission of Hearing Loss

Chromosomes—the bearers of genes, found in the cell nucleus. In humans, there are forty-six chromosomes; these occur in pairs, with one member of each pair from each parent.

Deoxyribonucleic acid (DNA)—double-helical structure composed of a sugar-phosphate backbone and four bases: adenine (A), guanine (G), thymine (T), and cytosine (C); carrier of genetic information.

Gene—the functional unit of heredity. Each occupies a specific location on a chromosome and is capable of reproducing itself exactly as the cells divide.

Mitochondria—small organelles located in the cytoplasm of cells; main source of cell energy; independent of the cell nucleus; possess their own DNA (mtDNA).

Autosomal dominant—inheritance of the condition is caused by a fully penetrant gene. When a single abnormal gene is present in either parent, each child has a 50 percent chance of inheriting the trait. Penetrance is a measure of a gene's ability to produce its effect in an individual: a fully penetrant gene will produce the effect 100 percent of the time, while a gene with decreased penetrance will produce the effect in a lesser proportion of individuals.

Autosomal recessive—two abnormal genes (one from each parent) are necessary for transmission. If both parents are carriers, each child has a 25 percent probability of inheritance.

Autosome—any chromosome that is not an X-chromosome or a Y-chromosome (i.e., a chromosome other than a sex chromosome). Of the twenty-three pairs of chromosomes in humans, twenty-two pairs are autosomal and the remaining pair is X-linked.

Sex-linked or **X-linked**—a gene located on the X-chromosome. The X-chromosome occurs singly in the nucleus of a male, who also has a Y-chromosome, and occurs twice in the female nucleus, which has no Y-chromosome.

Polygenic—transmission pattern in which multiple genes contribute to the manifested condition.

Heterozygous—a gene pair composed of different genes (carrier).

Homozygous—a gene pair composed of identical genes (affected individual).

Speech and Language Development in Early Childhood

Now that you have learned about developmental information regarding early childhood in general and the auditory system in particular, let's take a closer look at the development of speech and language. This is important information for the audiologist because speech and language development is closely tied to a child's hearing. Inquiring about age-appropriate developmental speech and language milestones is a critical part of an audiologist's role. Also, although formal assessment of speech and language development is not part of the scope of practice of the audiologist, speech and language screening is part of the audiologist's scope of practice, as is making appropriate referrals for comprehensive speech and language assessment. For these reasons, a basic understanding of developmental speech and language norms is included in this chapter. These norms are summarized in Table 8.6.

TABLE 8.6   Summary of Primary Language and Articulation Development in Young Children

Age	Language Skills	Speech Sounds Mastered
8–12 months	Follows simple commands Says first word Plays with sound	
12–18 months	Uses a variety of one-word utterances Uses "yes" and "no" Points to toys, people, clothing	
18 months–2 years	Uses a variety of two-word utterances Complies with simple spoken commands Identifies body parts	
2 years	200- to 300-word receptive vocabulary Names everyday objects Uses short sentences including some prepositions and some morphological markers	
3 years	Uses three- to four-word utterances Uses simple sentence structure (S-V or S-V-O) Follows two-step commands	Vowel sounds p, m, n, wh
4 years	Continued vocabulary growth and increased sentence complexity Increased skill at asking questions Retells stories accurately	b, d, k, g, f, j
5 years	Continued vocabulary growth Follows three-step commands Has 90% grammar acquisition	y, ng, d
6 years		t, r, l, sh, ch, & blends
7 years		v, th, s, z, & blends
8 years		th (voiced) & blends

As you review Table 8.6, you should be aware of a few key themes. First, note that although the beginnings of receptive language can be observed before 1 year of age, mastery of speech sounds takes much longer. In fact, it is not until after a child's fifth birthday that many speech sounds are fully mastered. Parents often bring a child in for audiological assessment because of concerns that the child's speech is "not clear." For example, consider the parents who come to the speech and hearing clinic with their 3-year-old, who is demonstrating the language skills noted in Table 8.6 but who "still can't say many sounds clearly." According to the norms provided, the child's language is developing appropriately and the child's lack of mastery of speech sounds is expected at this age. Audiologists often find themselves reassuring parents that the way a child's speech sounds (i.e., the child's articulation) is less important early in life than the child's language development (the child's ability to understand speech and, for example, to follow simple directions and to make his or her wants and needs known). However, the relationship between hearing loss and speech sound production must also be acknowledged.

What about the 3-year-old whose expressive language is limited to one-word utterances? Based on the information in Table 8.6, this is of concern because the typical 3-year-old exhibits utterances that are three to four words in length. This profile warrants comprehensive assessment by a speech–language pathologist, either independently or as part of a multidisciplinary team evaluation.

Finally, whenever audiologists are in doubt about what to recommend to parents about a child's speech production and/or language development, they should contact a speech–language pathologist for guidance or have the parent contact the therapist directly. Audiologists who do not work in a facility that also employs speech–language pathologists should establish positive working relationships with speech–language pathologists in their area. When any question exists regarding a child's speech–language development, audiologists should refer the child and family to a speech–language pathologist for consultation. In addition to formal assessment, the speech–language pathologist will make recommendations to promote speech and language development. Examples of such recommendations are included in Appendix A.

General Principles of Pediatric Audiological Assessment

From years of providing clinical audiology services to children, some broad principles have emerged that we believe are helpful in this work.

Principle #1. The audiological assessment should be structured so as to answer efficiently the particular question(s) that is/are being asked about the particular child. Although this is true for clients of all ages, it is especially true for pediatric clients because they may have limited abilities to perform the required task, remain on task for an extended period of time, or remain motivated to complete the testing. Clearly, behavioral assessment requires the child's attention and motivation to carry out specific tasks, but even physiological measures, such as immittance audiometry and otoacoustic emissions, require some degree of cooperation on the child's part (i.e., to remain still and relatively quiet). Failure on the audiologist's part to structure the test protocol based on the presenting questions/issues for a given child can result in inefficiency and can lead to not addressing the issues at hand.

Let's now discuss principle #1 in the context of one of the most commonly asked questions: Is this child's hearing adequate for normal speech and language development? Knowing the purpose of the evaluation, an audiologist must decide what specific tests should be done to answer that question. Often pure tones are used as part of this assessment. In order to improve efficiency, the audiologist may decide to forego threshold testing and instead may screen the child at various frequencies that are important to speech and language development. The advantages of using a pure tone screening are that it is much quicker than searching for threshold, often more reliable, and still answers the question at hand. As illustrated in Figure 8.3, the combination of pure tone information obtained in this way with results of speech audiometry yields the answer to the presenting question.

Principle #2. In structuring the audiological assessment to answer the specific question(s) about the particular child, the audiologist must factor in the child's age, temperament, and ability. These nonaudiological factors cannot be ignored because, regardless of the type of testing being done (except for perhaps testing done under sedation), obtaining audiological data requires that the child participate, to a greater or lesser extent, in the process. When attention is paid to the child's abilities and temperament and testing

FIGURE **8.3** **Combination of pure tone screening with speech audiometry.**

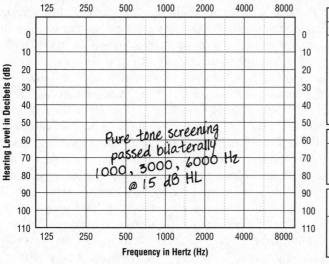

Ear	SRT	SDT	PTA	Test	Word Recognition Level/Percent Correct	MCL	LDL
Right		10		WIPI	40/100%		
Left		10		WIPI	40/100%		
Bone							
Sound Field							
Right Aided							
Left Aided							
Binaural Aided							

decisions are made with these in mind, the likelihood of success increases and the overall experience for the child, the parent, and the audiologist is improved.

To illustrate this point, consider the case of a typically developing 4-year-old child who was seen for audiological assessment due to recurring middle ear pathology. Although the child was 4 years of age, it quickly became apparent that he was very shy and initially hesitant to speak to or interact with strangers. In view of this, a decision was made to begin testing in the sound field, rather than under earphones. In addition, the initial task selected was to obtain a speech detection threshold using play audiometry, which would not require verbal responses. Note that our approach for other 4-year-olds could be very different, depending on the personality traits and abilities presented.

It should also be noted that information regarding a child's age is more helpful at some ages than others. For example, knowing that a child is 12 months of age is helpful because despite variability that exists in children of the same age, it is very likely that this 1-year-old will be able to participate in certain types of testing and will not be capable of participating in other types. In contrast, knowing that a child is 2 years old is less helpful because the variability among 2-year-olds is great. In this case, information about the child's ability and temperament will likely be more useful.

Principle #3. Multiple methods of assessment should be used to answer the question at hand. Because of the variety of behavioral and physiological assessment tools from which an audiologist can choose, it is good policy to collect information about the child's hearing from more than one source and then determine if these different sources are leading to the same conclusion. For example, the child who presents with air–bone gaps based on pure tone audiometry should also exhibit some type of abnormality on admittance test results. This congruence in data adds greatly to the reliability of the test findings and decreases the likelihood that the data have been influenced by child variables, such as a lack of attention to the task or an inability to understand the task directions.

Principle #4. Although multiple visits are often necessary to answer the presenting question, a "reasonable" time frame for making a diagnosis should be maintained. Any audiologist who works with children is aware that it may be necessary to see a child more than once to address completely the audiological question that has been posed. At the same time, it is also important to reiterate that undiagnosed and untreated hearing loss can have a disastrous effect on a child's speech–language development and learning. For this reason, decisions regarding the need for amplification or medical treatment must be made in a timely manner. The overarching goal of early hearing detection and intervention programs is consistent with Healthy People 2000 Objective 28.11, which includes diagnosing hearing loss by the age of 3 months and initiating habilitation by age 6 months. With this goal in mind, audiologists must use all of the resources available to them to diagnose hearing loss in children as early in life as possible so that the necessary remediation process can begin.

Special Role of Multidisciplinary Teams and Parents

Assessment and intervention for children with hearing loss requires building relationships among various teams throughout the child's life. In the period from birth to age 3, early-intervention program team members, with parents in a central role, work together toward agreed-upon outcomes to enhance the child's development. As the child becomes older, the preschool special education system (ages 3–5 five years) and later the educational system (5–21 years) will work with the child and family to plan and implement an appropriate educational program. The composition of the team will depend on the needs and preferences of the child with hearing loss and the family and may change over time. It is helpful to be aware of the laws and regulations that govern children's eligibility for services. The general information included later in this chapter should be supplemented by relevant information from state and local resources.

Service delivery to children with disabilities is part of the **Individuals with Disabilities Education Act (IDEA)**. IDEA is the federal law that governs Part C early intervention programs and Part B special education services. In addition to IDEA, **Section 504 of the Rehabilitation Act of 1973** contains language that is relevant to provision of services for students with hearing loss. Issues related to accessibility for individuals with hearing loss and other disabilities are addressed by the Americans with Disabilities Act. Table 8.7 contains information pertaining to delivery of audiological evaluations and/or services according to the provisions of relevant laws.

The classroom teacher(s) is in a unique position to observe changes in performance or behavior and to make recommendations that these be further explored.

Signs of possible hearing loss in students include:

- Academic achievement is below expectations for age/grade level
- Lack of attention to tasks/daydreaming
- Misunderstanding general information or directions
- Language skills (understanding language or producing language) below age/grade level

One helpful tool that can be used by a student's educators, including the classroom teacher, any resource teachers, or therapists is the **Screening Instrument for Targeting Educational Risk (SIFTER;** Anderson, 1989). This tool can be used both to identify and to monitor a student's classroom performance. It covers five general areas, including academics, attention, communication, class participation, and school behavior. The SIFTER is designed to flag those students who may be at educational risk due to hearing problems and is included in Appendix B.

For school-age children identified with hearing loss, a collaborative approach is recommended among the parents, student, educators, and related professionals. The minimum areas to be addressed include amplification options and modifications to enhance communication in the academic setting. The evaluation process should also include a speech–language evaluation to determine whether specific supports and services are needed and the frequency and intensity of such services. Table 8.7 contains information on federal legislation that is relevant to providing audiological services for school-age children.

The Assessment Process

The assessment of any age group, and perhaps children in particular, requires use of a combination of both behavioral and nonbehavioral tools. This chapter is arranged to

TABLE **8.7**   Laws Related to Providing Audiological Services

Law and Affected Age Group	Audiological Services	Documentation
IDEA PL 94-142 The Individuals with Disabilities Education Act (under the Office of Special Education Programs [OSEP]) Ages 5–21 years	Addressed in Section 300.16 of the Code of Federal Regulations (CFR) on Education, Title 34 (revision of July 1, 1997). Section 300.16 of the federal regulations defines *audiology* to include: i. Identification of children with hearing loss; ii. Determination of the range, nature, and degree of hearing loss, including referral for medical or other professional attention for the habilitation of hearing; iii. Provision of habilitative activities, such as language habilitation, auditory training, speech reading (lip reading), hearing evaluation, and speech conservation; iv. Creation and administration of programs for prevention of hearing loss; v. Counseling and guidance of pupils, parents, and teachers regarding hearing loss; and vi. Determination of the child's need for group and individual amplification, selection and fitting of an appropriate aid, and evaluation of the effectiveness of amplification.	Individualized Education Program (IEP)
IDEA PL 99-457 Ages 3–5 years (Part B of IDEA) were included as of the 1991–1992 school year; participation by states in provision of services to infants and toddlers (formerly Part H, now Part C of IDEA) is encouraged, but not required.	Audiological services included in the *Federal Register* for younger children are similar to those included in PL 94-142, addressing the identification, evaluation, and rehabilitation of hearing loss.	Individualized Family Service Plan (IFSP)

TABLE 8.7 *(continued)*

Law and Affected Age Group	Audiological Services	Documentation
Section 504 of the Rehabilitation Act of 1973 (under the Office for Civil Rights, U.S. Department of Education [OCR]) All ages	This section applies to all individuals to participate in school-sponsored programs or activities. For students in elementary, middle, and secondary education, Section 504 of the Rehabilitation Act provides that: "No otherwise qualified individual with handicaps in the United States, . . . shall, solely by reason of her or his handicap, be excluded from the participation in, be denied the benefits of, or be subjected to discrimination under any program or activity receiving Federal financial assistance. . . ." The definition of "handicapped person" under Section 504 is broader than the definition of "a child with a disability" under IDEA. In addition, under Section 504, a FAPE is defined as ". . . the provision of regular or special education and related aids and services that . . . is designed to meet the individual educational needs of handicapped persons as adequately as the needs of non-handicapped persons are met . . ." (34 CFR 104.33). If a child with hearing loss does not meet the eligibility requirements for special education services under IDEA, provision of adaptations to or modifications of regular education services to support the student's academic performance under Section 504 can be explored.	According to Section 504, provision of an IEP is one way to meet the FAPE requirement. Other documentation practices might include keeping a written record of the specific accommodations to be provided to a child. Practices may vary; seek direction from the specific school district for local policies and procedures for implementing Section 504 provisions.
The Americans with Disabilities Act (ADA) of 1990 All ages	Provides comprehensive civil rights protections to individuals with disabilities in the areas of employment, public accommodations, state and local government services, and telecommunications.	

Note: IDEA and Section 504 of the Rehabilitation Act address numerous issues, including, but not limited to: free and appropriate education (FAPE); least restrictive environment (LRE); compliance and enforcement, procedural safeguards (protections for parents' rights); evaluations; reevaluations; parental consent; composition of the multidisciplinary team; documentation; due process (procedures to be undertaken if there is a disagreement about the identification, evaluation, or educational placement of a child with a disability); and discipline of students with disabilities. Clinicians should be aware of relevant federal, state, and local laws, regulations, and policies and procedures that have an impact on service delivery.

Sources: Code of Federal Regulations on Education, Title 34-Education, IDEA 1997 Final Regulations (34 CFR Part 300). Available: www.ideapractices.org/regs/SubpartA.htm; Flexer, C. (1993). Management of hearing in an educational setting. In J. Alpiner and P. McCarthy (eds.), *Rehabilitative audiology: Children and adults.* Baltimore: Lippincott, Williams & Wilkins.

emphasize information regarding behavioral assessment of young children. Most of this information will be new to you, and for this reason it is the focus of this chapter. Physiological measures, which have been addressed in detail in Chapter 6, are included in the case examples in this chapter so that you will begin to understand how both behavioral and physiological tools are used together in hearing assessment.

It is important to note that although the development and use of physiological assessment tools with young children represent a very exciting and "high-tech" aspect of the field, audiologists must also possess skills that allow them to perform **behavioral tests of hearing.** There are three main reasons for this. First, although physiological measures, such as otoacoustic emissions and auditory brainstem testing, provide information regarding the integrity of certain structures that are important to the process of hearing, neither technique is a direct measure of hearing. Second, a number of conditions may compromise the results of these measures. For example, both otoacoustic emission and auditory brainstem testing are affected by the presence of middle ear pathology, a very common condition in children. Otoacoustic emissions testing also requires that the child remain relatively quiet. Similarly, beyond the newborn period, auditory brainstem testing often requires that the child be sedated. Finally, skill in performing behavioral testing is important because the increased use of physiological measures immediately after birth will result in greater numbers of young infants being referred for audiological assessment and management.

Students of audiology should also be reminded that the growing popularity of **universal newborn hearing screening programs** does not eliminate the need for ongoing monitoring of young children's responsiveness to auditory stimuli and consequently for comprehensive audiological assessment. Even those babies who have passed their mandatory screening should be afforded the same type of informal parental monitoring of auditory responsiveness and speech–language development that was done prior to the use of universal hearing screening programs. Keep in mind that the screening protocols used in newborn screening programs are designed to separate infants who need further audiological testing from those who do not; however, screening is not designed to provide specific threshold information or a complete picture of a child's hearing loss.

In view of this discussion, students of audiology should view the development of their skills in pediatric behavioral testing as an essential part of their training. Also, students of speech–language pathology must have an understanding of the various behavioral tools available in order to provide input to the audiologist regarding the preferred behavioral approach for a specific client. In addition, speech–language pathologists must be able to understand the meaning of behavioral audiological results in order to use these data in planning the child's therapy.

Case History

History taking is an important component of a pediatric audiological evaluation for a number of reasons. The information that can be derived from a comprehensive case history includes:

- Whether the child has factors that increase the possibility of hearing loss
- Clues about the possible etiology of hearing loss
- Other developmental concerns or issues to be addressed

- How the family views hearing loss
- Components of the test battery

Refer to Table 8.8 for sample case history questions and rationale for each. Note that several of the items on the case history were derived from the High Risk Register, which includes factors known to increase risk for permanent hearing loss in childhood, such as anoxia at birth, low birth weight, elevated bilirubin levels (jaundice), and family history of hearing loss.

In addition to providing insight about factors that may be contributing to a hearing loss, if identified, this information is critical to both the diagnostic audiological process and to the development of appropriate management strategies. Management strategies may be tied directly to audiological management or may involve referral to other professionals for additional evaluation. For further information, consult the **Joint Committee on Infant Hearing 2000 Position Statement,** which provides useful information related to infant hearing screening programs. The Developmental Index of Audition and Listening (DIAL), presented in Table 8.1, also provides useful information about milestones related to auditory skill development.

General Considerations in Pediatric Assessment

Three general considerations in testing young children's hearing are use of the sound field, minimum response levels, and choice of test stimuli.

The Sound Field

Up to this point, we have focused on air conduction testing performed in a sound-treated room, under earphones, as the primary behavioral method for obtaining information about hearing sensitivity in each ear. Although obtaining ear-specific information using earphones is the goal in testing all ages, it is not always possible with young children. Some young children may not tolerate earphones or may become so distracted by them that their ability to attend to the auditory signals is compromised. In these cases, an audiologist uses **sound field testing,** which refers to the presentation of signals through speakers that are mounted in the sound-treated booth. Illustrated in Figure 8.4 is an example of a sound field setup. Recall from our discussion in Chapter 4 that the room used is often a two-room suite, separated by a window. One side of the suite is the control room where the audiologist sits, and the other side is for the client. The child is seated on the chair, typically on the caregiver's lap, facing the window. The control side of the two-room suite is typically darkened so that the infant is unaware of the audiologist. Note also that there is a second observer in this room, preferably also an audiologist. Finally, note the two speakers mounted on the walls of the room and that to the side of each of these speakers is an animated toy. These can be illuminated by the audiologist and can be used to reinforce the child's responses to various types of auditory stimuli (e.g., tones, speech, and noisemakers).

We noted previously in our general discussion of infants that because of the maturity of cochlear and eighth-nerve structures at birth, the typical infant has hearing sensitivity that is within normal limits. However, the ability of infants to demonstrate their awareness to sound is limited to some extent by their **neurophysiological immaturity.** In other words, even though more objective measures, such as otoacoustic emissions and auditory

TABLE **8.8** **Components of Pediatric Case History**

Case History Question	Rationale
Identifying information (name, date of birth, address, telephone number, parents' names)	Record keeping/documentation and follow-up purposes
History (birth, medical, developmental)	
1. What did the baby weigh?	1. Birth weight under 3.3 pounds or 1,500 grams is a risk factor for hearing loss.
2. Apgar scores	2. Low Apgar scores suggest risk factors such as anoxia may have been present at the time of birth.
3. How many days was the baby in the hospital?	3. Extended hospitalization indicates that other factors related to hearing loss may be present.
4. Did the baby require any special care—either in the regular nursery or in the NICU?	4. Special care may include phototherapy for hyperbilirubinemia (jaundice), or oxygen, or intravenous medication, all of which signal risk factors.
5. Is there a history of infections either before or after birth?	5. In-utero infections such as cytomegalovirus, maternal rubella are risk factors; postnatal infections such as meningitis are associated with sensorineural hearing loss.
6. Is there a family history of hearing loss in childhood?	6. Another risk factor for hearing loss, which may be genetic or nongenetic.
7. Do you have concerns about your baby's hearing, speech/language development or general development?	7. Parental concerns should be considered regardless of whether the child has passed a newborn hearing screening because conditions may have changed and passing a newborn hearing screening does not preclude the development of late onset hearing loss or hearing loss due to recurrent otitis media.
8. Probe developmental milestones for development of motor and speech skills appropriate for the child's chronological age (e.g., how old was your child when she or he first sat up, crawled, walked, babbled, said their first word, etc.?).	8. Failure to develop age-appropriate motor skills (e.g., not sitting up at age 6 months) or speech skills (e.g., not babbling at age 9 months or stopping babbling) provide clues about the possibility of hearing loss and/or the need for other referrals to be made.
9. Have you received any other diagnostic information about your child?	9. Other conditions or syndromes may be present that are known to have hearing loss associated with them.
10. Has your child had ear infections?	10. Provides information about the possibility of conductive hearing loss, which may exist alone or in addition to sensorineural hearing loss.
11. If so, how many ear infections has your child had and when did they begin?	11. Provides insight regarding whether this is a chronic or occasional problem, the duration, and whether critical periods for speech–language development may be compromised.
12. How were they treated?	12. Provides insight regarding whether medications or surgery have been employed and whether referral has been made from the pediatrician/primary health care provider to a specialist (otolaryngologist).
13. Is there any other information you think is important for us to know?	13. Allows the parents/caregivers to fill in any information that may have been missed.

FIGURE **8.4** **Two-room audiological test suite typically used during behavioral testing of young children.**

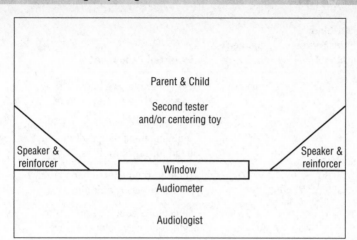

brainstem response testing, support the presence of normal hearing sensitivity very early in life, infants often lack the neurological development to coordinate neuromotor responses to auditory signals that are presented at threshold levels.

Hicks, Tharpe, and Ashmead (2000) conducted behavioral testing of 2- and 4-month-old infants and found that although thresholds could be obtained for the 4-month-old babies, the 2-month-old subjects were generally unresponsive to low- and moderate-intensity sounds and responded mostly at intensity levels that elicit startle responses. Also, Tharpe and Ashmead (2001) conducted a longitudinal investigation of infant auditory sensitivity using a behavioral testing procedure and found that responses of infants at 3 months of age were approximately 20 dB greater than adult thresholds; by 6 months of age, responses were 10 to 15 dB greater than the adult response.

In view of this information, at different ages and for different types of stimuli (e.g., speech, tones, noisemakers), infants and young children with normal hearing will exhibit different auditory responses. It is for this reason that some audiologists use a special set of norms when judging the responses of very young children. These are found in Table 8.9 and were adapted from McConnell and Ward (1967) by Northern and Downs (2002). Note that as children become older and more neurologically mature, they respond at softer levels. Hearing sensitivity is not improving, but their responsiveness to sound is improving. For most children, speech is the most salient of the presented stimuli because they have the most experience listening to speech and because it is a complex stimulus. As a result, they respond to speech at softer levels than to other stimuli.

Thresholds or Minimum Response Levels

Some controversy exists among audiologists as to whether behavioral testing can result in the measurement of very young children's actual thresholds or merely the lowest levels at which they exhibit a behavioral response to sound. If thresholds are being measured,

TABLE 8.9 Auditory Behavior Index for Infants: Stimulus and Level of Response*

Age	Noisemakers (Approximate dB SPL)	Warbled Pure Tones (dB HL)	Speech (dB HL)	Expected Response	Startle to Speech (db HL)
0–6 weeks	50–70	75	40–60	Eye widening, eye blink, stirring or arousal from sleep, startle	65
6 weeks–4 months	50–60	70	45	Eye widening, eye shift, eye blink, quieting; beginning rudimentary head turn by 4 months	65
4–7 months	40–50	50	20	Head turn on lateral plane toward sound; listening attitude	65
7–9 months	30–40	45	15	Direct localization of sounds to side, indirectly below ear level	65
9–13 months	25–35	38	10	Direct localization of sounds to side, directly below ear level, indirectly above ear level	65
13–16 months	25–30	30	5	Direct localization of sounds on side, above and below	65
16–21 months	25	25	5	Direct localization of sounds on side, above and below	65
21–24 months	25	25	5	Direct localization of sounds on side, above and below	65

*Testing done in a sound room.

Source: From Northern, J., & Downs, M. (2002). *Hearing in children* (5th ed.). New York: Lippincott, Williams & Wilkins. Reprinted by permission. McConnell, F., & Ward, P. (1967). *Deafness in childhood.* Nashville, TN: Vanderbilt University Press. Reprinted with permission.

this tells us about the child's auditory *sensitivity.* If, however, very young children respond at some level above their threshold (Martin & Clarke, 1996), we are limited to measuring **minimum response levels,** which tell us about auditory *responsiveness.* Some audiologists who believe that thresholds can be measured very early in life acknowledge that with age there is some slight improvement in very young children's responding due to increased attention and motivation (Diefendorf & Gravel, 1996).

Despite the lack of clear consensus on this topic, a review of the available information regarding threshold versus minimum response levels appears to support the following guidelines for testing very young children:

- Behavioral assessment of children from birth to 4 months of age is more a determination of auditory responsiveness, rather than hearing sensitivity. For this age group, responses to both speech and frequency-modulated (FM) tones can be very elevated (approximately 45–50 dB for speech and 70 dB to FM tones), compared to adult thresholds (i.e., 25 dB).

- Beyond 4–6 months of age, behavioral responses to speech stimuli should be noted at levels that are very similar to adult norms. Responses to FM tones may continue to be elevated until approximately 1.5 years of age.
- In all cases where elevated responses are noted, even when those responses are consistent with normative data, reassessment is recommended with the expectation that responses will improve with age.

Effectiveness of Test Stimuli

Speech is typically an effective stimulus for young listeners. Why, then, do audiologists attempt to use the less interesting pure tone or FM stimuli? The answer relates back to our discussion in Chapter 4 regarding the value of pure tone data. Remember that although speech is an effective stimulus for eliciting responses from the child, it does not provide audiologists with frequency-specific information. Recall from Chapter 5 that it is possible for a young child to respond at very normal levels to speech stimuli and still have a very significant hearing loss. The young child's response to speech at a given intensity level simply tells us that some portion of the speech spectrum is available to the child at that level. Note that we have said "some portion of the speech spectrum"; responses to speech alone do not provide information about how much of the speech spectrum is available, or about the configuration of a hearing loss, if present. To reiterate, interpretation of a normal response to speech stimuli must be made with caution, because it may mean simply that a very limited portion of the speech spectrum is heard at a normal intensity level; it clearly should not be interpreted as an indication that the child has "normal hearing."

In addition to the use of FM tones and speech stimuli, note also in Table 8.9 that noisemakers have been used. One of the reasons why noisemakers are appealing to the audiologist is that they produce complex signals that typically are effective in eliciting responses from infants. The limitation of noisemakers is the same as for speech stimuli: although effective in eliciting responses, information is not gained regarding what specific frequencies the child can and cannot hear. Like speech, the signal created by a noisemaker typically contains energy in many frequencies.

The above discussion highlights one of the many dilemmas facing audiologists who perform behavioral audiological assessments on children. The very stimuli that are most effective at eliciting responses from the child provide the least frequency-specific information, and the stimuli that do provide this information (i.e., pure tones or FM signals) are the least interesting to the child.

In view of the fact that collecting frequency-specific information is a critical part of the audiological assessment, how can the examiner minimize the difficulties noted above? One method is to use nonbehavioral methods of assessment to gain information about the child's ability to hear specific frequencies. For example, distortion product otoacoustic emissions can be used to obtain frequency-specific information on children who can sit quietly for the test and who do not have middle ear pathology.

Another practice among some audiologists in attempting to address this dilemma is to use narrow bands of noise, rather than pure tones or FM signals. As we noted in Chapter 4, **narrow-band noise** is a noise created by bandpass filtering that is centered at a specific audiometric frequency. The problem with using narrow bands of noise in the assessment of very young children is that the narrow bands produced by many audiometers are not as "narrow" as was once believed. So, for example, if the audiologist presents a 3,000-Hz narrow band of noise in the sound field and the child responds at a given intensity level, the audiologist cannot assume that information has been obtained about the child's hearing only at 3,000 Hz. If, in fact, that 3,000-Hz signal actually includes energy at frequencies lower and higher than 3,000 Hz, it is possible that the child's response to the signal reflects hearing ability at some other frequency. This can be particularly problematic in cases of high-frequency hearing loss, when the child responds normally to high-frequency narrow bands of noise because of the presence of lower-frequency energy within the signal's band of energy.

Another option that may be used by the audiologist is to replace the traditional speech stimuli with some type of filtered speech. A **filtered speech** task is one in which speech is presented through a device that allows only certain energy through. If a high-pass filter is used, high-frequency speech information is audible but low-frequency information is not included in the signal. Conversely, if a low-pass filter is used, low-frequency speech information is audible but high-frequency information is not. These types of modifications to speech can be useful in improving its frequency specificity and therefore its value to the audiologist.

Pediatric Test Techniques

This section includes specific test techniques for different age groups. Behavioral observation audiometry, visual reinforcement audiometry, and conditioned play audiometry are discussed.

Behavioral Observation Audiometry

Although its limitations are many and electrophysiological methods are superior in a number of ways, **behavioral observation audiometry (BOA)** is still used by audiologists as a behavioral method of assessing children's hearing up to 4 months of age. As the name suggests, this type of assessment involves careful observation of the infant's change in behavior in response to auditory stimuli. As is evident from Table 8.9, the stimulus levels used in testing children of this age category are rather intense. Also, expected responses include reflexive behaviors, such as eye blinking, change in sucking activity, or a startle response and orienting behaviors, such as eye widening or searching. During BOA testing the second observer is important because it may be difficult for the audiologist located in the control room to note the more subtle changes in the infant's behavior.

Remember, because the testing described above will most likely not be performed under earphones, the audiologist has gained information about the child's responsiveness to sound in only one ear. In other words, without earphones, the audiologist has not gained data regarding the right and left ears. Therefore, a child who responds well in the sound field could still have hearing loss in one ear. Finally, as has been addressed previously, perhaps the greatest concern regarding the use of BOA is that although it gives some information about the child's responsiveness to sound, it does not assess the child's threshold.

Visual Reinforcement Audiometry

In addition to challenges in audiological assessment of very young children created by the type of stimulus being used, reliable measurement of an infant's hearing is also made difficult by auditory habituation. **Habituation** is common in infants and refers to a reduction in the frequency and strength of a response as the novelty of the stimuli eliciting the response is decreased. In other words, as the audiological assessment proceeds and speech and tonal stimuli are repeated over and over, they lose some of their novelty and the child becomes less interested in them. This loss of interest is demonstrated by a lack of responsiveness, which obviously is problematic when attempting to assess hearing.

One way to deal with this phenomenon of auditory habituation is to alternate among the various test stimuli in order to maintain novelty. In other words, rather than presenting tonal stimuli for an extended period of time, the audiologist may choose to present speech for a brief period followed by tonal stimuli and then returning to speech. In some cases, renewed interest in the signal is created simply by changing from one test frequency to a different test frequency.

A very effective way to reduce habituation is to reinforce the child for appropriate responses to sound. This technique is referred to as **visual reinforcement audiometry (VRA)** and is most effectively used for children from approximately 5 months to 2 years of age. VRA relies on the child's ability to localize by turning toward the source of the sound. At this age, the child has matured enough that reflexive activity has decreased and the child can be conditioned to respond to sound.

How does this conditioning take place? One approach is first to pair sound with the visual reinforcement. The audiologist presents the auditory stimulus and simultaneously illuminates the toy. At this point, the child turns to observe the illuminated toy. After a few trials of this, the sound is presented, the child turns toward it, and is then reinforced with the lighted toy. This process of training the child to respond to the sound in order to receive reinforcement is referred to as **conditioning.** You may be familiar with the terms conditioning and reinforcement from your psychology coursework and may recall that a **reinforcement** is a positive consequence of some behavior that increases the likelihood that the behavior will occur again. As noted, this reinforcement reduces habituation and gives an audiologist a greater opportunity to obtain a range of responses from the child using a variety of stimuli. A child is conditioned to this task when random head movements are minimized and the child's head turning is elicited almost exclusively by the presentation of the auditory signal and is time-locked to the auditory signal.

When learning new tasks, reinforcement, as defined by Skinner (1983), is most effective when every correct response is reinforced. So, in the case of conditioning the child to localize, every time the child turns to the correct sound, the audiologist should reinforce that response. Research also indicates that once a behavior is established, **intermittent reinforcement** is actually more effective than **continuous reinforcement** because it increases the child's drive to be reinforced, which increases the desired behavior. Based on this information regarding reinforcement schedules, reinforcement during the conditioning phase should be after every correct response. Once the behavior is learned, some form of intermittent reinforcement should be used to keep the child responding for as long as possible.

When testing very young children it is quite helpful to have a second audiologist in the room with the child and parent. Although this is not always possible in work settings with limited personnel, the use of a second audiologist can greatly improve the reliability of the obtained data. Specifically, when VRA is used, this second audiologist serves the important function of keeping the child looking toward the midline when the child is not localizing sound. In other words, in order to obtain unambiguous responses to sound presented to the child's left and right sides, it is important that, when not responding to sound (between trials), the child is facing the midline. This second audiologist assists in this process by mildly (and, if possible, nonverbally) distracting the child, perhaps with some type of toy. The challenge here is to avoid too much distraction of the child because this can interfere with responsiveness to sound.

Another role of a second audiologist is to prevent parents from becoming so involved in the evaluation that they interfere with the testing. This is especially important if the child is seated on the parent's lap because some parents inadvertently provide cues to the child that sound is present. This is an obvious contamination of the testing and must be avoided. Some audiologists seat the child in a high chair to avoid communication between mother and child. In addition, the second audiologist often provides reassurance to parents in those cases when children are not responding to all of the signals being presented, but are still responding appropriately for their age.

Because most infants will have hearing that is within normal limits, it is logical for the audiologist to begin the testing process at intensity levels of 30 to 40 dB HL. As was the case for pure tone testing, audiologists use an ascending–descending approach to identify the lowest intensity level at which the child responds (usually in at least half of a series of trials). For example, when the child responds to a given signal, the audiologist decreases the intensity by 10 or 20 dB, presents this softer signal, and watches for localization. If a response is noted, another decrease in intensity results; if no response is observed, the signal is increased by 10 dB. When presenting signals, an audiologist should avoid presentation that is predictable and should use a sequence of auditory signals and brief periods of silence to ensure that responses are time-locked to the stimulus. Remember also that although VRA can be used successfully under earphones, there will be children who will not tolerate earphones and the testing will have to be done in the sound field.

The following two cases illustrate the use of VRA testing. The first case, illustrated in Figure 8.5, is an 8-month-old child whose speech detection threshold of 20 dB is within the norm. Responses to FM tones at 35 dB at 500 and 2,000 Hz and at 30 dB at 4,000 Hz are also within the norm for the child's age. Because earphone data were not collected, otoacoustic emission testing was also used to gain ear-specific information and was consistent with the normal findings. One of the important recommendations will be to pursue follow-up audiological testing to definitively rule out a mild hearing loss.

Contrast this with the case illustrated in Figure 8.6. This child is 16 months old, and responses to both speech and tones are not within the expected range for her age. This child appears to have a moderate to severe hearing loss. In this case, a test battery approach incorporating otoacoustic emission, auditory brainstem, and admittance test data should be used to provide further information regarding the type and severity of the loss. In this case, acoustic reflexes would be absent, and otoacoustic emissions would be absent, consistent with the degree of loss suggested by VRA. Further, absence of identifiable ABR waveforms at intensity levels less than 85 dB is consistent with this loss. Normal tympanometry suggests that the loss is likely to be sensorineural in nature.

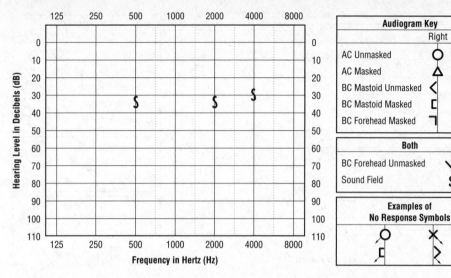

FIGURE **8.5** **Age-appropriate responses (using visual reinforcement audiometry) for an 8-month-old child.**

Audiogram Key	Right	Left
AC Unmasked	○	✕
AC Masked	△	□
BC Mastoid Unmasked	<	>
BC Mastoid Masked	⊏	⊐
BC Forehead Masked	⌐	⌐

Both	
BC Forehead Unmasked	Y
Sound Field	S

Examples of No Response Symbols	

Ear	SRT	SDT	PTA	Test	Word Recognition Level/Percent Correct	MCL	LDL
Right							
Left							
Bone							
Sound Field		20					
Right Aided							
Left Aided							
Binaural Aided							

Conditioned Play Audiometry

BOA and VRA are two common behavioral methods used by audiologists in obtaining audiological information on children from birth to 2 years of age. As children reach the age of 2 years and older, they can typically be conditioned to **play audiometry**. **Conditioned play audiometry (CPA)** is as a method of behavioral hearing testing in which responses to auditory signals are indicated by carrying out a predetermined play activity. For example, rather than require the child to raise a hand or push a response button, both of which are appropriate with adults but likely to be unreliable with very young children, play audiometry could involve dropping a block into a bucket or placing a plastic ring onto a post each time a tone is heard. Like VRA, play audiometry requires that the child be conditioned. Conditioning a child for play audiometry is typically done by pairing the tone and the response until the child carries out the play activity independently whenever the tone is detected.

FIGURE **8.6** **Results of visual reinforcement audiometry with a 16-month-old child suspected of having hearing loss.**

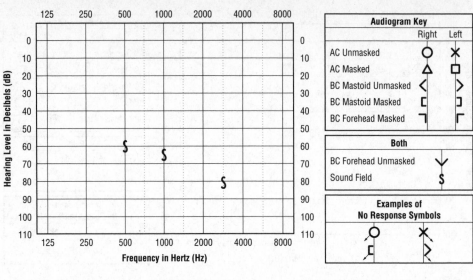

Ear	SRT	SDT	PTA	Test	Word Recognition Level/Percent Correct	MCL	LDL
Right							
Left							
Bone							
Sound Field		60					
Right Aided							
Left Aided							
Binaural Aided							

Before exploring a specific example of the use of play audiometry, it should be noted that a thorough understanding of play audiometric techniques is critical not only for the audiologist but also for the speech–language pathologist. As pointed out in Chapter 11, speech–language pathologists perform pure tone audiological screenings with a variety of individuals, including children. Play audiometry adds considerably to the reliability of such screenings. Also, some of the same play techniques that a speech–language pathologist uses with children can be used in screening adults who are not able to participate in behavioral testing using conventional test techniques. For example, speech–language pathologists employed in nursing homes and facilities for individuals with developmental disabilities will likely find these skills very valuable. Finally, speech–language pathologists can serve an important role in preparing the child for the audiological evaluation by working with the child on selected play audiometry tasks prior to the actual test visit. This advance practice can make the test session more efficient and successful.

Let's use a specific case example. As illustrated in Figure 8.7, Jason is a 2½-year-old who sits independently on the chair. His mother is seated behind him in the sound-treated booth and has been instructed that her purpose is simply to be a supportive presence in the room, but not to participate actively in the testing or prompt her son. One of the two audiologists performing the testing is seated at an angle in front of Jason, and the other audiologist is seated in the control room.

First, the audiologist provides a brief verbal explanation of the task. Although this can be useful to some 2-year-old children, this verbal explanation is not crucial. It is typically the conditioning that is about to take place that is most effective in establishing the bond between the stimulus and the response. An example of a typical verbal explanation is the following: "Jason, you are going to hear some whistles (or "birdy" sounds). When you hear the sound, drop the block in the bucket. Every time you hear the whistle, even if it's very far away, drop the block in the bucket." If audiologists choose to do so, they may also demonstrate this by dropping the block as a tone is presented.

Next, an audiologist places the earphones on Jason and puts her own earphones on in order to monitor the signals presented to the client. The audiologist then places a block in Jason's hand and gently places one hand over Jason's. This is referred to as hand-over-hand prompting. When a tone is presented through the earphones, the audiologist gently moves Jason's hand toward the bucket and prompts him to drop the block. Some form of reinforcement is given to Jason for the prompted response. This may be social reinforcement ("good listening!") or could include reinforcement by illuminating the toys that were described in VRA testing. This same hand-over-hand prompt can be repeated as necessary until Jason drops the block independently when the tone is presented.

Sometimes, depending on the particular child, it is necessary to fade the hand-over-hand prompting gradually. For example, if Jason responds appropriately to the tone when the audiologist's hand is placed over his but fails to respond when there is no

FIGURE **8.7**   **Test room setup for child and audiologist carrying out play audiometry.**

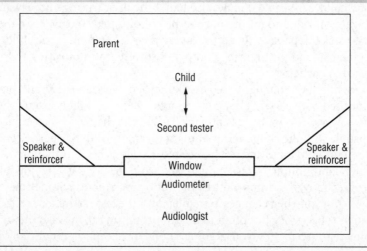

support, the audiologist may choose to tap Jason's hand very slightly when the tone is presented as a reminder of what he should do. This prompt can be faded even further by substituting the hand tap with a slight head nod. The point here is that some children will require that support be removed gradually before they can respond independently to the tones.

One of the most difficult aspects of play audiometry, especially for 2- and 3-year-old children, is waiting for the stimuli before responding. The reason for this is that children in this age category typically do not have well-developed behavioral inhibition skills. They have a block in their hand and they see an empty bucket, so it is logical to drop the block into it.

To assist the child with this waiting behavior, the audiologist sometimes places one hand in front of the child's. This barrier serves as a reminder to the child not to throw the block into the pail right away. When this technique is used during the conditioning phase, the audiologist removes the barrier as soon as the tone is presented and prompts the child to drop the block. Once the testing has begun, the audiologist keeps his hand in front of the child's, even when the tone is presented. A child who is conditioned to the task will move his hand over or around the man-made barrier and will drop the block.

Failure to be conditioned is not the only obstacle that the audiologist may face in using play audiometric techniques. A certain degree of motivation is required for play audiometry, and not all children will be motivated by the standard toys that the audiologist has in the clinic or by the traditional manner of performing play audiometry. Flexibility on the part of the audiologist is essential.

Two examples of this may be helpful. The first is a 4-year-old boy who refused to engage in play audiometry, despite prompting from his mother and the audiologist. After several unsuccessful attempts, the audiologist asked the mother what was motivating to the child and she noted his love of basketball. The audiologist then moved the empty bucket used in play audiometry to the opposite side of the room and asked how many points the child thought he could score by throwing the block into the "basket" when he heard the whistle. The child immediately responded to the challenge and carried out play audiometry without difficulty. It is important to note here that conditioning was very easy for the child; motivation was the issue.

A second child, a 3-year-old male, also had difficulty carrying out play audiometry and, once again, not due to an inability to be conditioned. In this case, the play audiometry task was too passive. By nature a very physical and energetic child, dropping blocks into the pail and putting rings onto a post were not motivating to him and he simply refused to participate.

To address this, the audiologist used the "knock it down" game. The audiologist made a tower comprised of five to six plastic blocks and when the child heard the "whistle" he knocked the tower down with great fanfare. This slight change in the activity to a task more compatible with the child's **temperament** meant the difference between obtaining behavioral responses to tones and not being able to collect this information.

Even after conditioning has been established and the child is carrying out play audiometry successfully, it is important to monitor performance. Sometimes reliability decreases with time or when changes in frequency or the test ear are made. If this occurs, reconditioning is necessary but often takes less prompting than was initially required. Also, ongoing reinforcement ("you're going a good job, keep listening"), and presetting

("I think there's another whistle coming, get ready") can be effective in maintaining re-

sponse reliability and the child's attention to the task. Finally, changing the toy used for play audiometry can have a very positive impact on reliability. Even though the task requirements have not changed, use of a novel toy can often reengage the child in the task.

Some children are hesitant to wear earphones and may even begin to cry when the phones are placed over their ears. In these cases, it is often useful to separate one of the earphones from the headband and play the "telephone game." The audiologist who is in the room with the child, or the child's parent, can hold the earphone to the child's ear and testing can proceed. It is important to remember to communicate to the audiologist in the control booth whether the right or left earphone is being used, to avoid inadvertently directing information to the earphone that is not being used or recording information incorrectly.

It should be clear at this point in our discussion that obtaining behavioral data on children in this age category can be challenging and requires the use of some special techniques. Because the degree of cooperation that the child will provide during the testing is unknown, it is important to structure the evaluation so that the maximum amount of information will be obtained in a brief period of time.

With this in mind, it has been our experience that it is more productive to obtain some frequency-specific information about each ear, rather than detailed information from one ear. Rather than test several frequencies in the right ear, it is recommended that the audiologist test one frequency in the right ear (one that will help to answer the particular question at hand) and then test that same frequency in the left ear. Because the reason for the referral is often to determine whether the child's hearing is adequate for normal speech and language development, beginning at 3,000 Hz is generally advisable. If the child remains motivated to respond to additional tonal stimuli, it is logical to fill in information at 2,000 and 4,000 Hz because of the significant contribution of information at these frequencies to speech intelligibility.

Conditioned Play Audiometry with Speech Stimuli

It should be noted that play audiometry can also be used for speech stimuli as well as for pure tones. In fact, because speech is a more appealing stimulus to children, it is sometimes useful to begin with a speech detection threshold using play audiometry and then follow it with pure-tone play audiometry. The very same toys and techniques described above could be used and, using the above case example, Jason would drop the block when he was told to "put it in" or when he heard "bababa." An ascending–descending approach would be used to identify the speech detection thresholds for each ear. Once the speech detection threshold (SDT) was obtained, Jason would hopefully have little difficulty transferring the conditioning he had received to the pure tone task. Note that for some children this transfer from a speech task to a tone task requires additional conditioning.

As has been discussed in detail in Chapter 5, the speech detection threshold provides less information regarding the child's hearing than the speech recognition threshold (SRT). For this reason, whenever possible, an SRT should be obtained. When testing children, a picture-pointing task is often useful in obtaining the SRT. Think for a moment about why this might be necessary. First, children who have been referred for audiological assessments often have delays in expressive language, which can interfere with their ability to repeat spondee words. Also, some children have normal language skills but poor articulation, making the words they say difficult to understand. Some of the children who are tested will be shy or reticent to speak during the test session. Often, these children are able to comply with all of the required tasks but are hesitant to verbalize. Finally, beginning with the SDT increases test reliability and efficiency by providing information to the audiologist about the accuracy of the pure tone responses being obtained.

Figure 8.8 shows an example of pictures from Auditec of St. Louis (1982) that can be used during SRT testing. Note that all of these pictures represent objects that are part of the child's environment and are likely to be familiar to the child. Because the audiologist is attempting to assess the child's speech understanding and not the child's vocabulary, it is best to have a series of pictures that represents items that are familiar to most young children. The audiologist should also be mindful of pictures that may be less familiar to certain ethnic or income groups, because these introduce test bias and should be avoided. During the SRT testing it is also important that the audiologist monitors the child's visual scanning ability to ensure that the child is reviewing all of the pictures before pointing.

As described in detail in Chapter 5, word recognition ability is another speech audiometry test that is carried out during audiological assessment. For the same reasons described above regarding the use of pictures during SRT testing, picture-pointing speech recognition testing is also very common. Note in Figure 8.9 an example of a picture plate from the Word Intelligibility by Picture Identification; or **WIPI,** test (Ross

FIGURE 8.8 Typical pictures used to obtain speech recognition threshold by picture pointing.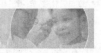

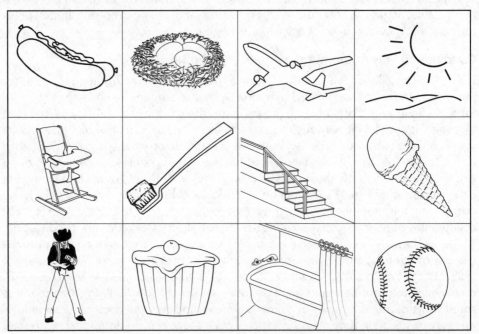

Source: Used with permission from W. F. Carver, Ph.D., Auditec of St. Louis.

FIGURE **8.9** **Sample items from the WIPI test.**

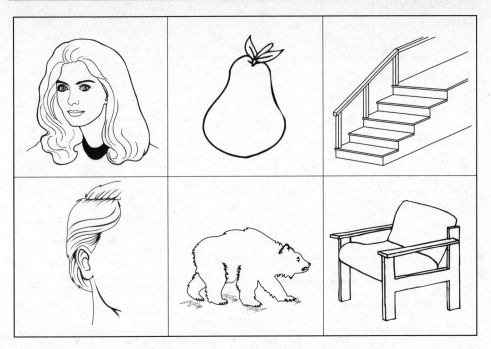

Source: Used with permission from W. F. Carver, Ph.D., Auditec of St. Louis.

& Lerman, 1970). Each of the pictures on the plate differs only slightly, requiring accurate perception of phonemes to identify the correct word. As noted earlier, the audiologist needs to be aware of vocabulary items that are not familiar to the child; parents can often be helpful in making these determinations. In addition to closed-set (picture-pointing) tests, there are also specific word lists for use with young children, such as the PBK-50 word list, discussed in Chapter 5. Figure 8.10 contains four case examples of assessments performed on young children. To develop your ability to read pediatric audiograms, examine each of the following audiograms and be sure that you understand what tests were done, how they were done, and how to interpret the findings. Once you have completed your interpretation, check your work by reading the information that follows.

The child represented in Case A did not tolerate earphones and cannot be conditioned to play audiometry. We know this from the audiogram because the "S" symbols used on the audiogram refer to the fact that responses to tones were obtained in the sound field and the examiner has checked VRA as the response technique. Pure tone responses support hearing that is within normal limits *in a better ear* at 500, 1,000, and 3,000 Hz. In other words, you cannot conclude that both ears have normal hearing sensitivity at the above-referenced frequencies because the child did not wear earphones during the test. A speech detection threshold was also obtained in the sound field and was within normal limits for at least one ear. Tympanometry supported normal middle ear pressure and admittance and acoustic reflexes were not tested.

FIGURE **8.10** **Four practice cases demonstrating various pediatric assessment techniques.**
Case A

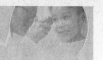

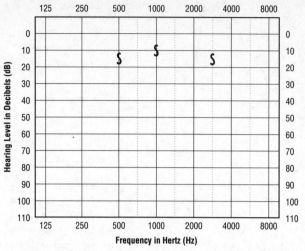

Test Technique: Conventional____ CPA____ VRA ✓ BOA____

Speech Audiometry

Ear	SRT	SDT	PTA	Test	Word Recognition Level/Percent Correct	MCL	LDL
Right							
Left							
Bone							
Sound Field		10					
Right Aided							
Left Aided							
Binaural Aided							

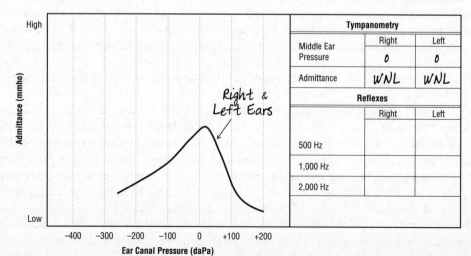

Tympanometry		
	Right	Left
Middle Ear Pressure	0	0
Admittance	WNL	WNL

Reflexes		
	Right	Left
500 Hz		
1,000 Hz		
2,000 Hz		

FIGURE 8.10 Four practice cases demonstrating various pediatric assessment techniques.
Case B

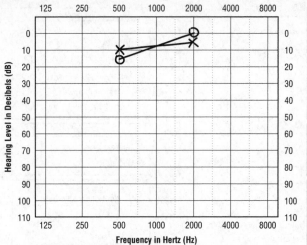

Test Technique: Conventional____ CPA____ VRA ✓ BOA____

Speech Audiometry

Ear	SRT	SDT	PTA	Test	Word Recognition Level/Percent Correct	MCL	LDL
Right		5					
Left		5					
Bone							
Sound Field							
Right Aided							
Left Aided							
Binaural Aided							

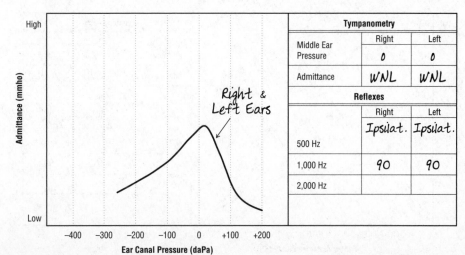

Tympanometry

	Right	Left
Middle Ear Pressure	0	0
Admittance	WNL	WNL

Reflexes

	Right	Left
500 Hz	Ipsilat.	Ipsilat.
1,000 Hz	90	90
2,000 Hz		

FIGURE **8.10** **Four practice cases demonstrating various pediatric assessment techniques.**
Case C

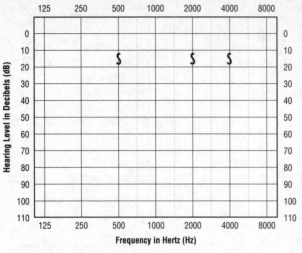

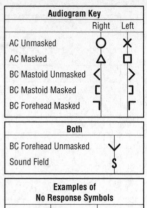

Audiogram Key		
	Right	Left
AC Unmasked	O	X
AC Masked	△	□
BC Mastoid Unmasked	<	>
BC Mastoid Masked	⊏	⊐
BC Forehead Masked	⊤	⊤

Both	
BC Forehead Unmasked	Y
Sound Field	S

Examples of No Response Symbols
O X

Test Technique: Conventional____ CPA ✓ VRA____ BOA____

Speech Audiometry

Ear	SRT	SDT	PTA	Test	Word Recognition Level/Percent Correct	MCL	LDL
Right							
Left							
Bone							
Sound Field	10			WIPI	45/10		
Right Aided							
Left Aided							
Binaural Aided							

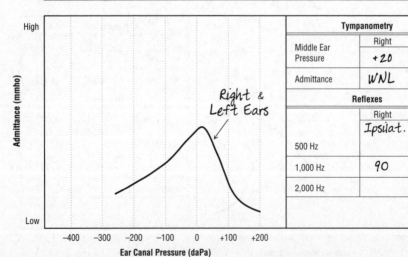

Right & Left Ears

Tympanometry		
	Right	Left
Middle Ear Pressure	+20	+20
Admittance	WNL	WNL
Reflexes		
	Right	Left
500 Hz	Ipsilat.	Ipsilat.
1,000 Hz	90	90
2,000 Hz		

FIGURE **8.10** **Four practice cases demonstrating various pediatric assessment techniques.**
Case D

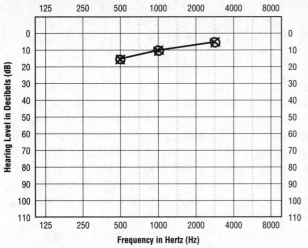

Test Technique: Conventional____ CPA ✓ VRA____ BOA____

Speech Audiometry

Ear	SRT	SDT	PTA	Test	Word Recognition Level/Percent Correct		MCL	LDL
Right	10			WIPI	45 /	10/10		
Left	5			WIPI	45 /	10/10		
Bone								
Sound Field								
Right Aided								
Left Aided								
Binaural Aided								

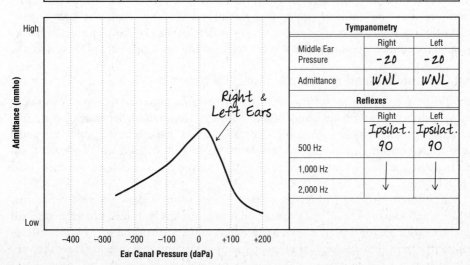

Tympanometry	Right	Left
Middle Ear Pressure	−20	−20
Admittance	WNL	WNL

Reflexes	Right	Left
500 Hz	Ipsilat. 90	Ipsilat. 90
1,000 Hz	↓	↓
2,000 Hz	↓	↓

In Case B, note that VRA is still the test technique, but this child did tolerate earphones. The "S" symbol that was used in Case A has been replaced with symbols for right and left ears for air conduction testing. Pure tone testing supports hearing that is within normal limits in each ear at 500 and 2,000 Hz. Note also that speech detection thresholds of 5 dB were obtained in each ear and are within normal limits. Tympanometry supports normal middle ear pressure and admittance with a 1,000-Hz screening reflex present bilaterally at 90 dB. The presence of a middle ear reflex contraindicates the presence of conductive involvement.

The child in Case C has moved beyond VRA testing and is able to be conditioned to play audiometry. The audiologist indicates this on the audiogram by checking CPA (conditioned play) on the line for test technique. Note also that the use of the "S" symbol indicates that the child does not wear earphones and that these play audiometry responses have been obtained in the sound field. Responses to tones support hearing that is within normal limits in at least one ear at 500, 2,000, and 4,000 Hz. The SRT of 10 dB is within normal limits and speech recognition ability is excellent (10/10) in at least one ear, when speech is presented at a conversational intensity level and a picture-pointing task is used. Tympanometry supports normal middle ear pressure and admittance with a 1,000-Hz screening reflex present bilaterally.

Finally, the child in Case D is tested through the use of conditioned play audiometry under earphones. This provides frequency specific data for each ear, which is often the ultimate goal of testing. Speech recognition thresholds of 10 dB in the right ear and 5 dB in the left ear are both within normal limits and speech recognition ability is excellent (10/10) bilaterally at conversational levels, using a picture-pointing task. All admittance findings are within normal limits bilaterally.

Masking and Young Children

When masking was discussed previously, it was noted that adult patients should be given verbal directions to disregard the masking signal and respond to the test signals. When masking is required during the testing of young children, it is often effective to simply direct the masking to the non-test ear while talking informally with the child but with no mention of the masking stimulus. After the masking signal has been activated for a brief period, instruct the child to carry out the play technique that was being used. Reconditioning the child may be necessary, but often by simply disregarding the masking signal the child understands that it is not relevant and responds only to the test signal.

What Constitutes Hearing within Normal Limits?

It should now be clear that what constitutes acceptable behavioral responses in very young children varies with age and with the different stimuli used. Separate norms, similar to those provided by Northern and Downs (2002), will likely be helpful to the audiologist in determining what response levels are acceptable when testing children from birth to approximately 2 years of age. Additional specific guidelines have been provided in this chapter.

For children who fall in the age range of older than 2 years and not yet adults, Northern and Downs (2002) recommend that hearing levels should not exceed 15 dB HL. Their rationale for this is that, unlike adults, children are in the very important developmental period of speech and language acquisition and they need to hear the very

321

•

Client-Specific
Protocols for
Audiological
Assessment of
Young Children

TABLE 8.10   Summary of Normal Hearing Criteria for Various Age Groups

Approximate Age	Speech Stimuli	Tonal Stimuli
Birth–4 months	45–50 dB	70 dB
4–8 months	20–25 dB	45–50 dB
1 year	10–15 dB	30–35 dB
1.5–2 years	10–15 dB	25 dB
2–18 years	0–15 dB	0–15 dB
Adult	0–25 dB	0–25 dB

Source: Northern, J., & Downs, M. (2002). *Hearing in children* (5th ed.). New York: Lippincott, Williams & Wilkins. Adapted by permission. F. N. Martin and J. G. Clarke. *Hearing care for children.* Published by Allyn and Bacon, Boston, MA. Adapted by permission of the publisher.

faint sounds contained in speech. Further, school-age children are constantly faced with the challenge of learning new information. In addition, although adults are able to "fill in" information that they may not hear with no loss of meaning, children do not have strong **top-down processing skills.** In other words, children rely very heavily on the message itself and less on the use of prediction ability, prior knowledge, or contextual cues in order to gain meaning. Therefore, even though an adult who has thresholds of 25 dB will likely receive a message presented at a conversational speech level without difficulty, a child with those same thresholds can have less than adequate access to the softer parts of that message, resulting in a less meaningful message.

Finally, for adults, as stated in Chapter 4, hearing at levels of 25 dB or less is generally viewed as within the normal range. Table 8.10 provides a summary of this discussion of normal hearing for various age categories.

Client-Specific Protocols for Audiological Assessment of Young Children

One of the questions that students commonly ask is what sequence of tests is most effective to determine the hearing status of a young child. Some texts attempt to answer this question by providing a rationale for performing a specific sequence of tests, often beginning with physiological measures, such as otoacoustic emission and admittance testing, and then moving to behavioral tests. The rationale for this protocol is that if diagnostic otoacoustic emission testing supports normal outer hair cells functioning, it is likely that hearing is within normal limits and that no middle ear pathology exists. Behavioral testing can then be used to verify the physiological data and to provide direct measurement of hearing sensitivity.

Although the protocol just described will be effective with some children, decisions about the sequence of tests and modifications of test techniques that will be most effective in assessing the hearing of young children must be made on a case-by-case basis. Let's now expand on this and some of the themes discussed in the beginning of this

chapter by examining Table 8.11, which illustrates our model of **client-specific protocols** for audiological assessment. Note that there are both known and unknown features
in the model. What does an audiologist know prior to the assessment? The audiologist
knows what question must be answered by the assessment. Very often, the question is "Is
this child's hearing within normal limits?" Another common question is, "Is this child's
hearing adequate for normal speech and language?" In addition, the audiologist knows
the kinds of tools or assets that are available at her work site to answer the question at
hand. The experience and training of the audiologist(s) is listed as a tool because this
will have a considerable impact on gathering information regarding the child's hearing.
Speech–language pathologists and other providers of pediatric services quickly become
knowledgeable about which audiologists have the needed creativity, patience, and training to work successfully with children.

The number of audiologists available to work on a given case is also listed under
"tools." In some settings, two audiologists are scheduled to work together on cases involving children under a certain age (e.g., 3 or 4 years old). In other settings, audiologists and
speech–language pathologists may work as a team to collect audiological information.
Although it is certainly possible for one audiologist to assess very young children, the use
of two audiologists would be viewed as an asset in answering the question at hand.

Certainly the equipment and tests that are at the disposal of the audiologist are
tools. The recent widespread use of otoacoustic emission testing is an example of a test
that has significantly enhanced the audiologist's ability to carry out efficient testing. Although assessment can certainly be performed without otoacoustic emission testing, facilities that do have access to this tool clearly have a powerful asset at their disposal.

Table 8.12 lists both behavioral and physiological tests that are commonly used in
the assessment of children. The column labeled "Information Obtained" provides a

---

TABLE 8.11   Client-Specific Protocols for Audiological Assessment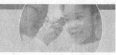

Known variables
    Question(s) to be answered by the audiological assessment:
        Does the child hear well enough to develop normal speech and language skills?
        Is there middle ear involvement?
        Is middle ear involvement interfering with the child's hearing ability?

    Tools available to the audiologist to answer the question(s):
        Experience of the audiologist
        Number of audiologists available to assess the child
        Types of audiological equipment/tests available to assess the child
        The audiologist's creative use of equipment and tests

Unknown child-centered variables
        Language skills/ability to follow directions
        Personality/temperament
        Cognitive skills
        Motivation
        Attending abilities
        Compliance level

Test	Method	Information Obtained	Comments
Speech detection threshold (SDT)	Visual reinforcement audiometry (VRA)	Some portion of the speech spectrum. If sound field is used, only assesses one ear.	VRA can be less reliable than CPA but is the behavioral test of choice for very young children and for individuals who have cognitive deficits.
SDT	Conditioned play audiometry (CPA)	See above.	Can be highly effective and is often the behavioral test of choice to begin the test session. Developmentally, it may be the test that is appropriate when child is too old for VRA.
Pure tones	VRA	Frequency-specific data. If sound field is used, only assesses one ear.	Can be less reliable than CPA. Habituation can be a problem for some children. Older children (by age 2 years) often do not perform the required localization task as well as younger children.
Speech recognition threshold (SRT)	Picture pointing	Some portion of the speech spectrum, mostly low frequencies. Provides more information than SDT because it requires understanding.	Requires some basic vocabulary and the ability to scan a series of pictures. Use of a closed set is typically easier than a verbal response.
SRT	Verbal	See above.	Requires that the client have sufficient intelligibility for the examiner to reliably judge his responses. Choose spondee words that are familiar to the client.
Pure tones	CPA	Frequency-specific information.	For young children obtaining frequency-specific information for each ear is often our ultimate goal.
Word recognition	Body parts identification	Some basic recognition of words that are not acoustically similar. If performance is good at a conversational level, can corroborate other normal findings.	Should only be used when more sensitive types of stimuli (e.g., monosyllables) are too difficult. Word recognition

(continued)

TABLE **8.12** (*continued*)

Test	Method	Information Obtained	Comments
Conversational questions	Some basic recognition of conversational questions. When	performed at conversational level, may give some information regarding functional impairment.	Questions can be provided by people who interact with the patient regularly. Can be useful in distinguishing between hearing loss and other cognitive impairments.
Word recognition	Monosyllables/picture pointing	Some portion of the speech spectrum; more high-frequency than SDT or SRT	Use of monosyllables makes the task more sensitive; use of a closed set makes the task easier than verbal response. Child must have sufficient vocabulary and visual scanning ability.
Word recognition	Monosyllables/verbal	See above.	Requires that the client can repeat back words with sufficient intelligibility that the examiner can make reliable judgments about understanding.
Admittance		Can provide information about the status of the middle ear and can be used to assess the consistency of other data obtained	
Otoacoustic emission		Can provide frequency-specific data for each ear regarding outer hair cell integrity. Also, if normal, can rule out middle ear pathology.	Although not a direct test of hearing, provides important information regarding integrity of structures that underlie hearing.
Auditory brainstem response		A combination of clicks and tone bursts can provide frequency-specific data for each ear regarding neural synchrony.	See above.

description of the type of information that each procedure provides and the "Comments" section gives guidance regarding the type of client that will likely benefit from a given test. It is important to note that although it may appear that the behavioral tests are ordered from developmentally easier to developmentally harder tasks, how difficult or easy a task is will depend on the particular child being tested. Despite the information that you have learned regarding the suitability of various techniques of testing used at various ages, audiologists must remember that age alone is not the determiner of what approach to use.

In addition to these known features of this model, there are also unknown features. These include the hearing status of the child and a number of child variables that will directly affect the testing process. For example, is the child's temperament one that will comply with the audiologist or will special measures to motivate the child be needed. Is the child capable of following directions or is this an area of difficulty? Does the child have the attending skills to maintain her focus on the tasks for an extended period of time? Will the child allow the audiologist to place earphones or a probe near or in her ears?

Because the answers to these questions will guide clinicians as to the most appropriate sequence of tests to be used with a particular child, within the very first few minutes of the case history interview an experienced audiologist will assess much of this information. When possible, some of this information can be obtained by collaboration with the child's teachers, speech–language pathologist, and service providers.

Consider Robert, age 3 years, who comes in to the clinic for audiological assessment. In the first few minutes of the case history interview the audiologist notes the following: (1) the child is clinging to his mother's leg and does not separate from her when asked if he would like to sit in his own chair; (2) when the audiologist pats the top of the child's head, he becomes upset and pulls away; (3) when asked if he can say the word *baseball,* the child does not respond; (4) when asked if the child has ever worn earphones at home, the mother reports that he has not; and (5) the mother notes that "we've had some trouble with him before at doctors' appointments."

Before we discuss how to begin testing this child, think back to the protocol that some texts recommend for young children: physiological measures followed by behavioral measures. If we followed this protocol, we would begin testing with otoacoustic emission testing or admittance, depending on the availability of equipment. How do you think the above child would react to this? Might this remind the child of his previous difficult experiences at his physician's office?

An approach based on the client-specific protocol in Table 8.11 would start with spending a few very important minutes making the child more comfortable in this unfamiliar environment. This can be accomplished by bringing both the child and his mother into the sound-treated booth and, using play audiometry, carrying out a speech detection threshold. Both the child and the mother can participate in throwing the blocks in the pail when directed to do so, and reinforcement can be provided by the illuminated toys that are mounted on either side of the speakers. Earphones are not used during this "warming-up" phase.

Advantages of this activity for Robert are that it is relatively easy and motivating, it does not involve use of earphones, and it does not require a verbal response. As is noted in Table 8.12, a speech detection threshold obtained in the sound field yields very limited information regarding the child's hearing. But at this point in the evaluation, our main goal is not to collect data but simply to help the child feel more comfortable. In most cases when we test children whose profile resembles Robert's, the speech detection threshold is simply the start of the data collection process.

Once the child has become more comfortable, the audiologist builds on the successful speech detection task. This can be accomplished by performing speech detection thresholds under earphones, in which case information about both ears is being collected. Another option is to collect pure tone information in the sound field through conditioned play audiometry and then adding earphones.

During the testing, the audiologist continually reviews the variety of tools he has at his disposal and, depending on the child's reactions and the question at hand, makes decisions about the most effective sequence of tests. In this way, the audiologist and the client together determine the child-specific protocol that is best suited to answer the question at hand. Note that even though the ultimate goal in addressing the question of whether a hearing loss exists is to obtain frequency-specific data for each ear, the process by which that goal is reached can be quite variable for different children.

The process of testing Robert is summarized in Table 8.13. Note that after using the speech detection threshold to desensitize Robert to the test situation, earphones were added and speech detection thresholds for each ear were obtained. Once comfortable with the earphones, Robert was conditioned to pure tone testing and data were obtained at 1,000 and 3,000 Hz. Also under earphones, Robert pointed to the pictures of the WIPI test and speech recognition was assessed. Finally, when Robert was very comfortable in the test situation, otoacoustic emission testing was used to corroborate the behavioral findings.

One of the themes that has been stressed in this text is collaboration. Cooperative interactions among a variety of professionals for the purpose of providing the best

TABLE 8.13   Client-Specific Protocol Developed in Assessing Robert

Test Chosen	Rationale
SDT in the sound field using play audiometry	Robert is fearful and shows resistance to having anything near his head or ears. This task will serve to desensitize him.
SDT under earphones using play audiometry	Robert is now more relaxed and tolerates earphones. Data collected is now ear specific. If wearing earphones was still problematic for Robert, they could be removed from the headband and one earphone could be held to his ear like a "telephone."
Pure tones (1,000 and 3,000 Hz) under earphone using play audiometry	Extend the above task to tones so that frequency-specific information is obtained in each ear.
Speech recognition under earphones using a picture-pointing task	Add in picture pointing to corroborate other findings.
Otoacoustic emission testing	This test is saved for last because Robert will likely view it as the most invasive. He is comfortable enough at this point to tolerate this well. It provides ear-specific and frequency-specific information that can corroborate other data. If normal, it rules out middle ear pathology.

clinical services possible have been urged. Our discussion of client-specific protocols extends this theme to include collaboration with the child and family. Too often, professionals share insights about clients without including the client in the process. Even though very young children may not have the ability to provide direct insights about themselves, an audiologist who works successfully with children will view the child as a wealth of information and will learn as much as possible from the child about the best way to sequence the audiological assessment. The most effective pediatric audiology services are those that involve direct collaboration between the audiologist and the child.

Let's examine a second case that illustrates the development of client-specific protocols in assessing children. Molly, age 12 years, has been diagnosed with developmental disabilities. Her estimated cognitive level is less than 2 years of age. Both receptive and expressive language skills are limited, which interfere with Molly's ability to follow even basic directions. During the case history interview the audiologist determines that Molly is comfortable with strangers and gives no negative reaction when the side of her head and ear are gently stroked.

As noted in Table 8.14, beginning with otoacoustic emissions may be well suited to Molly's situation because it is not likely to be upsetting to her and, if normal, can support normal outer hair cell functioning and the absence of middle ear pathology. Once this has been completed, behavioral tests can be attempted to obtain a direct measure of hearing. Because Molly's receptive and expressive language skills are weak, speech recognition testing is likely to be unreliable, even if a picture-pointing format is used. Beginning with

TABLE **8.14** **Client-Specific Protocol Developed in Assessing Molly**

Test Chosen	Rationale
Otoacoustic emission testing	Molly demonstrated no sensitivity to having her head and ear touched. This test will provide objective data about outer hair cell function and if normal will rule out middle ear pathology.
Speech detection thresholds under earphones using play audiometry	Although Molly tolerated the earphones with no difficulty, her cognitive limitations prevented conditioning to the play task.
Speech detection thresholds under earphones using VRA	Because the conditioning task (to play audiometry) appears to be beyond Molly's developmental level, the audiologist moves to a localization task. Molly is able to perform this task and ear-specific information about speech detection is obtained.
Pure tones under earphones using VRA	Success here provides a direct measure of frequency-specific information for each ear and can be compared to otoacoustic emission results for reliability check.

speech detection thresholds obtained under earphones using play audiometry may be an appropriate starting point. If Molly cannot be conditioned to this play task, the audiologist could then attempt to obtain speech detection thresholds under earphones using visual reinforcement audiometry (VRA) and observing Molly's localization to sound. If this is successful, pure tones can then be assessed in the same manner.

Molly's case highlights an important point. Audiologists should make use of information regarding a variety of characteristics of the child to guide the sequence of tests; they should not allow this information to impose unnecessary limitations on the testing process. For example, in this case, even if the examiner is told that Molly will not be able to follow the directions for play audiometry, the audiologist should still make an attempt to condition Molly's response to sound. In some cases, children demonstrate skills that are surprising to their parents and service providers.

It should be clear at this point that assessing the hearing of very young children can be challenging. The task of accurately assessing the hearing of children who present with a handicapping condition(s) can be equally challenging. Just as testing children involves general knowledge about developmental norms associated with various ages combined with very specific knowledge about the child, testing children with special needs requires knowledge about the general characteristics of various disability categories as well as information that is specific to the child being tested. This is fundamental to the information in Chapter 9 about assessment and management of other special populations.

Conveying Diagnostic Information to Parents

At the conclusion of the audiological evaluation, the diagnostic information that has been obtained about the child should be communicated to the parent(s) or caregiver(s). In addition to the verbal summary of results and recommendations, a written report will be generated to be disseminated to the parent(s), the child's physician or primary health care provider, and to other professionals who may be working with the child and family.

In general, professionals providing the results of diagnostic testing to families should ensure that the information is presented in a timely manner (preferably immediately following the test) and that the information is presented in a format that is understandable and useful to the recipient(s). Families should receive clear information about the test findings, what these findings mean related to the child's communication abilities, and what next steps, if any, should be pursued.

There will be times when the results of the test are perceived by the parents as "bad news." This perception on the part of parents is not limited to instances when the clinician is conveying information about severe to profound sensorineural hearing loss; rather, for some families, finding out their child has a relatively milder degree of hearing loss can be devastating. A diagnosis of profound sensorineural hearing loss may be perceived differently by deaf parents than by hearing parents, but clinicians should make no assumptions about the reaction a parent may have to receiving diagnostic information based on the parents' hearing status.

Grief over finding out the diagnosis of hearing loss is one possible reaction that parents may experience. Feelings of sadness, denial, and anger may be present. The now-familiar stages of the grieving process—denial, anger, bargaining, depression, and

329
•
Client-Specific
Protocols for
Audiological
Assessment of
Young Children

acceptance—may be present to varying degrees. Clinicians should recognize that these stages are not necessarily linear; in other words, people may not experience all stages or may experience them in a different progression. Also, grief can resurface with different life events, such as starting preschool or high school.

Although many reactions to the diagnosis of a permanent hearing loss in childhood are possible, there is agreement that the way the diagnostic information is conveyed has an effect on parents' ability to deal with their child's hearing loss. Studies that consider the reactions of parents of children with newly diagnosed hearing loss, as well as clinical experience, reveal some common themes regarding the needs of parents in this situation. Generally, parents want intervention to begin immediately once a hearing loss is confirmed. Providing accurate information is important to parents and it is important that clinicians foster realistic expectations and help the parents to have hope for the future. In addition to informing parents about the type and degree of hearing loss, amplification options, and so on (referred to as content counseling), clinicians must also be able to respond to parents' emotional reactions and concerns about the hearing loss and their ability to cope with it. This also may include providing support for the parents to make communication decisions and to help their child develop communication skills. David Luterman (1996) points out, when families do well, children will do well. Support and content counseling are discussed further in Chapter 12.

Genetic Counseling

When an infant or child is diagnosed with hearing loss, questions about the cause of the hearing loss naturally arise. On initial identification of a permanent hearing loss in childhood, referral is made for an otological evaluation to investigate the cause(s) of the hearing loss. This visit may include tests such as magnetic resonance imaging (MRI), blood work, and a comprehensive medical history and may or may not result in a definitive etiology (cause). In addition, referral for genetic counseling should be made. **Genetic counseling** involves providing information to parents about genetic factors causing the hearing loss and is intended to help families make informed decisions in the process of family planning. As more information about human genetics becomes known, families will have access to increasingly refined information about the cause(s) of hearing loss. Our role is to ensure that they have the opportunity to access this information.

Other Disabilities

Table 8.15 provides some general characteristics that are associated with various disability categories and how these can affect audiological assessment and rehabilitation. By combining the information included in Table 8.15 with the client-specific approach to diagnostics described above, the audiologist approaches the diagnostic task with both general and specific information. Once again, because the client-specific approach to testing is guided by the specific client being tested, it can be used effectively with all clients. This concept is also fundamental to assessment and intervention for special populations, discussed in the next chapter.

TABLE 8.15   Common Characteristics of Pediatric Disorders and Potential Effects on Hearing Assessment

Disorder	Relevant Features	Effects on Assessment
Mental retardation	Characterized by subaverage intellectual abilities and deficits in adaptive behavior. Impaired communication and social skills are common.	Difficulty with understanding may lead to use of more basic test techniques or reliance on physiological measures. Test protocol is determined not by the chronological age but by the child's demonstrated abilities with specific tasks.
Autism	Characterized by self-absorption; im-paired social relationships; decreased responsiveness to others and impaired language skills. Reduced cognitive skills are common as are decreased eye con-tact and repetitive patterns of behavior. Onset is prior to age 3 years.	Reduced cognitive skills and/or limited ability to interact socially may lead to use of more basic test techniques or more emphasis on pure tone rather than speech stimuli, or reliance on physiological (objective) measures. The audiologist should attempt to engage the child in the tasks at hand but this may be difficult. Children may engage in their own idiosyncratic behaviors.
Asperger syndrome	Commonly viewed as a higher functioning type of autism. IQ is typically normal. Although language is more age-appropriate, social language is impaired, as is affect. Social maladjustment is very common. Gait and coordination issues may be noted.	Should not interfere in any significant way. The audiologist should be respectful of the child's atypical social interactions.
Pervasive developmental disorder, not otherwise specified (PDD-NOS) (Adapted from *Diagnostic and Statistical Manual of Mental Disorders,* Fourth Edition [DSM-IV])	This diagnosis is consistent with the presence of a severe and pervasive impairment in the development of reciprocal social interaction or verbal and nonverbal communication skills where the criteria for other conditions are not met. Children diagnosed with PDD-NOS may exhibit characteristics of autism; however, they do not meet the specific diagnostic criteria for a diagnosis of autism, e.g., due to onset after age 3 years.	Inherent performance variability will necessitate an eclectic approach to evaluation. The specific test techniques, and whether these will be employed by one or two testers (audiologists), will depend on the child's abilities, determined through observation of the child, interaction with the child and trial and error using different test techniques.
Attention deficit hyperactivity disorder (ADHD)	In very young children, hyperactivity is common. Also, impulsivity, distractibility, and lack of behavioral inhibition are noted. Conduct and emotional disorders commonly coexist with this condition.	Use of two audiologists working together is strongly recommended because young children with this condition often require close monitoring and behavior control by one of the audiologists. Waiting for the auditory stimuli before responding will likely be challenging due to the impulsivity. Play techniques and physiological measures should be useful.

TABLE **8.15** (*Continued*)

Disorder	Relevant Features	Effects on Assessment
Conduct disorders	Can include a variety of behaviors including antisocial acts, noncompliance, verbal hostility, and defiance.	See comments above regarding use of two audiologists. In extreme cases, the audiologist should consult with parents/school staff regarding the need for additional personnel to accompany the child to the evaluation. The audiologist must demonstrate flexibility in attempting to devise tasks that the child will respond to.
Emotional disorders	Unlike conduct disorders in which the disturbance is directed to others, children with emotional disorders direct the disturbance inward in the form of anxiety and depression.	These children may demonstrate undue anxiety during the testing; may refuse to interact with the examiner; may cling to a parent. The audiologist needs to demonstrate empathy and patience in increasing the child's comfort level while gradually collecting the required data to answer the question at hand.
Cerebral palsy (CP)	Motor difficulties are the primary feature; may also include some mental retardation, hearing loss, and speech–language delays. There are various types of CP, which means the degree of rigidity and effect on upper or lower extremities varies with the individual.	Examine all motor tasks and modify them, as necessary to maximize success. For example, if play audiometry is used, avoid toys/objects that cannot be handled by the child. If the motor impairment interferes with speech and language production, use picture-pointing tasks or speech detection thresholds.
Down syndrome	This genetic disorder is commonly characterized by some degree of mental retardation, low muscle tone, and an increased incidence of middle ear pathology. Speech–language delays are common.	Assessment of middle ear status is critical due to the increased risk in this population. As with other cases of reduced cognitive and language skills, the audiologist should assess the child's ability with a given task and then move flexibly to an easier task, as necessary.

CHAPTER SUMMARY

This chapter presented general principles about testing young children and the specific tests available for this purpose. The use of a highly individualized approach to audiological assessment was emphasized. Detailed descriptions of test techniques were provided and applied to specific case examples. Information on embryonic development of auditory structures was presented and was integrated with management and counseling.

QUESTIONS FOR DISCUSSION

1. Compare and contrast the behavioral test techniques used in pediatric audiology, including BOA, VRA, and CPA.
2. Describe how clinicians can use information about the etiology (cause) of hearing loss to help children and families. Refer to Table 8.4 for examples.
3. Discuss how nonaudiometric variables have an impact on the sequence of the diagnostic audiological evaluation.
4. Develop a list of potential referrals that may be needed for a family of a child with a newly diagnosed sensorineural hearing loss.
5. What are signs of possible hearing loss in school-age students? How can you guide the classroom teacher in identifying and helping these students?

RECOMMENDED READING

Choo, D. (2002). The impact of molecular genetics on the clinical management of pediatric sensorineural hearing loss. *The Journal of Pediatrics, 140,* 148–149.

Diefendorf, A., & Gravel, J. (1996). Behavioral observation and visual reinforcement audiometry. In S. Gerber (Ed.), *The handbook of pediatric audiology.* Washington, DC: Gallaudet University Press.

Joint Committee on Infant Hearing. (2000, August). Year 2000 position statement: Principles and guidelines for early hearing detection and intervention programs. *Audiology Today, 12,* special issue, 7–27.

Luotonen, M., Uhari, M., Aitola, L., Lukkaroinen, A., Luotonen, J., & Uhari, M. (1998). A nationwide population-based survey of otitis media and school achievement. *International Journal of Pediatric Otorhinolaryngology, 43*(1), 41–51.

Madell, J. (1998). *Behavioral audiological evaluation of infants and younger chlidren.* New York: Thieme.

Northern, J., & Downs, M. (2002). *Hearing in children* (5th ed.). New York: Lippincott, Williams & Wilkins.

Oyer, H., Hall, B., & Haas, W. (2000). *Speech, language, and hearing disorders: A guide for the teacher.* Boston: Allyn & Bacon.

Shhallop, J. (2002). Auditory neropathy/dyssynchrony in adults and children. *Seminars in Hearing, 23*(3), 215–223.

Shprintzen, R. (2001). *Syndrome identification for audiology: An illustrated pocket guide.* Clifton Park, NY: Thomson Learning.

Shriberg, L., Flipsen, P., Thielke, H., Kwiatkowski, J., Kertoy, M., Katcher, M., et al. (2000). Risk for speech disorder associated with early recurrent otitis media with effusion: Two retrospective studies. *Journal of Speech, Language, and Hearing Research, 43*(1), 79–99.

Shriberg, L., Friel-Patti, S., Flipsen, P., & Brown, R. (2000). Otitis media, fluctuant hearing loss, and speech-language outcomes: A preliminary structural equation model. *Journal of Speech, Language, and Hearing Research, 43*(1), 100–120.

Sininger, Y. (2002). Identification of auditory neuropathy in infants and children. *Seminars in Hearing, 23*(3), 193–200.

Yoshinaga-Itano, C., Sedey, A., Coulter, D., & Mehl, A. (1998). Language of early and later identified children with hearing loss. *Pediatrics, 102,* 1161–1171.

REFERENCES

Anderson, K. L. (1989). *Screening Instrument for Targeting Educational Risk (SIFTER).* Austin, TX: Pro-Ed.

Auditec of St. Louis (personal communication with W. Carver, 1982). Speech Recognition Pictures.

Brunger, J., Matthews, A., Smith, R., & Robin, N. (2001, April). Genetic testing and genetic counseling for deafness: The future is here. *The Laryngoscope*, 715–718.

Code of Federal Regulations on Education, Title 34-Education, IDEA 1997 Final Regulations, (34 CFR Part 300). Available at www .ideapractices.org/regs/SubpartA.htm

Diefendorf, A., & Gravel, J. (1996) Behavioral observation and visual reinforcement audiometry. In S. Gerber (Ed.), *The handbook of pediatric audiology.* Washington, DC: Gallaudet University Press.

Flexer, C. (1993). Management of hearing in an educational setting. In J. Alpiner and P. McCarthy (Eds.), *Rehabilitative audiology: Children and adults.* Baltimore: Williams and Wilkins.

Hicks, A., Tharpe, A., & Ashmead, D. (2000). Behavioral auditory assessment of young infants: Methodological limitations or natural lack of auditory responsiveness? *American Journal of Audiology, 9,* 124–130.

Holmes, L. (1977). *Medical genetics in hearing loss in children* (pp. 253–265). In B. Jaffe (Ed.), *Hearing loss in children.* Baltimore: University Park Press.

Hood, L., Berlin, C., Morlet, T., Brashears, S., Rose, K., & Tedesco, S. (2002). Considerations in the clinical evaluation of auditory neuropathy/auditory dys-synchrony. *Seminars in Hearing, 23*(3), 201–208.

Joint Committee on Infant Hearing. (2000, August). Year 2000 position statement: Principles and guidelines for early hearing detection and intervention programs. *Audiology Today, 12,* special issue, 7–27.

Keats, B. (2002). Genes and syndromic hearing loss. *Journal of Communication Disorders, 35,* 355–366.

Luterman, D. (1996). *Counseling persons with communication disorders and their families* (3rd ed.). Austin, TX: Pro-Ed.

Martin, F., & Clarke, J. G. (1996). *Hearing care for children.* Boston: Allyn & Bacon.

Matkin, N. (1980). Adapted from "Screening Children for Communication Disorders," a project of the Robert Wood Johnson Foundation and University of Colorado Health Sciences Center, Denver.

McConnell, F., & Ward, P. (1967). *Deafness in childhood.* Nashville, TN: Vanderbilt University Press.

Northern, J., & Downs, M. (2002). *Hearing in children* (5th ed.). New York: Lippincott, Williams & Wilkins.

Palmer, C. V., & Mormer, E. A. (1998). *Developmental Index of Audition and Listening.* Pittsburgh: The University of Pittsburgh, Department of Communication Science and Disorders.

Paparella, M. (1977). Differential diagnosis of childhood deafness. In F. Bess (Ed.), *Childhood deafness: Causation, assessment, and management* (pp. 3–18). New York: Grune & Stratton.

Ross, M., & Lerman, J. (1970). A picture identification test for hearing-impaired children. *Journal of Speech and Hearing Research, 13,* 44–53.

Skinner, B. (1983). *A matter of consequences.* New York: Knopf.

Stach, B. (1997). *Comprehensive dictionary of audiology illustrated.* Halifax, Nova Scotia: Williams & Wilkins.

Stinckens, C., Ensink, R., Feenstra, L., Fryns, J., & Cremers, C. (1997). Non-syndromic dominant sensorineural hearing loss: From a few phenotypes to many genotypes. *International Journal of Pediatric Otorhinolaryngology, 38*(3), 237–245.

Tekin, M., Arnos, K., & Pandya, A. (2001). Advances in hereditary deafness. *The Lancet, 358,* 1082–1090.

Tharpe, A., & Ashmead, D. (2001). A longitudinal investigation of infant auditory sensitivity. *American Journal of Audiology, 10,* 104–112.

U.S. Department of Health and Human Services. (2000, January). *Healthy people 2010* (conference ed., in two volumes). Washington, DC: Author.

Yoshinaga-Itano, C., Sedey, A., Coulter, D., & Mehl, A. (1998). Language of early and later identified children with hearing loss. *Pediatrics, 102,* 1161–1171.

Zemlin, W. (1998). *Speech and hearing science: Anatomy and physiology.* Boston: Allyn & Bacon.

Appendix A
Suggestions for Parents of Children with Middle Ear Problems

The Importance of Talking

Talking to your child is necessary for his/her language development. Since children usually imitate what they hear, how much you talk to your child, what you say, and how you say it will affect how much and how well your child talks.

Look

Look directly at your child's face and wait until you have his/her attention before you begin talking.

Control Distance

Be sure that you are close to your child when you talk (no farther than 5 feet). The younger the child, the more important it is to be close.

Loudness

Talk slightly louder than you normally do. Turn off the radio, TV, dishwasher, etc., to remove background noise.

Be a Good Speech Model

- Describe to your child daily activities as they occur.
- Expand what your child says. For example, if your child points and says, "car," you say, "Oh, you want the car."
- Add new information. You might add, "That car is little."
- Build vocabulary, make teaching new words and concepts a natural part of everyday activities. Use new words while shopping, taking a walk, washing dishes, etc.
- Repeat your child's words using adult pronunciation.

Play and Talk

Set aside some time throughout each day for "play time" for just you and your child. Play can be looking at books, exploring toys, singing songs, coloring, etc. Talk to your child during these activities, keeping the conversation at his/her level.

Read

Begin reading to your child at a young age (under 12 months). Ask a librarian for books that are right for your child's age. Reading can be a calming-down activity that promotes closeness between you and your child. Reading provides another opportunity to teach and review words and ideas. Some children enjoy looking at pictures in magazines and catalogs.

Don't Wait

Your child should have the following skills by the ages listed below:

18 months: 3-word vocabulary.
2 years: 25–30-word vocabulary and several 2-word sentences.
2½ years: At least a 50-word vocabulary and 2-word sentences consistently.

If your child doesn't have these skills, tell your doctor. A referral to an audiologist and speech pathologist may be indicated. Hearing and language testing may lead to a better understanding of your child's language development.

Source: Matkin (1980). Reprinted by permission of Noel D. Matkin, Ph.D. Professor Emeritus, University of Arizona.

Appendix B
Screening Instrument for Targeting Educational Risk (SIFTER)

Student _____   Teacher _____   Grade _____

Date completed _____   School _____   District _____

The above student is suspect for hearing problems which may or may not be affecting his/her school performance. This rating scale has been designed to sift out students who are educationally at risk possibly as a result of hearing problems.

Based on your knowledge from observations of this student, circle the number best representing his/her behavior. After answering the questions, please record any comments about the student in the space provided on the reverse side.

1. What is your estimate of the student's class standing in comparison to that of his/her classmates?	UPPER 5	4	MIDDLE 3	2	LOWER 1	**ACADEMICS**	☐
2. How does the student's achievement compare to your estimation of his/her potential?	EQUAL 5	4	LOWER 3	2	MUCH LOWER 1		
3. What is the student's reading level, reading ability group or reading readiness group in the classroom (e.g., a student with average reading ability performs in the middle group)?	UPPER 5	4	MIDDLE 3	2	LOWER 1		
4. How distractible is the student in comparison to his/her classmates?	NOT VERY 5	4	AVERAGE 3	2	VERY 1	**ATTENTION**	☐
5. What is the student's attention span in comparison to that of his/her classmates?	LONGER 5	4	AVERAGE 3	2	SHORTER 1		
6. How often does the student hesitate or become confused when responding to oral directions (e.g.,"Turn to page . . .")?	NEVER 5	4	OCCASIONALLY 3	2	FREQUENTLY 1		
7. How does the student's comprehension compare to the average understanding ability of his/her classmates?	ABOVE 5	4	AVERAGE 3	2	BELOW 1	**COMMUNICATION**	☐
8. How do the student's vocabulary and word usage skills compare with those of other students in his/her age group?	ABOVE 5	4	AVERAGE 3	2	BELOW 1		
9. How proficient is the student at telling a story or relating happenings from home when compared to classmates?	ABOVE 5	4	AVERAGE 3	2	BELOW 1		
10. How often does the student volunteer information to class discussions or in answer to teacher questions?	FREQUENTLY 5	4	OCCASIONALLY 3	2	NEVER 1	**CLASS PARTICIPATION**	☐
11. With what frequency does the student complete his/her class and homework assignments within the time allocated?	ALWAYS 5	4	USUALLY 3	2	SELDOM 1		
12. After instruction, does the student have difficulty starting to work (looks at other students working or asks for help)?	NEVER 5	4	OCCASIONALLY 3	2	FREQUENTLY 1		
13. Does the student demonstrate any behaviors that seem unusual or inappropriate when compared to other students?	NEVER 5	4	OCCASIONALLY 3	2	FREQUENTLY 1	**SCHOOL BEHAVIOR**	☐
14. Does the student become frustrated easily, sometimes to the point of losing emotional control?	NEVER 5	4	OCCASIONALLY 3	2	FREQUENTLY 1		
15. In general, how would you rank the student's relationship with peers (ability to get along with others)?	GOOD 5	4	AVERAGE 3	2	POOR 1		

Source: Anderson, K. L. (1989). *Screening instrument for targeting educational risk (SIFTER)*. Tampa, FL: Educational Audiology Association. Reprinted by permission.

chapter 9

Assessment and Management of Special Populations

AFTER COMPLETING THIS CHAPTER, YOU SHOULD BE ABLE TO:

1. List the various types of special populations you might encounter in audiology practice.
2. For each of the populations noted, summarize their unique features and explain how each feature could affect the diagnostic and/or rehabilitation process.
3. Discuss how the use of "informed questions" can assist audiologists and other professionals in gaining relevant insight about the client without leading to stereotyped expectations.
4. Discuss the inconsistencies in audiometric data that suggest a nonorganic hearing loss may be present.
5. Understand why developing client-specific protocols is essential in the assessment of individuals who have special needs.
6. Understand how knowledge of multicultural issues facilitates a humanistic approach to providing audiological services.

The information in this chapter is designed to address how some of the primary characteristics of various populations of clients might influence the audiologist's ability to perform comprehensive assessment and aural rehabilitation. This information is clearly important to the audiologist because assessment and rehabilitation are critical roles of the audiologist, as is the provision of service to individuals who have special needs.

This information is equally relevant to speech–language pathologists, who serve as primary sources of referrals for comprehensive audiological assessment. Knowledge of audiological techniques and how a client's profile might interact with these techniques will facilitate better referrals and will allow the speech–language pathologist to provide greater insights to the audiologist regarding methods of effective assessment. In addition, although this chapter addresses comprehensive audiological assessment performed by an audiologist, much of the information can be combined with guidelines presented in Chapter 11 regarding the screening of individuals who are developmentally disabled, elderly, or who have neurological disorders.

Any discussion of special populations creates a dilemma: (1) How can we communicate that each client, regardless of medical, psychiatric, or educational label, is an individual person and should be treated as unique? and (2) How can we become knowledgeable about the types of disabilities that will be encountered in audiology practice in order to be more able to make prudent decisions regarding the most effective methods of assessment and rehabilitation? The answer to this dilemma may lie in the use of *informed questions*. What do we mean by informed questions? Specifically, audiologists, based on their knowledge of the issues and characteristics associated with a particular disability, should bring to their audiology work a series of relevant questions that will guide assessment and intervention. Note here that general knowledge of the disability area does not drive the audiologist's work. General knowledge can lead to stereotyped expectations that may not necessarily apply to the particular client at hand and should be avoided. General information is important, however, in that it can lead to specific and insightful questions about variables that can guide the audiologist. These variables have been described in our discussion of pediatric assessment and the use of client-specific protocols.

A brief example may illustrate. General information suggests that individuals who have had strokes often have had resulting language deficits. Knowing this, an audiologist asks a series of questions about language that are related to the client's ability to perform the tasks involved in the audiological assessment. The audiologist finds that although expressive abilities are impaired (including repeating), receptive skills are intact. The audiologist now can plan the assessment knowing that the client is likely to understand directions well and that word-repetition tasks will likely be difficult.

The use of informed questions requires that the audiologist know enough general information about various types of clients to generate relevant questions from this information. This chapter should be helpful in this regard. It also requires that the audiologist be willing to collaborate with others who have access to the answers to these questions.

The populations discussed in this chapter include individuals who are elderly, deaf, developmentally disabled, those who have neurogenic disorders, and those who have nonorganic hearing loss. The format of the information presented for the groups of clients is very similar, beginning with definitions and background information and then describing specifically how the characteristics of the client, or issues surrounding the disability, may affect the audiologist's ability to obtain reliable hearing assessment.

The Elderly

Information from the U.S. Bureau of the Census indicates that the number of individuals age 65 years and older is growing more rapidly than the rest of the U.S. population. Because hearing loss is a common problem in older individuals, this increase in the number of older citizens will have a noticeable impact on the delivery of health care, including hearing health care, in the coming years. Despite the projections that substantial numbers of people over the age of 65 will have a need for hearing health care services, this population is typically not a prime focus in preservice programs in communication disorders. It is not uncommon for clinicians to gain most of their experience in the assessment and rehabilitation of hearing loss in the elderly on the job. However, establishing the presence of hearing loss in the elderly is of prime importance in the differential diagnosis process, because other conditions, including **depression** and **dementia,** may be mistaken for hearing loss and vice versa.

Caring for the Elderly

Ageism may be defined as a generally negative view of the elderly. This attitude can stem from a variety of sources, including fear of the unknown, the value society places on youth and vitality, and fear of one's own aging/mortality. The study of aging and the problems of the aged is called **gerontology.** It is important that clinicians be aware of their own attitudes and beliefs and how these attitudes may influence care for older clients. It is also important that the client's birthdate does not disproportionately influence his or her hearing health care plan. For example, clients in their early nineties should not be discouraged from the purchase of a new hearing aid(s) on the basis of age. Rather, the client's communication status and individual needs should be the primary influence in the decision-making process.

When you think about aging, you may think of a process in which individuals experience a gradual decline in a variety of abilities. This is understandable because most of us know someone who, over time, has demonstrated a steady reduction in physical, sensory, and cognitive abilities. This has been the prevailing view of aging for many years.

An alternate view of aging was proposed by Smith (1989). This model of aging, referred to as the *terminal drop model,* is more positive and for many older individuals more representative of their functioning. The terminal drop model of aging states that many individuals in their seventies and eighties continue to perform successfully in a variety of physical and cognitive domains, just as they did in their forties and fifties, until some point where a sudden, steady decline occurs. This sudden decline is often brought about by an event that permanently impairs health.

Think again about the older individuals you know who are well into their seventies or even early eighties and who live independently, drive, attend social functions, and babysit their grandchildren. Certainly the second of these two models more accurately characterizes their process of aging.

It is important to remember that the terminal drop model applies to physical and mental abilities more than sensory abilities. This means that as individuals age, they are likely to experience a gradual loss of sensory abilities (e.g., hearing and vision). However, audiologists, speech–language pathologists, and other health care providers should not assume that cognitive and physical limitations will interfere with the older client's ability to perform the required assessment and rehabilitation procedures. Consistent with a humanistic philosophy of care, this should be determined on an individual basis.

The aging process affects all systems in the body, including the auditory and visual systems. The individual's memory, particularly short-term memory, and ability to perceive tactile sensation and pain may also be affected. Changes in these systems have a potential impact on the assessment and rehabilitation of hearing loss in older individuals. Hearing loss due to aging is called **presbycusis** and typically affects the higher frequencies, which are most important for speech intelligibility. In addition to the loss of hearing sensitivity, there is an accompanying decline in word recognition scores after age 60, generally by 13 percent per decade in males and by 6 percent per decade in females, according to the work of Chessman (1997).

Changes in the auditory system related to the aging process include the following:

• *Outer ear.* Loss of elasticity in cartilage, possibly resulting in **collapsing ear canals** (due to the force of the headband) during hearing testing. When screening or evaluating hearing, it is wise to check for collapsing canals before beginning work. This can be accomplished by viewing the ear canal with an otoscope and pressing on the pinna. If the ear canal collapses during this procedure, the clinician should employ a corrective action, such as use of insert earphones or pulling up and back on the pinna prior to placing the earphones, to avoid the need to retest. Collapsing ear canals should be suspected whenever high-frequency air–bone gaps are obtained.

• *Middle ear.* Arthritic changes in the middle ear bones (ossicles) and loss of elasticity in the tympanic membrane. Results of tympanometry may be stiffness-dominated; acoustic reflex data combined with comparison of air and bone conduction audiometric findings can provide useful information to rule out middle ear involvement in this instance. For example, if acoustic reflexes are present and the audiogram does not support air–bone gaps, conductive pathology is ruled out despite the tympanometric findings.

• *Inner ear.* Sensorineural hearing loss affecting the higher test frequencies, which results in misunderstanding of speech and reduced understanding of speech in noise. Benefit from amplification may be compromised depending on the extent of the reduction in word recognition ability that often accompanies presbycusis.

• *Eighth cranial nerve and neural processing.* Degenerative changes also take place in the central auditory system. These may include neural degeneration of the eighth cranial nerve (auditory nerve), the brainstem, and auditory association areas of the brain (cortex). These effects can compound the previously described peripheral effects, resulting in further decreases in word recognition ability and compromised benefit from aural rehabilitation.

The visual system also undergoes changes related to the aging process, as many people over the age of 40 know. Vision changes due to aging are called **presbyopia.** People generally require reading glasses, and may need large-print materials and more light to compensate for changes in the visual system. It is important to be mindful of these potential needs when providing written materials to support the hearing assessment and/or rehabilitation process. In addition, modifications to hearing aids may be necessary if clients cannot see the small markings on the devices. Rawool (2000) suggests that older clients use a magnifying glass to assist them in tasks related to hearing aid use and maintenance (e.g., routine cleaning of the hearing aid).

It should be noted here that many clients, including those in the elderly population, prefer to wear hearing aids that are small. It is the audiologist's responsibility to provide honest information to the client regarding his or her ability to function independently with the selected device.

Memory changes associated with aging vary from person to person. For those who experience memory loss, short-term memory is usually affected. Clinically, this may mean that additional time must be allotted, particularly during the initial phases of the hearing rehabilitation process, when new information regarding the hearing aids and their function and maintenance must be assimilated.

Some older individuals report decreased sensation, for example, in their fingers or fingertips. This may make various hearing aid-related tasks challenging, including inserting the hearing aid, changing the battery, and operating any switches on the hearing aid. A decrease in the ability to sense pain or discomfort may also occur. This is of concern because a new hearing aid or earmold that does not fit properly may cause irritation to the client's ear even though the client may be unaware of it. Solutions for this include instructions to the client and/or family members or caregivers to be aware of this possibility and to report any such irritation to the hearing aid dispenser promptly.

Studies have demonstrated that the characteristics of slowing and cautiousness have a different effect on the performance of elderly clients on tests using pure tone (Rees & Botwinick, 1984) versus speech (Gordon-Salant, 1986; McCarthy & Vesper, 2000) stimuli. Specifically, caution can cause elevated thresholds during conventional pure tone testing, but does not appear to have a similar effect during tests of word recognition ability. This information has implications for testing. First, beginning the assessment with the speech reception threshold and word recognition testing, rather than pure tones, may help the audiologist to obtain more accurate threshold information. Beginning with the more interesting speech stimuli gives the audiologist an idea of the degree of hearing loss, which then allows reinstruction of the client when the pure tone findings are elevated compared to the speech audiometry findings. Armed with this data, the clinician can proceed with the pure tone testing and provide reinstruction and encouragement if it is suspected that the pure tone data are suprathreshold.

The majority of elderly people live at home, either alone or with a spouse. The institutionalized elderly constitute a smaller proportion of the population; however, they are more likely to have a hearing loss, and the rehabilitation process is generally more complex for these individuals due to concomitant conditions such as dementia, vision loss, and reduced mobility/dexterity.

The changes noted above represent common changes that occur during the aging process. Unfortunately, a growing number of elderly individuals experience changes with aging that go beyond this. **Dementia** is the term used to refer to a group of (usually acquired) disorders of the central nervous system that progressively interfere with a person's cognitive functioning. **Alzheimer's disease,** a form of cortical dementia, commonly interferes with both memory and language skills, with eventual loss of all verbal abilities. Although different from the other neurogenic disorders described in this chapter (cerebrovascular accident and traumatic brain injury), many of the same suggestions for task modification will apply. Table 9.1 summarizes factors that can affect some elderly individuals, and potential effects on the diagnostic and rehabilitative audiological processes.

Audiological assessment for the elderly can take place in traditional settings (i.e., in the clinical setting in a sound-treated test suite) or in nontraditional settings (i.e., the patient's living room, or a treatment room in a health care facility). The ASHA (1997) guidelines for audiology service delivery in nursing homes note that "an experienced audiologist can apply standard procedures in nonstandard settings to attain a complete picture of a resident's current hearing status and audiologic rehabilitation needs" (p. 17). This document further discusses screening, audiological assessment, and intervention for individuals in home care and institutional settings.

An individualized approach to hearing rehabilitation should be employed. Jerger et al. (1996) discuss the subject of monaural versus binaural hearing aids for older adults, and indicate that for some older adults, one hearing aid may actually be better than two. They add that some older patients report too much confusion of sounds with two hearing aids. The lesson from this is that, although most people do better with two hearing

TABLE 9.1 Factors Affecting Some Elderly Individuals and Potential Effects on Hearing Evaluation and Aural Rehabilitation

Factor	Effects on Hearing Evaluation	Effects on Aural Rehabilitation
Ageism	Bias toward client by the audiologist and/or family, caregivers	Biased recommendations, may include failure to recommend amplification or to explore the full range of available options
Auditory Collapsing canals	False conductive hearing loss; solutions: careful placement of supra-aural earphones or use of insert earphones	May have an impact on earmold/hearing aid fit; care should be taken during earmold impression making
Middle ear stiffness	False indication of middle ear pathology; solutions: cross-check with other data including air and bone conduction results and acoustic reflexes	
Decreased word recognition ability		May limit potential benefit from amplification; implications for counseling regarding expectations from AR
Vision	Can interfere with assessment if picture pointing task is attempted and/or if comparing auditory alone with auditory + visual conditions	Modify hearing aid to accommodate reduced vision; possible impact on size of hearing aid selected; enlarge any written materials provided to patient
Memory	Can interfere with client's ability to respond consistently to pure tones; play techniques may be helpful	Provide written information regarding the hearing aid and include family members or caregivers in rehabilitation sessions
Decreased body sensation		May affect ability to control small dials, switches on hearing aid; consider use of automatic circuitry; also, reduced awareness of ear discomfort related to earmold and/or hearing aid fit
Skin changes		Silicone materials used for making earmold impressions may cause irritation; use alternate material if necessary
Slowing and cautiousness	Begin with speech audiometry rather than pure tones; need careful monitoring of intertest agreement	Similar effects may be present during behavioral testing to verify hearing aid benefit

aids, this is not a universal finding. Since there will always be exceptions, it is important to treat people individually and to listen to what the patient and family or caregivers say on hearing aid follow-up visits before making final decisions on the hearing aid arrangement.

Individuals Who Are Deaf

Even though the definition of deafness is straightforward from an audiometric point of view, many other factors must also be taken into consideration when addressing the communicative needs of deaf individuals. Some of these factors include the general communication skill of the individual and their family, the family and individual cultural view of deafness, the age of onset of hearing loss, the amount of residual hearing, and the presence of other disabilities, including cognitive status.

Definitions

Students in audiology and speech–language pathology programs often ask about the distinction between the terms *deaf* and *hard of hearing*. The traditional audiometric interpretation is that hearing impairment that is 90 dB or greater on the audiogram constitutes **deafness; hard of hearing** is generally defined as hearing thresholds that are less than 90 dB, but not within the normal range.

When considering the distinction between the categories *deaf* and *hard of hearing*, it is far more important to consider an individual's functional communication skills than to focus on an arbitrary decibel value. With this in mind, differentiating between the categories deaf and hard of hearing should be viewed in terms of the degree to which an individual uses manual or oral/aural systems for communication.

The word *oral* refers to the process of producing speech and language for communication; the word *aural* refers to auditory reception of this information. Individuals who have normal hearing and those who are hard of hearing usually rely on the **oral/aural** mechanism as their primary means of developing speech language; secondarily they use the visual modality. In other words, with the exception of people who are deaf, it is mainly through speaking and listening that communication occurs. In those instances when a person watches the speaker's face or lips to gain additional information, the visual modality is providing supplemental information.

Based on the definitions provided, individuals who are deaf typically rely primarily on the visual modality for language acquisition and use. Because of the degree of their hearing loss, the visual modality, usually through sign language, provides the primary communication input, and the auditory mechanism provides secondary cues.

Two audiograms are shown in Figure 9.1, illustrating the differences described between hearing impairment and deafness. Note that the person who is hard of hearing, depicted in Audiogram A, has a severe sensorineural hearing loss. Despite this, the aided thresholds (marked "A" on the audiogram) reveal considerable benefit from amplification and further suggest that this person, even with this degree of hearing loss, will have access to many of the phonemes of our language. Because of this, this individual is likely to develop speech and language *primarily* using the oral/aural systems. Of course, other individuals with this audiometric profile may use a more manual or combined ("Total Communication") approach.

FIGURE 9.1 **Audiograms depicting hard of hearing (A) and deafness (B).**

Audiogram A

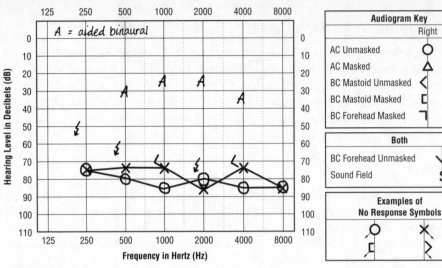

Audiogram B

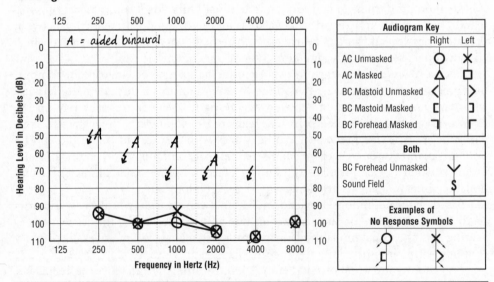

Contrast this with Audiogram B, in which the hearing thresholds are greater than 90 dB bilaterally. Note that even with good amplification, the aided responses do not provide this person with access to most of the phonemes in our language. With this limited access to the speech signal, it is likely that language develops primarily through use of manual communication. In some cases, cochlear implantation, discussed in Chapter 12, provides additional access to the speech signal. This increased access may or may not result in a change in communication approach.

Communication Mismatch

Individuals who are deaf may consider **American Sign Language** (ASL) as their native language. ASL is not only a different mode of communication (signed rather than spoken); it also is a different language from oral English. ASL has its own unique syntax and conveys information through movement of the hands, arms, face, and body. Rather than being processed sequentially, like English, ASL is processed spatially, and allows for communication of complete ideas with single signs. In contrast, **Manually Coded English** (MCE) systems (e.g., Seeing Essential English, Signing Exact English) are based on the structure of English using manual forms. While SEE differs from oral English in form, ASL differs from oral English both in form and in language. Some deaf individuals use a communication approach referred to as **Total Communication.** In this methodology, any and all means of communication are used, including aural (e.g., hearing aids), manual (gestures, signs, body movement), and oral (speech) systems. Summarized in Table 9.2 are some of the various communication approaches used by individuals who are hard of hearing and deaf.

The fact that individuals who are deaf will most likely use a language different from English, and/or a nonspoken mode of communication, presents audiologists with a mandate to interact successfully with these clients. One way to do this is to make arrangements for a sign language interpreter to accompany the client to the evaluation. ASL is a language that is distinct from English, and it is rare that an audiologist who is not regularly working with individuals who are deaf will be fluent in this language. Use

TABLE 9.2 **Summary of Primary Communication Approaches for Individuals Who Are Deaf**

Communication System	Description
American Sign Language (ASL)	Considered by most deaf individuals to be their native language. Uses a different grammar than oral English. Communicates concepts rather than individual words. Uses facial and body movement. Is processed spatially.
Manually Coded English (MCE)	English in manual form. Signs correspond to English words, and the syntax is the same. Includes English morphemes. Variations of MCE are Seeing Essential English and Signing Exact English.
Pidgin Sign English (PSE)	Combines aspects of ASL with MCE. For example, may use ASL signs in English word order. May include more English morphemes than ASL.
Total Communication	Uses all modes of communication (e.g., sign, speech delivered through amplification, writing, gestures). Designed to provide multisensory information for communication.

of a sign language interpreter is perhaps the most efficient way to solve this language difference and is required under the Americans with Disabilities Act (ADA) legislation.

Despite the value of using an interpreter for audiology evaluations, the reality is that there will be many times when a client who is deaf arrives for evaluation without an interpreter. The audiologist then needs to determine which methods of exchanging information will be most effective. Sometimes writing can be used, but it should be noted that **prelingually deafened** individuals typically have reading skills that do not exceed the fourth-grade level. For this reason, the audiologist should make every attempt to use basic vocabulary and sentence structure. Lip reading is sometimes helpful with individuals who are deaf and, along with basic gestures, may give the client enough information to understand the audiologist. Also, the audiologist should have at least a basic knowledge of selected signs so that these can be used for the most frequently occurring topics during an audiology assessment. If the audiologist is not fluent with sign language and the client's reading skills are poor, interpreter services should be obtained so that the client will be able to receive all the information needed regarding the results of the testing and recommendations, and will be able to ask questions and make contributions to the overall rehabilitation plan.

Cultural Mismatch

In addition to the likely difference in language or language modes confronting the audiologist and the client, there may also be a **cultural mismatch** that must be accommodated. The student who is new to the field of communication disorders, and particularly to issues of deafness, may be unfamiliar with these two differing perspectives on deafness: one that deafness is a disability (in this case the word *deaf* is spelled with a lowercase *d*) and the other, common among individuals who are born deaf, that deafness is not a disability but rather a cultural difference (in which case the word **Deaf** is spelled with a capital *D*). Individuals who hold the cultural view of deafness describe ASL as a minority language that does not rely on audition and view their deafness as the source of their culture. They do not view deafness as a disability. The cultural view of deafness is common in cases in which the parents, and sometimes other relatives, are also deaf. In fact, in households in which both parents are deaf, the news that the newborn baby is also deaf is typically met with great joy.

This concept tends to be difficult for many hearing people to understand. How could a hearing loss that exceeds 90 dB on the audiogram not constitute a disability? How could reading levels that are equivalent to those of a fourth-grade student not constitute a disability? Is it really possible that news that a child is deaf is an occasion for celebration? One of the reasons this concept tends to be difficult is that many of us who have chosen to work in the helping professions have been trained in a disability model. We have learned about normal development and have been taught to intervene in ways that make abnormal conditions more like normal. A good example of this is the use of hearing aids. By amplifying sounds, we provide individuals who have abnormal thresholds with greater access to sound to help them function more like hearing individuals. Another, more controversial, example is cochlear implant surgery. This is described in Chapter 12. Although widely seen by hearing individuals as an attempt to "help" the individual who is deaf, cochlear implants are often viewed by those who hold the cultural view of deafness as a dangerous and misguided attempt to change someone who does not need to be changed.

How does this information regarding the two views of deafness potentially impact the audiologist's work in assessment and rehabilitation? First, audiologists must be cautious not to impose their view of deafness on the client. Clinicians must expend the necessary time and effort to understand how clients view themselves and how the audiologist might be helpful. Too often in the helping professions the clinicians presume that they know what clients need. For example, if one were not knowledgeable about the cultural perspective of deafness, it would seem logical that a person with profound hearing loss would need powerful hearing aids. But this is logical only if clients agree that hearing is important and valuable to their own self-perception. Many deaf individuals do not choose to wear amplification because they believe that ASL gives them a language system that is quite successful. Similarly, even though hearing clients often view the cochlear implant as a major breakthrough in improving the communication skills of clients, this perspective does not hold up if one's perspective is that deafness is culture.

Other Factors

Now that we have discussed communication and cultural factors associated with deafness that can affect the work of audiologists, let's examine how other factors may influence the success or failure of audiological assessment and rehabilitation. These factors are age of onset, the degree of residual hearing, the presence of other disabilities, and cognitive status. Table 9.3 provides a summary of the essential points of this discussion.

Age of Onset

As discussed earlier, individuals who are born deaf or who become deaf early in life (prelingual deafness) experience dramatically greater disruption in their oral communication skills compared to those whose hearing loss occurs after the initial development of speech and language (**postlingual deafness**). For example, children who have normal hearing until the age of 2 and then become deaf perform significantly better on measures of oral English skills compared to those whose hearing loss occurred prior to age 2 years.

In view of this, the audiologist working with a client who is deaf is well advised to inquire about the age of onset of the hearing loss. In cases in which the hearing loss is postlingual, the client is likely to use oral English as the primary means of communication and may be able to carry out standard audiological tests, including speech audiometry and pure tones. Depending on the length of time the client has had this hearing loss, the client may experience reduced articulation skills, which may require the use of picture pointing in the assessment of speech recognition.

In terms of rehabilitation, the person who is postlingually deafened is likely to use hearing aids successfully and to view the audiologist and the aural rehabilitation process in positive terms. Because they once had normal hearing, these clients are unlikely to view their deafness as part of their culture.

Degree of Residual Hearing

As we have noted previously, the degree of **residual hearing** in individuals described as deaf can vary greatly. As noted in Figure 9.2, audiogram A represents a person with thresholds of 90 dB across all frequencies from 250 to 4,000 Hz. Audiogram B in Figure 9.2 represents what is commonly referred to as a **corner audiogram,** with residual hearing primarily in the low-frequency ranges. Even though both of these hearing losses can be

TABLE 9.3   Factors Related to Assessment and Rehabilitation for Individuals with Deafness

Relevant Features	Impact on Assessment	Impact on Rehabilitation
View of deafness	If considered culture, the audiologist may be viewed by the client with skepticism.	If viewed as a culture, the client may not view rehabilitation as necessary. The client may choose not to wear hearing aids and will likely be satisfied with ASL. The client may object to cochlear implant procedures.
Communication mode	If ASL, interpreter services may be required. If SEE, the audiologist should know some basic signs. If oral English, the client is more likely to be able to carry out the standard audiology tests but may need picture-pointing tasks rather than word repetition. Assessment of client's use of lipreading cues is recommended.	If ASL, may not see the need for rehabilitation. If oral English, may be more invested in rehabilitation.
Age of onset	Individuals who are deafened after having had normal hearing during initial period development of speech and language development are more likely to use oral English. See comments noted for communication mode.	The postlingually impaired individual will be more likely to rely on audition and will therefore view the audiologist and rehabilitation as relevant to his/her life.
Degree of residual hearing	The greater the residual hearing, the more likely the client will be able to understand words for speech audiometry. Intelligibility may be poor but picture-pointing should help.	The greater the residual hearing, the greater the benefit from amplification and the more invested in amplification the client is likely to be. Those with little residual are usually better candidates for cochlear implants.
Presence of other disabilities	Physical disabilities can interfere with the clients ability to scan and point to pictures, use response button, and carry out play audiometry techniques. Depending on the type/degree of the physical disability, testing modifications must be made.	Some disabilities interfere with use of hearing aids. Newer, more automatic, self-adjusting devices may be appropriate. Assessment of degree of home support is essential.
Cognitive status	Reduced cognitive skills may lead to use of the more basic tasks on the audiology test continuum. Sound field VRA using speech may represent the most basic level of assessment.	Very reduced cognitive skills may prevent the client from using the amplified information (e.g., is it meaningful to the client?). Because the client may not be able to understand the rehabilitation. instruction, assessment of degree of home support is essential.

FIGURE 9.2 **Audiograms depicting deafness with considerable residual hearing (A) and deafness with minimal residual hearing (B).**

Audiogram A

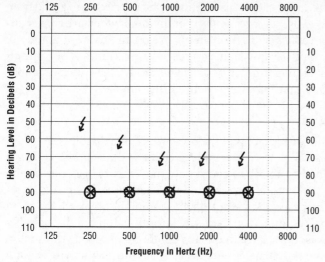

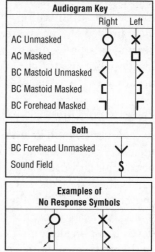

Audiogram B

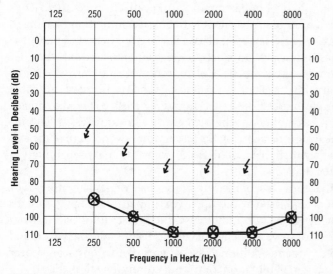

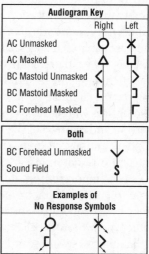

described by the term *deafness,* these two people obviously have different degrees of residual hearing. During assessment, the person with audiogram A will be more likely to understand words and will therefore be more likely to perform speech reception threshold testing. If speech intelligibility is poor, word repetition will likely be unsuccessful but picture-pointing tasks could be successful. Recognition of monosyllables is more difficult than understanding of spondee words, so speech recognition testing may be more challenging for the client, although use of pictures could be successful here.

The person with audiogram B may not be able to understand spondee words. If this is the case, speech awareness thresholds can be attempted and should correspond roughly with the low-frequency hearing.

In terms of rehabilitation, the individual who has greater residual hearing is likely to receive greater benefit from hearing aids. This may motivate the person in audiogram A to pursue amplification and to use it more regularly. Individuals who have corner audiograms tend to receive less overall benefit from amplification and may opt not to use hearing aids, preferring some type of sign language as their primary means of communication. Because the client in audiogram B is less likely to receive benefit from amplification, he is more likely to be a candidate for a cochlear implant.

Presence of Other Disabilities

Audiologists should be mindful of the fact that the presence of one disability increases the likelihood of a second disability. If, for example, a client with deafness also has a neurological disorder affecting her ability to coordinate movements of her arms and hands, the audiologist may need to modify the method the client uses for signaling a response to tones. Rather than using a response button, the audiologist may ask the client to nod her head or give a verbal response (e.g., "yes," or "I hear it"). If the audiologist believed that play audiometry was the best technique for obtaining pure tone thresholds, care would have to be taken that the client's ability to carry out the play activity was not hindered by physical limitations.

In terms of rehabilitation, physical impairments can negatively affect the client's ability to use amplification. For example, for a client with physical limitations, having to adjust the volume wheel of a hearing aid or even place a hearing aid in the ear may pose unreasonable challenges. These physical factors need to be taken into account when decisions regarding rehabilitation are being made. Collaboration with others who know the client well and are familiar with the client's surroundings and the degree of available support is essential. For example, one question that should regularly be asked by an audiologist is whether the client has family or other caregivers who could assist with insertion and removal of the hearing aid, changing the battery, and overall care of the aid. Understanding the supports that are in place allows audiologists to make rehabilitation suggestions that have a greater chance of succeeding.

It is important to note that some disabilities are more observable than others. For example, physical impairments tend to be readily apparent; impairments in visual skills may be less obvious. The challenge for the audiologist is to collect information from others who know the client well, observe the behaviors of the client in the diagnostic and rehabilitative sessions, and recommend additional assessments if other obstacles appear to be interfering with assessment, rehabilitation, or overall communication abilities.

Cognitive Status

Although there is nothing inherent in deafness that causes cognitive deficits, there is still the possibility that cognitive deficits may coexist with deafness. Most experts believe that the minimum IQ score for normal cognition is 85 on typical IQ tests (e.g., Wechsler, Stanford-Binet). During assessment, individuals who are deaf and have low IQ scores will likely need additional supports in the form of conditioned play audiometry in order to complete the audiological assessment successfully. Depending on the degree of cognitive impairment, the audiologist may have to rely on tasks that are more basic. In cases of significant cognitive impairment, rehabilitation instruction may not be understood by the client, and the value of amplification may be in doubt because of the client's lack of understanding of incoming information. Refer to the information presented in this chapter on working with developmentally disabled adults.

Finally, it should be noted that although the relevant features discussed in this section are described separately, they present themselves in combinations in real clients. For example, a client who has a prelingual hearing loss, minimal residual hearing, holds a cultural view of deafness, and uses ASL fluently may regard the practice of audiology with skepticism and have little use for regular audiological assessment and rehabilitation services. Conversely, a client who is postlingually deafened, presents with greater residual hearing, and who uses oral English will most likely view regular testing and hearing-aid checks as valuable. Finally, a client who has deafness along with little residual hearing and somewhat reduced cognitive skills may be difficult to test and receive minimal assistance from auditory rehabilitation services. Other rehabilitation services, however, such as vocational rehabilitation to assist with job placement, may be of significant benefit to the client.

Adults with Developmental Disabilities

Definition

It is important to remember that no two individuals are alike. This is true of adults with and without disabilities. There are attributes that characterize developmental disabilities that are included in the definition of developmental disabilities in the Developmental Disabilities Assistance and Bill of Rights Act of 1990, which follows. The term **developmental disability** means a severe, chronic disability of an individual 5 years of age or older that:

1. Is attributable to a mental or physical impairment or combination of mental and physical impairments
2. Is manifested before the individual attains age 22
3. Is likely to continue indefinitely
4. Results in substantial functional limitations in three or more of the following areas of major life activity: self-care, receptive and expressive language, learning, mobility, self-direction, capacity for independent living, and economic self-sufficiency
5. Reflects the individual's need for a combination and sequence of special, interdisciplinary, or generic services, supports, or other assistance that is of lifelong or extended duration and is individually planned and coordinated, except that such term, when applied to infants and young children means individuals from birth to age 5, inclusive, who have substantial developmental delay or specific congenital or acquired conditions with a high probability of resulting in developmental disabilities if services are not provided

A significant opportunity for collaboration among caregivers, paraprofessionals, and professionals is presented when adults with developmental disabilities are referred for audiological evaluation or consultation. As you know, in many instances developmental disabilities coexist with a variety of other conditions requiring creative interactions among professionals. This is one of the many reasons why clinical preparation of speech–language pathologists and audiologists should include a rich variety of clients and settings.

The following scenario is not an uncommon one and serves to illustrate a number of important points, including the necessity of communication among all members of a team to achieve the most favorable outcomes for each patient/client.

You are about to greet your third client for the day, a 40-something adult male (we'll call him Jack) with developmental disabilities. Jack has a severe motor disability, including both **spastic** and **athetoid cerebral palsy,** and uses a wheelchair. He is a new client, and the information you have is limited to Jack's identifying information, his previous diagnoses (significant motor disability and mental retardation), and what you can observe. From your observations, Jack does not appear to be able to speak, and his speech–language skills are not addressed in the chart. The individual transporting Jack to this appointment does not know him well and does not know how to communicate with Jack. As you bring Jack to the sound-treated room for his hearing test, several colleagues ask whether you will need assistance during testing.

Think about the client-specific protocol we have described and the types of tests you might use in assessing Jack's hearing sensitivity. In addition, refer to Table 9.4 for a summary of key issues. Will you start with an SRT or an SAT? How will you approach pure tone testing? Will conventional testing be possible? If conditioned play is needed, will Jack's severe motor involvement preclude holding/releasing a stick or poker chip? If VRA is used, does Jack have the motor control to turn his head toward the sound source? Will he be able to be conditioned? What information would help you with the answers to these questions?

Information about Jack's cognitive status and his speech–language skills, including his receptive and expressive abilities, would provide insight into how to approach his hearing evaluation. For example, does he have a consistent yes/no response? Will he understand the test directions? Does Jack use an **augmentative alternative communication (AAC)** device, and if so, was it brought to the test session? Does Jack become frustrated in challenging or different situations or environments? Without this information, the clinician must go through a process of "trial and error" to arrive at the optimal test technique—the one that best fits the client's abilities.

In the scenario just described, it would be reasonable to assume that a second tester would be needed to help this client perform the tasks required of him during audiological testing. It would be reasonable to begin with an SAT since we have observed that Jack's vocalizations are not intelligible. It would be reasonable, given the available information, to wonder how to accomplish word recognition testing, since picture pointing does not appear feasible due to the degree of motor involvement and the fact that Jack's vocalizations are not intelligible.

All of these assumptions would be reasonable but in Jack's case were incorrect. Now let's picture a scenario in which the audiologist receives the relevant information from the client's speech–language pathologist. As a result, testing decisions are informed as follows: Jack is diagnosed with mild mental retardation, secondary to his severe motor disability. He uses a head pointer and communication board to indicate his wants and needs. He can read and has a large vocabulary. His receptive language skills are good

TABLE 9.4 Adults with Developmental Disabilities

Relevant Features	Impact on Hearing Evaluation	Impact on Aural Rehabilitation
1. Cognitive status	Need to combine the available information with a functional assessment of the client's ability to perform audiological test tasks; in general, begin with the most challenging task, dropping back to less challenging tasks.	The potential benefit from amplification or other assistive technology should be considered by the rehabilitation team. In some instances, e.g., profound mental retardation, the team may conclude that amplification does not improve functional communication status in a measurable way and recommend discontinuation of amplification.
2. Behavioral issues	May affect degree of cooperation with tasks required for completion of behavioral testing. Desensitization to the test environment may be effective. Use of less demanding test tasks may be necessary.	Gradual introduction of the hearing aid or assistive listening device may be effective. If behaviors that are destructive to the hearing aid or other assistive listening device persist, use of such devices may require direct supervision.
3. Tactile defensiveness	If significant, may prevent use of earphones and/or probe tip for immittance testing. Potential helps may include using a hand-held earphone; client may prefer having someone familiar holding the earphone to his or her ear. Use of screening immittance equipment may make it possible to obtain information about middle ear status.	May affect the client's ability to tolerate an assistive listening device. Gradual desensitization may be effective.
4. Communication status	The client's verbal skills, presence of yes/no response are factors in determining which test tasks will yield reliable information. Clients with limited expressive language skills and good receptive skills may succeed with a picture-pointing task for SRT and/or word recognition testing. More basic behavioral tasks, such as an SAT, will be used for clients with limited receptive and expressive language skills.	Clients with an auditory/aural vs. manual mode of communication may benefit differently from amplification.
5. Motor skills	Significant motor involvement may interfere with or preclude use of conditioned play techniques; alternatives may include eye gaze or behavioral observation audiometry.	Significant motor involvement may interfere with or preclude independent insertion/removal of amplification devices and/or adjustment of controls.

and he will easily understand the directions for his hearing test. He has sufficient vocal control to say or approximate "yes" each time he hears a tone. His visual acuity is normal and he will be able to point to pictures using his head pointer, which is stored in the bag attached to the back of his wheelchair. There are no known behavioral issues; Jack is cooperative and enjoys meeting new people.

Armed with this information, the hearing test can proceed smoothly and without "guesswork." Pure tone testing can be completed in the conventional manner, using the verbal "yes" response. An SRT can be obtained using pictures and a picture-pointing response; word recognition scores can be obtained in the same manner. There are no behavioral issues or tactile defensiveness, so the tools needed for obtaining audiological data, such as the earphones, the otoscope, and the probes for middle ear analysis (admittance testing) can be employed.

If this critical information had not been available, at a minimum, testing would not have proceeded smoothly, and at worst, assumptions about Jack's abilities would have prevented the clinician from getting as much information about his hearing as possible.

In summary, it is critical that the communication status of adults with developmental disabilities be conveyed to the audiologist when referrals for audiological evaluations are made. This information may be provided by a variety of people, including the client, or people associated with the client, such as family members, professionals, and paraprofessionals. If an individual or individuals who are knowledgeable about the client cannot be present for the appointment, written documentation should be forwarded either ahead of time or should accompany the client. The type of information needed by the audiologist includes:

- The client's cognitive status
- The client's receptive and expressive language abilities
- Whether the client is verbal or nonverbal
- Whether the client speaks or uses an augmentative/alternative communication (AAC) device/general mode of communication
- Whether the client has an established yes/no response
- Whether the client's response to sound has been successfully conditioned
- Any previous hearing test results
- Behavioral issues and "triggers" (e.g., tactile defensiveness, low tolerance for new situations)
- Things the client likes (e.g., music, positive reinforcement, a calm manner, minimal distractions)

Preparation for the test session, which may take a number of forms, such as clearing away unnecessary or potentially distracting items from the test room, having appropriate reinforcers available, planning extra time to practice the tasks required during testing, or scheduling with two testers available if necessary can only be accomplished if information about the client is transmitted to the audiologist prior to the appointment time. Preplanning enables the audiologist to make the best use of clinical time. This can be critical in test situations where a limited attention span necessitates obtaining the most essential test data first and either going without information considered less essential or rescheduling to "fill in" missing information on another day.

There will be audiologists who will read this recommendation for prior information and will view it as unrealistic given the busy schedules that many audiologists maintain in everyday clinical work. Our response is that this information can be obtained in numerous ways—on the same day as the evaluation from those accompanying the client, either verbally or through notes. This situation provides an opportunity for education of caregivers and therapists and collaboration with all team members to obtain the most complete picture of each client's auditory skills.

In general, testing for adults with developmental disabilities should begin with the highest-level tasks (conventional test techniques with the signals presented through earphones) and drop back to less challenging tasks if the client does not evidence the skills needed for conventional testing. If conditioned play audiometry is employed, age-appropriate "props" should be used, such as poker chips, as opposed to more pediatric props.

Occasionally it will not be possible to obtain reliable behavioral audiological data to establish the hearing status of a developmentally disabled individual. If this is the case, alternative techniques such as otoacoustic emissions or brainstem auditory evoked response testing can be employed to assess auditory system function. See Chapter 6 for additional information on these tests. Whatever technique is used, it is important to provide useful, functional information about the client's auditory status to the people who interact with him or her on a regular basis.

Additional Considerations

When testing hearing sensitivity in adults with significant developmental disabilities, it is not unusual to note a discrepancy between the responses obtained to pure tone versus speech stimuli. The speech signal is generally more salient and more interesting to the client, resulting in a "better" response to the speech signal. This can make interpretation of behavioral responses challenging, since there are no normative data similar to those used in testing the birth to 2-year-old population that can be applied. Also, there is no definitive protocol for interpretation of discrepancies between clients' responses to pure tone and speech stimuli. Some audiologists deal with this issue by applying pediatric norms to adults with developmental disabilities. This can be problematic, however. Because these individuals are adults and their auditory experience is different from that of the birth–2 population, these pediatric norms are not applicable in this circumstance. A test battery approach is recommended, using behavioral and objective measures as needed to provide the most complete information about the client's auditory status.

Management Plans

Recommendations for frequency of evaluations and/or reevaluations for this population are included in Appendix A. If the adult with a developmental disability is found to have a hearing loss requiring amplification, aural rehabilitation should be pursued on a trial basis contingent on medical clearance. It will be important to establish with the client and caregivers the importance of properly caring for and maintaining amplification devices. Occasionally, behavior issues require attention so that aural rehabilitation can be successful. For example, if the client does not tolerate wearing a hearing aid or other assistive listening device, a program of gradual desensitization may work.

Sometimes behavior management does not bring about the desired results, and amplification devices can only be used while the client is under direct supervision. This solution is less than ideal, but may be necessary if all else fails.

There are times when the client's caregivers report no noticeable benefit from the use of amplification. This may be related to numerous factors including behavioral issues described above or severely reduced cognitive skills that preclude the client's meaningful appreciation or use of amplified sound. In these instances it is reasonable to discontinue hearing aid use, but only after collecting input from all team members. It is important to document the specific input that resulted in this decision. In these cases, use of the communication strategies noted in Appendix B can be helpful. In addition, the use of assistive listening devices that may be more acceptable to the client can be explored.

People with Neurogenic Disorders

Consider the following scenario. Early in your audiology career, you are asked to evaluate a gentleman of about 70 years of age who has suffered a stroke. You are not given any details about the man's condition; being new to the field, you do not know enough to ask. Upon entering his hospital room, you find your client sitting in a wheelchair ready to be brought downstairs for his hearing test. You introduce yourself. The client extends his left hand and you shake hands firmly. Then you notice that his right hand and arm are in some type of support and that he does not seem to have use of them.

As you make your trip downstairs to the speech and hearing department, you ask the gentleman how long he has been at the hospital. Without hesitation he responds: "Well, the frapper is all that really matters so that's what you do." At first you think you have misheard him, but then you realize you did not when he comments to one of the nurses at the nurses station that "I dollared him with the frapper." You also began to realize that your lack of knowledge about this man's neurological condition will likely cause some difficulties and that you are heading into this evaluation very unprepared.

As your trip to the speech and hearing department continues, you realize that in addition to not being able to express himself so that others can understand him, this client also has minimal understanding of what you are asking. This becomes apparent during the actual assessment. The patient is not able to carry out instructions to raise his hand when he hears the tone or to say "yes" in response to tones. Attempts to have the patient perform word repetition tasks are equally unsuccessful. After about 30 minutes of attempts, you bring the patient back to his room so that he will not miss his next scheduled therapy. What would have happened if you learned information about this patient's functional strengths and weaknesses prior to the assessment? You could have factored this information into your assessment and increased the chances of obtaining some important information about his hearing in the scheduled session.

Audiologists need to know much more than audiology in order to be successful. As the above vignette illustrates, a lack of understanding of who the patient is and what his strengths and limitations are can undermine any audiologist. On the other hand, a willingness to learn about your client and to seek out information from those people who already know a lot about him increases the likelihood of success.

Although a variety of **neurogenic disorders** of communication exist, this section will briefly describe two: stroke or **cerebrovascular accident (CVA)** and **traumatic brain** injury (TBI). In addition to exposing you to some general information about these disorders, specific characteristics of each will be discussed relative to obtaining reliable hearing assessment and performing aural rehabilitation.

Relevant Anatomy and Physiology for Stroke and TBI

A detailed treatment of the anatomy and physiology of the **central nervous system (CNS)** that supports this discussion of audiological assessment of individuals who have neurogenic disorders of communication is beyond the scope of this text. Instead, a summary of key facts related to this discussion is provided. The largest part of the brain, referred to as the **cerebrum,** is composed of two halves, called cerebral hemispheres. Each of these two hemispheres is divided into the four lobes of the brain, which are depicted in Figure 9.3. The relevant structure and function for the lobes of the brain are described in Table 9.5. The temporal and frontal lobes play essential roles in speech and language, with understanding primarily a function of the **temporal lobe** and production is primarily a function of the **frontal lobe.** The frontal lobe is also involved in executive functions (e.g., memory, problem solving, inhibition, self-regulation, planning) which influence emotional mediation, personality, and pragmatic language abilities.

- The left and right hemispheres do not perform the same functions, with the left side of the brain primarily processing verbal information and the right side more suited to visual-spatial information (in most people).
- The brain's nourishment (oxygen and glucose) is carried by the blood. Because the brain is unable to store these nutrients, it is essential that it receive an uninterrupted blood supply. There are two main sources of blood supply to the brain: the carotid artery and the vertebral artery. Because the **carotid artery** supplies the scalp, face, and frontal lobe, disruption here is likely to have a negative impact on speech, language, and hearing function.

FIGURE 9.3   **Lobes of the brain.**

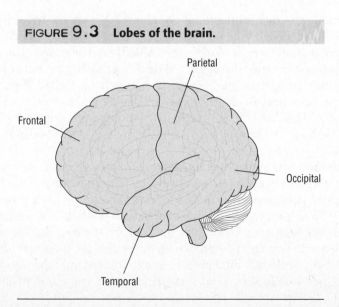

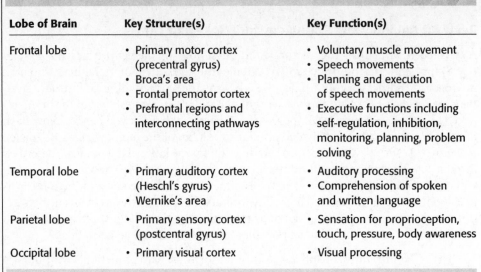

TABLE 9.5	Relevant Structure and Function for the Lobes of the Brain	
Lobe of Brain	**Key Structure(s)**	**Key Function(s)**
Frontal lobe	• Primary motor cortex (precentral gyrus) • Broca's area • Frontal premotor cortex • Prefrontal regions and interconnecting pathways	• Voluntary muscle movement • Speech movements • Planning and execution of speech movements • Executive functions including self-regulation, inhibition, monitoring, planning, problem solving
Temporal lobe	• Primary auditory cortex (Heschl's gyrus) • Wernike's area	• Auditory processing • Comprehension of spoken and written language
Parietal lobe	• Primary sensory cortex (postcentral gyrus)	• Sensation for proprioception, touch, pressure, body awareness
Occipital lobe	• Primary visual cortex	• Visual processing

• The **peripheral nervous system** is made up of the spinal nerves and the cranial nerves. The spinal nerves attach to the spinal cord, transmitting sensory information to the higher brain centers and bringing motor information from these higher centers to muscles. Cranial nerves originate from the brainstem, and many of these nerves (e.g., vagus, hypoglossal, facial, etc.) are closely related to production of speech.

Stroke

A more technical term that is often used synonymously with the term *stroke* is **cerebrovascular accident (CVA)**. When a person has a cerebrovascular accident, he or she usually experiences some type of blockage of a blood vessel or an actual break of one. In either case, the blood supply is disrupted and neurological damage, either temporary or permanent, is likely to occur. Strokes are very common in the United States. In fact, they are the third leading cause of death, after heart disease and cancer. Strokes are much more common in adults over the age of 65 and are more common among African Americans, and individuals who have a history of heart disease, high blood pressure, obesity, and/or diabetes.

One of the most common outcomes of stroke is **aphasia,** which is language impairment due to brain damage. Audiologists working with individuals who have aphasia should know that these clients may be divided into two groups: those with fluent aphasia and those with nonfluent aphasia. **Fluent aphasia** is typically characterized by lots of language produced with good articulation and syntax. The language, however, is often vague and filled with jargon. Individuals with fluent aphasia often have auditory comprehension deficits, making it difficult for them to understand others and themselves. **Nonfluent aphasia,** on the other hand, is characterized by sparse output and difficulties with prosody, articulation, and syntax. Individuals with nonfluent aphasia often have normal to near-normal understanding of spoken information. This distinction can be helpful to the audiologist because it can influence the types of audiological tasks that are more or less likely to be successful in yielding reliable information.

In addition to aphasia, a number of other features are associated with stroke and can affect reliable hearing assessment. These are summarized in Table 9.6. Note that, in addition to knowing whether the patient's aphasia is categorized as fluent or nonfluent, the audiologist should also have some awareness of whether motor speech disorders

TABLE 9.6   Features Associated with Stroke and Potential Impact on Reliable Hearing Assessment

Relevant Features	Impact on Hearing Assessment
Fluent vs. nonfluent aphasia	Individuals with fluent aphasia are more likely to have auditory comprehension deficits which interfere with overall understanding of task directions. These individuals may do better with gestural methods of task demonstration (e.g., show them that they are to put the block in the pail when they hear the sound). Nonfluent individuals will likely understand more but will not be able to provide detailed case history information.
Overall auditory comprehension	This is one of the primary questions that the audiologist must ask prior to assessing the patient. As noted above, for patients who have auditory comprehension deficits, demonstration of how to carry out the pure tone task will likely be more successful than verbal instruction. Also, the audiologist should inquire as to whether the patient is able to answer basic yes/no questions and carry out basic commands. Finally, information about the client's reading skills may be useful.
Presence of motor speech and nonspeech disorders	Both dysarthria and apraxia are likely to interfere with the client's ability to repeat words upon command and carry out directions. With prompting, the client may be able to produce automatic speech, like counting or the alphabet. If picture pointing tasks are used, the audiologist must watch for comprehension deficits, difficulty scanning the pictures, and motor deficits interfering with the pointing response.
Left- vs. right-sided damage	Damage to the left side of the brain will result in greater language disruption than right-sided damage. Right-sided damage may have a greater effect on visual-spatial skills, possibly interfering with picture-pointing tasks.
Emotional state	The audiologist must always be sensitive to signs of depression. Also, some clients experience agitation, which may necessitate support from staff during the hearing assessment.

exist. The presence of such disorders will likely interfere with word repetition tasks, which are part of the audiological assessment.

It is important to note that sometimes individuals who have **apraxia** are able to produce speech that is of a very automatic nature. For example, although they will likely have difficulty repeating back spondee words presented, they may be able, with prompting, to sing "Happy Birthday" or recite the alphabet. This may allow the clinician to use these automatic-type responses to assess basic reception of speech information.

If any type of word repetition is problematic for the client, the audiologist will likely want to try to use picture-pointing tasks. However, the success of these will depend on the client's overall auditory comprehension. Also, audiologists should be mindful that the client may also have some gross motor difficulties that make picture pointing problematic.

Another distinction that could be relevant is whether the stroke was on the left or right side. Because language is processed primarily in the left hemisphere, individuals who suffer left-sided strokes generally have greater language impairment than those who suffer right-sided strokes. Consistent with the anatomy discussed previously, patients with right-sided strokes are more likely to have greater visual-spatial deficits, which could interfere with picture-pointing tasks.

The emotional state of the client is clearly important to this discussion. If the client is experiencing depression, she may not be motivated to participate in the audiological assessment. If the client is agitated, the audiologist may want to request that someone who knows her and has earned her trust accompany her and assist throughout the evaluation.

Traumatic Brain Injury

Traumatic brain injury (TBI) may be defined as a traumatic insult to the brain that can result in impairment in the physical, intellectual, emotional, social, or vocational functioning of an individual (Brain Injury Association of America, 2007). TBI is the leading cause of death and disability among children and young adults in industrialized nations (Annegers, 1983). Unlike strokes, which are much more common in the elderly, TBI is much more common in adult or young adult males, especially those with a history of risk taking.

Audiologists who have some experience with TBI will acknowledge that this is a very heterogeneous group of clients. For example, compare the following cases. A high school football player suffers a brain trauma but does not lose consciousness (or loses it for a very short period of time) and experiences only temporary symptoms of difficulty concentrating and memory problems. The second individual is involved in a car accident and sustains a head injury, which results in a period in which he is completely unresponsive to external stimuli (e.g., a comatose state). Eventually he becomes conscious but experiences lifelong disruption of his speech and language abilities, some loss of motor function, and changes in personality, all of which leave him dependent on others in order to carry out activities of daily living. It is this second individual who will pose unique challenges to the audiologist who is asked to carry out reliable assessment of hearing.

Because TBI can result in language impairment, **dysarthria,** and apraxia, much of the information noted in Table 9.6 regarding stroke should also apply to this discussion of TBI. There are, however, some important differences between the two disorders that require audiologists to seek out some different types of information.

Regarding language, there is agreement among experts that individuals who have sustained serious trauma to the brain often exhibit language that does not make sense in the given situation or relative to the topic at hand. In addition, auditory comprehension deficits are common, which interfere with the client's ability to understand verbal directions about how to respond during the hearing assessment. Refer to Table 9.6 for strategies to assist with this.

Audiologists may also benefit from knowing whether the damage to the brain affected a limited, specific area (referred to as *focal damage*) or whether the damage was broader in nature (referred to as *diffuse damage*). Strokes, in general, cause focal damage, but TBI may cause focal or diffuse damage. The person whose TBI was the result of a sharp object penetrating the skull will likely suffer primarily focal damage. On the other hand, the person whose TBI was the result of a car accident will likely suffer diffuse damage. As the car accident occurs and the frontal lobe makes impact with some hard surface (e.g., the dashboard, the steering wheel), specific damage occurs. In addition, however, the subsequent continuing movement of the person's body in different directions results in the brain's continuing contact with the skull, which leads to multiple sites of injury. In cases such as these, where there is diffuse damage, the challenges to those working with the client will be greater.

Cognitive changes are very common following serious TBI. Two of the most frequently reported of these are reductions in attention and memory. Some clients who are in the initial stages of recovery are only able to sustain attention for seconds at a time. It should be noted that hearing assessment requires that the individual be able to sustain attention on the same task (e.g., pure-tone play audiometry) for extended periods of time. Also, some memory deficits are so severe that the client may not be able to remember a word that has just been presented. Investigating the status of the client's attention and **short-term memory** before the evaluation will help the audiologist plan an approach to the audiological evaluation for maximum efficiency.

Finally, it should be pointed out that many clinicians working with individuals who have experienced TBI use various scales to assist in identifying the person's level of cognitive functioning. A review of these scales leads logically to a series of specific questions that the audiologist might consider prior to assessment. This information will be helpful in determining what will likely be the best initial approach for assessment. Questions for consideration include the following six:

1. Is the patient responsive to external stimuli? If yes, are those responses consistent?
2. Does the patient respond differently to different stimuli?
3. Can the client respond to simple commands. If yes, are those responses consistent?
4. Is the client agitated? If yes, are appropriate support personnel available to assist with the evaluation?
5. For approximately how long can the client sustain his or her attention to a task? Does distractibility interfere with task performance?
6. Will memory difficulties interfere with the client's ability to repeat back words and remember the directions for the tasks at hand?

Answers to these questions, combined with information about the previously discussed issues related to TBI, can then be viewed in conjunction with the continuum of audiological tests already discussed. The audiologist can then make a reasonable plan for effective and efficient assessment of the individual with TBI.

Individuals with Nonorganic Hearing Loss

Definition of Terms

When an audiologist identifies hearing loss during an audiometric examination, there is typically some underlying physical basis for it. For example, as we have discussed, if conductive hearing loss is identified, this can be traced to some disorder of the outer and/or middle ear. If sensorineural hearing loss is noted, some problem likely exists in the cochlea or eighth cranial nerve.

Nonorganic hearing loss refers to reported hearing loss (based on the responses given by the patient) that does not have any underlying organic basis. Other terms that are often used to mean the same thing include **pseudohypacusis** and **functional hearing loss.** You may be wondering how this type of hearing loss could arise. One example of a nonorganic hearing loss is the patient who, for some unknown psychological or emotional reasons, does not respond at normal threshold levels, even though the auditory system is intact. Sometimes the term **psychogenic hearing loss** is used in such cases. This term should be used cautiously, because audiologists are not trained to make psychological diagnoses. A related but different term is **malingering,** which refers to a deliberate falsification of results. Note here that of the terms mentioned so far, malingering carries with it judgment about the client's actions and implies that the client is intentionally falsifying his or her responses.

Motivation for Pseudohypacusis

Students are typically curious when discussing the fact that some people would intentionally give false results during a hearing test. One of the first questions they ask about this is "Why would someone do this?" The answer varies with, among other factors, the age of the person. Pseudohypacusis in children is often related to a need for gaining attention, usually from a parent or parents. Also, children who are having difficulty in school sometimes see exaggerating a hearing loss as a way to receive more support.

Pseudohypacusis in adults can be due to the potential for financial gain. For example, some industrial companies pay employees a lump-sum monetary award based on the degree of hearing loss they have. The greater the hearing loss, the larger is the compensation check. This policy is designed to compensate individuals who have suffered work-related hearing loss, but it is not difficult to see how this could actually motivate people to be dishonest.

Audiological Evaluation

The audiological evaluation in cases when pseudohypacusis may occur begins the same way other evaluations would begin—with the case history. One of the first things the audiologist should note in adults is whether the case involves some sort of compensation. By noting this, the audiologist is not prejudging the client, but will use this information as a reminder to carefully monitor all test findings to be sure that they are internally consistent. This should be done during every audiological evaluation, but it becomes even more important in cases when motivation to exaggerate or feign hearing loss may exist. During the case history, the audiologist talks with the adult client in a conversational manner.

Although the audiological testing has not yet begun, the audiologist is already getting some impression of the client's ability to understand conversational speech. Adults with potential nonorganic or functional hearing loss during the test situation often respond to conversational questions posed during the case history interview with ease. On the other hand, some adults with nonorganic hearing loss may show exaggerated listening behaviors during the case interview, such as asking for frequent repetition or cupping their hand behind their ear. For those individuals who respond without difficulty during the case history, it is not uncommon for their behavior to change and their responsiveness worsen once they enter the sound-treated booth. This may be due to the fact that, once in the booth, the client becomes aware that she is being tested and is cued to present herself as someone who does not hear well. This contrast between auditory behavior during the interview and in the booth can be an indication of potential pseudohypacusis.

Summarized in Table 9.7 are the patterns observed during behavioral hearing assessment and admittance testing for a client with unilateral nonorganic hearing loss. Although there is no one audiometric configuration associated with nonorganic hearing loss, this unilateral case is presented as a way to illustrate several important principles. Referring to the audiogram in Figure 9.4, note that the right ear is within normal limits at all frequencies, but the left ear appears to have a severe hearing loss. One internal test inconsistency that signals potential nonorganic hearing loss is the lack of crossover by air conduction. Remember from our discussion in Chapter 4 that once the signal in the poor ear exceeds the bone conduction threshold in the good ear by approximately 40 dB, part of the signal directed to the poor ear will be picked up by the good ear. In other words, in cases of a unilateral severe hearing loss the unmasked thresholds in the poor ear initially appear at levels less than severe because of the influence of the better ear, resulting in a "shadow curve." It is through masking that the audiologist effectively removes the good ear from the test and then notes the drop in thresholds in the poor ear. In cases of unilateral pseudohypacusis, the reported thresholds in the poor ear are often severe or even profound even though the good ear is unmasked. This pattern can occur only if sound did not cross over to the opposite ear.

Referring again to Figure 9.4, note also the lack of agreement in the left ear between the speech recognition threshold (SRT) and the three-frequency pure tone average. The SRT of 50 dB is more than 30 dB greater than the left pure tone average of 83 dB. Recall from our previous discussion of speech audiometry that consistency between the pure tone average and SRT is achieved when the two measures are within 10 dB of each other. Typically, when agreement is not achieved, the SRT is better than the pure tone threshold.

Do we believe that the SRT of 50 dB in Figure 9.4 in the left ear is reliable? In order to assess this, the audiologist may choose to assess the client's speech recognition ability at 50 dB. Recall that in the typical test situation, the audiologist adds 35–40 dB to the SRT, or in some cases uses the person's most comfortable level (MCL), in order to establish a presentation level for testing speech recognition that is well above threshold. This is necessary because speech recognition is a suprathreshold task. Referring back to Figure 9.4, how should you interpret the client's excellent word recognition ability at 50 dB (i.e., her supposed threshold)? We said that speech recognition is a suprathreshold task and we note that this client has excellent speech recognition ability at a given level of 50 dB. Is it likely that this level of 50 dB is truly her threshold? No. If the patient is able to understand one-syllable words with excellent accuracy at 50 dB, then 50 dB is likely to represent a suprathreshold level for this individual rather than a threshold level.

TABLE 9.7 Patterns Observed in Assessment of Unilateral Nonorganic Hearing Loss

Test Feature	Pattern Noted	Comment
Case history	Client may perform well during case history interview and then demonstrate exaggerated difficulties understanding in the sound booth.	The client often does not think about the the fact that during the case history, audiologist is obtaining some general information regarding ability to hear.
Configuration of the loss	No one pattern is associated with nonorganic hearing loss. When the loss is unilateral and severe, crossover is not seen (even though the good ear is unmasked).	Once the tone in the bad ear exceeds the bone conduction level in the good ear by about 40 dB, crossover is likely.
SRT/pure tone relationship	The SRT and pure tone average should be within 10 dB of each other. Often, the SRT will be considerably better than the pure tone average.	When assessing the SRT, use an ascending approach. This is likely to provide results that are closer to threshold.
Word recognition ability	Sometimes assessing word recognition ability at a threshold level (and finding that it is good to excellent) is effective in establishing nonorganic hearing loss.	Remember that word recognition is a suprathreshold task. A client who does well at his or her reported threshold level raises concern that the reported threshold is not his or her true threshold.
Acoustic reflex/pure tone relationship	Once a cochlear hearing loss exceeds 80 dB, the likelihood of observing acoustic reflexes decreases dramatically. Present reflexes are often noted with severe or even profound hearing loss in cases of nonorganic hearing loss.	Students should review carefully information regarding hearing loss and acoustic reflexes in order to understand this pattern.
Stenger Screening	A positive result occurs when the client fails to respond to a tone in the bad ear, even though there also is a tone in the good ear at an intensity level that is above the admitted threshold. Failure to respond supports nonorganic hearing loss.	This screening test should be done routinely in all cases of unilateral hearing loss.

You may be wondering at this point why a person with a functional hearing loss would repeat monosyllabic words correctly if she is attempting to feign a hearing loss. The answer to this question probably lies in the client's perception of the loudness of the stimuli being presented. Because 50 dB is not a soft level, and because it is difficult for clients to equate the loudness of speech stimuli with the loudness of tonal stimuli, clients with nonorganic hearing loss sometimes respond to speech at suprathreshold levels even though admitted pure tone responses are much worse than that. In other cases, clients are observed to make atypical errors during speech audiometry.

FIGURE 9.4 **Pattern of audiometric results for a client with pseudohypacusis.**

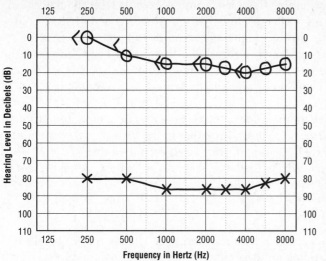

Speech Audiometry

Ear	SRT	SDT	PTA 5 - 2	Test	Word Recognition Level/Percent Correct	MCL	LDL
Right	10		13	NU6	45 / 100%		
Left	50		83	NU6	50/92%		
Bone							
Sound Field							
Right Aided							
Left Aided							
Binaural Aided							

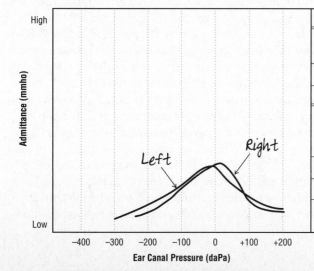

Tympanometry

	Right	Left
Middle Ear Pressure	0	– 20
Admittance	WNL	WNL

Reflexes

	Right	Left
	Ipsilat.	Ipsilat.
500 Hz	85	85
1,000 Hz	85	90
2,000 Hz	90	90

Related to this point about the client's perception of the loudness of the stimuli, most audiologists have learned that when presenting pure tones and speech to a client with a potential nonorganic hearing loss, it is advisable to use an ascending technique. In other words, rather than beginning the test at a suprathreshold level and descending to find threshold, it is often more effective to begin at a faint level and increase gradually until the client responds. This technique will certainly not guarantee that the response obtained will be the client's true threshold, but it will deny the client the opportunity to hear what louder stimuli sound like. It will limit the information she has about the scale of intensity being used, which may promote her responding closer to threshold.

During admittance testing the audiologist tests overall middle ear function through use of tympanometry and acoustic reflexes. Note that in the left ear of the case under discussion, acoustic reflexes are present at normal levels even though a loss of 80 dB is being reported. As you have already learned, the likelihood of reflexes being present in an ear with hearing levels of 80 dB is negligible.

Additional Audiometric Tests

The reader should note that thus far it is by examining the consistency of results obtained in the conventional audiological battery that an audiologist establishes that a potential nonorganic hearing loss exists. The next step is for the audiologist to obtain reliable estimates of the person's true thresholds. One way to do this is to explain to the client that the information that she has provided thus far is not consistent and that perhaps she did not completely understand the instructions. This gives the client an opportunity to respond reliably during the second test. With children, sometimes the parents can be told of these inconsistencies and can be asked to talk with their child in order to reinforce the importance of accurate responses.

If these efforts are not successful, an audiologist can use some additional, more specific tests. First, the Stenger is a test that can be helpful. The **Stenger test** is based on the principle that if two tones of the same frequency are presented to the two ears simultaneously, only the louder one will be perceived. It can be used as a screening in cases when unilateral nonorganic hearing loss is suspected. To apply the **Stenger principle,** consider once again the audiogram in Figure 9.4. A client has an admitted threshold of 5 dB HL at 1,000 Hz in the right ear, and of 100 dB HL in the left ear. The audiologist simultaneously introduces a 1,000-Hz tone to the right ear at 15 dB HL and to the left ear at 90 dB HL, with the instruction to the client: "Say yes when you hear a tone." What response would you expect from the client? If the original results are true, the client will say yes because she hears the tone presented to the right ear (a negative Stenger). If the original results are not true, the client hears only the louder tone in the left ear and does not respond because he does not want to admit hearing in the left ear (a positive Stenger). The Stenger screening should be applied routinely in cases of unilateral hearing loss.

Although the Stenger screening can be useful in indicating the presence of pseudohypacusis, it does not provide information about the client's true thresholds. This type of information may be obtained by obtaining Minimum Contralateral Interference Levels (MCIL). Also based on the Stenger principle, these levels can be obtained in the following manner:

1. Present a tone to the good ear at 10 dB above the true threshold (i.e., 10 dB SL). Because the tone is only in the good ear, the patient should respond.
2. Simultaneously present a tone to the bad ear at 0 dB HL and present the 10 dB SL tone to the good ear.
3. If the client responds, the level of the tone in the bad ear is raised in 5 dB steps until the client stops responding. The tone in the good ear remains unchanged.

The lowest level at which the client responds to the tone in the bad ear is the MCIL. This level is likely to be within (no greater than) 20 dB of the client's threshold. Remember, obtaining minimum contralateral interference levels is based on the Stenger principle: The client stops responding when the tone in the bad ear is heard loudly enough that he is no longer aware of the tone in the good ear.

Also, as discussed in Chapter 6, both **otoacoustic emissions (OAEs)** and **auditory brainstem testing (ABR)** can be used to estimate hearing thresholds. OAE specifically assesses the response of cochlear hair cells to auditory stimulation. ABR, using latency–intensity protocols combined with frequency-specific tone bursts, can also be effective in determining accurate hearing thresholds.

Assessment and Management

At this point we can summarize some guiding principles for assessment of all individuals, including individuals who may present with pseudohypacusis. We also can include some ideas that might add to the effectiveness of the assessment.

First, observe all possible inconsistencies during the audiological session. These include: (1) behavioral inconsistencies between the case history interview and the actual test situation, (2) the presence of a unilateral hearing loss that appears without crossover to the better ear, (3) an SRT that is not within 10 dB of the pure tone average, (4) speech recognition that is good to excellent when testing at the admitted threshold, and (5) acoustic reflexes that are present in an ear with thresholds that are in the severe or greater range.

As noted, reinstruction should be used in order to notify the client that you are aware of the inconsistent test results, as well as to provide him with an opportunity to respond at threshold. Sometimes it is advisable to reschedule the client and begin fresh on another day. When these efforts are not successful, tests such as ABR and OAEs can be used to obtain threshold data.

Regardless of whether threshold data are obtained, it is important that the person's inconsistent response pattern be reported. For example, on more than one occasion we have seen children who feign hearing loss on a hearing test who also have a history of reporting various other medical symptoms that cannot be verified with testing. These children may be attempting to gain needed attention and may be undergoing unnecessary medical testing in this effort. By alerting the parents and the pediatrician to the noted pattern of behavior, the audiologist is potentially expediting the process of understanding the underlying issues. The audiologist is not judging the child, but is helping others to understand the child better, which leads to providing the child with whatever help he may need. In all cases, the results should be reported in an objective and factual manner, pointing out the internal discrepancies that do not allow a firm conclusion about the individual's hearing status to be drawn. Also, at all times these clients, like all clients, should be treated with kindness and respect.

Patient Counseling and Report Writing

One of the more challenging but important aspects of dealing with pseudohypacusis involves transmitting the results to the client and, in cases involving children, to the client and their parent(s). Even though this can be difficult, audiologists should not avoid the responsibility that they have to communicate what they have observed in as objective a manner as possible. For example, if after attempting to achieve consistency through re-instruction and encouragement by the audiologist, an adult client presents pure tone data that are not in agreement with speech measures (e.g., pure tone average is not within 10 dB of the SRT) or data that are not consistent with acoustic reflex findings (reflexes are present in an ear with a severe hearing loss), the audiologist should communicate to the client that the data are not internally consistent and that meaningful interpretation of these results will not be possible. It is also important to state clearly in the written report that internal consistency was not achieved and that reevaluation or additional testing (e.g., otoacoustic emissions, ABR) is necessary. Remember that the focus of this discussion with the client is on the data obtained, not on the client's behavior or on any personal feelings the audiologist may have about the client's performance on the tests.

Communication of this information can be more challenging when the client is a child because parents sometimes interpret the report of lack of consistency as a negative judgment of their child. This obviously can interfere with the rapport between the parents and the audiologist. In other cases, parents may react with anger directed toward the child. In either case, it is important for the audiologist to attempt to maintain positive interactions, while simultaneously communicating directly about the data. It is often helpful for the audiologist to recommend additional tests that can be administered to answer the questions at hand regarding hearing sensitivity.

Multicultural Issues

Ethnicity

An **ethnic group** is a group of individuals who share common bonds based on such things as the country from which their ancestors came, their race, their religious practices, the language that they speak, their social customs, and their behavior patterns (Gollnick & Chinn, 1994). A review of Census Bureau statistics reveals that the number of U.S. citizens who are part of ethnic (minority) groups has increased from 9 million in 1900 to 87 million today (U.S. Census Bureau). The increasing diversity of the U.S. population has already had wide-ranging ramifications on many aspects of society, including our economy, our politics, and our worldview.

Our work as providers of health and educational services is also influenced by the diversity of our clients. Speech–language pathologists have had to address issues of diversity in dealing with the features and characteristics of nonstandard forms of English and in understanding that these language differences do not represent language deficits. In addition, administration of bilingual speech and language evaluations has become more and more common over the past decade.

Audiologists too have become more sensitive to issues of diversity in conducting assessments. In fact, ASHA (2005) notes that ethical standards of the association require that audiologists consider their own possible cultural biases in order to avoid allowing these biases to interfere with interactions with clients from other cultures. Audiologists also must be open to collaborating with and making referrals to other professionals when this is necessary. Arranging for a translator (either formally or informally by using a family member) when necessary so that all test instructions and recommendations are clearly understood should be routine clinical practice. Recorded speech audiometry test materials are available in Spanish and in other languages and should be used when appropriate.

Audiologists should also be aware of relevant research on this topic. For example, Ramkissoon and colleagues (2002) found that digit pairs more effectively assessed speech thresholds of nonnative speakers of English compared to traditionally used CID words. Also, Nelson (2005) and colleagues found that noise and reverberation had a greater negative effect on native Spanish-speaking children who were learning English as a second language compared to a group of their English-only-speaking peers.

Although progress is being made in our efforts to meet the needs of all of our clients, audiology services that are both scientific and humanistic require that our knowledge about people from various ethnic groups extend beyond language barriers and include less obvious barriers such as those created by differences in verbal and nonverbal communication style, concepts of time, and attitudes toward health (Wyatt, 2002).

Table 9.8 summarizes potential cross-cultural differences to consider when working with minority families. Think about the issues raised in this table in the context of an audiologist who is working with a minority family. The audiologist has just identified a hearing loss in the 6-year-old child. As the audiologist presents information to the parents, they sit silently and for the most part avoid eye contact. When the audiologist asks questions to assess their understanding of the information, they respond in a manner that the audiologist has difficulty interpreting. Although the audiologist expresses a desire to outline some options for intervention, the family does not appear motivated to operate on a time line.

This scenario should illustrate the importance of gaining increased understanding of how people of different cultures assimilate information. If the audiologist made use of some of the concepts outlined in Table 9.8, she may have modified her delivery to accommodate the needs of the family and may have been less perplexed by their reaction in the clinical setting.

Social Class

In addition to ethnicity, social class plays an important role in human behavior. Social class may be determined by factors including annual income, occupation, and years of education. These three factors are commonly used by the federal government to determine socioeconomic status (SES). Although members of any group of people may have a reduced SES, significantly more African American, Hispanic American, and Native American families find themselves classified in this way.

As summarized by Biehler and Snowman (1997), this means that more members of these three minority groups experience poorer health and less adequate health care and are more likely to have a single head of household. In addition, children in these cultures are less likely to be motivated to do well in school and are more likely to suffer reduced self-esteem. These same children may suffer from learned helplessness as a result of the repeated failures that they have experienced (Seligman, 1975). This information has significant implications for counseling and management of hearing loss in traditionally underserved populations.

TABLE 9.8   Potential Cross-Cultural Differences to Consider When Working with Minority Families

Potential Source of Difference	Majority Perspective	Minority Perspective
Verbal communication/ discourse	A verbal approach is generally viewed more positively.	Silence may be valued (e.g., Navajo culture); in some cultures children are taught to speak when spoken to and to provide minimum information.
	A certain degree of pause time is expected between conversational turns; interrupting is generally not viewed positively.	Less pause time is appropriate in certain cultures; multiple speakers may speak simultaneously and interruptions are acceptable as long as they add to the relevant discussion (e.g., African American culture).
	Direct communication is highly regarded; an indirect communication style is often viewed as evasive.	An indirect style of communication is preferred in some cultures (e.g., Asian Americans). Direct communication may be viewed as rude.
	During discussions, periods of active listening are employed.	In African American cultures, for example, discussions require active verbal participation; lack of such participation may be viewed as deliberate attempt to conceal information.
	In discussions, the emphasis should be on objective "truths"; a "rational" approach is valued.	In African American cultures, for example, effective arguments include emotional appeals that include personal beliefs.
Nonverbal communication	Eye contact is viewed positively; lack of eye contact often suggests a "pragmatic" language problem; may be viewed as indicator of nonattention, disrespect.	In some cultures (e.g., African American, Asian American, Latino), diverted eye gaze is a way of expressing attention and respect.
Concept of time	Efficiency is praised and rewarded.	Some cultures are less bound by time (e.g., Hispanic Americans, Native Americans) and may value deliberation more than expediency.
Attitude toward health, health care, and the medical establishment	Communication disorders are typically viewed as responsive to intervention; parents seek out competent professionals for guidance.	Forms of illness or disability may be viewed as a blessing from God, a punishment for previous sins, or may be ignored completely. Recommendations made by professionals may be viewed with skepticism, and the potential effectiveness of intervention may be doubted.

Source: Wyatt (2002).

CHAPTER SUMMARY

This chapter has provided detailed information about different populations that are encountered in clinical audiology practice. Students of audiology and speech–language pathology are urged to take responsibility for knowing general information about the various types of clients they may encounter and to use this information to ask specific questions about the client that can guide the assessment and often the rehabilitation as well. It is the audiologist's positive and productive collaborations with the speech–language pathologist, others who know the client well, and of course, the client, that make audiological assessment and rehabilitation most effective.

A humanistic approach to audiology views clients, regardless of their medical, psychiatric, or educational labels, as individual persons who should be treated as unique. Students of audiology should avoid relying solely on general knowledge about populations, which can lead to stereotyped expectations that may not necessarily apply to the particular client at hand. Rather, they should become knowledgeable about the types of disabilities that will be encountered in an audiology practice in order to develop a series of relevant questions that will guide assessment. In addition to the theme of collaboration, we have also stressed the need for the audiologist to make every attempt to gain as much information as possible during the audiological evaluation. Toward this goal, we have provided some specific suggestions that we believe will be effective in reducing obstacles that result from various disabilities. These suggestions, combined with the continuum of audiological tests discussed, should be valuable resources for the audiologist. Although this chapter addresses comprehensive assessment performed by the audiologist, this information, combined with information in Chapter 11 regarding screenings, should be most useful to speech–language pathologists who screen individuals with various disabilities. Finally, this chapter included a review of multicultural issues, which apply to both new and experienced audiologists, and raised awareness of the potential influence of cultural bias on assessment and intervention.

QUESTIONS FOR DISCUSSION

1. Considering what you have learned about neurogenic disorders, think about the gentleman described earlier in the chapter who has suffered a stroke. Write down what you know about his condition and what indicators you used to determine this.
2. For the same client, list specific strategies you would use to assess his hearing.
3. Why do you believe that these strategies will be successful?
4. Compare and contrast your role as a clinician for clients with a cultural view of deafness versus clients who view deafness as a disability.
5. What are the audiological and nonaudiological factors that cue the clinician to the possibility of nonorganic hearing loss?
6. Discuss how knowledge of multicultural issues facilitates a humanistic approach to providing audiological care.

RECOMMENDED READING

Council for Exceptional Children. www.cec
.sped.org/index.html

Hardman, M., Drew, C., & Egan, M. (2002).
*Human exceptionality: Society, school, and
family.* 7th ed. Boston: Allyn & Bacon.

Paul, P. (2000). *Language and deafness.* Clifton
Park, NY: Delmar Thomson Learning.

Weinstein, B. (2000). *Geriatric audiology.* New
York: Thieme.

Worall, L., & Frattali, C. (2000). *Neurogenic communication disorders: A functional approach.*
New York: Thieme.

REFERENCES

American Speech-Language-Hearing Association (ASHA). (1997, Spring). Guidelines for
audiology service delivery in nursing homes.
ASHA, 39(Suppl. 17), 15–29.

American Speech-Language-Hearing Association (ASHA). (2005). Cultural competence.
ASHA supplement, 25, in press.

Annegars, J. F. (1983). The epidemiology of
head trauma in children. In K. Shapiro (Ed.),
Pediatric head trauma (pp. 1–10). Mt. Kisco,
NY: Futura.

Biehler, R., & Snowman, J. (1997). *Psychology
applied to teaching* (8th ed.), New York:
Houghton Mifflin.

Brain Injury Association of America. (2007).
www.biausa.org. Accessed April 2007.

Centers for Disease Control. (2001). *Traumatic
brain injury in the United States: A report to
Congress.* Available at: www.cdc.gov/ncipc/
pub-res/tbicongress.htm

Chessman, M. (1997). Speech perception by
elderly listeners: Basic knowledge and implications for audiology. *Journal of Speech-
Language Pathology and Audiology, 21,*
104–110.

Developmental Disabilities Assistance and Bill of
Rights Act of 1990. Title 42, U.S.C. 6000-6083.
U.S. Statutes at Large, 104, 1191–1204.

Gollnick, D., & Chinn, P. (1994). *Multicultural
education in a pluralistic society* (4th ed.).
New York: Merrill.

Gordon-Salant, S. (1986). Effects of aging on response criteria in speech recognition tasks.
Journal of Speech and Hearing Research, 29,
155–162.

Jerger, J., Chmiel, R., Wilson, N., & Luchi, R.
(1996). Hearing impairment in older adults:
New concepts. *Journal of the American Geri-
atrics Society, 43,* 928–935.

McCarthy, P., & Vesper, S. (2000). Rehabilitative
needs of the aging population. In J. Alpiner &
P. McCarthy (Eds.), *Rehabilitative audiology
in children and adults* (3rd ed., pp. 402–434).
New York: Lippincott, Williams & Wilkins.

Nelson, P., Kohnert, K., Sabur, S., & Shaw, D.
(2005). Classroom noise and children learning through a second language: Double jeop-
ardy? *Language, Speech, and Hearing Services
in Schools, 36*(3), 219–229.

Rawool, V. (2000, October). Addressing the special needs of older adult clients. *The Hearing
Review, 7,* 38–43.

Rees, J., & Botwinick, J. (1971). Detection and
decision factors in auditory behavior of
the elderly. *Journal of Gerontology, 26*(2),
133–136.

Seligman, M. (1975). *Helplessness: On depression, development, and death.* San Francisco:
Freeman.

Smith, M. (1989). Neurophysiology of aging.
Seminars in Neurology, 9, 64–77.

U.S. Census Bureau. *U.S. Census 2000.* From
www.census.gov. Accessed April 2007.

Wyatt, T. (2002). Assesing the communicative
language backgrounds. In D. Battle (Ed.),
*Communication disorders in multicultural
populations* (3rd ed.). Boston: Butterworth-
Heinemann.

Young, C., Colmer, S., & Holloway, A. (1978). *A
hearing conservation plan for individuals
with developmental disabilities: A proposed
model.* Poster session at the Illinois Speech
and Hearing Association Convention,
Chicago.

373
•
Appendix B:
Communication
Strategies for
Use with
Individuals with
Developmental
Disabilities

Appendix A
Considerations for Hearing Assessment and Case Management of Individuals Who Have Developmental Disabilities*

• Because the incidence of hearing loss is greater in individuals who have other developmental/medical issues, individuals with developmental disabilities should be monitored closely for hearing loss, either through screenings or diagnostic evaluations.

• Depending on the data that can be obtained regarding the client's hearing ability, screenings may be sufficient to address the presenting question(s) regarding the client's hearing status. In some cases, screenings carried out by the speech–language pathologist will not yield sufficient data. These individuals should be seen by the audiologist for diagnostic assessment.

• Diagnostic assessment should employ whatever means necessary to answer the presenting question(s) regarding the client's hearing status. This includes both behavioral and more objective measures. Decisions regarding the most appropriate protocol for testing an individual client should be made based on the client's unique set of personal traits and abilities. Collaboration with staff and support personnel is crucial.

• In order to monitor both hearing and middle ear function, use of tympanometry is recommended, particularly in children with developmental disabilities and in those individuals with developmental disabilities who are at risk for conductive hearing loss due to middle ear pathology (e.g., cleft palate, Down syndrome, craniofacial anomalies).

• Unless more frequent screening is required under law or regulations, or mandated by the presence of a medical condition, formal monitoring should be done yearly or every other year. Ongoing informal monitoring (for changes in behavior or functional communication ability) should be done based on training provided to staff and support personnel by the speech–language pathologist and/or audiologist.

*Updated and adapted from Young and colleagues (1978).

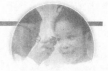

Appendix B
Communication Strategies for Use with Individuals with Developmental Disabilities

• Gain eye contact before communicating with the client.
• Speak in an articulate manner at a conversational intensity level, or slightly above.
• Avoid shouting, since this will distort the auditory signal.
• Combine the use of gestures and body language with spoken language.
• Move away from or reduce background noise when feasible.

- Use vocabulary that is familiar to the client and an appropriate sentence length.
- Slow the rate of presentation.
- Become familiar with any augmentative alternative communication (AAC) devices that may be used by the client.
- If you are misunderstood, rephrase rather than repeating the original message.

chapter 10

(Central) Auditory Processing Disorders

AFTER COMPLETING THIS CHAPTER, YOU SHOULD BE ABLE TO:

1. Describe the historical development of tests of central auditory processing.
2. Summarize criticism of use of tests of auditory processing for assessment of learning difficulties.
3. Describe the role of the speech–language pathologist in making appropriate referrals for central auditory processing testing.
4. List candidacy requirements for tests of auditory processing.
5. Describe four broad categories of auditory processing tests and their purposes.
6. Make appropriate intervention recommendations based on specific test results.

(Central) Auditory Processing Disorders in School-Age Children

As noted in Chapter 3 of the text, the auditory system is composed not only of the outer, middle, and inner ear—**peripheral auditory system**—but also includes a complicated neural system consisting of the brainstem and brain. This portion of the auditory system is referred to as the **central auditory system.** This system is responsible for directing and coding the auditory information from the cochlea to the higher brain centers.

In recent years, some audiologists have offered comprehensive testing of auditory processing targeted particularly at children who exhibit auditory-based difficulties in school. Although this testing has met with considerable controversy, ASHA (2004) includes it in the audiologist's scope of practice and also includes aspects of remediation in the scope of practice for the speech–language pathologist.

Some confusion does exist regarding the use of the terms *central auditory processing disorder* and *auditory processing disorder.* The Consensus Conference for the Diagnosis of Auditory Processing Disorders in School-Aged Children (Jerger & Musiek, 2000) objected to the term, *central auditory processing disorder (CAPD)* and suggested that it be replaced with *auditory processing disorder (APD).* ASHA (2005) recommended continued use of (central) auditory processing disorder, or (C)APD, but added that the two terms could be considered synonymous. In this chapter (C)APD is used.

Maturation and Plasticity of the Central Auditory System

It is important for the students of audiology and speech–language pathology to appreciate that at birth, the peripheral auditory system is quite developed, with even very young babies being able to discriminate fine differences between phonemes. The same is not true of the central auditory system. In fact, there are parts of the system that are still developing in young adults at 20 years of age. It should also be noted that development of the central auditory system proceeds from brainstem to cortical areas. In other words, the structures of the brainstem develop earlier than those parts of the auditory system that are part of the cerebral cortex. Think for a moment about the types of activities that a newborn is typically involved in: sleeping, crying, sucking, and having bowel movements. Remember that the newborn relies on brainstem functioning for all of these activities—in fact for their very survival—and therefore it is logical that this part of the central system would develop early.

Another important point regarding maturation of the central auditory system is that maturation of the system, in large part, involves **myelinization** of the system. *Myelin* is an insulating sheath that covers nerves and enhances the speed with which neuronal communication occurs. It makes up the white matter of the brain. The **corpus callosum** is the structure responsible for interhemispheric transfer of neural information and is largely composed of myelin.

Not only is the young central auditory system immature, it is also viewed as "plastic," referring to its ability to adapt to internal and external events. For example, in the unfortunate case of a young child who has had a stroke, recovery is noticeably more rapid and more pronounced (compared to the adult case) because of the central nervous system's ability to reorganize. This adaptability allows nondamaged areas to assume functions that would have been performed by the damaged areas. Auditory deprivation also illustrates the concept of plasticity: lack of auditory input causes abnormalities in the shape, size, and function of the structures of the central auditory system.

Nature and Development of Tests of (Central) Auditory Processing Disorder (CAPD)

Prior to the development of advanced imaging techniques, tests of auditory processing were used to determine the location of neurologic abnormalities (e.g., tumors) in the central auditory system of adults. These original tests date back to the 1950s and 1960s and almost exclusively involved speech stimuli, based on the assumption that in order to assess the integrity of higher (central) auditory centers simple tonal stimuli would not be sufficient. In addition, these speech stimuli were degraded in some way (e.g., filtering, competition, compression, etc.) in order to reduce the redundancy of the signal, thereby further enhancing the diagnostic effectiveness of the stimuli in identifying central lesions. Today, because of technology such as computerized axial tomography (CT) scans, magnetic resonance imaging (MRI) equipment, and positron emission tomography

(PET) scans, use of behavioral tests of auditory processing for site-of-lesion purposes is less common in audiology practice. However, these tests (and other more recent tests) are now being used by some audiologists to assess the functional auditory strengths and weaknesses of children who, despite normal hearing sensitivity, have difficulty with auditory-based tasks. The newer tests of auditory processing typically make minimal linguistic demands so that performance can be attributed to auditory-perceptual skill.

This more recent use of auditory processing tests to measure the functional auditory processing of children has met with considerable criticism. One problem with the reliability of tests of auditory processing is that factors such as age, ongoing changes in the central auditory system, and variable attention can affect test performance. Because of this, few current tests of auditory processing have adequate information regarding test–retest reliability.

The validity of tests of auditory processing is more established than reliability. One way to establish that a particular test of auditory processing is valid is to demonstrate that individuals with known auditory processing disorders perform poorly on the test. Musiek, Gollegly, and Baran (1984) reported that children with suspected auditory processing disorders demonstrated test results that were consistent with the patterns exhibited by children who had confirmed central auditory system lesions.

Another criticism of this testing is related to the inevitable difficulty that arises when we attempt to measure something as complex as auditory processing. The relative contributions of the peripheral auditory system, language, cognition, motivation, and attention to auditory processing are not fully understood, so questions arise as to whether the construct of auditory processing is a meaningful one. As noted by Jerger and Musiek (2000), one of the primary challenges that audiologists face in the assessment of auditory processing disorders is the fact that a number of childhood disorders exhibit similar behaviors and some of the current audiological tests do not effectively differentiate these disorders.

Cacace and MacFarland (1998) question the rationale for evaluating (C)APD in school-age children using only auditory tasks. They argue that it is more logical to employ tasks that tap auditory and other (e.g., visual) perceptual skills to prove or disprove the presence of a specific auditory processing disorder.

Despite these criticisms, ASHA recognizes the existence of (C)APD and includes assessment of the auditory processing system as part of the scope of practice of the audiologist (ASHA, 2004) and intervention as the responsibility of both the audiologist and speech–language pathologist (ASHA, 2001). ASHA (2005) also states that regardless of the exact nature of the processing deficit, most people who experience difficulty processing spoken language are likely to benefit from interventions designed to improve access to acoustic signals and to enhance language competence. ASHA adds that techniques which improve language competence will probably also improve the auditory processing of language, and techniques that improve auditory processing are likely to have a positive impact on language in general.

Definition

An ASHA (2005) technical report states that (C)APDs refer to difficulties in the perceptual processing of auditory information in the central nervous system as demonstrated by poor performance in one of more the following skill areas: (1) sound localization; (2) auditory discrimination; (3) auditory pattern recognition (ability to analyze acoustic events over time); (4) auditory performance in competing acoustic signals; and (5) auditory performance with degraded acoustic signals (e.g., signals in background noise, signals in which some frequencies have been removed).

Screening for (Central) Auditory Processing Disorders

It would be an inefficient use of both time and money to refer large numbers of children for comprehensive tests of auditory processing based simply on observed difficulty in the classroom. One of the reasons for this is that the symptoms of an auditory processing disorder frequently resemble symptoms of other disorders. For example, the child who demonstrates difficulty following oral directions and requires frequent repetition of information and prompting could have any of the following: a sensorineural hearing loss; a fluctuating conductive hearing loss related to otitis media with effusion; undiagnosed language deficits; an undiagnosed learning disability; undiagnosed cognitive deficits; a disorder of attention; or a lack of motivation. There are additional possible explanations for this child's difficulties, but the point here is that a referral for (C)APD testing should not be made until some method of screening has been employed to determine if the student is at risk for this disorder.

The report of the Consensus Conference on the Diagnosis of Auditory Processing Disorders in School-Aged Children (Jerger & Musiek, 2000) recommended the development of a screening procedure specifically for school-age children that could take the form of either a test, a questionnaire, or a combination of these two. The conference also suggested that screening by test should include dichotic digit and gap detection measures. Screening by questionnaire should assess evidence of difficulty in (1) hearing/understanding in background noise or reverberant settings, (2) understanding speech that is degraded, (3) following oral directions, and (4) identifying and discriminating speech sounds.

One commonly used questionnaire is the Children's Auditory Performance Scale (CHAPS), developed by Smoski, Brunt, and Tanahill (1998). This behavioral questionnaire assesses auditory function using a rating scale of +1 to −5. Teachers and parents are asked to rate the child on six listening conditions by comparing them to other children of similar age and background; a rating of +1 indicates less difficulty, whereas −5 indicates severe difficulty. The listening conditions are (1) noise, (2) quiet, (3) ideal, (4) multiple inputs, (5) auditory memory/sequencing, and (6) auditory attention span.

The SCAN test (Keith, 1986, 2000), which may be used as a diagnostic or screening tool, is commonly used by audiologists and contains subtests that assess understanding of low-pass filtered words, auditory figure-ground abilities, and understanding of competing words. It can be administered by audiologists or by nonaudiologists in a quiet room using a CD player. Because this tool has been criticized due to a lack of test–retest reliability (Amos & Humes, 1998) and reduced validity when used outside the test booth (Emerson et al., 1998) decisions to refer a child for further testing should not be based on SCAN findings alone.

Bellis (2003) believes that screening for (C)APD requires a collaborative, multidisciplinary team (e.g., audiologist, speech–language clinician, teacher, psychologist) who collect data in order to gain an understanding of a child's strengths and weaknesses and to develop an auditory profile. By assessing overall cognitive, language, and achievement abilities prior to any decision to administer a (C)APD test battery, the presence of more global difficulties that might explain the student's presenting problems might be discovered, making (C)AP tests unnecessary. Table 10.1 summarizes some of the types and sources of information that might be relevant in screening for (C)APD.

TABLE 10.1 Data Collection Sheet for Determining the Need for Comprehensive Assessment of CAP

Type of Information	Primary Source(s)	Common Pattern(s)
Auditory behavior	Fisher's Auditory Problems Checklist Children's Auditory Performance Scale (CHAPS) Questionnaire SIFTER Scale Observations of parents/teachers Selective Auditory Attention Test (SAAT) Screening Test for Auditory Processing Disorders (SCAN)	Says "what?" often Needs directions repeated Auditory distractibility Reduced performance in noise/groups Reduced performance on screening tools
Academic	Report card Individualized Education Plan (IEP) Achievement tests Observations of parents/teachers	Reduced ability in reading, spelling, writing Average to above average ability in math Better with "hands-on" learning Difficulty with note taking
Language	Speech–language report Teachers Parents Observations of parents/teachers	Decreased language skills, sometimes on basic language or sometimes only on higher-level language use
Cognitive/mode of learning	Psychoeducational report Observations of parents/teachers	Better performance than verbal IQ score More of a visual mode of learning
Medical	Physician's reports Audiologist's reports	History of otitis media

Important Role of the Speech–Language Pathologist in Screening

According to ASHA (2002a, 2002b), nearly 60 percent of certified speech–language pathologists are employed by schools and only 10 percent of audiologists are so employed. Because of this disparity in numbers between the two types of professionals, speech–language pathologists often take on a critical coordination role in the screening of children suspected of having auditory processing deficits. For example, it is often the speech–language pathologist who administers the SCAN, guides the classroom teacher in completing the relevant auditory questionnaire, and making careful observations about the child's auditory behaviors. The speech–language pathologist also coordinates a review of the child's academic profile for indications of difficulties in auditory-based areas such as reading, spelling, and understanding in adverse listening conditions.

In addition, the speech–language pathologist administers a number of important language tests that provide essential information regarding receptive and expressive oral language skills, higher-level cognitive-linguistic abilities, and auditory perceptual skills. Table 10.2 lists some of these tests. Note that in addition to tests which assess language, speech–language pathologists may also administer tests of auditory perceptual skills. Comparing a student's performance on tests that tap auditory perceptual abilities and those that tap language abilities can assist in determining if a referral for (C)AP testing is appropriate. For example, if the child in question performs poorly on all of the tests that tap auditory perceptual skills and performs age-appropriately on the tests that assess true language abilities, the breakdown is likely to be more in the auditory perceptual area and referral for (C)AP testing would appear appropriate. If however, as is

---

TABLE 10.2 Speech–Language and Auditory Perceptual Tests Commonly Used in Assessing Students at Risk for (C)APD

Speech and Language Tests
- Peabody Picture Vocabulary Test III
- Expressive Vocabulary Test
- Oral and Written Language Scales
- Language Sample/Narrative Analysis
- Woodcock Reading Mastery Test—Revised
- Test of Early Written Language—2
- Goldman-Fristoe Test of Articulation
- Illinois Test of Psycholinguistic Abilities—3
- Clinical Evaluation of Language Fundamentals (CELF)—3

Auditory Perceptual Tests
- Lindamood Auditory Conceptualization Test
- Test of Auditory Processing Skills Revised
- Language Processing Test
- Comprehensive Test of Phonological Processing
- The Listening Test
- The Auditory Processing Abilities Test

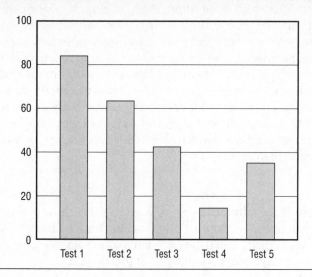

FIGURE 10.1 Comparison of performance on speech and language tests with either primary auditory or primary language loading.

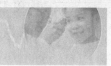

381
•

Peripheral
Audiological
Assessment and
Candidacy for
Testing

Test Performance for Jimmy on
five tests of auditory-language

Test 1: Auditory Load
Test 2: Auditory Load
Test 3: Language Load
Test 4: Language Load
Test 5: Language Load

illustrated in Figure 10.1, the child performs well on those auditory perceptual tasks and has difficulty on the linguistic tasks, a comprehensive assessment of language may be the most appropriate first step.

Peripheral Audiological Assessment and Candidacy for Testing

Once it has been determined that a comprehensive assessment of a child's auditory processing abilities is warranted, the child is scheduled to see an audiologist who will first assess peripheral hearing sensitivity. At a minimum, the audiologist will include pure tone air and bone conduction testing, speech recognition thresholds, word recognition testing, and immittance testing, including ipsilateral and contralateral acoustic reflexes and acoustic reflex decay.

Although some tests of auditory processing can be administered with hearing loss, many audiologists require that the child have normal hearing in order to be a candidate for auditory processing testing. Other commonly used candidacy requirements include: (1) minimum of 7 years of age, (2) near-normal to normal IQ, (3) no greater than a moderate language impairment, and (4) sufficient attentional abilities to perform the assessment tasks. The logic of these candidacy requirements is simple: diagnosis of auditory processing difficulties is complicated when other factors that might negatively impact the child's ability to perform the tasks are present.

(Central) Auditory Processing Assessment

Parents and members of allied professions often ask how the tests that are included in the auditory processing battery differ from those administered during the hearing test. The answer to this is two-fold. First, because tests of auditory processing involve information that is degraded in some way (e.g., different stimuli are presented to each ear simultaneously, background noise is added), they give us a better understanding of how the child performs in the classroom setting, where many of these same conditions exist. Second, simple auditory stimuli, such as tones presented to one ear at a time, or words presented without competition, may be effective for peripheral auditory assessment but are not very effective at assessing the integrity of the central auditory system. Auditory processing assessment requires use of signals that have less redundancy and greater involvement of **contralateral neural pathways.**

The Assessment Process

The first part of the assessment is the administration of a detailed case history form, which may be sent to the parents a few weeks prior to the evaluation. The parents are asked to provide information about their child that is relevant to the evaluation. A sample of one such form is provided in Appendix A at the end of this chapter.

Behavioral Tests of Auditory Processing and Implications for Remediation

Although efforts have been made (Jerger & Musiek, 2000) to identify a minimum test battery that would provide reliable and valid measures of auditory processing disorders, a lack of consensus currently exists in the literature regarding the specific tests that should constitute this battery. ASHA (2005) notes that there are currently four types of behavioral auditory processing tests that can be administered. These are described briefly below along with implications for children who have difficulty on them and possible intervention steps. This information is summarized in Table 10.3. There are also objective tests of the auditory system that may have potential for use in assessment of central auditory processing skills. These are described in Chapter 6 on electrophysiologic tests, and include the middle and late auditory evoked potentials and mismatch negativity.

Tests of Temporal Processes

The word *temporal* refers to time and these tests tap the listener's ability to correctly perceive the order or sequence of auditory stimuli. The stimuli often used are tones of varying frequency or of different durations. Individuals who have difficulty with these tests may miss the suprasegmental/prosody cues used in our language *(per*mit versus per*mit)* and may require speech–language services in the form of prosody training to remediate this. Whenever possible, the language stimuli used in such activities should be chosen in collaboration with the classroom teacher so that carryover to other settings will be enhanced.

Tests of Dichotic Listening

Dichotic tasks involve presentation of different information simultaneously to each ear. If a patient is asked to repeat back everything that is presented, the auditory process assessed is **binaural integration.** Many audiologists use the Staggered Spondaic Word (SSW) test to assess this. The patient is asked to repeat two compound words, which are

TABLE 10.3   Four Types of Behavioral Auditory Processing Tests

Type of Test	Site of Lesion Assessed	Auditory Process	Symptoms
Dichotic			
Dichotic digits	Brainstem, auditory cortex, corpus callosum	Binaural integration	Difficulty in group or noisy settings
SSW	Brainstem, cortex	Binaural integration	Difficulty in group or noisy settings
Competing sentences	Neuromaturation, language processing	Binaural separation	Selective attention deficits
Temporal			
Frequency patterns	Cerebral hemispheres, interhemispheric transfer	Frequency discrimination, temporal ordering, linguistic labeling, working memory	Difficulty recognizing and using prosodic features of speech
Duration patterns	Cerebral hemispheres, interhemispheric transfer	Duration discrimination, temporal ordering, linguistic labeling	Difficulty recognizing and using prosodic features of speech
Monaural low-redundancy			
Low-pass filtered	Brainstem, cortical	Auditory closure	Reduced ability to "fill in" missing auditory information
Time compressed	Primary auditory cortex	Auditory closure	Reduced ability to "fill in" missing auditory information
Speech in noise	Possibly low brainstem, cortical	Auditory closure	Reduced ability to "fill in" missing auditory information
Binaural interaction			
Alternating speech	Possibly low brainstem	Binaural interaction	Reduced ability to detect signals in noise
MLD	Brainstem	Binaural interaction	Reduced ability to detect signals in noise
Binaural fusion	Low brainstem	Binaural interaction	Reduced ability to detect signals in noise

Source: Assessment and Management of Central Auditory Processing Disorders in the Educational Setting, From Science to Practice, 2nd edition, by Bellis. 2003. Adapted with permission of Delmar Learning, a division of Thomson Learning: www.thomsonrights.com. Fax 800-730-2215.

presented in a partially overlapping manner to both ears. The manner of presentation results in four test conditions, so that there are left and right noncompeting conditions and left and right competing conditions, as follows:

UP STAIRS

DOWN TOWN

If "up" is presented to the right ear, "up" and "town" are the two noncompeting conditions, while "stairs" and "down" constitute the competing test conditions.

The Competing Sentences test is also dichotic, but in this case the patient is asked to repeat back only the information presented to one ear, while ignoring the information in the other ear. The auditory process assessed by the Competing Sentences test is **binaural separation.** As summarized in Table 10.3, difficulty on dichotic tests is often associated with difficulty understanding speech in group or noisy settings. Enhancing the signal-to-noise ratio is often helpful in these cases, as well as teaching the child more efficient attending skills and building up language skills.

There are a number of ways to enhance the signal-to-noise ratio of an environment. One way is first to evaluate the environment and then to carry out steps to cut down on the noise levels and reverberation. Classrooms with a number of soft (i.e., sound-absorbing) surfaces are typically less reverberant. Additional information regarding classroom modifications is found in Chapter 12.

The most effective way to enhance the signal-to-noise ratio is through the use of an **FM device.** Traditionally used with children who have hearing loss, several companies now make FM units for children who have normal hearing but who need an enhancement of the signal over the background noise. Such devices have been shown not only to improve attending abilities but also to enhance word identification skills and academic success. Please refer to Chapter 12 for details regarding the use of personal and sound field FM systems. A significant advantage of such devices is that because of the location of the microphone, which is worn just inches below the mouth of the speaker, the important speech information is enhanced but the various background noise common in classrooms is not. It is also important to remember that only FM devices made specifically for individuals who have normal hearing should be used with normal hearing children. Selecting, calibrating, and fitting FM devices for children with identified auditory disorders is the responsibility of a licensed audiologist.

Tests of Low Redundancy Monaural Speech

As the name implies, these tests involve speech information that is delivered to one ear and that has been altered in such a way that the signal being sent to the auditory system is less redundant than normal. Clients are instructed to repeat what they hear even though they may be uncertain of the word. As a result, word understanding is compromised. An example of a low-redundancy monaural speech test is the Speech-in-Noise test. The low redundancy is a result of masking of the primary signal by the noise. Once again, the client is required to repeat words, this time in the presence of noise.

Individuals who perform poorly on these tests may benefit from auditory closure activities to foster their access to incomplete auditory information. Such activities may include teaching the child to use context cues in attempting to figure out a missing word from a sentence. Because auditory closure skills are related to a person's vocabulary building up vocabulary and language in general is an important intervention step for children with deficits on low-redundancy tests. Use of FM technology may also be useful for students with deficits in this area.

Tests of Binaural Interaction

Like dichotic tests, these tests involve presentation of stimuli to each ear. The difference here is that for tests of binaural interaction the stimuli are presented in a sequential manner, rather than simultaneously. Another variation of these tests involves presentation of part of a total message to each ear, requiring the child to combine the two parts for understanding. As noted on Table 10.3, difficulties here (especially on the MLD) would warrant first ruling out neurological pathology. Because difficulties here are associated with decreased ability to detect information in noise, improving the signal-to-noise ratio is also recommended.

As you have most likely noted as you reviewed the information on Table 10.3 concerning intervention suggestions, current attempts to remediate auditory processing deficits address the specific auditory skills believed to be important to the processing of auditory/linguistic information, the higher-order processes involved in language understanding and effective use of comprehension strategies, and efforts to improve the listening environment. This combined approach is believed to be the one that has the greatest chance of being effective and, as noted previously, requires a collaborative effort among professionals, parents, and the child.

Buffalo and Bellis Models

Rather than interpreting results of (C)AP tests individually, some researchers, like Katz (1992) and Bellis (2006), recommend analyzing patterns of performance to determine what category of (C)APD emerges. The advantage of this approach is that the diagnosed deficits are tied to functional communication and learning difficulties that can then lead to specific types of intervention. These two classification approaches are summarized on Tables 10.4 and 10.5.

Final Remarks: (Central) Auditory Processing as a Useful Construct

If you were asked to go into a fourth-grade classroom and measure the degree of motivation of each of the students you would most likely find this task quite challenging. Why? Because motivation is not easily measured. A person's motivation can be related to a number of other phenomena and is something that we typically infer, rather than directly measure. Motivation, like auditory processing, is a construct that has been developed to help us to understand and explain human behavior. Even if there were no construct that we referred to as "motivation," teachers would still take note of the fact that some children are enthusiastic about their work and approach it with energy and a positive attitude; others do all that they can to avoid doing their work. By creating a construct, we are able to make our observations about human beings more concrete.

Perhaps the most famous of all constructs is the construct of "intelligence." This construct resulted from early researchers' and educators' observations that some children learned new information and could apply it to new situations with ease, whereas

TABLE 10.4   (C)APD Categories of the Buffalo Model

Category	Speech/Language and Academic Implications
Decoding (DEC)	Receptive language, particularly morphology Word-finding errors Prosody errors Oral and written discourse errors Articulation errors: /r/ & /l/ Slow responder Reading and spelling deficits Poor understanding of directions Weak on written tests Minimal oral discussions Difficulty with group listening
Tolerance-fading memory (TFM)	Expressive language weakness: cluttering Inconsistent articulation Receptive language weakness: Discourse errors: oral and written Poor attention span Distractible Reading comprehension weaknesses Weak short-term memory Poor direction following Poor handwriting Impulsivity Poor motor planning
Integration (INT)	Word-finding problems Receptive language errors involving morphology and syntax Expressive language errors: oral and written Extremely slow responder Poor phonetic skills Poor sound–symbol relationships Severs reading and spelling problems Very poor handwriting Difficulty with multimodal tasks
Organization (ORG)	Discourse errors: oral and written Sequencing Listener perspective Sequencing errors Disorganization

Source: Larry Medwetsky, in M. Gay Masters, N. A. Strecker, & J. Katz, "Memory and Attention Processing Deficits." *Central Auditory Processing Disorders.* Published by Allyn and Bacon, Boston, MA. Copyright © 1998 by Pearson Education. Reprinted by permission of the publisher.

others struggled to do so. The construct of intelligence has become so established in our society that many fail to think of it as a construct and think that it is something that we directly measure with intelligence tests. In fact, intelligence tests measure mostly verbal skills and, to some extent, visual-motor skills. Some experts believe that intelligence is far more multifaceted than this and includes skill in music and movement.

The important point here with respect to our discussion of (central) auditory processing is that auditory processing, like a number of other man-made constructs, is not

Subtype	Presumed Site of Dysfunction	Auditory and Associated Symptoms
Auditory Decoding Deficit	Primary auditory cortex (left hemisphere)	Difficulties in speech–sound discrimination, speech-in-noise, reading and spelling (word attack skills), foreign language learning, phonological awareness. May complain of auditory fatigue in challenging listening environments. Verbal poorer than performance IQ. Preserved sight-word reading skills, visual–spatial processing, and nonlanguage-based abilities (e.g., math calculation). Benefit from addition of visual or multimodality cues.
Prosodic Deficit	Right hemisphere	Difficulties in comprehension of prosodic elements of speech, reading and spelling (sight word skills), pragmatics. Speaking or reading voice may be monotonic. Associated right-hemisphere symptoms include math calculation and visuo-spatial difficulties, difficulties with topic maintenance, poor sequencing abilities. Performance IQ may be poorer with verbal IQ.
Integration Deficit	Corpus callosum	Difficulties in any task requiring interhemispheric cooperation, including linking linguistic and prosodic elements of speech, understanding speech in noise, and reading/spelling (association of written symbol with corresponding speech sound). Performance IQ and verbal IQ equal, with deficits in task-specific areas. Bimanual coordination and other interhemispheric difficulties may be present, but auditory deficits are primary. Addition of visual or multimodality cues may confuse rather than clarify.

Source: Bellis, T. (2006). Interpretation of APD test results. In T. Parthasarathy (Ed.), *An Introduction to Auditory Processing Disorders in Children.* Mahwah, NJ: Lawrence Erlbaum. Reprinted with permission.

perfect but is a way to help us to better understand human behavior. The auditory processing construct specifically attempts to give us insight into why some individuals who have normal hearing sensitivity are unable to understand incoming auditory/linguistic information in the presence of adverse listening conditions (e.g., background noise, rapid presentation rate, etc). Just as is the case when attempting to measure motivation, assessment of auditory processing is not easy and will require ongoing research and study in order to improve current methods. But the difficulties posed in measuring the construct do not imply that the construct is not meaningful or useful. It simply means that we must increase our efforts to find ways to accurately assess (C)APD, which will lead to more effective methods of remediation for children and adults.

CHAPTER SUMMARY

This chapter presented an overview of the nature of auditory processing, including the relevant anatomic structures, screening approaches, candidacy for testing, and common tests used in the assessment process. Various remediation strategies were discussed.

QUESTIONS FOR DISCUSSION

1. Compare the early use of tests of auditory processing with more recent use.
2. Describe controversies surrounding currently used (C)APD test batteries.
3. List and discuss four candidacy requirements for auditory processing testing.
4. Describe the role of the speech–language pathologist in identifying individuals who should be referred for auditory processing evaluations.
5. List and briefly discuss five remedial strategies to assist students diagnosed with an auditory processing disorder in the classroom.

RECOMMENDED READING

American Speech-Language-Hearing Association (ASHA). (1996). Task Force on Central Auditory Processing Consensus Development. *American Journal of Audiology, 5,* 41–54.

Baran, J. (2002). Managing auditory processing disorders in adolescents and adults. *Seminars in Hearing, 23,* 327–335.

Bellis, T. (1996). *Assessment and management of central auditory processing disorders in the educational setting.* San Diego: Singular.

Bellis, T. (2002). Developing deficit-specific intervention plans for individuals with auditory processing disorders. *Seminars in Hearing, 23,* 287–295.

Chermak, G., & Musiek, F. (2002). Auditory training: Principles and approaches for remediating and managing auditory processing disorders. *Seminar in Hearing, 23,* 297–308.

Educational Audiology Association. www.edaud.org

Flexer, C. (1999). *Facilitating hearing and listening in young children.* San Diego: Singular.

Halling, D., & Humes, L. (2000). Factors affecting the recognition of reverberant speech by elderly listeners. *Journal of Speech, Language, and Hearing Research, 41,* 414–431.

Jerger, J. (2001). Asymmetry in auditory function in elderly persons. *Seminars in Hearing, 22*(3), 255–268.

Koehnke, J., & Besing, J. (2001). The effects of aging on binaural and spatial hearing. *Seminars in Hearing, 22*(3), 241–253.

Masters, M. G., Stecker, N., & Katz, J. (1998). *Central auditory processing disorders: Mostly management.* Boston: Allyn & Bacon.

Schneider, B., & Pichora-Fuller, M. (2001). Age-related changes in temporal processing: Implications for speech perception. *Seminars in Hearing, 22*(3), 227–239.

Task Force on Central Auditory Processing Consensus Development. (1996, July). Central auditory processing: Current status of research and implications for clinical practice. *American Journal of Audiology, 5*(2), 41–54.

Tremblay, K., & Kraus, N. (2002). Auditory training induced asymmetrical changes in cortical neural activity. *Journal of Speech, Language, and Hearing Research, 45*(3), 564–572.

REFERENCES

American Speech-Language-Hearing Association. (2001). Scope of practice in speech–language pathology. Rockville, MD: Author.

American Speech-Language-Hearing Association. (2002a). *2002 omnibus survey caseload report: Practice trends in audiology.* Rockville, MD: Author.

American Speech-Language-Hearing Association. (2002b). *2002 omnibus survey caseload report: SLP.* Rockville, MD: author.

American Speech-Language-Hearing Association. (2004). Scope of practice in audiology. *ASHA Supplement, 24,* in press.

American Speech-Language-Hearing Association. (2005). (Central) auditory processing disorders. Available at www.asha.org/members/deskref-journals/deskref/default

Amos, N. E., & Humes, L. E. (1998). SCAN test-retest reliability for first- and third-grade children. *Journal of Speech, Language, and Hearing Research, 41*, 834–845.

Bellis, T. (2003). *Assessment and management of central auditory processing disorders in the educational setting.* San Diego: Singular.

Bellis, T. (2006). Interpretation of APD test results. In T. Parthasarathy (Ed.). *An introduction to auditory processing disorders in children.* NJ: Lawrence Erlbaum Publishers.

Cacace, A., & McFarland, D. (1998). Central auditory processing disorder in school-aged children: A critical review. *Journal of Speech, Language, and Hearing Research, 41,* 355–373.

Emerson, M. F., Crandall, K. K., Seikel, J. A., & Chermak, G. (1998). The use of SCAN to identify children at risk for CAPD: Response to Keith. *Language, Speech, and Hearing Services in Schools, 29(2),* 118–119.

Jerger, J., & Musiek, F. (2000). Report on the consensus conference on the diagnosis of auditory processing disorders in school-aged children. *Journal of the American Academy of Audiology, 11,* 467–474.

Katz, J., Stecker, N., & Henderson, D. (1992). *Central auditory processing: A transdisciplinary view.* Boston: Mosby Year Book.

Keith, R. (1986). *SCAN: A screening test for auditory processing disorders.* San Diego: The Psychological Corp.

Keith, R. (2000). *SCAN-C: Test for Auditory Processing Disorders in Children-Revised.* San Antonio: The Psychological Corp.

Masters, M. G., Stecker, N., & Katz, J. (1998) *Central auditory processing disorders: Mostly management.* Boston: Allyn & Bacon.

Musiek, F. E., Gollegly, K., & Baron, J. (1984). Myelination of the corpus callosum and auditory processing problems in children: Theoretical and clinical correlates. *Seminars in Hearing, 5,* 231–242.

Smoski, W. J., Brunt, M. A., & Tannahill, J. C. (1992). Listening characteristics of children with central auditory processing disorders. *Language, Speech, and Hearing Services in Schools, 23,* 145–149.

389
•

Appendix A:
Sample Case
History Form
for Auditory
Processing
Evaluation

Appendix A
Sample Case History Form for Auditory Processing Evaluation

Central Auditory Processing Evaluation History Form

I. Identifying Information

Name: _____   DOB: _____

School: _____   Grade: _____

Teachers: _____

Referring physician _____

Parent(s) names: _____

II. Reason for Referral

_____

_____

_____

_____

III. Your Child's *Current* Educational Program

(Describe any services s/he receives (e.g., speech therapy, resource room assistance) and the frequency of these services (e.g., once a week, three times a week).

_____

_____

_____

_____

IV. Results of Any Other Diagnostic Testing Completed for Your Child within the Past Two Years

Bring results of psychoeducational testing, IQ scores, speech/language evaluations, attention deficit screenings, or any other assessments to your appointment.

V. Educational History

Please list any other schools your child has attended (including preschool, if applicable):

_____

_____

Did your child receive any services as a preschooler?　　Yes _____　　No _____
(e.g., specialized preschool program, speech therapy, PT, OT). Please describe:

_____

_____

Did your child skip or repeat any grades? _____

Has your child experienced any difficulties learning classroom materials?

Yes _____　　No _____

If yes, in what subjects? _____

Has your child's teacher approached you with information or concerns regarding your child's performance?　　Yes _____　　No _____

VI. Hearing History

Is there a history of ear infections?　　Yes _____　　No _____

If yes, please describe the following:

Approximate number per year and at what ages: _____

Method of treatment (medications, surgery): _____

_____

Were pressure-equalization tubes inserted?　　Yes _____　　No _____

If yes, at what age(s)? _____

Has your child had a hearing evaluation?　　Yes _____　　No _____

Briefly describe the test results: _____

_____

Is there a family history of hearing loss?　　Yes _____　　No _____

VII. Other

Please add any additional information you wish to include:

_____

_____

_____

_____

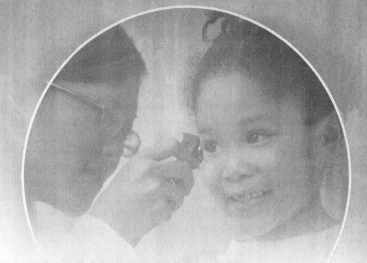

chapter 11

Screening

AFTER COMPLETING THIS CHAPTER, YOU SHOULD BE ABLE TO:

1. Define the term *screening.*
2. Compare and contrast the medical and educational screening models.
3. Apply the terms *sensitivity* and *specificity* to a discussion of screening effectiveness.
4. Define *reliability* and *validity* and describe their importance in the screening process.
5. List at least six decisions that have to be made before embarking on a screening program, and summarize the major relevant issue for each.
6. Create a chart that summarizes screening procedures across the life span, beginning with infancy and continuing through old age.
7. Understand the difference between the information to be conveyed after hearing screening versus after diagnostic audiological evaluation.

The Scope of Practice in Audiology (ASHA, 2004) and Scope of Practice in Speech–Language Pathology (ASHA, 2001) both include audiological screenings. For this reason, this chapter is an important one. Further, audiologists and speech–language pathologists are dedicated to improving the communication abilities of all people, and it is often through audiological screenings that individuals with hearing loss can begin the process of receiving the needed intervention.

Up to this point, you have learned about **diagnostic audiometry.** When a comprehensive battery of tests is done for purposes of making a diagnosis, we are using the most effective tools at our disposal to determine whether a disease or condition (in this case hearing impairment) is present. In addition, information may be collected that will be useful in the planning of rehabilitation. For example, the word recognition testing that an audiologist does during routine audiological assessment can provide insight as to how the client will do with hearing aids or how he is currently functioning when speech is presented at conversational levels.

In screening, less information is collected. A screening tool is used to separate those individuals who are most likely to have a hearing loss from those who are not likely to have a loss, so that the former group can be referred for further (i.e., diagnostic) testing.

As with many other clinical activities that audiologists and speech–language pathologists perform, guidance in administering hearing screening programs can be found in multiple places, including ASHA guidelines, ANSI standards, and federal and state laws and regulations. In some instances, ASHA guidelines and state regulations may differ, in which case the clinician should adhere to the regulatory requirements in effect in the locality.

Definitions and Models

Nicolosi, Harryman, and Kresheck (1989) define **screening** as "any gross measure utilized to separate those who may require specific help in a specific area, such as language, hearing, articulation, fluency, and voice, from those who obviously do not need any help" (p. 233). ASHA (1997c) defines **audiological screening** performed by audiologists as "a pass/fail procedure to prevent or detect early auditory impairment, disorder, and disability to identify individuals who require further audiologic assessment and/or treatment or referral for other professional services" (pp. 1–32).

Medical Model versus Educational Model

Kenworthy (1993) describes two different approaches to screening, including the medical/epidemiological approach and the educational approach. In the medical approach, the disease or condition for which an individual is screened should lend itself to a binary outcome (either pass or refer), and the condition should exist primarily in isolation. An educational approach differs in that the focus is broader. Also, "the focus is programmatic and is aimed at establishing a continuum of services rather than a single test/treatment protocol. The process is generally referred to as identification and incorporates such elements as case finding (screening), tracking, referral, follow-up, and advocacy, particularly public education" (p. 54). Students of communication disorders will see throughout the following discussion of screening for hearing loss that an educational approach to screening, with particular attention to outcomes, has greater applicability to both the identification and management of individuals with communication disorders. It is important to move beyond the outcome of the screening and be able to answer the critical questions—what happened to the individuals who did not pass the screening, and did they receive the help they needed?

Before deciding to screen individuals for a specific disorder, some commonly accepted principles should be understood:

- The disorder has some negative effect on the person and consequently has a negative effect on society.
- There must be a follow-up test (i.e., the diagnostic test battery) that will have great accuracy in determining the presence or absence of the disorder.

Effective treatments should be available for those individuals who ultimately are determined to have the disorder. In the case of conductive hearing loss, medical treatments are available. In cases of sensorineural hearing loss, hearing aids do not treat the hearing loss, in the sense that they do not alter the presence of hearing loss. They do, however, represent an intervention that can reduce many of the negative effects of hearing impairment.

- Because screenings typically involve large numbers of participants, it is important that the screening be easy to administer, quick, and reasonable in price.
- Screening programs should be evaluated to determine their effectiveness and cost efficiency.

This last principle of evaluating the effectiveness of the screening is extremely important and requires greater discussion. Let's say that a screening tool has been devised to determine which individuals are likely to have a certain disease or condition. During the course of a day, 100 people are screened. As expected, some of the people who are screened will fail the screening and some will pass. How do you know whether the screening is accurate and effective? What other information must you have in order to determine this? You need to compare the number of people who fail the screening with the number of people who truly have this condition. You also need to compare the number of people who pass the screening with the number of people who do not have the condition. How do you find out who truly has the condition? Determining if a person truly has a disorder is the purpose of the diagnostic test.

In order to evaluate a new screening tool, you could take the 100 people who have just been screened and have them all receive a complete diagnostic evaluation. Then, you could compare the findings of the diagnostic test with the results obtained using the new screening tool.

Looking at Figure 11.1, you can see that even though the individuals who were screened either passed or were referred (failed), there are actually four possible outcomes when both a screening and diagnostic test are administered to a group of individuals. Box A represents the number of individuals who failed the screening and were found to have the condition when given the diagnostic test. Developers of screening tools hope that this number is large. The larger this number is, the more accurate is the screening tool. There were 10 of these individuals. Now take a look at box D. Like box A, this box provides information regarding the accuracy of the screening tool, because it represents the number of individuals who passed the screening and were found not to have the condition after the diagnostic evaluation. There were 80 of these individuals.

Sensitivity and Specificity

Two important concepts related to screening are sensitivity and specificity. **Sensitivity** refers to how effective the screening tool is at picking out those individuals who have the disorder. Looking again at Figure 11.1, we see that a total of 13 individuals were found through the diagnostic test to have the disorder (box A + box C), and the screening tool correctly identified 10 of them. So, the sensitivity of the screening tool is 10/13 or 77 percent.

What about **specificity**? This refers to how effective the screening tool is at passing individuals who do not have the disorder. Looking again at Figure 11.1, note that a total of 87 individuals were found by the diagnostic test to be free of the disorder (box B + box D), and the screening tool correctly identified 80 of them. So, the specificity of the screening tool is 80/87 or 92 percent.

The relevance of sensitivity and specificity is illustrated in the following scenario. Imagine for a moment that you go to your physician for your annual physical exam. Your physician recommends that you have blood drawn as a way of

FIGURE **11.1** **Tetrachoric (2 x 2) table used to monitor effectiveness of a screening instrument.**

screening you for certain types of diseases. Let's also assume for discussion purposes that the screening has very high sensitivity but only moderate specificity.

Think about some of the issues surrounding the screening results. If you are a person who has one of these undetected diseases, the high sensitivity of the screening measure will most likely result in a **positive finding** ("positive" in medical terms means that you have the condition) and early detection. (A **negative finding,** in medical terms, means that you do *not* have the condition.) The high sensitivity of the screening was to your benefit. But what if you are free of the disease? The moderate specificity of the screening method means that the blood test sometimes yields positive results in individuals who are completely healthy. A **false positive screening result** means that you failed the screening even though you will pass the diagnostic test. The number of people with a false positive result is represented in box B. What are the consequences here? First, the individual is now worried about his health for no reason. Second, if large numbers of people are referred for diagnostic testing based on inaccurate screening results (i.e., overreferral) health care costs rise and the credibility of the screening tool, the person administering the screening, and sometimes the entire profession associated with the screening is reduced.

Again considering the above scenario, would it be better to have a test that has less sensitivity and more specificity? Not necessarily. Less sensitive tests will miss more individuals who have the condition, and this will result in **false negative screening results** (see box C for the number of individuals with false negative results). False negatives occur when individuals pass the screening even though they do have the disorder. Obviously, this leads to underreferral, which can prevent individuals from receiving needed treatment.

Calculation of false positive and false negative rates is relatively simple. The **false positive rate** is the number of false positives divided by the total number of normal individuals (i.e., those who did not have the disorder based on the diagnostic test). So, referring again to Figure 11.1, you divide 7 (box B) by 87 (box B + box D) for a rate of 8 percent. Similarly, the **false negative rate** is the number of false negatives divided by the total number of abnormal individuals. This number is 3 (box C) divided by 13 (box A + box C) for a rate of 23 percent.

Finally, using the above information, let's calculate the **prevalence** of the disorder, which refers to the number of cases in the population. We noted above that the total number of cases being studied was 100 and also that the total number of individuals who tested positive for the disorder (based on the diagnosis) was 13. Therefore, the prevalence of this disorder is estimated to be 13 percent (13/100).

Reliability and Validity

You may recall from previous courses that **validity** refers to the degree to which a measuring instrument (e.g., a test or a screening) measures what it purports to measure. There are a number of different types of validity, with construct validity being perhaps the most important. **Construct validity** refers to the extent to which the results of the measuring tool are consistent with what is known about the construct.

Let's look at a specific example related to hearing. If a new screening tool is developed for the detection of hearing loss and administered to a group of school-age children in a regular educational setting and also to a second group of elderly individuals in a nursing home setting, you would expect that more of the subjects in the second group would fail the screening. Why? Because one of the things that you know about the

construct of hearing is that as people get older they are more likely to have hearing loss. **395**
If results from the screening are not consistent with this, it is possible that the screening
tool lacks construct validity; it may not be measuring what it was intended to measure.

Reliability is another aspect of the measuring tool, and it refers to the consistency
with which the tool measures whatever it is intended to measure. For example, if a language test is administered to a preschool child on Monday and then readministered one
week later, it is expected that the child's performance would be about the same. If there
is a significant change in the child's score, it may be due to a lack of reliability of the test
instrument. In other words, the change is not due to any real change in the child, but
rather is due to the lack of stability of the tool.

The screenings that speech–language pathologists and audiologists perform for detection of hearing loss must be both reliable and valid. One way to promote validity of
the screening instrument is to choose screening tools that match the client's age and
ability. For example, using a pure tone screening tool to assess the hearing of an infant
is problematic, because failure of the infant to respond could be related to a number of
variables (e.g., maturation, attention) that are not related to the infant's hearing. This is
an example of a lack of validity because the screening device is not measuring what it
purports to measure.

Reliability can be affected by factors such as the clarity of the directions and the
level of the background noise. If pure tone screening is administered to a preschooler on
a day when the screening room is quite noisy, the child may fail. If the same preschooler
is rescreened when the room is quieter, the child may pass. This lack of stability is not related to any change in the child, but rather is due to a lack of reliability in the screening
protocol. Similarly, if the directions given to the person being screened are not clear, the
person's performance on the screening may be unstable.

The last point that should be made regarding reliability and validity is that a screening tool that lacks reliability also lacks validity. In other words, if the screening tool
yields unstable results, it is not measuring what it is intended to measure. Reliability is
a necessary criterion for a tool to be valid. It should also be noted, however, that just because a tool is reliable does not mean that it is valid. The following example may help
illustrate this reliability–validity relationship. Assume for a moment that a decision was
made to use the color of a person's hair to screen for hearing loss. All those with blond
hair would automatically fail the screening and those with brown hair would pass.
Because we would all consistently identify the same individuals as passing or failing the
screening, we would achieve near 100 percent reliability. However, because hair color is
not an indicator of hearing loss, our measure would not be valid.

Decisions about the Screening Protocol

Decisions that have to be made prior to carrying out hearing screenings and how those
decisions might impact some of the terms you have just learned about are discussed in
this section.

Have I Obtained the Necessary Permission to Carry Out the Screening?

Depending on the site where the screening is taking place and any statutory requirements that might govern the screening protocol, it may or may not be necessary to

obtain written consent prior to performing the screening. Such consent is commonly an issue when children are being screened and is provided by the parent or legal guardian. In some cases, such as universal newborn hearing screening, consent for the screening may be included in the general hospital admission consent signed by the parent. If the screening takes place in a different setting, for example, an outpatient clinic, the conventions and protocols for permission used in the clinic would be followed. Preschool screenings, on the other hand, often do require that parents provide specific permission. For these and other populations, because of the great variability from state to state and from facility to facility, anyone conducting screenings should take the time to consult existing guidelines and make decisions based on the available information.

Where Will the Screening Be Performed?

Remember that in most cases, hearing screenings are not done in acoustically controlled environments, such as a sound-treated booth. Speech–language pathologists in schools and school nurses have long struggled to find reasonably quiet environments in which to carry out pure tone screening. Think for a moment about our discussion in Chapter 2 regarding masking of sounds by background noise. If noise levels in the screening environment are not sufficiently reduced, individuals being screened may not hear the tones being presented at the screening level and will fail the screening even though they have normal hearing. This constitutes a false positive result and leads to overreferral. It is the responsibility of the professional who is conducting the screening to educate the appropriate administrators (e.g., school principal, hospital vice president) about the importance of a quiet environment for screenings.

There are standards for the maximum permissible noise levels in rooms where air conduction screenings take place. These are available through ANSI (1999). In the ideal situation, the noise levels would be measured with a sound level meter in order to determine if the room was suitable for testing. In the real world, however, the rooms that are chosen for screenings will not have had a noise analysis and the screener will have to make subjective decisions about the room's suitability. How might this be done? First, screeners can place the earphones over their own ears and present the signals at the screening level at the various frequencies. Assuming a screener has normal hearing levels, if the tones cannot be heard, the noise levels are too high. At this point a decision has to be made. Should the screening level be increased, or should efforts be made to find a quieter room? Considering the issues of sensitivity and specificity, finding a quieter room (or making modifications to the existing room) is preferable.

Noise is an issue that must be considered in most screening situations. In addition to pure tone screening, other screening tools such as otoacoustic emissions used for infant hearing screening are vulnerable to external noise. Some tests, such as the auditory brainstem response and immittance measures, are less influenced by environmental noise, but are affected by internal noises generated by the infant (e.g., sucking or muscle movement). Regardless of the noise source(s) (e.g., internal or external), individuals conducting screenings must be aware of the potential effect of noise on screening outcomes.

What Will the Pass/Refer Criteria Be?

When a screening protocol is devised, decisions have to be made regarding what constitutes a "pass" and what constitutes a "refer." These decisions are made based on the need to keep both sensitivity and specificity as high as possible. In other words, pass/refer criteria are determined so that the maximum number of individuals with the disorder will fall into the "refer" category and the maximum number of individuals who do not have the disorder will fall into the "pass" category.

It is important to remember that if we use a screening level that is too intense, we decrease the sensitivity of the screening because individuals who have hearing loss may pass. Conversely, using a screening level of insufficient intensity decreases the specificity because individuals who have normal hearing are likely to fail. Also, the choice of screening level interacts with the quality of the acoustic environment. One of the most common mistakes made during screenings is to increase the intensity of the tones in order to compensate for the noise level. The problem here is that the greater the intensity of the tone, the greater is the chance that a person who truly has a hearing loss will pass the screening. This creates an inherent lack of sensitivity in the screening and leads to **underreferrals.** Let's take a look at a case example illustrating this.

Carlita, age 4 years, has a flat sensorineural hearing loss with thresholds of 25–30 dB HL bilaterally. Because of poor room acoustics, she is given a screening at a level of 35 dB HL. Carlita passes the screening, and her mild sensorineural hearing loss goes undetected. She continues to make slow progress in articulation therapy, and her preschool teacher notes that she does not seem to have good attending skills.

What Specific Frequencies Will Be Screened?

Another pitfall to avoid in screenings involves the specific frequencies that are included in the screening. For example, ASHA (1997a) does not recommend including 500 Hz in the screening for this reason. Inclusion of 500 Hz in a screening that is not conducted in a sound booth decreases the specificity of the screening because individuals who do not have a hearing loss often fail the screening, leading to overreferrals. If the screening does take place in a sound-treated booth, 500 Hz may be included. ASHA guidelines tend to emphasize the middle to higher frequencies and deemphasize the lower frequencies, in part because of the problem noted detecting lower frequencies in less-than-ideal screening settings but also because of the critical role of the high-frequency consonants to speech and language development.

What Equipment Will Be Needed for the Different Populations to Be Screened?

The specific equipment that is used during the screening will, of course, depend on the population being screened and the specific purpose of the screening. For example, if you are screening infants, a pure tone audiometer will certainly *not* be the test of choice. Instead, otoacoustic emissions or auditory brainstem responses will likely be employed. Regarding the issue of what you are screening for, keep in mind that for some populations screenings are done not only for purposes of identifying individuals who are likely to have hearing loss, but also to identify outer and/or middle ear disease. In these cases, some combination of hearing screening equipment and immittance equipment will be needed. Bone conduction testing is not part of screenings because the **ambient noise** levels of the uncontrolled acoustic environment would make it unreliable.

Let's think for a moment about the populations for whom screening for outer/ middle ear disease would be most important. If you said preschoolers, you were correct.

This is due in part to the effects of fluctuating conductive hearing loss on speech and language development. Also, children who already have sensorineural hearing loss need close monitoring for conductive pathology, as do children who are at particular risk for **middle ear effusion** (e.g., children who have craniofacial abnormalities, children with cleft lip or palate).

Let's take a look at a case study illustrating the value of tympanometry in a screening. Michael, age 3 years, is screened for hearing loss using a portable audiometer. On the day of the screening, Michael has bilateral otitis media. Presume now that we have a crystal ball and can see Michael's true audiogram. This audiogram is provided in Figure 11.2. Note that Michael's air conduction thresholds are 20 dB at all frequencies and his bone conduction thresholds are between −5 and 0 dB HL. If, due to the noise level of the room, a screening level of 25 dB is used (rather than 20 dB recommended by ASHA) and we do not include tympanometry in our screening, what is the outcome? Michael passes the screening even though he is not hearing within normal limits and certainly not up to his potential. This represents a sensitivity problem with the screening. If, on the other hand, we include tympanometry, what happens? Michael will not pass the screening because the tympanograms will likely identify some type of middle ear dysfunction. Instead of being passed, Michael will be monitored, and if the abnormal tympanograms persist, he will be referred to his physician.

Is My Equipment in Calibration?

It is important in this chapter to reemphasize the role that calibration plays in screenings. Remember that screenings are often done in locations outside of the clinic or

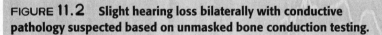

FIGURE 11.2 Slight hearing loss bilaterally with conductive pathology suspected based on unmasked bone conduction testing.

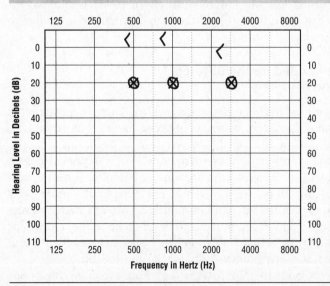

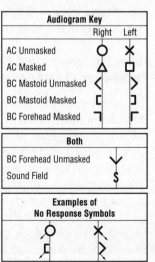

hospital or private practice. This means that the portable equipment that is being used has been transported, and this can compromise calibration more quickly than for equipment that is not moved around. Also, school administrators should be reminded of the importance of calibration of pure tone audiometers so that funding for annual calibration of equipment will be allocated. Remember that the reliability and validity of any screening done with faulty equipment is questionable. In general, calibration is done on an annual basis. At a minimum, calibration should be done in accordance with the manufacturer's specifications.

Let's think now about sensitivity and specificity and issues of calibration. Consider the audiometer that is producing too little sound pressure. For example, when the attenuator dial reads 20 dB, the sound pressure at the eardrum is 10 dB less than it should be. What effect does this have? It decreases the specificity of the screening, because individuals who do not have a hearing loss will fail the screening. Another way to say this is that the screening has become too sensitive, so much so that it is not distinguishing between those who have and those who do not have a problem. The uncalibrated audiometer can also produce too much sound pressure. In this case, the screening's sensitivity suffers because individuals who have hearing loss may be able to pass the screening.

In addition to ensuring that annual calibration is done, subjective calibration is a useful procedure that can be done immediately prior to the screening. In the absence of a sound level meter, the clinician conducting the screening places the earphones over her ears and assesses the integrity of the equipment by monitoring the following:

- Is the tone heard when the interrupt button is depressed?
- Do the "right" and "left" buttons deliver the tone to the corresponding ears?
- In addition to the tone, are additional, unwanted sounds (e.g., static) present?
- As the attenuator dial is adjusted, is there a corresponding increase or decrease in intensity?
- As the frequency dial is adjusted, is there a corresponding increase or decrease in frequency?
- Do changes in frequency and intensity occur in a linear fashion, or are there large changes in the stimuli with small changes on the dial?

As noted in Chapter 4, calibration applies not only to the audiometer but also to the test environment. Unlike comprehensive audiological assessment, in which the client is in a sound-treated booth, screenings are often done in acoustically uncontrolled environments. This increases the likelihood that background noise could interfere with the client's ability to hear the tones presented. However, remember that screenings do not involve threshold searches and therefore noise levels do not have to be as controlled as they have to be for threshold testing. Also, bone conduction testing is not part of screenings, so once again noise levels do not have to be quite as controlled. Because it is rare that actual room noise levels will be measured with a sound level meter, the individual conducting the screening should use his or her own judgment about the feasibility of conducting screenings in a given room.

The reader is directed to Table 11.1 for a summary of the various factors commonly encountered in screenings and how they affect sensitivity, specificity, and referral decisions.

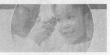

TABLE 11.1   Factors Commonly Encountered in Screenings That Affect Sensitivity, Specificity, and Referral

Problem Encountered	Effect on Sensitivity or Specificity	Effect on Referral Decision
Excessive room noise	Decreases specificity	Overreferral
Screening level of insufficient intensity	Decreases specificity	Overreferral
Screening level that is too intense	Decreases sensitivity	Underreferral
Inclusion of 500 Hz when not in sound-treated booth	Decreases specificity	Overreferral
Uncalibrated audiometer that produces too little sound pressure	Decreases specificity	Overreferral
Uncalibrated audiometer that produces too much sound pressure	Decreases sensitivity	Underreferral
Omission of tympanometry in screening preschoolers	Decreases sensitivity	Underreferral

How Should the Results of the Screening Be Recorded and Interpreted?

Appendix A shows suggested content to assist in the development of forms that might be used to record the results of the various screenings. A typical form is provided in Appendix B. Remember, because you are not collecting threshold information during the screening, you do not record screening information directly on the audiogram. Let's say, for example, that you have just screened a 3-year-old and he passed the screening at 20 dB at 1,000, 2,000, and 4,000 Hz. If you use the air conduction symbols associated with air conduction testing, you are communicating to the reader that 20 dB represents the softest level at which the child can hear the tones at these frequencies. However, this is not what we have tested, because you did not investigate whether the child was able to hear at levels softer than 20 dB. That would have required some type of ascending–descending pure tone test technique that is not part of the screening process. Illustrated in Figure 11.3 are two examples of audiograms with screening results. Note that in example A, the screener has incorrectly reported screening level data as threshold data. In example B, the audiologist has made it clear to the reader that responses to tones at 20 dB were screening levels only.

A sample recording form for screenings with the adult population is found in Appendix B. This form can also be adapted for preschool and school-age clients. At a minimum, a screening form should include the client's name, the date of the screening, the screening levels, the frequencies assessed, whether the client has passed or failed, and recommendations. Typically, for those who fail a screening, recommendations include a rescreen or a referral to an audiologist for comprehensive assessment. As discussed, in some cases a medical referral is made.

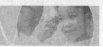

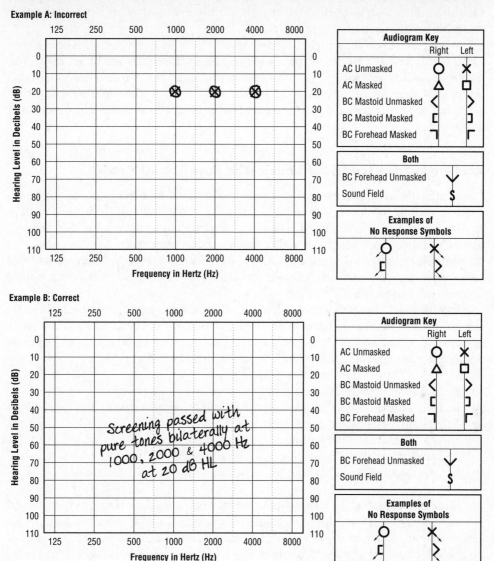

FIGURE 11.3   Correct and incorrect ways of reporting screening results on the audiogram.

Example A: Incorrect

Example B: Correct

Screening passed with pure tones bilaterally at 1000, 2000 & 4000 Hz at 20 dB HL

In addition to correct recording of the results on the designated form, it is often necessary for audiologists and speech–language pathologists to describe the screening findings in written form or verbally (e.g., at a meeting). In these cases, it is important not to overinterpret the screening findings. How might one overinterpret? One common way to do this is to claim, based on the screening, that the child has "normal hearing." Why is this statement not justified when only screening data have been collected? First, "hearing" is more than merely perception of tones at different frequencies. As you know, it also involves reception and recognition of speech stimuli. Second, a limited number of frequencies are tested in the screening, and it is possible that hearing loss exists at frequencies not screened. In addition, it is important to note that the screening represents a point in time, and does not allow us a prediction as to what will happen in the future. This is an important point for practitioners involved in newborn hearing screening programs to keep in mind.

What type of wording might be better when a pure tone screening has been done? "Jane Smith passed a 20-dB HL pure tone screening at frequencies 1,000, 2,000, and 4,000 Hz. No further testing is recommended at this time." For an individual who passed middle ear screening, the report might indicate that "results of middle ear function screening met the criteria for passing the screening. No further testing is recommended at this time."

Am I Prepared to Screen Individuals Who Have Special Needs?

Many individuals who have special needs will be able to participate in a conventional screening protocol without difficulty. For those individuals who may have developmental/cognitive deficits that interfere with their ability to perform the screening, a speech–language pathologist or audiologist should be prepared to use the special play audiometric techniques described in Chapter 8. Although these techniques appear to be very simple, they are extremely valuable and can make the difference between a reliable screening and an unreliable one.

In addition, Chapter 9 provides detailed information regarding comprehensive assessment of various populations. Much of this information can be applied to the screening process. A summary of the key issues raised in Chapter 9 and that might need to be addressed when screening individuals who have special needs are

- Reduced cognitive skills, often affecting memory and attention
- Reduced language skills, interfering with overall comprehension of task instructions
- Behavioral issues that interfere with task compliance
- Tactile defensiveness preventing use of earphones or probe insertion
- Reduced motor skills, interfering with conditioned play audiometry
- Emotional upset brought about by a new situation and/or new demands

Generally, conditioning an individual to respond during a hearing screening should not take more than a few minutes. In those cases where a conditioning bond cannot be established in a short time and a reliable screening cannot be obtained, referral should be made to an audiologist, particularly one who has experience working with individuals who have special needs.

How Will Costs Associated with the Hearing Screening Be Handled?

The specific answer to this question will vary depending on the age of the population to be screened, the setting of the screening, and whether the screening is mandated. Before initiating a screening program, it is important to investigate potential funding sources. Examples of funding sources include public (e.g., state, county, school district), private (e.g., insurance, personal payment), or grant monies allocated to provide screening to certain populations that may be at risk for a condition or are underserved. Finally, in some cases, an agency may donate its time and expertise as an in-kind service.

General Screening Components

Some general screening considerations that can apply to all clients are discussed here. These include otoscopy, earphone placement, presenting pure tones, and making recommendations.

Nondiagnostic Otoscopy

First, explain to the client that you will be examining his or her ears. After completing nondiagnostic otoscopy, record on the screening form your findings using the following guidelines:

Observation	*Written Remarks*
None to minimal wax	Clear
Moderate wax, eardrum visible	Some wax noted; not occluded
Significant wax, eardrum not visible	Occluded

If the ear canal is occluded or nearly occluded, the screener should recommend wax removal. The screening can still be done, and if the client passes, the results may be viewed as reliable but the recommendation for wax removal should still be made. If the client fails the screening, a reevaluation after wax removal should be recommended. For individuals who have difficulty doing the screening and who require greater amounts of support, it may be better to delay the screening until after the wax is removed.

Individuals who have limited experience using an otoscope may be uncertain about what they are viewing. For example, it is easy to mistake the canal wall for wax blockage. In addition to wax, the examiner should look for inflammation, blood, or obvious drainage. Be sure to seek out the opinion of a colleague or supervisor if there is any question about the status of the client's external ear.

Instructions and Earphone Placement

Before performing the testing, give instructions to the client. These will vary with the amount of support the client requires. For individuals who require minimal support in carrying out the screening, give the following instructions:

> You are going to hear a series of tones. Every time you hear the tone, please raise your hand [or say "yes"]. Some of these tones may be faint; remember, even if the tone is very soft, I still want you to raise your hand [or say "yes"]. It doesn't matter which ear you hear the tone in, just raise your hand [or say "yes"] when you hear it.

For individuals who require greater amounts of support to complete the screening successfully, refer to techniques in Chapter 8 on conditioned play audiometry as well as Chapter 9 on assessment of special populations.

When placing the earphones, be sure that the earphones are directly over the ears and that you adjust them so that they are comfortable for the client. If necessary, have the client remove earrings and eyeglasses before putting on the earphones. Some clients rely heavily on visual/facial cues for reinforcement during the screening; with these clients, try to let them leave their glasses on.

Administering the Screening

Depending on the client, you may want to do a few practice tones (which can be either steady or pulsing) and be sure the client responds appropriately. To do this, set the earphones on the table next to the client. Turn the attenuator dial of the audiometer up to 100 dB and present the tone at 1,000 Hz. (Remember, the earphones are *not* on the client at this point.) If the client responds appropriately, begin the actual screening by placing the earphones on the client and setting the attenuator dial to the screening level. If the client does not respond to this stimulus, prompt the client physically (if he is using the hand-raising response) or verbally (if he is using the verbal response). Do this several times to be sure the client is responding reliably. The client who needs minimal to no support in doing the screening will now be able to respond reliably to the tones. During the screening, monitor response reliability and reinstruct and/or re-prompt, as needed.

Remember not to be too predictable in the pattern of tone presentations. Be sure to pause every once in a while (e.g., every 2 to 3 seconds) to be sure the client is waiting for the stimulus before responding.

Occasionally during a screening, the examiner will go back to those test frequencies at which the client failed the screening and obtain what is referred to as the client's **first level of response (FLR)** as described by Doyle (1997). This is done using an ascending approach, moving up in intensity in 5-dB steps beginning at the screening level and ending when the client responds. Remember that this is not threshold testing, because that requires an acoustically controlled environment and a standardized threshold search procedure.

The logic in pursuing the FLR is that a client who fails at 30 dB may hear at that frequency at 35 dB, which constitutes a mild hearing loss; or the person may hear at that frequency at 80 dB, which constitutes a severe loss. By obtaining the FLR for the failed frequency, we have more information about the degree of hearing loss and perhaps about how much the loss will interfere with the person's communication abilities. Even when the FLR is obtained, the examiner is still performing a hearing screening and the true thresholds will have to be established by a licensed audiologist in a sound-treated room in the context of a full audiological assessment.

Making Recommendations

Recommendations made based on audiological screenings typically include, but are not limited to, the following:

- Wax removal by physician
- Referral to physician due to _____
- Rescreening in _____ weeks/1 year
- Refer to audiologist for full audiological evaluation
- Use of communication strategies

It is important for the nonaudiologist to remember that just because a client is unable to be screened does not mean that he will not be able to participate in a comprehensive audiological assessment. In addition to speech audiometry, which many clients can perform, an audiologist has use of tools such as otoacoustic emissions and evoked potentials, which do not require active participation from the client.

Screening Protocols across the Life Span

Early Identification of Hearing Loss in Infants

History of Newborn Hearing Screening

Newborn infants are screened for a variety of conditions, including inborn metabolic disorders, genetic, and infectious conditions. Generally, public health programs target conditions for which early identification and intervention can lead to improved outcomes for those who are found to have the condition. Hearing loss fits the criteria for conditions that warrant newborn screening, because the timing of intervention for hearing loss can lead to a significant reduction in the potential disabilities associated with hearing loss in affected infants.

Various individuals and organizations have recognized the need for and importance of early identification of hearing loss in infants. Early efforts to identify infants with hearing loss included the development of a **high-risk register** for hearing loss. This work helped to raise awareness of factors that are associated with hearing loss. Such risk factors, now called indicators, include anoxia, low birth weight, elevated bilirubin levels, family history of hearing loss, intrauterine infections, and craniofacial anomalies. However, the presence of risk factors, or indicators, falls short in identifying all infants with communicatively and educationally significant hearing loss. Analysis of data on newborn hearing screening suggests that approximately 30 percent of infants who have hearing loss do not exhibit risk factors (Kileny & Lesperance, 2001). Through the years, a variety of screening techniques have been developed to detect hearing loss early in life, including the use of high-risk registers, behavioral observation, and automated tests such as the Crib-o-gram. The **Crib-o-gram** used a motion-sensitive device placed in the infant's crib to record the infant's response to sound but was found to lack reliability.

Although these early efforts were important attempts to identify infants with hearing loss, they were not well suited to the task of universal newborn hearing screening. For example, in order to perform **behavioral observation audiometry** (BOA) reliably, a sound-treated booth equipped with calibrated speakers is necessary. This is clearly impractical for screening large numbers of infants prior to their discharge from the hospital nursery.

Current Recommendations for Newborn Hearing Screening

The Joint Committee on Infant Hearing (JCIH) was formed in 1970 and has periodically issued position statements about newborn hearing screening, taking into account relevant research findings and reflecting the "state of the art" at the time. The JCIH includes representatives from the following organizations: the American Academy of Audiology; the American Academy of Otolaryngology—Head and Neck Surgery; the

American Academy of Pediatrics; the American Speech-Language-Hearing Association; the Council on Education of the Deaf, whose member organizations include the Alexander Graham Bell Association for the Deaf and Hard of Hearing, the American Society for Deaf Children, the Conference of Educational Administrators of Schools and Programs for the Deaf, the Convention of American Instructors of the Deaf, the National Association of the Deaf, and the Association of College Educators of the Deaf and Hard of Hearing; and the Directors of Speech and Hearing Programs in State Health and Welfare Agencies. The JCIH Year 2000 Position Statement includes principles and guidelines for early hearing detection and intervention programs and is a valuable resource for those involved in, or considering involvement in, newborn hearing screening initiatives (JCIH, 2000).

Recommended Screening Techniques

The JCIH Year 2000 Position Statement includes eight principles considered by the writers to be the foundation for effective early hearing detection and intervention systems. The first principle provides that all infants have access to hearing screening using a physiological measure. Both the Joint Committee on Infant Hearing and the American Academy of Pediatrics include otoacoustic emissions and auditory brainstem response as techniques that are appropriate for use in newborn hearing screening programs.

Rationale for Early Detection of Hearing Loss

Students of communication disorders know that the earlier hearing loss is detected and intervention is initiated, the better. According to the American Academy of Pediatrics Task Force on Newborn and Infant Hearing (1999), "significant hearing loss is one of the most common major abnormalities present at birth, and, if undetected, will impede speech, language and cognitive development" (p. 527). The goals of early hearing detection and intervention programs are to screen all infants by age 1 month, identify hearing loss by age 3 months, and begin early intervention services for infants with hearing loss and their families by age 6 months, according to *Healthy People 2010* Objective 28.11 (DHHS, 2000). This has become known as the "1-3-6 rule" and it provides a useful context for considering the relative success or failure of newborn hearing screening programs. In the larger context, newborn hearing screening should be considered one element in an effective **universal newborn hearing screening** program. In addition to the initial hearing screening, the other elements of an effective program include tracking and follow-up of infants who do not pass the screening, identification of hearing loss, intervention for infants with hearing loss and their families, and evaluation of the screening program. Collaboration is an essential ingredient in a successful newborn hearing screening program. One important relationship is the partnership between the child's physician/health care provider and parents, sometimes referred to as the child's "medical home." Other important relationships include partnerships between the family and the audiologist, speech–language pathologist, and teacher of the deaf and hard of hearing, among others. Figure 11.4 summarizes the American Academy of Pediatrics' (AAP) universal newborn hearing screening, diagnosis, and intervention guidelines, which are important for pediatric medical home providers and other professionals involved in newborn hearing screening programs.

FIGURE **11.4** **Universal newborn hearing screening, diagnosis, and intervention guidelines for pediatric medical home providers.**

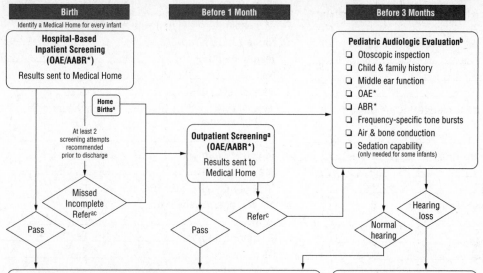

Birth	Before 1 Month	Before 3 Months

Identify a Medical Home for every infant

Hospital-Based Inpatient Screening (OAE/AABR*)
Results sent to Medical Home

Home Births[a]

At least 2 screening attempts recommended prior to discharge

Missed Incomplete Refer[ac]

Pass

Outpatient Screening[a] (OAE/AABR*)
Results sent to Medical Home

Pass

Refer[c]

Pediatric Audiologic Evaluation[b]
- ❑ Otoscopic inspection
- ❑ Child & family history
- ❑ Middle ear function
- ❑ OAE*
- ❑ ABR*
- ❑ Frequency-specific tone bursts
- ❑ Air & bone conduction
- ❑ Sedation capability
  (only needed for some infants)

Normal hearing

Hearing loss

Ongoing Care of All Infants[d] from the Medical Home Provider
- Provide parents with information about hearing, speech, and language milestones
- Identify and aggressively treat middle ear disease
- Provide vision screening and referral as needed
- Provide ongoing developmental surveillance and referral to appropriate resources
- Identify and refer for audiologic monitoring infants who have the following risk indicators for late-onset hearing loss:
  — Parental or caregiver concern regarding hearing, speech, language, and/or developmental delay
  — Family history of permanent childhood hearing loss
  — Stigmata or other findings associated with a syndrome known to include a sensorineural or conductive hearing loss or eustachian tube dysfunction
  — Postnatal infections associated with sensorineural hearing loss including bacterial meningitis
  — In utero infections such as cytomegalovirus, herpes, rubella, syphilis, and toxoplasmosis
  — Neonatal indicators—specifically hyperbilirubinemia at a serum level requiring exchange transfusion, persistent pulmonary hypertension of the newborn associated with mechanical ventilation, and conditions requiring the use of extracorporeal membrane oxygenation
  — Syndromes associated with progressive hearing loss such as neurofibromatosis, osteopetrosis, and Usher syndrome
  — Neurodegenerative disorders, such as Hunter syndrome, or sensory motor neuropathies, such as Friedreich ataxia and Charcot-Marie-Tooth disease
  — Head trauma
  — Recurrent or persistent otitis media with effusion for at least 3 months

Report to State EHDI Program
Every child with a permanent hearing loss

Refer to IDEA* Part C
Coordinating agency for early intervention

Medical & Otologic Evaluations
To recommend treatment and provide clearance for hearing aid fitting

Pediatric Audiologic
Hearing aid fitting and monitoring

Advise family
About assistive listening devices (hearing aids, cochlear implants, etc.) and communication options

Before 6 Months

Continued enrollment in IDEA* Part C
(transition to Part B at 3 years of age)

Medical Evaluations To determine etiology and identity related conditions
- ❑ Ophthalmologic (annually)
- ❑ Genetic
- ❑ Developmental pediatrics neurology, cardiology, and nephrology (as needed)

Pediatric Audiologic Services
- ❑ Behavioral response audiometry
- ❑ Ongoing monitoring

*OAF = Otoacoustic Emissions
ABR = Auditory Brainstem Response
AABR = Automated Auditory Brainstem Response
IDEA = Individualism with Disabilities Education Act

Notes:
(a) In screening programs that do not provide Outpatient Screening, infants will be referred directly from Inpatient Screening to Pediatric Audiologic Evaluation. Likewise, infants at higher risk for hearing loss, or loss to follow-up, also may be referred directly to Pediatric Audiologic Evaluation.

(b) Part C of IDEA* may provide diagnostic audiologic evaluation services as part of Child Find activities.

(c) Infants who fail the screening in one or both ears should be referred for further screening or Pediatric Audiologic Evaluation.

(d) Includes infants whose parents refused initial or follow-up hearing screening.

Source: Reprinted by permission of the American Academy of Pediatrics.

(continued)

FIGURE **11.4** (*continued*)

Appropriate Referrals

1. Audiologist knowledgeable in pediatric screening and amplification

Name: _____

Telephone number: _____

Fax: _____

Date of referral: _____

2. Otolaryngologist knowledgeable in pediatric hearing loss

Name: _____

Telephone number: _____

Fax: _____

Date of referral: _____

3. Local early intervention system

Name: _____

Telephone number: _____

Fax: _____

Date of referral: _____

4. Family support resources, financial resources

Name: _____

Telephone number: _____

Fax: _____

Date of referral: _____

5. Speech/language therapy and/or aural rehabilitation therapy

Name: _____

Telephone number: _____

Fax: _____

Date of referral: _____

6. Sign language classes if parents choose manual approach

Name: _____

Telephone number: _____

Fax: _____

Date of referral: _____

7. Ophthalmologist knowledgeable in co-morbid conditons in children with hearing loss

Name: _____

Telephone number: _____

Fax: _____

Date of referral: _____

8. Clinical geneticist knowledgeable in hearing impairment

Name: _____

Telephone number: _____

Fax: _____

Date of referral: _____

9. Equipment vendor(s)

Name: _____

Telephone number: _____

Fax: _____

Date of referral: _____

10. State EHDI coordinator
    http://www:infanthearing.org/status/cnhs.html

Name: _____

Telephone number: _____

Fax: _____

Date of referral: _____

11. AAP Chapter champion http://www:medicalhomeinfo
    .org/screening/Champions%20Roster.pdf

Name: _____

Telephone number: _____

Fax: _____

Date of referral: _____

12. Family physician(s)

Name: _____

Telephone number: _____

Fax: _____

Date of referral: _____

National Resources

Alexander Graham Bell Association for the Deaf and Hard of Hearing (AG Bell)
202/337-5220
www.agbell.org

American Academy of Audiology (AAA)
800/AAA-2336
www.audiology.org

American Academy of Pediatrics
www.aap.org

American Society for Deaf Children
717/334 722
www.deafchildren.org

American Speech-Language-Hearing Association (ASHA)

800/498-2071
www.asha.org

Boys Town Center for Childhood Deafness
www.babyhearing.org

Centers for Disease Control and Prevention
www.cdc.gov/ncbddd/ehdi

Cochlear Implant Association, Inc.
202/895-2781
www.cici.org

Families for Hands and Voices
303/300-9763
www.handsandvoices.org

Laurent Clerc National Deal Education Center and Clearinghouse

at Gallaudet University
www.clerccenter.gallaudet.edu/InfoToGo

National Association of the Deal (NAD)
301/587-1788
www.nad.org

National Center on Hearing Assessment and Management (NCHAM)
www.infanthearing.org

National Institute on Deafness and Other Communication Disorders
www.nidcd.nih.gov

Oberkotter Foundation
www.oraldeafed.org

The primary role of the speech–language pathologist will most likely begin after the initial screening and diagnostic audiological evaluation(s), when an audiological diagnosis has been made. This role is a critical one, and may include providing information to families of newly diagnosed infants with hearing loss about a host of issues. The speech–language pathologist may provide information on the range of communication and parent training options that are available. It will be important for the speech–language pathologist to have skills in functioning on a team that includes the parents, health care provider, audiologist, and other early interventionists (special educator; teacher of the deaf and hard of hearing; ear, nose, and throat physician, etc.).

The speech–language pathologist will be called on to share an abundance of information and resources with the members of the multidisciplinary team. As new born hearing screening programs become a reality in more and more states, a basic understanding of the types of screening techniques typically employed in newborn hearing screening will also be helpful to the practicing speech–language pathologist. Specialists in communication disorders should know the two main screening techniques used—otoacoustic emissions and automated auditory brainstem responses—and should understand what these tools can and cannot tell us about the human auditory system.

Otoacoustic Emissions and Automated Auditory Brainstem Responses

Otoacoustic Emissions (OAEs). Evoked otoacoustic emissions are defined as sounds generated in the cochlea in response to auditory stimuli, which can be measured in the ear canal and arise from activity of outer hair cells. OAEs were discovered by David Kemp in 1978. There are three types of evoked otoacoustic emissions, defined by the type of stimulus used to elicit them:

1. **Distortion product OAEs**—elicited by presenting two tones to the ear
2. **Transient evoked OAEs**—elicited by presenting a transient, or brief, stimulus to the ear, such as a click
3. **Stimulus frequency OAEs**—elicited by presenting a single tone to the ear

The first two types of OAEs listed, distortion product OAEs and transient evoked OAEs, are the most widely used in newborn hearing screening applications. **Spontaneous OAEs,** the fourth type of OAE, do not require a stimulus; rather, this type of OAE can be measured in the ear canal without presenting a stimulus. The drawback to clinical use of spontaneous OAEs is that they are present in only about 50 percent of normal ears. Thus, absence of a spontaneous OAE may or may not be correlated with a deficit in the peripheral auditory system/cochlea.

Otoacoustic emissions are obtained using a probe that is placed in the ear canal. The presence of an emission is contingent on normal outer and middle ear function. Compromised function in the ear's conducting mechanism (e.g., due to fluid or debris remaining in the ear canal after birth or due to a fluid-filled middle ear) will cause the OAE to be obscured. Otoacoustic emissions provide information about the integrity of the auditory system up to the cochlea (inner ear), excluding the auditory nerve. OAEs are thought to reflect activity of the outer hair cells within the cochlea. Since they do not tell us information about the auditory nerve, OAEs may be referred to as a "preneural event." The presence of an OAE is consistent with normal auditory system function up to the cochlea. OAEs are typically absent when hearing thresholds exceed 30 dB.

Transient evoked OAEs are sensitive to the frequency range 1,000–3,000 Hz, which, as you know, contains important information for speech recognition. Transient evoked OAEs are commonly used in newborn hearing screening programs. Distortion product OAEs are the product of two stimulus frequencies that are introduced into the ear canal simultaneously and have a mathematical relationship to one another (2f1 – f2), where f2 is the higher of the two primary tones in the two-tone stimulus. They can reflect various frequencies depending on the stimuli presented. Gorga et al. (2000) found that distortion product OAE measurements in neonates and infants provided useful information at 2,000, 3,000, and 4,000 Hz, and were less reliable at 1,000 Hz due to the effects of noise.

Auditory Brainstem Response.   The **auditory brainstem response (ABR)** reflects information about auditory system function including the inner ear, auditory nerve, and lower brainstem pathways. This is also an evoked response, and can be elicited by presenting brief stimuli, such as clicks, to the ear. Other stimuli, such as tone pips, are sometimes used. The ABR can be described as a brain wave or electrical potential that is generated when the ear is stimulated with sound. Auditory brainstem responses were described by two different groups of workers in the early 1970s: Jewett and Williston (1971) and Lev and Sohmer (1972). They are recorded through the use of surface electrodes and depend on computer averaging techniques that help to extract the signal, or the response being sought, from other ongoing brain activity and outside influences such as movement or muscle activity.

Use of OAE or ABR, either alone or in combination, has made it possible to conduct universal newborn hearing screening without having to rely on risk indicators or behavioral responses to sound. A large, multicenter research study was conducted by Susan Norton and colleagues (2000) to look at the efficacy of the three main screening techniques—automated ABR, distortion product OAE, and transient evoked OAE. Results obtained on newborns using these screening techniques were compared with results of follow-up behavioral testing when the babies were between 8 and 12 months of age. This allowed for confirmation of the screening results. All three screening tools were shown to be effective and reliable for use in newborn hearing screening.

Each of these techniques has advantages and disadvantages relative to use in newborn hearing screening. For example, OAEs are generally faster to administer, but may be contaminated by the presence of debris or fluid in the ear canal in infants 24–48 hours of age. ABRs require the use of more "disposables," such as the pads that secure the electrodes to the scalp, which can result in higher costs for administering the screening. Noise in the environment or from the infant can affect the test time and outcomes for both techniques, with OAE generally more susceptible to the influence of ambient room noise.

Incidence of Hearing Loss

The process of developing and implementing a hearing screening program includes consideration of numerous factors, including the incidence of the target disorder or condition, how the screening will be done, and the type of follow-up that may be needed.

In the case of newborn hearing screening, it is important to know the number of infants expected to be identified with significant hearing loss for program monitoring and evaluation purposes. Additionally, it is important to be aware of the possibility of later-onset hearing losses. This information helps clinicians to educate parents of infants who will receive newborn hearing screening and personnel who are or will be involved in newborn hearing screening efforts.

The incidence of permanent, severe hearing loss in infants is 1 to 3 per 1,000, with an estimated additional 3 infants per 1,000 if moderate degrees of hearing loss are included, according to figures from the American Speech-Language-Hearing Association (1999). Since the goal of infant hearing screening is to find those infants with permanent hearing loss, it is important to be aware of these figures. What might this mean for a hearing screening program in which a hospital screens infants for hearing loss prior to discharge? Could the hospital screen the first 500 infants and have all the babies pass the screening? Since 1 to 3 per 1,000 infants are expected to have a permanent hearing loss, it is quite possible that the first 500 screenings completed in the well-baby nursery would not result in the identification of any infants with hearing loss. Do you think it would be important for the staff and administrators of the hospital to be aware of this information? Yes, because this knowledge is critical to program management and evaluation efforts. Clearly, if half of the babies did not pass the screening, troubleshooting would be needed to determine the reason(s) for so many unexpected screening failures.

Expectations will be different for screening failures in a **neonatal intensive care unit (NICU)**. Data from the New York State Newborn Hearing Screening Demonstration Project (Prieve et al., 2000) compared screening failures in the well-baby nursery (WBN) and the NICU, and showed that the prevalence of hearing loss varies with nursery type. Specifically, the prevalence of permanent hearing loss in the NICU population was 8/1,000; in the WBN, the prevalence of permanent hearing loss was approximately 1/1,000. Thus, hospital staff screening infants in the NICU would expect to find more babies with permanent hearing loss. In this case, finding that 500 consecutive infants passed the hearing screening would be unlikely.

Protocols and Screening Levels

Sensitivity and specificity remain among the important factors in selecting screening protocols for this population. Although no screening tool is perfect, the goal should be to identify as many infants at risk for significant hearing loss as possible, while minimizing overreferrals or "false alarms." Limiting overreferrals for follow-up screening is a major concern. Data from the Norton et al. (2000) multicenter study and the New York State Universal Newborn Hearing Screening Demonstration Project (Prieve et al., 2000) suggest that the use of a two-stage inpatient screening protocol (two screenings prior to discharge) in newborn hearing screening programs can reduce the number of infants who are referred for additional testing. Generally, refer rates of 8 to 10 percent can be anticipated if infant hearing screening is done using OAEs alone. Use of OAE followed by an ABR for those infants who do not pass the initial screen results in referral rates of 3 to 5 percent.

Specific selection of pass and fail (refer) criteria for each technique will also have an impact on the number of babies who pass or do not pass the hearing screening. Defining the stimulus parameters for use in newborn hearing screening has been a challenge. This is due in part to the available equipment, and evolving information about correlations between results of objective (electrophysiologic or otoacoustic) measures to behavioral measures of hearing. The stimulus parameters used by Norton et al. (2000) were as follows:

Transient evoked OAE—stimulus was an 80-dB SPL click

Distortion product OAE—stimulus was $L1 = 65$ and $L2 = 50$ dB SPL

AABR—stimulus was a 30-dB nHL click

The authors concluded that these techniques and the specified screening parameters worked well as predictors of permanent hearing loss of 30 dB or greater. This was determined by comparing screening results with confirmatory diagnostic tests completed when the infants were between 8 and 12 months corrected age. The "gold standard" applied was behavioral testing (visual reinforcement audiometry) at 8–12 months corrected age. Although no technique performed perfectly, both OAE and ABR were found to be reliable screening tools. Use of a two-stage protocol, as mentioned earlier, was an effective way to reduce the referral rate. This is important because a high referral rate will result in infants and families pursuing unnecessary follow-up screening and/or diagnostic testing, in addition to the worry and anxiety that are associated with a positive screening outcome.

Interpretation of Results and Conveying Screening Information

Training screeners in the performance of newborn hearing screening should address how information is to be conveyed to the parents of infants following the screening. Ideally, parents should receive information about their baby's hearing screening as soon after the screening as possible. For example, this is a prime opportunity to educate families of infants who pass the screening about monitoring their child's language and speech development, or signs that suggest that their child is experiencing an intermittent conductive hearing loss or a late-onset permanent hearing loss. Families of infants who do not pass the initial screening must be provided with information about follow-up, including the importance of follow-up and how to go about obtaining follow-up. Procedures should be developed to ensure that parents get the information they need and have an opportunity to ask any questions they have. Involving the infant's primary health care provider is an important part of this process.

The number of states participating in newborn hearing screening in the United States is growing. Screening of infants prior to discharge from the hospital is the most common approach, and a variety of personnel may be engaged in the conduct of newborn hearing screening. Such personnel may include nurses, audiologists, or trained technicians, or paraprofessionals. The techniques used for newborn hearing screening include otoacoustic emissions and (automated) auditory brainstem response. It has been shown that in most newborn hearing screening programs, fewer referrals occur after the first 6 months to 1 year of program operation. Factors in reducing the referral rate include refining screening protocols, increased experience of the personnel performing the screening, and controlling for environmental factors such as noise.

Newborn Hearing Screening Follow-up

Newborn hearing screening programs must be viewed in a broader sense, beyond the actual performance of the screening. The program must include providing follow-up diagnostic audiological evaluations for those infants who do not pass the screening, for aural habilitation for those infants who are identified with permanent hearing loss, and for evaluation of the overall program to determine whether the original goals are being met or if modifications are needed. Work by Yoshinaga-Itano et al. (1998) showed that infants with hearing loss who received intervention early (by age 6 months) had age-appropriate language outcomes through age 3 years. The American Academy of Pediatrics Task Force on Newborn and Infant Hearing (1999) includes tracking and follow-up as integral parts of programs designed for early identification of hearing loss. Program evaluation will likely include data collection and analysis to determine whether the infants that do not pass the screening are ultimately identified and provided with appropriate early intervention services.

Follow-up after newborn hearing screening has not kept pace with performance of the screening itself. The Centers for Disease Control and Prevention (CDC) track newborn hearing screening data, compiling reports from states about their newborn hearing screening programs. Data from a 2004 CDC report (www.cdc.gov/ncbddd/ehdi/2004/DIPS_2004_final.pdf) indicate that just below 49 percent of babies referred for a diagnostic audiological evaluation had received one. Primus (2005) points out that a successful newborn hearing program is one in which identified individuals receive appropriate follow-up audiological services. What are some barriers to effective follow-up after newborn hearing screening? Nemes (2006) summarizes a number of barriers to getting infants from a failed newborn hearing screening to a diagnostic audiological evaluation, including:

- A shortage of pediatric audiologists with the necessary skills for evaluating young infants and fitting them with hearing aids
- Insufficient training in working with young infants in professional education programs for audiologists
- Inadequate data management systems in some states to effectively track and manage failed screenings
- Lack of effective services for young children diagnosed with milder degrees of hearing loss
- Lack of information among physicians on the referral process for infants with suspected hearing loss
- Insufficient education of families about the consequences of late-identified hearing loss.

Efforts are under way on multiple fronts to eliminate these barriers to successful newborn hearing screening programs. For example, curricula in audiology preparation programs are being updated to include training in the audiological assessment and hearing aid fitting techniques necessary for working with young infants. The Joint Committee on Infant Hearing is developing a new position statement that will focus on follow-up (diagnostic testing and intervention) for young children who fail an initial hearing screening. The resources section at the end of this chapter contains the Web address for the JCIH and several other organizations that have been closely involved in developing and improving early hearing detection and intervention (EHDI) programs.

All clinicians working with infants and toddlers and their families must understand what newborn hearing screening results tell us, what the results of diagnostic testing mean, and how to facilitate obtaining hearing habilitation services in the community. Program requirements may vary somewhat depending on the specific requirements of the state or municipality in which people live. Generally, early intervention programs require primary referral sources, such as physicians, nurses, speech–language pathologists, and other professionals, who have identified an infant or toddler at risk of a disability to make a referral to early intervention unless the parent objects. In order for EHDI programs to be successful, clinicians must familiarize themselves with the referral requirements and protocols in their area so that valuable time is not wasted when an infant is at risk for, or is suspected of having, a hearing loss. The lead agencies and Part C Coordinators (Part C of the Individuals with Disabilities Education Act is the federal law that governs early intervention programs) for early intervention systems in each state are available at www.nectac.org, which is the Web site of the National Early Childhood Technical Assistance Center.

It is well established that, in the absence of universal newborn hearing screening, the average age of identification of permanent childhood hearing loss can be over 2 years of age. Since no screening is perfect and we cannot account for late-onset or progressive hearing losses with newborn hearing screening, professionals must remain vigilant in their efforts to ensure that all children with hearing loss are correctly identified as early as possible. Speech–language and audiology professionals are uniquely qualified to make appropriate referrals for screening or formal diagnostic testing and to inform and educate parents and professionals of other disciplines about communication milestones and communication development. In short, even with widespread newborn hearing screening, clinicians must remember that some children with hearing loss may come to our attention through different avenues. Another important point is that screening results represent a point in time, and do not exclude the possibility of hearing loss, either transient or permanent, at a later age.

It is important for speech–language pathologists and other professionals to keep this information in mind when they receive referrals of young children due to concerns about development. Screening in the field of communication disorders frequently results in more than a binary (pass/refer) outcome. In other words, rather than obtaining a yes or no result with a straightforward treatment decision, professionals in the field of communication disorders are often faced with multiple decisions when they conduct screening. Even when the child passes a particular screening, it is not unusual for clinicians to conclude that additional referral(s) may be warranted. Sometimes these conclusions are the result of careful listening to parents' concerns or of observations of the child made during the screening process. Some of these decisions may include referrals to other disciplines to rule out, for example, motor involvement or developmental delay. Audiologists conducting preschool hearing screenings may make observations about the speech of children during the screening process and refer those children for speech/language screening or evaluation.

Preschool Screening

Even though universal newborn screening is rapidly becoming the norm nationally, there will unfortunately still be children who will have unidentified hearing loss in the preschool years. These children may have progressive losses that were originally slight enough that they were able to pass initial screenings, or they may have late-onset losses that did not develop until some time after birth. For these reasons it is important that screenings be in place at different times in a child's life. It is equally important for parents to continue to monitor their child's responsiveness to auditory stimuli (even if an initial screening has been passed) and to follow up on any suspected hearing loss.

If you think back to Chapter 7 and our discussion of otitis media and Eustachian tube dysfunction, you will remember that preschoolers are at great risk for this middle ear condition that can create conductive hearing impairment. Because the preschool period is one of tremendous language and cognitive growth, it is important to ensure that the child's hearing sensitivity is adequate for these purposes. A child with fluctuating conductive hearing loss is at risk for disruption in the development of these areas.

Middle ear infection (otitis media) is the most common disease in early childhood (Northern & Downs, 2002). It is estimated that 75 percent of all 2-year-old children have experienced a temporary conductive hearing loss at some time in their life due to this condition. Thirty-three percent of children in the general population and 80 percent of children attending day care centers have had at least three episodes of otitis media by the age of 3 years (Denny, 1984; Preliner, Kalm, & Harsten, 1992; Teele, Klein, & Rosner, 1984).

Sensorineural hearing loss is less common in preschoolers than conductive hearing loss but nonetheless does occur. In fact, the milder degrees of congenital sensorineural hearing loss and unilateral sensorineural hearing losses are typically still not identified at 3 years of age. It has been established that even milder degrees of hearing loss can interfere with the language and academic growth of the child.

Testing Protocol

For preschoolers, a combination of equipment will be required, including a pure tone audiometer, an otoscope, and a **tympanometer.** In cases when the screening is done at a site such as a preschool or day care center, portable equipment may be necessary. Let's discuss each of these briefly.

For children between the ages of 3 and 5 years, ASHA (1997a) recommends pure tone testing under earphones at 1,000, 2,000, and 4,000 Hz at 20 dB HL. Note that 500 Hz is not included because it increases the chance of false positive findings, as discussed previously. Also note that two of the three frequencies included in the screening protocol are high frequencies, reflecting the important goal of ruling out a loss in this range that will likely interfere with speech and language development. Remember that the pure tone part of the screening is for purposes of identifying peripheral hearing loss.

In order to identify outer and middle ear pathology, the screening includes case history data, otoscopy, and tympanometry (middle ear screening). If case history or otoscopy reveal any of the following, a referral for medical examination is urged, according to ASHA (1997a):

- Drainage from the ear
- Ear pain
- Structural anomalies of the ear that were not previously identified
- Ear canal abnormalities (e.g., wax impaction, blood, foreign body, atresia, stenosis)
- Eardrum abnormalities or perforations

It should be noted that many audiologists refer to otoscopy as **nondiagnostic otoscopy,** because its purpose is not to diagnose, but rather to identify gross structural abnormalities or blockage. Otoscopy is also necessary whenever tympanometry is done, because it is not safe to insert a probe into the ear canal without first examining the canal.

Regarding tympanometry, ASHA (1997a) suggests that medical referral be made if a flat tracing is noted in the presence of a large equivalent ear canal volume reading. Remember that this combination can suggest a perforation of the eardrum. The exception to this is the case in which a functioning pressure equalization (PE) tube exists, because an open tube will also create a large volume reading. ASHA also recommends that **peak compensated static acoustic admittance** and **tympanometric width** be the measures used in the tympanometric screening. Specifically, if static admittance is too low or tympanometric width is too wide, the child has failed the screening and a rescreen should be arranged. See Table 11.2 for normative data. You can also refer to the

TABLE 11.2 Middle Ear Screening Guidelines		
Aspect of Screening	**Referral Criteria**	**Recommendation**
Case history/otoscopy	Ear drainage Ear pain Structural abnormalities of the ear (not already identified and known to a physician) Abnormalities of the ear canal or eardrum (not already identified and known to a physician)	Refer for medical examination
Tympanometry Ear canal volume	If greater than 1.0 cc and the tympanogram is flat	Refer for medical examination (unless a pressure equalization tube is present or if a known eardrum perforation exists for which the client is already under the care of a physician).
Peak compensated static admittance	Infants: less than 0.2 mmho 1 year to school age: less than 0.3 mmho 6 years and older: less than 0.4 mmho (when using ± 400 daPa for compensation)	Refer for rescreen; if rescreen is failed, refer for medical. Subsequent to medical, rescreen or pursue diagnostic assessment to monitor middle ear function. If rescreen is passed, monitor middle ear status through subsequent rescreening.
Tympanometric width	Infants: greater than 235 daPa 1 year to school-age: greater than 200 daPa	Refer for rescreen; if rescreen is failed, refer for medical. Subsequent to medical, rescreen or pursue diagnostic assessment to monitor middle ear function. If rescreen is passed, monitor middle ear status through subsequent rescreening.

Source: Based on ASHA (1997a) and American Academy of Audiology (1992).

ASHA (1997a) *Guidelines for Audiological Screening* for additional information regarding recommended initial tympanometric screening test criteria.

Recording and Interpretation of Data

Refer to previous sections for information regarding appropriate wording and to Appendix A for suggested content for forms used to report screening findings.

Combined Screenings

Sometimes, clinicians of various disciplines will work together on combined hearing and speech–language screenings with preschoolers, or hearing screenings combined with another type of developmental screening. This is certainly a logical combination, because preschoolers are in the midst of a period of great cognitive, developmental, and language growth, all of which may be affected by their hearing status. Just as the hearing screening should meet certain standards for reliability, validity, sensitivity, and specificity, other screening tools chosen as part of the screening must also conform to some standards. Remember, whenever we administer brief tests (a necessity when screening), reliability may suffer. Examples of screening tools that may be useful for the speech–language component of a combined speech–language–hearing screening for preschoolers are

- Preschool Language Scale—4
- Brief spontaneous language sample
- Goldman-Fristoe Test of Articulation
- Brief oral-motor exam

Screening for School-Age Children

Background and Rationale

Regardless of the age of the population being screened, the reason for screening must be clear so that program evaluators can determine whether the goals of the program have been met. In the case of hearing screening for school-age children, one program goal is ensuring that these children are hearing normally so they can function optimally in the auditory-verbal environment of most classrooms. Without access to the auditory-oral language of the classroom, children in school are at a considerable disadvantage. In addition to identifying and ensuring appropriate care for students with hearing loss, other program goals can include communication of information to teachers of students with hearing loss and providing accommodations to assist those students.

Incidence

It is helpful for program planners to know the expected incidence of the target condition(s) of the screening program. The incidence of hearing loss in the school-age population may be considered for the two main types of hearing loss—conductive and sensorineural. ASHA (1993) includes figures suggesting that the incidence of hearing loss in children from birth to age 18 years may be as high as 5 percent. Conductive hearing loss and the associated mild to moderate hearing loss is most common in early childhood and can continue until the child reaches the age of 8 to 10 years. Sensorineural hearing loss is estimated to affect 10 per 1,000 students. The incidence of hearing loss in students in special education programs is higher than in the general school population. In recognition of this, program planners may choose to incorporate more frequent screening for this group. Other conditions, such as (central) auditory processing disorders, discussed in Chapter 10, can have an impact on a student's academic performance. If the goal of screening is to rule out the need for further auditory processing evaluation, the screening technique should be selected with this in mind. For purposes of this discussion, ruling out peripheral hearing loss will be the primary focus.

Interface between Audiology and Speech–Language Pathology

ASHA's *Preferred Practice Patterns for the Profession of Audiology* (1997c) includes a section (01.0) on audiological screening (as performed by an audiologist). Relative to school-age children, this section specifies that children should have their hearing screened annually from kindergarten to third grade and then in seventh and eleventh grades, with additional screening if concerns arise. Children with known hearing loss often receive annual audiological reevaluation and therefore do not participate in the school hearing screening schedule. Section 01.0 includes additional information, such as safety and health precautions, and recommends that universal precautions be followed.

For children in this age group, conventional audiometric techniques are typically employed during screening, and conditioned play audiometry (CPA) techniques may be used as needed. ASHA recommends that screening be done at 20 dB HL in the frequency region 1,000–4,000 Hz. The purpose of air conduction screening is to establish whether additional hearing testing is warranted. Passing the air conduction screening suggests that the student has peripheral hearing sensitivity in the normal range for the selected frequencies, which provide important components of the speech signal.

Screening procedures may differ somewhat depending on policies of a particular state or school district. Policies and procedures should address who will conduct the screening, the applicable pass/refer criteria, documentation, and follow-up procedures. ASHA's (1997a) *Guidelines for Audiological Screening,* Hearing Impairment—School-Age Children, 5 through 18 Years, can be referred to for additional details on this topic.

In addition to the protocols recommended by professional organizations for clinicians specializing in communication disorders, state departments of education may have developed policies and procedures for hearing screening programs in schools under their jurisdiction. For example, the topics that might be included in such policies and procedures include the purpose of the school hearing screening program, the legislative background, specific information about who should receive hearing screening, and how often screening should occur. The screening procedure may also be specified, including procedures for follow-up and informing parents and teachers of the results. Clinicians should be aware of the particular policies and procedures in effect in the school district where they work.

Tympanometry

If the purpose of screening is to discover hearing loss, air conduction screening is the method of choice for school-age children. If, however, detection of middle ear disorders is the goal of screening, then use of tympanometry is the preferred method. Clearly, if the purpose of screening is to identify both hearing loss and middle ear disorders, a combination of pure tone screening and tympanometry should be employed. The incidence of middle ear dysfunction is known to peak in early childhood, so tympanometry is often included in screening of young children. Screening programs for school-age children are less likely to incorporate tympanometric screening as a routine; however, program planners may opt to include tympanometry for certain populations with known risk indicators such as a history of otitis media or learning disabilities. Examples of indicators that warrant including tympanometric screening are found in Table 11.3.

Whether the equipment used for tympanometric screening has diagnostic capability or only screening capability, program planners should establish pass/refer criteria and a plan for management for those students who do not pass the middle ear screening. Specific components of the screening should include a brief history, otoscopy, middle ear screening via tympanometry, documentation of findings, and recommended follow-up. Great care must be taken to design the screening protocol in a way that the number of overreferrals to health care providers is kept to a minimum. For example, use of a two-stage screening protocol, with the follow-up screening following the initial screening by 6 to 8 weeks, can effectively reduce the number of referrals for medical follow-up. Specific techniques for conducting tympanometry and interpretation of the results obtained are presented in detail in Chapter 6.

Role and Responsibilities of the Speech–Language Pathologist

The speech–language pathologist in the school is in a unique position to assist in identifying children with suspected hearing loss and helping them obtain hearing screening to confirm or rule out the need for further audiologic evaluation. Collaboration with classroom teachers is one way to accomplish this goal. Anderson's (1989) **Screening Instrument for Targeting Educational Risk (SIFTER)** is a tool that can be used to open a dialogue between the speech–language pathologist and the classroom teacher, and can be helpful in identifying students who are at risk for hearing loss. The SIFTER asks the observer to rate a student's classroom performance in five areas—academics, attention, communication, class participation, and school behavior. Students found to have indicators of difficulty can then be referred for hearing screening and/or other appropriate screening or evaluation.

ASHA's *Preferred Practice Patterns for the Profession of Speech–Language Pathology* (1997d) includes a section (01.0) on audiological screening as performed by speech–language pathologists that defines screening and further clarifies the role of the speech–language pathologists in conducting hearing screening. In this context, screening

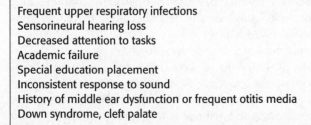

TABLE 11.3 Indicators That Tympanometric Screening Should Be Included

Frequent upper respiratory infections
Sensorineural hearing loss
Decreased attention to tasks
Academic failure
Special education placement
Inconsistent response to sound
History of middle ear dysfunction or frequent otitis media
Down syndrome, cleft palate

is defined as "a pass/fail procedure to identify individuals who require further audiologic assessment or referral for other professional and/or medical services" (p. 56).

ASHA (1997d) further specifies that speech–language pathologists are limited to pure tone air conduction and screening tympanometry for initial identification and/or referral purposes. Further, ASHA requires that documentation by the speech–language pathologist performing hearing screening should contain "a statement of identifying information, screening results, and recommendations, including the need for rescreening, assessment, or referral" (p. 56). The recommended content is summarized in Appendix A.

Training Screening Personnel

Personnel conducting hearing screening for school-age children may include audiologists, speech–language pathologists, and school nurse–teachers. Depending on the regulations governing the conduct of hearing screening in a particular locality, other individuals may be permitted to perform hearing screening in the schools with the appropriate training. From the preceding discussion of screening protocols, it can be seen that training of personnel performing hearing screening in the schools should address the following:

- Knowledge of risk indicators for hearing loss
- Signs of hearing loss
- Procedures used for screening (including the location and how to administer the screening)
- Familiarity with the equipment used for screening (pure tone audiometer and/or acoustic admittance/tympanometry equipment)
- Health and safety precautions
- Criteria for passing/failing the screening
- Documentation of screening results
- Follow-up procedures for students who fail the screening, including notification of parents and educators or "next steps"

In addition to the general screening guidelines in this chapter, general guidance on conducting hearing screening and practical information on pitfalls to avoid in screening are included in Table 11.4 for reference purposes.

Audiological Screening of Adults

The ASHA (1997a) guidelines for adult hearing screenings are divided into three sections: screening for hearing disorders, screening for hearing impairment, and screening for hearing disability. The section that follows briefly describes these three screening protocols as used with noninstitutionalized adults.

Hearing disorders include otological or anatomic abnormalities of the ear and are screened using a case history and otoscopy. As expected, the suggested case history (found in Appendix B), includes questions concerning potential medical issues, such as presence of dizziness, ear pain or drainage, unilateral hearing loss, and tinnitus. The screening is failed, and an immediate medical referral is made, if the client responds positively to any of these items and has not yet informed his or her physician about

TABLE 11.4 Pitfalls to Avoid in Hearing Screening and Immittance Screening

Hearing Screening Pitfalls

Child observing dials. This should be avoided at all times, because children will respond to the visual cues. The most appropriate position to seat the child is at an oblique angle, so the tester and audiometer are out of the child's peripheral vision.

Examiner giving visual cues (facial expression, eye or head movements, etc.).

Incorrect adjustment of the head band and earphone placement. Care must be taken to place the earphones carefully over the ears so that the protective screen mesh of the earphone diaphragm is directly over the entrance of the external auditory canal. Misplacement of the earphone by only 1 inch can cause as great as a 30–35 dB threshold shift.

Vague instructions.

Noise in the test area.

Overlong test sessions. The screening should require only 3–5 minutes. If a child requires significantly more time that this, the routine screening should be discontinued, and a short rest taken. If the child continues to be difficult to test, play conditioning should be used.

Too long or too short a presentation of the test tone. The test stimulus should be presented for 1–2 seconds. If the stimulus is for a shorter or longer time that this, inaccurate responses may be obtained.

Immittance Screening Pitfalls

Clogged probe and probe tip. The probe and probe tips must be kept free from earwax.

Probe tip too large or too small. Each ear canal is different and may require a different-sized probe tip. Utilization of the correct size for each child will avoid possible errors.

Head movement, swallowing, or eye-blinks. The child should be kept still during testing, as a sudden abnormal movement during testing may be interpreted as a reflex.

Probe tip against ear canal wall. The probe tip must be inserted directly into the ear canal, and when the canal is not straight, the tip must be kept away from the canal wall.

Debris in ear canal. The ear canal should be inspected before testing to ensure that it is clear.

Source: Northern, J., & Downs, M. (2002). *Hearing in children* (5th ed.). New York: Lippincott, Williams & Wilkins. Reprinted by permission.

them. A referral is also warranted if the tester notes any physical abnormality or cerumen blockage during otoscopy.

You may be thinking that admittance (tympanometry) would be a valuable tool in the screening of hearing disorders. ASHA (1997a) states that because of the low incidence of middle ear pathology in adults, admittance should not be substituted for visual inspection of the ear. Some audiologists do add a tympanometric screening to the above protocol.

The second aspect of audiological screening for adults is to screen for hearing loss. Remember that the purpose of this is to identify those individuals who are in need of further audiological assessment. ASHA (1997a) recommends use of a 25-dB intensity level and inclusion of the frequencies 1,000, 2,000, and 4,000 Hz. A referral is made if the client fails any one frequency in either ear.

The final aspect of audiological hearing screening in adults is to screen for **hearing disability,** which refers to how the hearing impairment interferes with the client's ability to carry out those activities that are important in his life. These may include social, vocational, or educational activities, to name just a few. Hearing disability is typically screened using some type of inventory, questionnaire, or survey. ASHA provides pass/refer criteria for one such instrument (Hearing Handicap Inventory for the Elderly—Screening Version; Ventry & Weinstein, 1983) reproduced in Appendix C. It is important that in choosing instruments, clinicians attend carefully to the psychometric properties of the tool, including reliability and validity.

Before moving to the next section of this discussion, a distinction should be made between the screening of adults and the screening of the elderly. This distinction is important because hearing loss increases with age, and we do not want our screening to result in referral of large numbers of individuals who do not present with a hearing handicap. In fact, despite ASHA's recommendation to screen adults using a 25-dB intensity level, Schow's (1991) research suggests that use of an intensity level of 25 dB when screening the elderly may result in overreferrals.

Based on the available evidence, it appears reasonable to use a combination protocol that includes hearing handicap scales and pure tones in the 30- to 35-dB range as a first approximation. It may also be useful to give the client's report of hearing handicap primary importance (over the pure tone findings) as a way to limit referrals to those clients who report true hearing handicap.

Related to avoiding overreferrals, it should be noted that a strong correlation exists between hearing sensitivity at 2,000 Hz and the degree of hearing handicap. Based on early studies of filtered speech and clinical observation, it is clear that individuals who have good hearing at 2,000 Hz, even if hearing loss exists at frequencies above 2,000 Hz, perform relatively well on speech recognition tasks if the listening environment is quiet. This is important to note, because it reinforces the point that some clients will fail their hearing screening but will not necessarily be experiencing difficulty hearing in quiet environments. Referral to an audiologist may not be essential for these clients.

Another distinction that is important when discussing the audiological screening of adults is the distinction between individuals who are institutionalized and those who are not. We have just described protocols for noninstitutionalized individuals. According to the ASHA *Guidelines for Audiology Service Delivery in Nursing Homes* (ASHA, 1997b), the vast majority of individuals who reside in nursing homes are funded through Medicaid, and this federal funding requires that the facilities complete a form entitled the Minimum Data Set for Nursing Home Resident Assessment and Care Screening (MDS). Included on this form are questions regarding a variety of issues pertaining to the client's physical health and emotional well-being, as well as questions regarding the client's perception of his or her hearing ability and use of amplification. Further, ASHA recommends that the person conducting the screening make observations about the client's need to have questions repeated, the family's perception of hearing difficulty, and client's complaints of ear pain. Although ASHA guidelines emphasize the use of pure tone screening, they also acknowledge that this is not always possible in nursing home settings, and state that problems on the MDS are sufficient to trigger referral for comprehensive audiological assessment.

In cases where audiological screenings are performed in nursing home settings, the likelihood that special techniques, such as play audiometry, will be required increases. Consult Chapter 8, where play audiometry is discussed, and Chapter 9, where characteristics of different populations and potential effects on hearing assessment are reviewed.

Finally, it is important to make a brief comment about the use of children's materials and activities with adult populations. It is crucial that the examiner be sensitive to the fact that the client, although having difficulty performing the tasks involved in hearing screening, may be acutely aware that the materials she is being asked to use are more commonly used with children. Although most clients typically do not display negative reactions to this, it remains important for the examiner to monitor client reactions and to communicate respect to the client in as many ways as possible. For adults who need greater amounts of support during hearing screening, use of more concrete materials and activities is not offensive as long as the client believes that the examiner respects him.

CHAPTER SUMMARY

This chapter presented information on screening for hearing loss in people of all ages. The nature of screening was discussed, including relevant concepts such as sensitivity, specificity, overreferral, and underreferral. Screening techniques for infants, preschoolers, school-age children, adults, and the elderly were addressed. Principles to remember and decisions to be made when embarking on a screening program were discussed relative to audiologists and speech–language pathologists. The importance of tracking and follow-up were emphasized.

QUESTIONS FOR DISCUSSION

1. Discuss the reciprocal relationship that exists between sensitivity and specificity. Include the advantages and disadvantages of high sensitivity and high specificity.
2. Construct a table in which you compare and contrast the screening protocols for individuals of different ages.
3. List five things that parents of infants who have received newborn hearing screening should know.
4. Discuss three ways to improve newborn hearing screening follow-up.
5. Differentiate the information provided through screening versus information obtained through a diagnostic evaluation.
6. Discuss five clues that might alert a classroom teacher that a student may have hearing loss.

RECOMMENDED READING

American Speech-Language-Hearing Association Audiological Assessment Panel 1996. (1997). *Guidelines for audiological screening.* Rockville, MD: ASHA.

Joint Committee on Infant Hearing. (2000, August). Year 2000 position statement: Principles and guidelines for early hearing detection and intervention program. *Audiology Today, 12,* special issue.

Lankford, J., & Hopkins, C. (2000). Ambient noise levels in nursing homes: Implications for audiometric assessment. *American Journal of Audiology, 9,* 30–35.

Ventry, I., & Weinstein, B. (1983). Identification of elderly people with hearing problems. *ASHA, 25,* 37–42.

Spivak, L. (1998). *Universal newborn hearing screening.* New York: Thieme.

Additional Resources

The following organizations have additional information about newborn hearing screening programs, also known as early hearing detection and intervention (EHDI) programs:

The National Center for Hearing Assessment and Management (NCHAM): www.infanthearing.org

The Joint Committee on Infant Hearing (JCIH): www.jcih.org

Health Resources and Services Administration (HRSA)/Maternal and Child Health Bureau: http://mchb.hrsa.gov

Centers for Disease Control and Prevention (CDC): www.cdc.gov

REFERENCES

American Academy of Audiology. (1992). *Audiologic guidelines for the diagnosis and treatment of otitis media in children.* McLean, VA: Author.

American Academy of Pediatrics Task Force on Newborn and Infant Hearing. (1999). Newborn and infant hearing loss: Detection and intervention. *Pediatrics, 103,* 527–530.

American Academy of Pediatrics. (2002). *Universal newborn hearing screening, diagnosis, and intervention: Guidelines for pediatric medical home providers.* Elk Grove Village, IL: Author.

American National Standards Institute (ANSI). (1999). Maximum permissible ambient noise for audiometric test rooms ANSI S3.1-1999. New York: Author.

American Speech-Language-Hearing Association (ASHA). (1993). Guidelines for audiology services in the schools. *ASHA, 35*(Suppl. 10), 24–32.

American Speech-Language-Hearing Association (ASHA). (1996a, Spring). Scope of practice in audiology. *ASHA, 38*(Suppl. 16), 12–15.

American Speech-Language-Hearing Association (ASHA). (1996b, Spring). Scope of practice in speech–language pathology. *ASHA, 38*(Suppl. 16), 16–20.

American Speech-Language-Hearing Association Audiological Assessment Panel 1996. (1997a). *Guidelines for audiological screening.* Rockville, MD: Author.

American Speech-Language-Hearing Association (ASHA). (1997b, Spring). Guidelines for audiology service delivery in nursing homes. *ASHA, 39*(Suppl. 17), 15–29.

American Speech-Language-Hearing Association (ASHA). (1997c). *Preferred practice patterns for the profession of audiology.* Rockville, MD: Author.

American Speech-Language-Hearing Association (ASHA). (1997d). *Preferred practice patterns for the profession of speech–language pathology.* Rockville, MD: Author.

American Speech-Language-Hearing Association (ASHA). (1999). Facts on hearing loss in children. Available at: www.asha.org /infanthearing/facts.htm

Anderson, K. (1989). *Screening Instrument for Targeting Educational Risk (SIFTER).* Austin, TX: Pro-Ed.

Denny, F. (1984). Otitis media. *Pediatric News, 18,* 38.

Doyle, J. (1997). *Audiology for the speech–language pathologist.* London: Whurr.

Gorga, M. P., Norton, S. J., Sininger, Y. S., Cone-Wesson, B., Folsom, R. C., Vohr, B. R., Widen, J. E., & Neely, S. T. (2000). Identification of neonatal hearing impairment: Distortion product otoacoustic emissions during the perinatal period. *Ear and Hearing, 21*(5), 400.

Jewett, D., & Williston, J. (1971). Auditory evoked far fields averaged from the scalp of humans. *Brain, 4,* 681–696.

Joint Committee on Infant Hearing (JCIH). (2000, August). Year 2000 position statement: Principles and guidelines for early hearing detection and intervention programs. *Audiology Today, 12,* special issue, 7–27.

Kemp, D. (1978). Stimulated acoustic emission from the human auditory system. *Journal of the Acoustic Society of America, 64,* 1386–1391.

Kenworthy, O. (1993). Early identification: Principles and practices. In J. Alpiner & P. McCarthy (Eds.), *Rehabilitative audiology: Children and adults.* Baltimore: Williams & Wilkins.

Kileny, P., & Lesperance, M. (2001). Evidence in support of a different model of universal newborn hearing loss identification. *American Journal of Audiology, 10*(2), 65–67.

Lev, A., & Sohmer, H. (1972). Sources of averaged neural responses recorded in animal and human subjects during cochlear audiometry. *Archives Klin Exp Ohren Nasen Kehlokopfheilkd, 201,* 79–90.

Lichtenstein, M., Bess, F., & Logan, S. (1988). Diagnostic performance of the hearing handicap inventory for the elderly (screening version)

425

•

**Appendix A:
Sample Content to
Include in Forms
for Reporting
Hearing Screening
Results**

against differing definitions of hearing loss. *Ear and Hearing, 9,* 209–211.

Nemes, Judith. (2006). Success of infant screening creates urgent need for better follow-up. *The Hearing Journal, 59*(4), 21–28.

Nicolosi, L., Harryman, E., & Kresheck, J. (1989). *Terminology of communication disorders: Speech-language-hearing* (3rd ed.). Baltimore: Williams & Wilkins.

Northern, J., & Downs, M. (2002). *Hearing in children* (5th ed.). New York: Lippincott, Williams & Wilkins.

Norton, S., Gorga, M., Widen, J., Folsom, R., Sininger, Y., Cone-Wesson, B., Vohr, B., & Fletcher, K. (2000). Identification of neonatal hearing impairment: Summary and recommendations. *Ear and Hearing, 21*(5), 529–535.

Preliner, K., Kalm, O., & Harsten, G. (1992). Middle ear problems in childhood. *Acta Otolaryngologica Supplement, 493,* 93–98.

Prieve, B., Dalzell, L., Berg, A., Bradley, M., Cacace, A., Campbell, D., DeCristoforo, J., Gravel, J., Greenberg, E., Gross, S., Orlando, M., Pinhiero, J., Regan, J., Spivak, L., & Stevens, F. (2000). The New York State Universal Newborn Hearing Screening Demonstration Project: Outpatient outcome measures. *Ear and Hearing, 21*(2).

Primus, Michael A. (2005) Newborn hearing screening follow-up: The essential next step. *The Hearing Review,* 18–19.

Schow, R. (1991). Considerations in selecting and validating an adult/elderly hearing screening protocol. *Ear and Hearing, 12*(5), 337–347.

Teele, D., Klein, J., Rosner, B., & The Greater Boston Otitis Media Study Group. (1984). Otitis media with effusion during the first three years of life and development of speech and language. *Pediatrics, 74,* 282–287.

U.S. Department of Health and Human Services (DHHS). (2000, January). *Healthy people 2010* (conference ed., in two volumes). Washington, DC: Author.

Ventry, I., & Weinstein, B. (1983). Identification of elderly people with hearing problems. *ASHA, 25,* 37–42.

Yoshinaga-Itano, C., Sedey, A., Coulter, D., & Mehl, A. (1998). Language of early- and later-identified children with hearing loss. *Pediatrics, 102,* 1161–1171.

Appendix A
Sample Content to Include in Forms for Reporting Hearing Screening Results

ASHA (1997a) provides information on documentation of screening results, and specifies that documentation should contain a statement of identifying information; impairment, disorder, and disability screening results; and recommendations, including the need for rescreening, audiological assessment, counseling, or referral.

The companion document regarding audiological screening performed by speech–language pathologists indicates that documentation should include a statement of identifying information, screening results, and recommendations including the need for rescreening, assessment, or referral (ASHA, 1997a).

Newborn Hearing Screening

Name _____

Date _____

Technique(s) Used _____

Results: Right Ear _____   Left Ear _____

Recommendations

☐ Review of findings by physician/health care provider

☐ No further testing is recommended at this time

☐ Rescreen in _____ weeks

☐ Refer for diagnostic audiological evaluation

☐ Refer for early intervention services

Request results from referrals and/or any follow-up screening or assessment

Screener's name, contact information

Preschool Hearing Screening

Name _____

Date _____

Technique(s) Used _____

Results: Right Ear _____   Left Ear _____

Recommendations

☐ Review of findings by physician/health care provider

☐ No further testing is recommended at this time

☐ Rescreen in _____ weeks

☐ Refer for diagnostic audiological evaluation

☐ Refer for other evaluation (e.g., speech–language evaluation)

Screener's name, contact information

School-Age Hearing Screening

Name _____

Date _____

Technique(s) Used _____

Results _____
_____
_____

Recommendations

☐ Review of findings by physician/health care provider/educational team

☐ No further testing is recommended at this time

☐ Rescreen in _____ weeks

☐ Refer for diagnostic audiological evaluation

Screener's name, contact information

Reporting forms for hearing screening vary in appearance, but should contain certain common elements. The client's name and date of the screening must be recorded. Screening results should be reported as pass/fail and the recommended next steps for follow-up, if applicable, should be clearly indicated.

Although the specific criteria for passing/failing the screening do not necessarily appear on the form, these should be recorded in the policies and procedures of the oversight agency for reference and monitoring purposes. Those conducting hearing screening programs should also maintain records of equipment calibration.

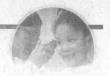

Appendix B
Hearing Screening (Adults)

Name _____ Date _____

Birth Date _____ Age _____ Gender: M F

Screening Unit/Examiner _____ Calibration Date _____

Case History—Circle Appropriate Answers

Do you think you have a hearing loss?	Yes	No
Have hearing aid(s) ever been recommended for you?	Yes	No
Is your hearing better in one ear?	Yes	No

If yes, which is the better ear?   Right   Left

Have you ever had a sudden or rapid progression of hearing loss?	Yes	No

    If yes, which ear?   Right   Left

Do you have ringing or noises in your ears?	Yes	No

    If yes,   Right   Left   Both

Do you consider dizziness to be a problem for you?	Yes	No
Have you had recent drainage from your ear(s)?	Yes	No

    If yes,   Right   Left

Do you have pain or discomfort in your ear(s)?	Yes	No

    If yes,   Right   Left

Have you received medical consultation for any of the above conditions?	Yes	No

PASS   REFER

Visual/Otoscopic Inspection

PASS   REFER   Right   Left

Referral for cerumen management _____ Referral for medical evaluation _____

Pure Tone Screen (25 dB HL)   (R = Response, NR = No Response)

Frequency	1000	2000	4000 Hz
Right Ear			
Left Ear			

PASS   REFER

Hearing-Disability Index

Score: HHIE-S _____   SAC _____   Other _____   Score _____

PASS   REFER

Discharge

_____ Medical Examination   _____ Counsel

_____ Cerumen Management   _____ Audiologic Evaluation

Comments _____

_____

Patient Signature _____ Date _____

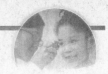

Appendix C

Hearing Handicap Inventory for the Elderly

Screening Version (HHIE-S)

Please check yes, no, or sometimes in response to each of the following items. Do not skip a question if you avoid a situation because of a hearing problem. If you use a hearing aid, please answer the way you hear without the aid.

E = emotional   S = social   No response = 0   Sometimes = 2   Yes = 4

		Yes	Sometimes	No
E	1. Does a hearing problem cause you to feel embarrassed when you meet new people?			
E	2. Does a hearing problem cause you to feel frustrated when talking to members of your family?			
S	3. Do you have difficulty hearing when someone speaks in a whisper?			
E	4. Do you feel handicapped by a hearing problem?			
S	5. Does a hearing problem cause you difficulty when visiting friends, relatives, or neighbors?			
S	6. Does a hearing problem cause you to attend religious services less often than you would like?			
E	7. Does a hearing problem cause you to have arguments with family members?			
S	8. Does a hearing problem cause you difficulty when listening to TV or radio?			
E	9. Do you feel that any difficulty with your hearing limits or hampers your personal or social life?			
S	10. Does a hearing problem cause you difficulty when in a restaurant with relatives or friends?			
Score_____				

HHIE-S Score Interpretation (Lichtenstein, Bess, & Logan, 1988)

Raw Score	Handicap Range	Posthoc Prob. Of Hearing Impairment
0–8	No handicap	13%
10–24	Mild-moderate handicap	50%
26–40	Severe handicap	84%

Source: Ventry, I., & Weinstein, B. (1983). The Hearing Handicap Inventory for the Elderly: A new tool. *Ear and Hearing, 3,* 128–134. Reprinted by permission.

chapter 12

Helping Individuals with Hearing Loss

AFTER COMPLETING THIS CHAPTER, YOU SHOULD BE ABLE TO:

1. Describe a model of aural rehabilitation that includes both the assistive technology and services required to support individuals with hearing loss.
2. Describe five broad steps in the hearing aid amplification process, from initial assessment through counseling/follow-up.
3. Compare various styles of hearing aids and various features of hearing aids and evaluate their potential usefulness for different clients.
4. List various types of assistive devices that are available and describe their appropriateness for clients with various audiometric/communication profiles.
5. List possible causes and describe potential interventions for tinnitus.
6. Distinguish between content counseling and support counseling and describe various theories of counseling that might be used with individuals who have hearing loss.
7. List and define three coding strategies used in the speech processor of a cochlear implant.
8. Discuss advantages and disadvantages of the following cochlear implant/hearing aid arrangements: bimodal listening, combined electric and acoustic stimulation (EAS), and bilateral cochlear implants.

L earning the mechanics of audiological evaluation consumes the majority of time and effort for students in introductory audiology courses. Knowledge of the normal and disordered auditory system, appropriate tests and test techniques, and how to interpret data obtained during the evaluation process are all critical to providing accurate diagnostic evaluations. One purpose of a diagnostic evaluation is to define or quantify the type (nature) and degree of hearing loss. The next link in the chain between diagnostics and rehabilitation is to consider how the identified hearing loss affects the life of the individual in our care. Although other chapters provide information about intervention, this entire chapter on intervention is included to emphasize the importance of moving forward from diagnostics to intervention.

The effect of a hearing loss on an individual's life will differ depending on a variety of factors, including, but not limited to, the person's listening demands, vocation, family constellation, personality, and degree/type of hearing loss. In fact, it is not uncommon for individuals with similar audiograms to report very different communication effects or handicaps. The hearing handicap associated with hearing loss can be related to speech and language skill development or maintenance, academics, and psychosocial development. Feelings of isolation or withdrawal may occur as a result of hearing loss at any age. Hearing loss can be mistaken for, or coexist with, any number of other conditions, such as attention deficit hyperactivity disorder, a language learning disability, autism spectrum disorders, mental retardation, or dementia.

The number of possible communication disorders related to hearing loss, and the highly individual nature of these effects, makes it necessary to consider input from multiple sources in order to develop a rehabilitation plan that best suits each client. Effective aural rehabilitation will involve the efforts of the client, the client's family, audiologists, speech–language pathologists, and related professionals aimed at common, agreed-upon goals.

Model of Aural Rehabilitation

An accurate diagnostic audiological evaluation is certainly one of the core elements that must exist to effectively help people with hearing loss. Also, additional assessments, which make use of multiple resources and are targeted at the selection of appropriate device(s) and strategies, are also required in order to improve communicative function.

Federal Assistive Technology Definitions

Hearing aid and aural rehabilitation services may be viewed as part of a broader category of assistive technology. Two relevant definitions are contained in the Assistive Technology Act of 1998 (PL 105-394): Assistive Technology Device and Assistive Technology Service. The Technology Act of 1998 says that **assistive technology device** means "any item, piece of equipment, or product system, whether acquired commercially, modified, or customized, that is used to increase, maintain, or improve functional capabilities of individuals with disabilities." The term **assistive technology service** "means any service that directly assists an individual with a disability in the selection, acquisition, or use of an assistive technology device." Assistive technology services are further defined to include:

- The evaluation of the assistive technology needs of an individual with a disability, including a functional evaluation of the impact of the provision of appropriate assistive technology and appropriate services to the individual in the customary environment of the individual
- Services consisting of purchasing, leasing, or otherwise providing for the acquisition of assistive technology devices by individuals with disabilities
- Services consisting of selecting, designing, fitting, customizing, adapting, applying, maintaining, repairing, or replacing assistive technology devices
- Coordination and use of necessary therapies, interventions, or services with assistive technology devices, such as therapies, interventions, or services associated with education and rehabilitation plans and programs

- Training or technical assistance for an individual with disabilities, or, when appropriate, the family members, guardians, advocates, or authorized representatives of such an individual
- Training or technical assistance for professionals (including individuals providing education and rehabilitation services), employers, or other individuals who provide services to, employ, or are otherwise substantially involved in the major life functions of individuals with disabilities

It is not an accident that assistive technology devices and services are both included in the federal Assistive Technology Act of 1998. Similar definitions are included in the **Individuals with Disabilities Education Act (IDEA)** final regulations. People familiar with assistive technology, either as consumers or dispensers, are aware that unfortunately these devices sometimes end up in dresser drawers or closets, often because of a failure to pair assistive devices with the services needed to teach individuals how to optimize use of the device in their daily lives.

Aural rehabilitation can be considered a blend of providing device(s) and service(s) with the goal of improving overall communicative function for an individual with a hearing loss and their family. Depending on the nature of the hearing loss, initiating aural rehabilitation generally involves consultation with general physicians or otolaryngologists to obtain medical or otological clearance for use of amplification. For most individuals with sensorineural hearing loss, medical clearance for amplification is provided by their general physician. In cases of conductive involvement, medical management is a primary focus. If amplification is being considered, otological clearance is sought. It should also be noted that sometimes individuals with a conductive hearing loss, for example, due to otosclerosis, opt to pursue use of amplification instead of a surgical intervention. In such cases, once otological clearance has been documented, proceeding with the aural rehabilitation process, selecting technology, and providing services to support the client's adaptation to and use of that technology is an appropriate course of action. An overview of the process from diagnostic audiology through rehabilitation assessment and intervention is illustrated in the flow chart in Figure 12.1.

Obtaining Aural Rehabilitation Services

Resources

Those serving clients who may need aural rehabilitation should be aware of community resources for obtaining such services. These may include hospital-based hearing and speech clinics, college- or university-affiliated hearing and speech clinics, Veterans Administration hospitals, audiologists in private practice, and general physicians' or specialists' (e.g., otolaryngologist) office.

Hearing Aid Amplification

In describing a process by which a person pursues amplification as part of an overall rehabilitation program, it should first be pointed out that there is great variability among audiologists in this process. Efforts to produce guidelines that audiologists can follow have resulted in some clear themes, however, including valid audiological assessment, treatment planning, hearing aid selection, verification and validation, hearing aid orientation, and counseling and follow-up (AHSA 1997). Each of these steps is addressed in this chapter.

FIGURE 12.1 **An overview of the process from diagnostic audiology through rehabilitation assessment and intervention.**

Considerations for Helping Individuals with Hearing Loss

Identification/Diagnosis of Hearing Loss

Factors Influencing the Rehabilitation Process

Intrinsic	Extrinsic	Potential Collaborators
Motivation	Community resources	Family members
Personality/temperament	Listening environment(s)	Primary health care provider
Cognitive ability	Noise	Teacher
Age	Distance	Related educators
Health	Reverberation	Audiologists
	Classroom acoustics	Speech–language pathologists

Resources to Help Individuals with Hearing Loss

Devices	Services	Verification/Validation
Hearing aids	Hearing aid orientation	Real ear measures
Assistive listening devices	Speech–language consult	Aided behavioral testing
Assistive devices	Communication training	Client questionnaires
Cochlear implants	Speechreading	Client journal or daily log
Middle ear implants	Auditory training	
Vibrotactile devices	Communication strategies	
	Hearing loss prevention	
	Plan for follow-up	

Audiological Assessment

Case History

You will recall that when a client visits the audiologist for a hearing evaluation, a case history interview is performed. As summarized in Table 4.3, many of the questions in the case history are designed to provide insight into the nature of the hearing loss. In addition, a number of the questions relate directly to the client's level of difficulty understanding speech. Question 1, which asks the reason for the client's visit to the audiologist, is a way to determine if the client's primary concern is a medical one (a sudden unexplained hearing loss, drainage from the ears, etc.) or one that may involve amplification. Question 2, which asks if the person believes that he or she has a hearing problem, is important because many people with hearing loss are unaware that they have a problem. This can occur because family and friends routinely raise the level of their voices to compensate for the person's hearing loss, or because the person is in denial about it. Working with clients to better appreciate the hearing loss they have can be a challenge for the audiologist. Question 5 clearly addresses possible aural rehabilitation needs of the client. This question attempts to pinpoint those areas where the client is having the greatest communication difficulty. Finally, question 10 asks specifically whether the person is wearing hearing aids, and the client's level of satisfaction with them.

It is important during the case history phase of the assessment that audiologists attempt to gain insight into not only the factual information presented by the client but also the client's emotional response to having a hearing loss. Because audiologists deal with hearing loss every day, it is easy to treat it as a routine matter. For people who are just realizing that their hearing is impaired and that this impairment is interfering with their life in some way, this is far from a routine matter. In fact, in some cases it can be devastating. As we discuss later in this chapter in the section on counseling, failure to acknowledge the emotional aspect of the client's hearing loss will inevitably interfere with the audiologist's effectiveness and the client's satisfaction.

Importance of Audiological Data

Pure tone testing provides information about the degree of hearing loss, which is an important factor in determining the overall amount of gain (amplification) a hearing aid must deliver in order to improve a client's ability to understand speech. In addition, the pure tone thresholds form a particular pattern, referred to as the slope or configuration of the hearing loss, and this shape is a factor in determining which frequencies will need to be amplified and to what degree, as well as the number of channels that might be necessary. Pure tones can also be used to calculate the **dynamic range,** which is defined as the difference in decibels between a client's hearing threshold and his or her threshold of discomfort. When the dynamic range is measured for pure tones, it is done at various frequencies that are important for hearing speech sounds. The advantage of determining the pure tone dynamic range for various frequencies is that a client may have a normal dynamic range at some frequencies but a significantly reduced range at others. You will recall from Chapter 5 that a reduced dynamic range can make the hearing aid fitting process more challenging. Finally, pure tone thresholds provide information regarding differences between the two ears in cases of unilateral or asymmetrical hearing loss.

The role of speech audiometry is described in detail in Chapter 5. As summarized in Table 5.2 of that chapter, word recognition can be particularly important in the aural rehabilitation process because it can provide the audiologist with information about how well the client understands speech that is presented at conversational levels, at his/her most comfortable listening level (MCL), and when background noise is introduced. The dynamic range can also be calculated using speech by calculating the difference between the client's SRT and UCL.

Following the hearing evaluation, presuming that there are no medical concerns that must first be addressed (e.g., conductive or suspected retrocochlear pathology), the audiologist consults with the client, and often with members of the family or other significant people in the person's life, to gain insight into the degree to which the client might be a candidate for amplification and motivated to use it. Candidacy decisions are facilitated by the use of certain established tools, such as the Self Assessment of Communication Function (SAC), the Significant Other Assessment of Communication (SOAC), the Denver Scale of Communication Function, the Communication Profile for the Hearing Impaired (CPHI; Demorest & Erdman, 1986) and the Hearing Handicap Inventory for Adults (HHIA; Newman et al., 1990).

Treatment Planning

In the **treatment planning** stage, the audiologist and the client, along with other significant people included by the client, jointly address specific communication priorities of the client. These priorities are important because they become the basis on which the client will judge the success or failure of the hearing aid fitting. If the client does not receive sufficient guidance and counseling at this stage of the process, he may assume that amplification will accomplish goals that the audiologist knows are not reasonable. In addition to setting priorities, treatment planning also includes discussing the cost of amplification and agreeing on a sequence of events in cases when amplification is one of a number of rehabilitation steps to be pursued.

Hearing Aid Selection

Basic Definitions of Hearing Aids and Related Terms

A **hearing aid** may be defined as an electronic device consisting of a microphone, amplifier, and receiver, used to amplify sound and deliver it to the user's ear. Let's examine each of these three components of all hearing aids.

The **hearing aid microphone,** which is located on the outside of the hearing aid so that it can pick up acoustic energy (i.e., sound waves) in the air, converts this acoustic energy into electrical energy. Because of its role in changing energy from one form to another, microphones are also often referred to as transducers. Next, the electric signal reaches the amplifier and, as expected, the **hearing aid amplifier** increases the intensity of the electric signal. Keep in mind that the human ear does not process electric signals, so these must be converted back into acoustic energy. This is done by the **hearing aid receiver**. These three essential components of hearing aids are illustrated in Figure 12.2.

An important distinction should be made at this point between air conduction and bone conduction hearing aids. Consistent with our use of the term throughout the text, **air conduction hearing aids** direct amplified sound through the outer and middle ears to the cochlea. This is typically accomplished by placing an earmold that is coupled to a hearing aid directly into the ear canal or by placing a custom-made hearing aid into the ear canal. Various styles of air conduction hearing aids are described in the next section with pictures included in Figure 12.3. In contrast, **bone conduction hearing aids** make use of an oscillator placed on the mastoid area to route amplified sound directly to the cochlea, without involvement of the outer and middle

FIGURE **12.2** **Essential components of a conventional hearing aid.**

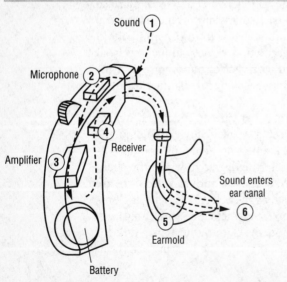

ears. Unless otherwise specified, use of the term *hearing aid* typically refers to air conduction aids.

You should also have a basic understanding of the difference between analog (from the word *analogous*) and digital (from the word *digit*) hearing aids. Both analog and digital circuits are illustrated in Figure 12.4. Note that in an **analog hearing aid,** the acoustic signal entering the hearing aid creates "patterns of electrical currents or voltages . . . [that are] analogous (similar) to those of the acoustic (sound) input" (Venema, 2006, p. 149). Through the action of the receiver, these currents are converted back into acoustic energy (i.e., sound). In a **digital hearing aid,** an analog-to-digital converter changes the electricity into numbers, which can then be manipulated, converted back to an analog signal (by the digital-to-analog converter), and then converted into an acoustic signal. The rationale for carrying out this conversion to numbers is that these numbers can then be easily manipulated by the computer to meet the client's gain, frequency response, and output needs more precisely. The extreme flexibility associated with digital amplification is typically not possible with analog instruments. The vast majority of hearing aids sold today are digital.

During the **hearing aid selection** process, decisions regarding both the electroacoustic and nonelectroacoustic characteristics of the hearing aids are made.

FIGURE **12.3** **Various styles of air conduction hearing aids.**

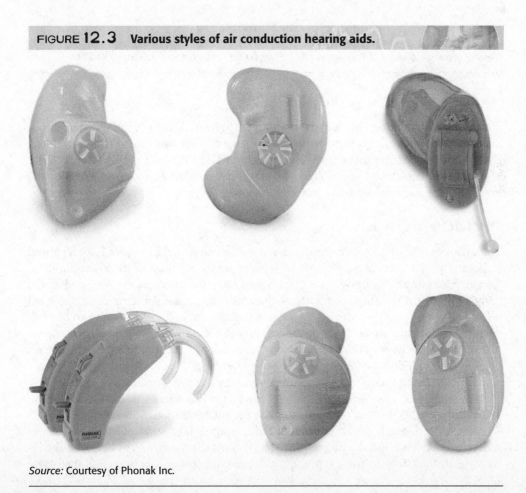

Source: Courtesy of Phonak Inc.

FIGURE **12.4**   **Comparison of analog and digital hearing aid circuits.**

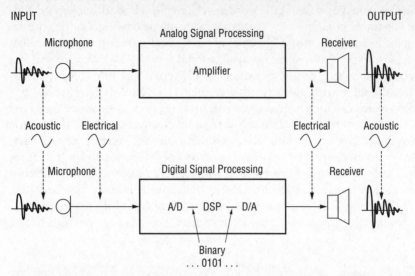

Source: *Compression for Clinicians,* 2nd edition, by Venema. 2006. Reprinted with permission of Delmar Learning, a division of Thomson Learning: www.thomsonrights.com. Fax 800-730-2215.

Electroacoustic hearing aid characteristics refer to hearing aid output characteristics, including the gain, frequency response, and maximum output of the aids. **Non-electroacoustic hearing aid characteristics** include decisions such as the style and color of the aids, whether the client will have a user-adjusted volume control or an automatic one. Let's examine some of these factors.

Styles of Hearing Aids

The various styles of air conduction hearing aids are depicted in Figure 12.3. It should be noted that the hearing aid style name is based on the location of the microphone of the aid. For example, the body aid is so named because the microphone is located on the body, typically on the chest. Similarly, the behind-the-ear aid's microphone is located behind the ear. In general, the larger the hearing aid, the more effective it can be with more severe hearing losses. The clinician's role is to provide honest and balanced information about the devices that are most appropriate for each client based on the client's hearing loss, individual listening needs, and preferences. The audiologist should provide the client with accurate information about which style(s) of aids will have the best chance of being effective for his listening needs, and at the same time, must remain flexible because clients will not wear aids that they deem cosmetically unacceptable.

When hearing aids were first introduced in early 1900s, body and behind-the-ear styles were available and the body-worn style was more powerful than the behind-the-ear style. By the 1970s, in-the-ear hearing aids became more widely used. Full shell-style in-the-ear aids are the largest of the in-the-ear styles; the half-shell, low-profile, and in-the-canal style are progressively smaller versions. In the 1980s, deep-canal aids (also referred to as completely in-the-canal aids or CICs) were introduced. Because these aids fit deep into the ear canal, they are cosmetically appealing. A helpful trend in hearing aid technology is the increasing availability of smaller behind-the-ear hearing aids, which combine cosmetic appeal with the flexibility to meet a wide range of audiometric needs. Specifically, these smaller behind-the-ear aids offer flexible gain and output and compatibility with other assistive devices, discussed later.

Although choice of hearing aid style can be made based solely on the degree of power required, it is much more common for this decision to be made in part based on audiological variables and in part based on the cosmetic appeal of the aid. In addition, choice of hearing aid style can be based on practical matters, such as the ease with which the device can be inserted into the ear canal. Experience working with older people suggests that behind-the-ear hearing aids can be difficult to insert because the client first has to insert the earmold and then place the aid itself over the pinna. Also, if the aid has a volume control, it also is located behind the ear, and adjusting it has to be done without accidentally pushing the aid from its location. Full-shell, in-the-ear aids, on the other hand, tend to be easier to insert, and if a volume wheel exists its location allows for easier manipulation. With older individuals, smaller in-the-ear aids, such as canal hearing aids, can pose difficulties because they may be too small for the client to handle.

Disadvantages of in-the-ear aids can include the common problem of wax building up and clogging the receiver. Although audiologists counsel clients to clean the sound bore area to prevent wax-related problems and manufacturers work to develop effective wax collectors, this problem remains a big one. Because behind-the-ear aids have a mold that goes into the ear and the mold can be removed from the aid and easily cleaned, behind-the-ear fittings do not have this problem.

All in-the-ear fittings, especially very small styles, can also have the disadvantage of not having enough room for special features or controls that might be helpful to the client. Remember that for all in-the-ear hearing aids, the size of the aid is determined by the size of the person's ear. If the audiologist is fitting a person with a small ear who wants to have an in-the-ear aid, options that might be helpful to the client may not fit on the aid. In addition, smaller hearing aids generally have less capability for use with other assistive technology, discussed later in this chapter.

Monaural versus Binaural Fitting

Years ago, before the value of **binaural** (both ears) hearing was clearly established, the question of whether to fit a client with one or two hearing aids was a prominent one in the decision-making process. Now that the benefits of binaural amplification are more clearly understood and documented, this question is less perplexing. In most cases, individuals who have hearing loss in each ear that interferes with communication ability should wear hearing aids in each ear. There are a number of reasons for this recommendation.

First, when both ears are amplified, the sound from each ear fuses together at the level of the brainstem, resulting in a 3-dB increase in gain compared to wearing a monaural aid. This phenomenon is referred to as **binaural summation** and means that by wearing two aids, the audiologist is able to provide more usable gain for the client.

Second, when both ears are amplified the brainstem is more able to separate speech information from background noise. This is referred to as **binaural squelch** and is supported by the common complaint of individuals who have hearing loss in one ear: difficulty understanding speech in noisy environments.

Third, use of binaural amplification (versus a single hearing aid) allows the client to localize sounds. **Localization** refers to a person's ability to locate the source of a sound. This requires that both ears work together, because localization relies on different time and intensity cues that result from the arrival of sound to each ear at different times. As noted above, individuals who have unilateral hearing loss commonly report an inability to localize.

Lastly, when both ears are amplified the head-shadow effect is eliminated. Examine the audiogram in Figure 12.5. Note that this person has a mild-to-moderate bilateral symmetrical sensorineural hearing loss. If the client chooses to obtain a hearing aid only for the right ear, sound directed to the left ear will have to cross over the head in order to be received by the aided ear. In the process of crossing the head, the intensity of the sound is reduced, usually by 12–16 dB in the higher frequencies, which are important for understanding speech. Consequently, this client will regularly turn the aided ear toward the speech information. The **head-shadow effect,** which refers to the attenuation of sound as it crosses from one side of the head to the other, is something that is resolved with a binaural fitting.

Despite the clear benefits of binaural amplification, there are times when it is necessary/appropriate to fit only one ear (**monoaural** amplification). Unfortunately, one of the reasons for monaural fittings is that many clients, especially those on a fixed income, cannot afford two hearing aids. Many insurance carriers do not cover hearing

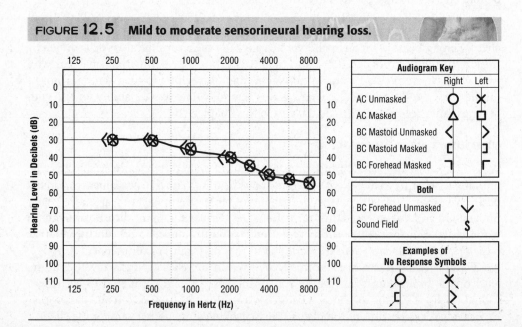

FIGURE **12.5** **Mild to moderate sensorineural hearing loss.**

aids, nor does Medicare, the federal health care program for individuals 65 years of age and older.

Electroacoustic and Acoustic Options

We have seen that hearing aids have different features, shapes, and sizes on the outside. The components inside each device may differ as well, but there are some common elements in all hearing aids. Hearing aids can be measured against standards developed by the American National Standards Institute (ANSI) to ensure that they perform as they are designed and intended to. Certain electroacoustic characteristics form the basis for measuring the performance of hearing aids. The major characteristics are gain, frequency response, and output.

The **gain** of the hearing aid can be defined as the overall amount of amplification, measured in decibels (dB). The **frequency response** of the hearing aid is simply the gain delivered at specific frequencies. This response can be changed by the audiologist and is part of a process of signal shaping that is often necessary to give the client an amplified signal that is acceptable. Most manufacturer specifications include a frequency response curve, which is a graph of the amount of gain a hearing aid supplies at each frequency, usually in a range from 500 Hz to 6,000 Hz. **Selective amplification** means that some frequencies will receive greater amounts of amplification than others. This makes intuitive sense because the degree of hearing loss offers differs at various frequencies. **Output limiting** is related to providing hearing aid users with comfortable amplification. Hearing aids do not amplify to infinity and there are some primary ways in which the output of the hearing aid is limited.

Another important term to introduce at this point in our discussion is the **hearing aid test box,** illustrated in Figure 12.6. This device is a sound-treated box in which measurements are made of specific characteristics of hearing aids. Because the goal is to measure the output of the hearing aid, also located in the box is a speaker that produces sounds. As described previously, the hearing aid microphone amplifies the sound, which is then delivered to the receiver. In this measurement system, the receiver is attached to a **2-cc coupler,** which is used to connect the hearing aid to an electroacoustic analyzer. In this way the hearing aid's output is measured.

The input signal that is presented from the speaker and the position of the volume control of the hearing aid are chosen based on the particular measurement being made. For example, some measurements provide data about the hearing aid's gain for conversational speech. For such measures, the volume control is positioned to simulate typical use by the client and the input signal approximates conversational speech (i.e., 65 dB SPL). Conversely, if we are interested in measuring the maximum amount of amplification that the aid will deliver, the volume control is set to the maximum position (referred to as full-on gain) and the input signal used is very intense (e.g., 90 dB). Today, digital hearing aids include advanced features such as automatic directional microphones, digital noise suppression, and multichannel compression, all of which can be measured in the test box.

Electroacoustic Options—Frequency Response

One of the important decisions to be made when fitting hearing aids is how the amplified signal will be shaped or modified. Let's think about why this shaping is important.

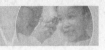

FIGURE **12.6**   **Illustration of the main components of a hearing aid test system.**

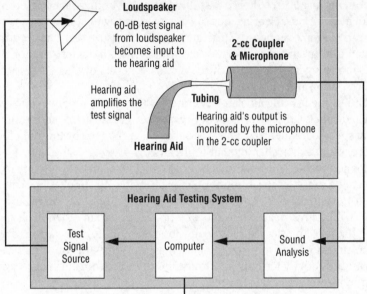

Hearing Aid Test Box

Loudspeaker

60-dB test signal
from loudspeaker
becomes input to
the hearing aid

**2-cc Coupler
& Microphone**

Hearing aid
amplifies the
test signal

Tubing

Hearing aid's output is
monitored by the microphone
in the 2-cc coupler

Hearing Aid

Hearing Aid Testing System

| Test Signal Source | Computer | Sound Analysis |

The output from the hearing aid is compared to the input signal,
and the results are shown on a screen and/or printout.

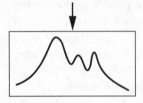

Source: Gelfand, S. (2001). *Essentials of audiology* (2nd ed.). New York: Thieme. Reprinted by permission.

Consider the audiogram in Figure 12.7. This person has a relatively flat sensorineural hearing loss, which at least theoretically requires some amplification at all frequencies. Assume that this client is fitted with hearing aids and reports that speech is loud enough but not clear. She also reports that she is receiving too much amplification of background sounds and unwanted noise. Does the audiologist conclude that this aid is not appropriate for this client? The answer to this question is no, because for most hearing aids the signal can be shaped in some way to match the particular needs of the client.

In the past, shaping or modification of the amplified signal of the hearing aid was accomplished through use of potentiometers. A **potentiometer** is a resistor that allows changes to be made in the current of the hearing aid. If the particular change being made affects the frequencies that are amplified, the potentiometer is referred to as a **tone**

FIGURE **12.7**   **Flat sensorineural hearing loss.**

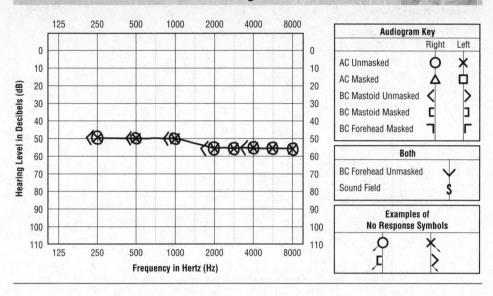

control. If the potentiometer affects the maximum amount of amplification produced by the hearing aid when a very intense signal is introduced, that potentiometer is referred to as an **output limiter.** A **volume control** is also an example of a potentiometer because manipulation of it changes the degree of resistance to the current of the hearing aid.

In the past, adjusting a potentiometer was accomplished by manipulating an external trimmer using a screwdriver; today such shaping is accomplished by computer. Further, because the vast majority of today's hearing aids are digital, shaping the signal no longer involves variable resistors, but rather is accomplished by signal processors that carry out mathematical operations on a digital version of the signal. The exact mathematical operation depends on the type of shaping that is being performed (Vonlanthen & Arndt, 2007).

How does the audiologist monitor changes that are being made to the amplified signal? In the past, audiologists referred extensively to specification guidelines (often called "specs") produced by the hearing aid manufacturers. For example, examine the graph depicted in Figure 12.8. On this frequency–response graph, the horizontal axis depicts frequencies and the vertical axis depicts gain, which is the degree of amplification. Note also that there are two different curves on the graph, one labeled N and the other H. In comparing these two graphs, note that the N response produces gain at all of the frequencies from 200 to 5,000 Hz. When the potentiometer is adjusted to the H response, note that there is a decrease in the low-frequency gain. The exact decrease in low-frequency amplification can be calculated by subtracting, for example, the degree of gain at 500 Hz when the potentiometer is set to N, compared to the degree of amplification when the potentiometer is set to H.

Today, rather than refer to specification sheets, audiologists monitor the changes they make to the amplified signal on their personal computer, which is equipped with

FIGURE **12.8** **Frequency–response graph depicting the effects of an N-H tone control.**

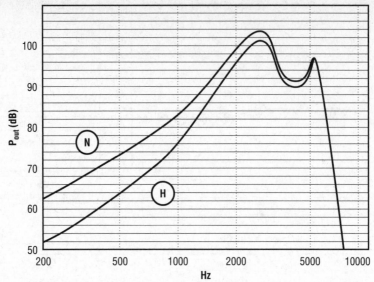

some type of programming interface and loaded with hearing instrument manufacturer adjustment software. HI-PRO is a commonly used interface that enables a hardware connection between the computer and the hearing aid(s) being programmed. More recently, NOAHlink has been developed to allow wireless communication between hearing aids and a computer using Bluetooth technology.

Acoustic Options for Modifying the Frequency Response

This discussion of electroacoustics must also include information regarding earmolds and earmold acoustics. An earmold is a coupler or fitting that is made by the audiologist from an ear impression of the client's ear. The earmold is designed to fit comfortably in the client's ear and to conduct sound into the ear from the hearing aid. A related term is **earmold acoustics,** which refers to the acoustical changes that occur to the output acoustic signal by the characteristics of the tube or channel through which the signal travels. In fact, the amplified acoustic signal entering the ear can be altered considerably by the characteristics of the earmold of a behind-the-ear aid or the shell of an in-the-ear aid.

As illustrated in Figure 12.9, earmolds can be ordered in various styles based on the desired acoustic effect. These styles include the popular **skeleton earmold,** characterized by an open space in the concha area to improve the mold's appearance; the **shell mold,** which lacks the open space in the concha and is often used when very powerful hearing aids are being fit; and the **receiver earmold,** which has a metal or plastic snap adapter inserted into it so that an external receiver, like that used in a body aid, can be coupled to it.

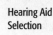

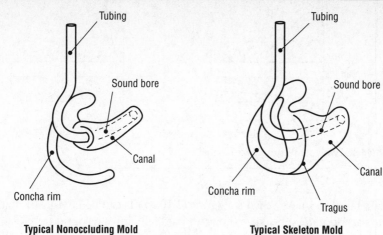

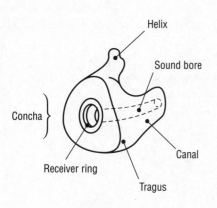

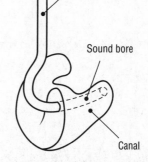

Typical Nonoccluding Mold

Typical Skeleton Mold

Typical Standard Mold

Typical Shell Mold

Source: Reprinted with permission of Microsonic.

Note also that earmolds with a full canal are often referred to as **occluding molds** because they fill the ear canal. **Nonoccluding earmolds** tend to introduce much less material into the ear canal and therefore leave it more open or unoccluded. They also do not significantly alter the natural resonance of the ear canal. Open earmolds have traditionally been most appropriate for individuals who have mild hearing losses or very normal hearing in the low- to middle-frequency range.

In some cases, an open mold is desirable but not possible due to concerns about **acoustic feedback,** which results from reamplification of sound that leaks out (through the vent) from the hearing aid receiver and is picked up by the hearing aid microphone. In these cases, an opening or **vent** can be placed in the earmold to reduce at least some

FIGURE **12.10**   **Comparison of parallel and diagonal earmold vents.**

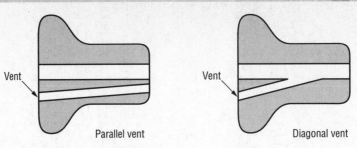

Source: Reprinted with permission of Microsonic.

of the canal occlusion. As noted in Figure 12.10, vents can be parallel or diagonal. **Parallel vents** are so named because they run parallel with the sound bore of the hearing aid, making them less likely to produce feedback. **Select-a-vent systems,** illustrated in Figure 12.11, are commonly used because of they allows quick and easy variation in the vent size.

To more fully illustrate some of these points, note the hearing loss depicted in Figure 12.12. This client has hearing well within normal limits at 250 and 500 Hz but has

FIGURE **12.11**   **Depiction of two variable venting systems.**

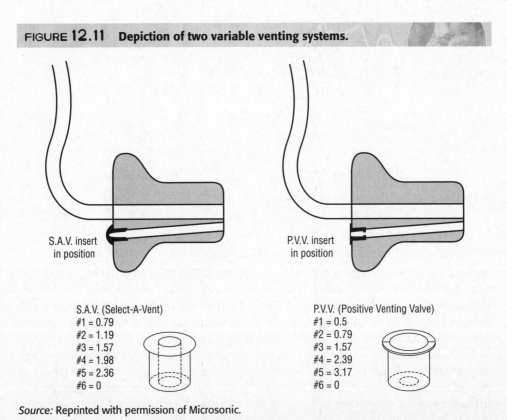

Source: Reprinted with permission of Microsonic.

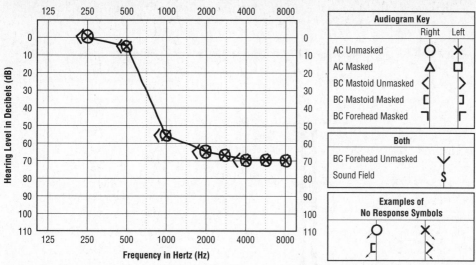

FIGURE **12.12** **Sloping sensorineural hearing loss with normal low-frequency hearing.**

considerable hearing loss beyond this. The frequencies beyond 250 and 500 Hz will require considerable amplification, and for this reason it would have been necessary in the past to avoid the use of any vent, except perhaps for a very small one, in order to avoid acoustic feedback caused by the sound escaping from the earmold. If a larger vent was used, traditional measures to control the resulting feedback might have included reducing the high-frequency gain and notched filtering. Both of these steps result in reduced gain in the very frequencies where the client most needs amplification. Even if decreased feedback were achieved, decreased audibility of speech sounds would also be likely.

New technology utilizes digital phase cancellation to control feedback. Rather than reducing gain, phase cancellation involves canceling the feedback by introducing an additional signal that is out of phase from the signal creating the feedback. Although this technology does not result in complete cancellation of feedback, it does allow more gain at the mid- to high frequencies before feedback occurs and often also allows this to occur with an increased vent. Such improvements in feedback control have led to increased interest in open hearing aid fittings, which are discussed later in the chapter.

The Horn Effect

We noted previously in our discussion of frequency–response graphs that when a tone control is adjusted from the N setting to the H setting, we are not increasing the high frequencies. Rather, we are decreasing the lows. We also noted that this can improve the high-frequency response of the aid by reducing the likelihood that upward spread of masking will occur.

Although the high frequencies cannot be increased electronically, they can be extended acoustically, by "belling" the end of the earmold or the hearing aid. Sometimes this process is referred to as the **horn effect**.

One common way of employing the horn effect with earmolds is to use a Libby horn. Examine the earmold in Figure 12.13 and note first the tubing that runs through the earmold, bringing the sound from the hearing aid to the ear. Note also that although the diameter of the tube that is attached to the earhook of the hearing aid is 2 mm, it

FIGURE **12.13** **Influence of horn effect on frequency response.**

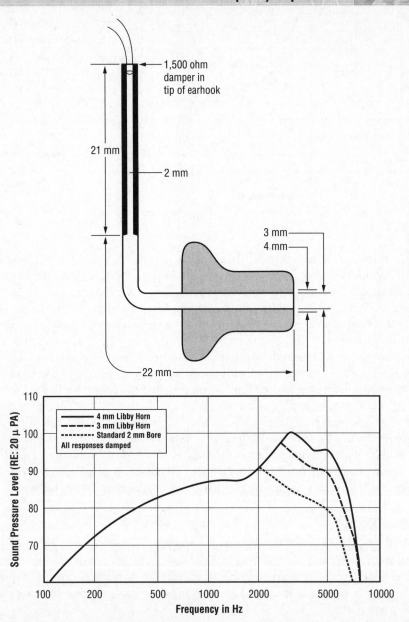

Source: Reprinted with permission of Microsonic.

then increases to 3 or 4 mm, creating the horn effect. (In cases where the client's ear canal cannot accommodate a 4-mm tube, a 3-mm Libby horn can be used.)

Now, examine the frequency–response graph in Figure 12.13, which compares the standard earmold (2-mm-diameter tubing at the earhook and continuing through the earmold) with the 3-mm Libby horn and the 4-mm Libby horn. With the standard mold, the frequency response of the hearing aid begins to drop off at approximately 2,000 Hz. The high-frequency response is extended considerably into the higher frequencies with both of the Libby horns.

Maximum Output

All hearing aids include an output limiting system to ensure the user's comfort in the presence of intense sounds. One general way to limit the output of a hearing aid is through peak clipping; the other general way is the use of compression. In this section, the mechanisms of peak clipping and compression are explained, along with advantages and limitations.

Examine the graph in Figure 12.14. Note that in this graph the maximum output of the hearing aid is depicted as a function of frequency. Examine the output graph and determine the maximum intensity that this aid will produce at 500 Hz. Then do the same for 2,000 Hz. If you determined values of 120 and 122 dB SPL, you are correct.

Knowing the maximum output of a hearing aid is very important. Consider the client who has a severe hearing loss bilaterally and is wearing powerful hearing aids binaurally. Each aid has an overall gain of 45 dB SPL. When average conversational speech, which is the input signal, is delivered to the aid, the resulting output signal is

FIGURE 12.14   Maximum power output graph.

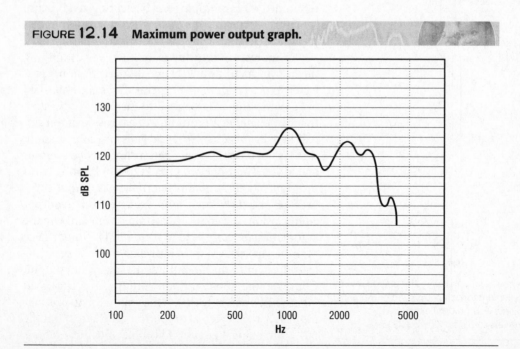

110 dB SPL. This value is the result of boosting a 65 dB SPL conversational signal by 45 dB SPL (65 + 45).

Now consider what happens when the client is walking outside and a large truck drives by. If the input signal from the truck is 80 dB SPL, what is the signal that reaches the client's ear? If you calculated 145 dB SPL, you are correct (80 + 65 dB). In order to understand this more fully, let's introduce the term *linear amplification*. As shown in Figure 12.15, **linear amplification** refers to a hearing aid circuit that provides equal gain for all input intensity levels (Venema, 2006). This means that there is a one-to-one relationship between the output signal (the sound resulting from the amplification) and the input signal (the sound being amplified). The problem with linear amplification is that it often does not provide adequate amplification for soft sounds and often provides too much amplification for loud sounds. This problem with loud sounds can be addressed by limiting the maximum output of hearing aids. In particular, if the client has a reduced dynamic range, he will most likely need a hearing aid that limits the maximum output. Otherwise, loud sounds will be amplified to a point that exceeds their uncomfortable level and the client will not be able to use the amplification being provided effectively.

Peak clipping removes amplitude peaks at specific levels so that those peaks do not reach a level that is uncomfortable for the client. For example, examine Figure 12.15 and note that if a given hearing aid has a gain of 60 dB, an input signal of 20 dB is amplified to a level of 80 dB, and an input signal of 40 dB is amplified to a level of 100 dB. Note, however, that an intensity level of 100 dB does not exceed 120 dB because the hearing aid automatically becomes saturated and goes into the peak-clipping mode. Figure 12.16 provides an example of a maximum output curve of a hearing aid that allows reduction of the saturation level by use of a potentiometer. Peak clipping has been criticized because it removes some of the signal, which can result in distortion and reduced speech understanding.

Compression limiting is another way of limiting the hearing aid output and one that is commonly preferred to peak clipping. In general, this is accomplished by "compressing" the signal into the person's dynamic range by changing the amount of gain as the input signal changes. Once a hearing aid goes into compression, there is not a one-to-one relationship between output and input. There are two broad types of limiting compression. The first type is referred to as output compression and the other is input compression. In **output compression,** the volume control is located before the automatic gain control (AGC) circuit. The importance of this is that the volume control of the hearing aid affects the gain of the aid but not the maximum output. Compare the three output compression curves in Figure 12.17 and note that as the volume control is manipulated, the degree of amplification changes but the output remains the same. This type of compression is

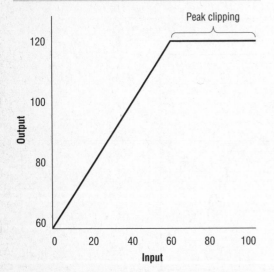

FIGURE **12.15 Typical input/output graph for linear amplification.**

Source: Compression for Clinicians, 2nd edition, by Venema. 2006. Reprinted with permission of Delmar Learning, a division of Thomson Learning: www.thomsonrights.com. Fax 800-730-2215.

FIGURE 12.16 **Maximum output responses with minimum
and maximum peak clipping.**

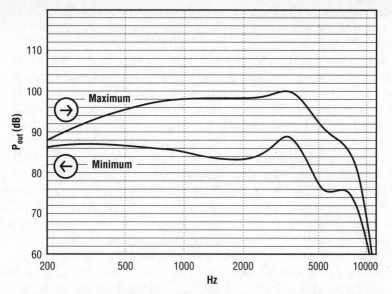

FIGURE 12.17 **Input/output graphs and circuit illustrations
comparing the effects of the volume control in input and output
compression instruments.**

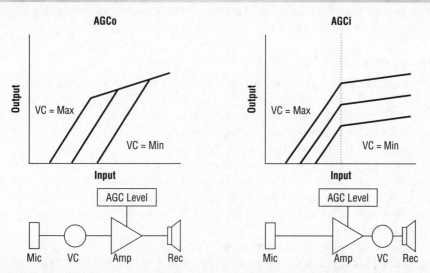

Source: Compression for Clinicians, 2nd edition, by Venema. 2006. Reprinted with permission of
Delmar Learning, a division of Thomson Learning: www.thomsonrights.com. Fax 800-730-2215.

typically used with individuals who have severe hearing loss and a reduced dynamic range. The reason for this is that output compression will prevent increases in volume of the hearing aid from resulting in increases in the maximum output of the aid. Note also on this graph that gain is linear until a certain "kneepoint" is reached. The **kneepoint** is the point on the curve where the slope changes; this represents the intensity level at which compression "kicks in."

Another important term that should be understood in this discussion of output limiting is compression ratio. Once the hearing aid is in compression, it compresses the signal to a certain degree. The **compression ratio** refers to the relationship, in decibels, between the input signal and the resulting output signal. It was noted previously that in linear amplification this relationship is 1:1. When compression is used the ratio can be quite high. For example, if a hearing aid had the potential to significantly limit the maximum output of a hearing aid, it could have a compression ratio of 6:1. This would mean that for every 6 dB of input, the output increases by only 1 dB.

Based on the above information, a hearing aid with output compression may act in the following manner: amplify in a linear fashion, producing 1 dB of output for every 1 dB of input and then, at some point determined by the setting of the compression kneepoint, change the input–output relationship (referred to as the compression ratio) for purposes of fitting the amplified signal into the client's dynamic range.

The second type of compression limiting is **input compression**. With this type, the volume control affects both the gain and the output because the volume control is located after the AGC circuit. Examine Figure 12.17 again, this time looking at the curves for input compression. Note that the lowest curve, reflecting the lowest volume control setting and the least amount of gain, also has the lowest output. Conversely, the top curve reflects the most volume, the most gain, and the highest output. Input compression is typically used with individuals who have mild to moderate hearing losses because they usually have less recruitment and therefore a larger dynamic range. Because of these factors, these individuals are less likely to have problems with amplified signals exceeding their discomfort levels.

Wide Dynamic Range Compression

Use of **wide dynamic range compression** (WDRC) is a very different application of compression and represents another development that has changed the way hearing aids are fitted. With wide dynamic range compression, the threshold kneepoints are much lower (e.g., 40 dB) and the degree of compression is much less (e.g., 2:1 ratio). This type of compression is not intended to protect the person from sounds that become too loud, but rather is used as a way to increase the gain for soft sounds. In fact, as the compression threshold is decreased, the gain for soft sounds increases. Because soft high-frequency sounds make up an essential group of consonant sounds in our language, use of wide dynamic range compression can be particularly helpful in improving speech understanding.

Finally, it should be noted that some wide dynamic range hearing aids use both wide dynamic range compression and compression limiting. Soft sounds are amplified based on where the threshold kneepoint is set (referred to as the lower kneepoint) and loud sounds are prevented from becoming too loud because sounds that exceed the upper kneepoint are compressed. See Figure 12.18 for an illustration.

FIGURE 12.18 Input/output graphs comparing traditional compression limiting and wide dynamic range compression.

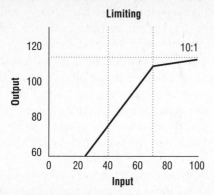
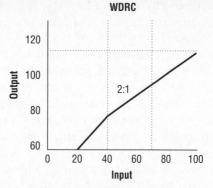

Source: Compression for Clinicians, 2nd edition, by Venema. 2006. Reprinted with permission of Delmar Learning, a division of Thomson Learning: www.thomsonrights.com. Fax 800-730-2215.

Recent Developments

The Digital Age

The beginning of the "digital era" of hearing aids began in the mid-1990s but by 1998 only 5 percent of all hearing aid sales in the United States were digital products. Today, less than one decade later, survey data reveal that 90 percent of all hearing aids sold are digital. This growth in sales of digital hearing aids is likely due to a number of advantages that digital hearing aids have over other hearing aids including: the ability to capture more incoming speech information and less noise; increased fitting flexibility, allowing the audiologist to tailor amplification to the client's particular audiometric configuration; increased feedback reduction capabilities; and greater options for using various compression limiting approaches within a given channel. Survey data also reveal that dispensers of hearing aids believe that they can better satisfy their patients with digital products compared to analog hearing aids (Kirkwood, 2005).

Hearing Aids and Noise

One of the most frequent complaints from individuals who wear hearing aids is that they continue to have difficulty understanding speech when in a background of noise (Kirkwood, 2005). Typically, hearing aid microphones are **omnidirectional,** meaning that they pick up sound coming from different directions with nearly equal sensitivity. This means that sounds coming from the sides, the back and the front are all amplified to nearly the same degree. The signal-to-noise ratio can become quite poor in noisy settings with omnidirectional microphones.

A **directional microphone** is more sensitive to sounds directed from the front, compared to sounds coming from other directions. This allows speech information that is directed to the client to be amplified more than the extraneous information that is to her side and behind her. This can improve the signal-to-noise ratio significantly. In fact, use of directional microphones can result in as much as a 6-dB improvement in the signal-to-noise ratio.

Currently, directional microphones may be activated either manually or automatically. In manual activation, the user of the hearing aid pushes a button in order to change the microphone from the omnidirectional mode to the directional mode. Automatic directional microphones do not require manual activation. Another feather on directional microphones is a fixed or adaptive **polar plot**. A polar plot refers to a depiction of the directional characteristics of a hearing aid microphone. In a fixed situation, the polar plot remains the same even though the separation between the speech and the noise may change. In the adaptive situation, the polar plot changes in response to the relationship between the location of the noise and the location of the speech.

In addition to the use of directional microphones, technology is also available to digitally reduce noise; this is referred to as **digital noise reduction technology.** This technology allows the hearing aid to monitor the incoming signal to determine whether it is speech or noise. The hearing aid makes these decisions regarding the nature of the incoming signal by monitoring changes in amplitude. This is based on the fact that speech has a more variable amplitude than noise, which tends to be more steady-state. Research suggests that digital noise reduction technology may improve the listener's comfort when communicating in a background of noise, which could lead the listener to become less stressed, more attentive, and less fatigued in such situations. Research does not currently support the goal of increased speech intelligibility using digital noise reduction circuitry.

FIGURE **12.19** **Delta open amplification system.**

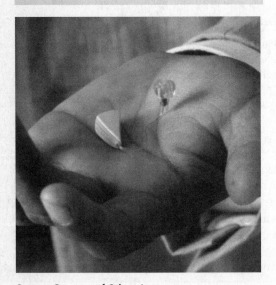

Source: Courtesy of Oticon Inc.

Open Fittings

Increased control of feedback combined with miniaturization and use of digital signal processing have resulted in resurgence in the use of open fittings with discrete behind-the-ear hearing aids. One such example is found in Figure 12.19. The hearing aid is placed behind the ear and is attached to a thin tube that hooks over the ear and attaches to a small ear bud, which comes in various sizes. One of the major advantages of open fittings is that a custom mold is not required and the client can obtain the hearing aid on the day that he receives the hearing evaluation. In addition, the thin tube/miniature hearing aid unit sitting behind the ear is cosmetically appealing for first-time users and baby boomers who are hesitant to wear more noticeable hearing aid products. In addition to achieving the goal of avoiding occlusion by keeping the ear canal open, the listener maintains 15 to 20 dB of natural amplification that occurs due to the resonance characteristics of the ear canal. Making open fittings even more appealing is the fact that most of these products include directional microphones to allow increased speech intelligibility in background noise settings. Finally, it should be noted that improved sound quality is often reported with open fittings, most likely due to the fact that the signal arriving at the ear drum is a combination of unaided low frequencies which enter the ear canal bypassing the ear bud and amplified high-frequency sounds.

Telephone Use

Many users of hearing aids report that their ability to understand speech over the telephone is decreased compared to their ability to understand live speech. They also report that speech understanding over their cell phone is reduced compared to their landline phone. Use of the telephone is very important, especially when we think about the fact that many hearing aid users are elderly and rely on the phone to maintain social interactions and in cases of emergency.

In 1947, Lybarger developed the T-coil to reduce the feedback issues that were occurring as the telephone receiver was placed near a hearing aid. Although in some cases the use of a traditional telecoil is successful, a number of problems have been noted, including overall reduced output and limited speech understanding; interference from other electrical equipment, which creates a buzz that interferes with speech understanding; lack of information regarding the exact position in which to hold the telephone for best speech reception; difficulties in operating manually activated telephone switches; and increased use of cell phones, many of which are incompatible with hearing aids.

Today, a number of developments are helping individuals with hearing loss converse over the telephone. First, the automatic telephone switch has been developed. As the receiver of the telephone is placed near the hearing aid, the induction field generated by the telephone automatically engages a switch in the hearing aid and changes it from the microphone position to the telephone position. In addition, many hearing aids contain telephone coils that are programmable, allowing for flexible programming of the gain and frequency response to improve speech understanding. Also, in July of 2003, the Federal Communications Communication Commission (FCC) mandated that the mobile telephone industry must design telephones that are compatible with hearing aids and that by 2008 half of all the mobile phones produced must be compatible with hearing aids. Finally, the use of Bluetooth technology may be particularly useful for individuals who have difficulty on the phone. Bluetooth technology is discussed later in this chapter.

Wireless Technology

Think for a minute about the fact that today it is possible to use your computer with a wireless mouse, a wireless printer, and a wireless keyboard. You also are able to obtain wireless Internet access. New developments in wireless technology represent a huge leap forward compared to the early days when children in schools using auditory trainers were connected by cables and cords to their teachers. Early FM technology allowed this communication between teacher and student to become wireless and other technologies have also been useful in this capacity. For example, infrared technology and the use of loop systems have also allowed wireless communication. The problem with these systems is that they tend to pick up interference from various sources in the environment, which degrades speech quality.

Fortunately for individuals who have hearing loss, it now appears that experts in the fields of telecommunication and consumer electronics have joined forces with experts in hearing aids and assistive listening devices to create a series of devices that best utilize these emerging technologies. This unique collaboration should help individuals with hearing loss to benefit from all of the information accumulated by these various areas of study, and lead to improvements in the listener's ability to understand speech, particularly in noisy situations and over distances.

Perhaps the most commonly mentioned technology related to wireless communication is **Bluetooth technology,** which is a short-range wireless digital communication standard used to carry audio information or data from one device to another (Yanz, 2005). Bluetooth technology can be used in computer applications, telephone applications, entertainment systems, and personal digital assistants (PDAs) without the use of wires, connectors, or plugs. Bluetooth technology provides a clean, clear digital signal because it is less vulnerable to sources of interference, such as the electrical noise that affects FM technology. The Bluetooth signal is extracted from the noise and only the signal is transferred and amplified. Bluetooth technology also tends to minimize battery consumption.

Bluetooth technology is the technology used in the NOAH-Link, which allows wireless programming of hearing aids. As noted in Figure 12.20, a clients' hearing aid is connected to the NOAH-Link medallion which is worn around the client's neck. Without any wire connection between that medallion and the computer, the audiologist is able to program the aids. This technology affords greater flexibility to audiologists, especially when they make site visits outside of the office. This technology allows greater freedom of movement for both the patient and the audiologist. Bluetooth technology is also being used in brainstem equipment to permit brainstem testing without having the patient attached to the equipment by cords and cables. This application could be particularly important when testing babies or individuals who are difficult to test.

Perhaps the major application of Bluetooth technology for individuals who have hearing loss is assisting them in using the telephone. As depicted in Figure 12.21, a cell phone with Bluetooth technology can be set to automatically recognize the Bluetooth transmitter and as the telephone rings the client can receive that call by simply activating his transmitter, rather than placing the telephone to the ear. This can occur because the conversation is directed to FM receivers, which are attached to his behind-the-ear hearing aid. He does not need to touch the telephone except to dial.

Ear Molds

As you will recall, ear molds are a very important part of the hearing aid fitting process because of the role they play in retention, comfort, controlling feedback, and shaping the acoustic signal. Recently, more attention has been paid in the literature to the

FIGURE **12.20** **Noah medallion.**

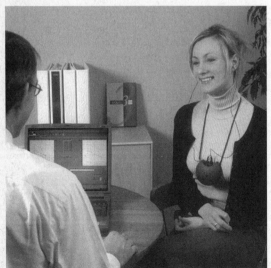

Source: Courtesy of HIMSA Inc.

ear canal as dynamic, and it is now viewed as a changing environment. This is based on recent research (Oliveira et al., 2005) that studied the effects of opening and closing the jaw on the volume of the cartilaginous portion of the ear canal.

You will recall that the cartilaginous portion is the portion between the first and second bend of the ear canal. When the mouth is opened, the volume of the canal increases as the condyle of the jaw moves forward, pulling the cartilage in front of the ears; conversely, when the person bites down, the condyle moves closer to the ear canal compressing the cartilage and causing the ear can volume to decrease. Oliveira and colleagues found that in a significant number of the patients studied, a considerable difference in volume between the two ears was noted as the jaw was opened and closed. This may account for the number of clients who report discomfort or poor fitting from one of their two hearing aids, particularly when they are chewing, smiling, or yawning. The researchers also suggest that the problems noted with ill-forming ear molds may not be related to a poor ear mold impression, but rather due to lack of attention to these volume differences. One potential solution to this problem has been to make ear mold impressions with the patient's jaw opened, using a mouth prop (Pirzanski, 2006). Oliveira and colleagues (2005) believe that new, compliant, otoplastic materials need to be developed that will more readily adapt to these changing ear canal dynamics.

Another recent development regarding ear molds has to do with the scanning of ear mold impressions into a computer and sending them via e-mail to the manufacturer.

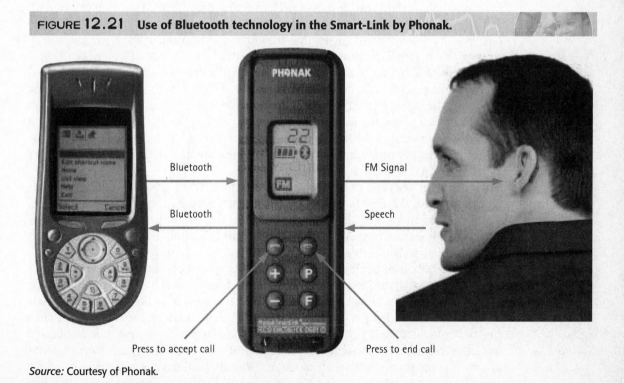

FIGURE 12.21   **Use of Bluetooth technology in the Smart-Link by Phonak.**

Bluetooth

FM Signal

Bluetooth

Speech

Press to accept call

Press to end call

Source: Courtesy of Phonak.

This process has become more common in the last 5 years by the major hearing aid manufacturers and has the advantages of eliminating the need to mail the ear mold and the possibility that the mold will become damaged or change shape/size during shipping. This process (referred to as laser sintering) requires a special scanning device, connected to a personal computer, to scan the impressions into 3D digital models. These models are then saved in a special file and e-mailed to the manufacturer. Some authorities believe that eventually ear mold impressions will no longer be necessary because technology will exist to scan the ear directly into the computer and the ear mold will be built from those digital images.

Verification

Verification is the next stage in the process of hearing aid fitting and is defined as "measures made to determine that the hearing aids meet a set of standards . . . including basic electroacoustics, cosmetic appeal, comfortable fit, and real-ear electroacoustic performance" (ASHA, 1997, p. 127). This step begins when the hearing aids have arrived at the audiologist's office. Perhaps the first aspect of this process that can be carried out is **electroacoustic verification.** This can be assessed by performing a series of measures in the hearing aid text box and comparing the data obtained with the specifications ("specs") provided by the manufacturer. AHSA (1997) notes that ANSI Standards S3.22 and S3.42 should be consulted in performing these measures. A subjective listening check should also be carried out at this stage of the process to ensure that the quality of the sound is consistent with expectations and is free of any gross distortion or evidence of malfunction. Once the hearing aids are in the client's ears, the audiologist should perform a visual inspection to ensure that they fit properly and that the client can insert, remove, and manipulate controls with relative ease.

Also during this verification stage the audiologist determines that the targets used during the hearing aid selection stage have been met. Based on ASHA (1997) guidelines, this should be accomplished through **probe microphone testing.** Figure 12.22 includes a diagram of a probe microphone system. This system involves insertion of a small probe microphone into the ear canal close to the eardrum. Using a speaker placed to the side of the client to produce sound, the system measures the change in sound pressure at the eardrum in the aided condition.

Despite the importance of establishing that the hearing aids are producing the appropriate gain and output, survey data suggest that real ear probe microphone testing, which has been commercially available for about the last 15 years, is not used extensively by audiologists. In fact, only about one-third of audiologists in the United States routinely perform probe microphone testing.

A review of the recent literature on probe microphone testing reveals a focus on the use of speech signals at various input levels. Specifically, recommended input levels are soft, average, and loud in order to ensure that soft speech is audible, average speech is comfortable, and loud signals do not exceed the listener's uncomfortable levels. Referring to Figure 12.23A, B, C, and D, note that these four graphs represent data collected using the Audioscan, a commercially available probe microphone system. Note that, unlike the audiogram, the graphs are based on SPL, with soft sounds at the bottom of the graph and intense sounds at the top. In graph A, 0 dB is represented by the dotted line

FIGURE **12.22** **Depiction of real ear measurement system.**

457

•

Verification

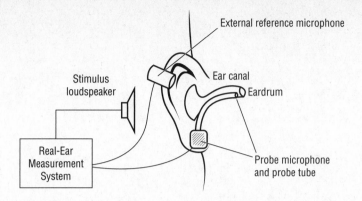

Probe Tube System with a Hearing Aid in Place

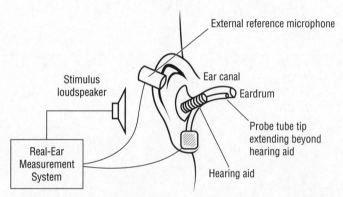

Source: Gelfand, S. (2001). *Essentials of audiology* (2nd ed.). New York: Thieme. Reprinted by permission.

on the lower portion of the graph, the patient's hearing thresholds are in the middle of the graph represented by circles, and the patient's discomfort levels are denoted by asterisks toward the top of the graph. As Smirga (2004) notes, in order for the output of the hearing to be both audible and tolerable, it must produce energy that falls within these two boundaries.

Note next in graph B the introduction of speech stimuli demonstrated by the hatched area. The speech signal is soft (55 dB SPL). Note also that there are three lines, which make up the hatched area. The bottom and top lines represent the softest and loudest components of soft speech respectively, sometimes referred to as L1 and L70. The middle line of the hatched area is the long-term average speech spectrum for soft speech. Note also in graph B that the middle line of the hatched area falls just above the client's threshold, ensuring that soft speech will be audible.

In graph C, average speech is presented (70 dB SPL), and you will note that the softest components of average speech (L70) are close to the patient's thresholds, ensuring

FIGURE **12.23** **Probe microphone testing using speech at various input levels.**

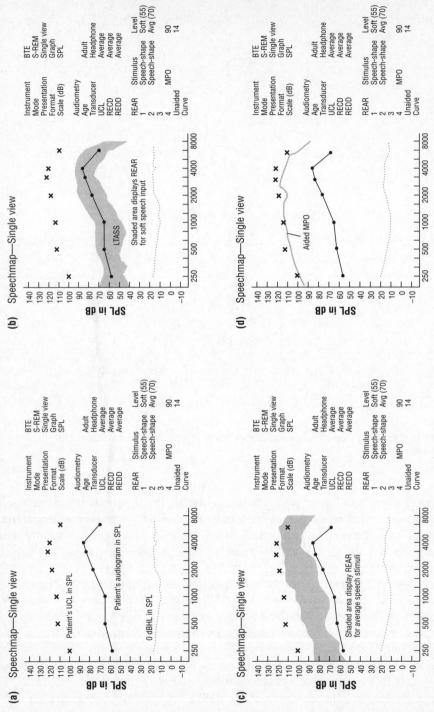

(a) Speechmap—Single view

(b) Speechmap—Single view

(c) Speechmap—Single view

(d) Speechmap—Single view

Source: Smriga, D. (2004). How to measure and demonstrate four key digital hearing aid performance features. *The Hearing Review,* 30–38. Reprinted by permission.

that average speech will be maximally audible to the patient. Note also that the loud components of average speech (L1) do not reach the patient's discomfort level.

Finally, graph D presents data obtained when 85 dB tone bursts are delivered to the hearing aid, ensuring that the output produced does not exceed the patient's discomfort level.

We noted previously that few dispensers routinely use real ear measures to verify hearing aid fittings, instead relying on software predictions made by hearing aid fitting software. Although these software programs are very helpful for making adjustments to hearing aids, they are simulations of gain and output measures for different inputs and are not consistent with real ear aided values. Reliance on software values may lead to under amplification at certain frequencies and over amplification at other frequencies. The obvious advantage of using real ear measures over software predictions is that real ear measures represent actual SLP values for that individual client.

Validation

In addition to verification, audiologists also need to validate that the hearing aids which have been fit to the client are helping the person in the real world. This process of validation may be defined as a determination of whether "the disability has been reduced and that appropriately established goals have been addressed" (ASHA, 1997, p. 128). This is important for a number of reasons. First, validation is a way to determine whether the client's particular concerns are being addressed by the hearing aids. Also, validation allows audiologists to compare the performance of a given client with other client's in the practice. Validation is also important in that it is a way to monitor the overall performance of the practice with respect to meeting clients' needs with amplification. As insurance companies require increasing documentation in order to provide coverage for aural rehabilitation services, validation is becoming an even more important aspect of the fitting process. And finally, performing validated outcome measures is consistent with the important focus in the literature on using evidence-based data to drive clinical decision making.

Despite the importance of performing validation measures, survey data suggest that only about one-third of audiologists use standardized outcome measures to validate hearing aid performance. These same surveys suggest that the two most commonly used outcome measures are the COSI (Client Oriented Scale of Improvement) and the APHAB (Abbreviated Profile of Hearing Aid Benefit). The COSI (Dillon, James, & Ginis, 1997) was developed at the National Acoustics Lab in Australia and requires clients to identify five listening situations that pose difficulties to them and then rank these listening situations in order of importance. Comparisons are then made at the pre- and post–hearing aid fitting. The APHAB, which was developed by Cox and Alexander (1995), consists of twenty-four items that are scored in four different subscales: ease of communication, reverberation, background noise, and adversiveness. The questions are rated on a 7-point scale from "never" to "always."

Finally, the Hearing Instrument Manufacturer's Software Association (HIMSA) created a NOAH-3 module that collects, stores, and retrieves APHAB and COSI data. This module can be downloaded from www.himsa.com and is free to audiologists who are registered on NOAH-3.

Implantable Hearing Aids

In addition to cochlear implants, discussed in detail later in this chapter, there are three basic types of implantable hearing devices: bone anchored hearing aids (BAHA) middle ear implantable hearing devices (MEIHDs), and auditory brainstem implants (ABI). The name of each of these aids is based on the location of the receiver (output transducer). For the BAHA, this would be the temporal bone, behind the ear; for MEIHD, the receiver is implanted in the middle ear cavity, usually on the ossicular chain; for ABI the location would be the brainstem at the level of the cochlear nucleus. Each of these devices provides options to eligible clients for whom where hearing aids no longer provide sufficient assistance. Figure 12.24 shows two implantable hearing aids.

Bone Anchored Hearing Aid (BAHA)

Just as is the case with bone conduction hearing aids described earlier, the BAHA stimulates the cochlea by bone conduction for those clients who cannot wear air conduction aids (e.g., chronically draining ear, postoperative ear abnormalities, congenital atresia). The difference between the BAHA and the traditional bone conduction aid is that the BAHA is secured directly to the mastoid via a surgically implanted screw. An abutment is attached to the screw and the BAHA snaps onto this. This eliminates the potential problem of discomfort or ulcers developing on the mastoid area caused by wearing the

FIGURE **12.24** **Middle ear implantable hearing device (MEIHD) and bone anchored hearing aid (BAHA).**

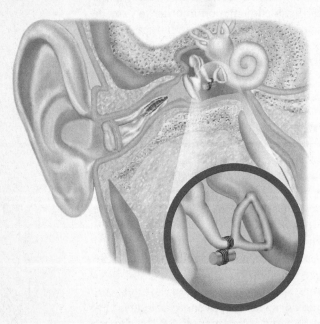
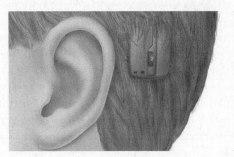

Sources: Left, courtesy of SOUNDTEC. Right, courtesy of Cochlear Limited.

headband required with traditional bone conduction aids. The BAHA received FDA approval (for adults) in 1996 and was introduced in the United States in 1997. Research by Wazen and colleagues (1998, 2001) supports improved speech recognition and hearing handicap scores.

In addition to having some medical or anatomical issues that warrant use of a BAHA, candidates should also report positive benefits during preoperative sound field testing using the BAHA attached to a special headband. Clients should also have the necessary manual dexterity to use the device and to keep the surgical site clean. They also should be free of psychological/psychiatric issues that could interfere with the successful use of the device. Another, more recent, application of the BAHA is for single-side deafness. Traditionally, CROS hearing aids have been used with these clients to route speech from the poor ear to the better ear. Implanting the BAHA on the poor ear has been shown to be an effective way to route information to the better ear, thereby improving overall communication performance.

Middle Ear Implantable Hearing Device

Although digital hearing aids have some clear advantages over analog aids and user satisfaction with the digital aids in on the rise, problems with feedback, occlusion, and comfort persist for some clients. Middle ear implantable hearing devices (MEIHD) were designed to address these issues. As described by Spindel (2002), MEIHDs use a microphone, amplifier, and processor that are similar to those in conventional hearing aids. With MEHIDs, however, the amplified vibrational energy that would typically be directed to the cochlea via the outer and middle ear systems is sent directly to the ossicles using an implanted vibrational transducer. Although the magnet that attaches to the ossicles is implantable, MEIHDs also have an external coil that may be placed either behind or in the ear, depending on the model. Completely implantable devices are not yet available commercially in the United States. MEIHDs were approved by the FDA for adults in 2000 and are appropriate for clients who have up to a severe cochlear hearing loss.

Auditory Brainstem Implant (ABI)

ABI was developed for individuals with Neurofibromatosis type II (NF2). These clients often exhibit bilateral acoustic neuromas. Upon removal of the tumors, profound hearing loss may exist in each ear. Because cranial nerve VIII is often compromised in these clients, cochlear implantation is not feasible. ABI uses an implanted electrode and an external sounds processor to send electrical simulation of the auditory neurons of the cochlear nucleus in hopes of improving the client's ability to detect or understand incoming speech information.

Hearing Aid Orientation

Two federal agencies, the Federal Trade Commission (FTC) and the Food and Drug Administration (FDA), have oversight of hearing aid–related issues. The FTC monitors the sales practices of hearing aid dispensers and vendors. Because hearing aids are considered medical devices, the FDA enforces regulations that deal with their manufacture and sale. States may have their own regulations governing how hearing aids are sold and who may dispense them, including the education, training, and licensure or certification requirements for hearing aid dispensers.

Hearing aids may be dispensed with a **trial period,** which enables consumers to try their custom-made devices for a specified period of time with a return option if the hearing aids prove unsatisfactory. Generally, such a trial period will have certain terms attached. For example, the dispenser may retain a small percentage of the purchase price of the hearing aid(s) if they are returned within the agreed-upon time frame. In addition, it is not uncommon for adjustments or modifications to hearing aids to be made at no additional charge, either by the dispenser or by the manufacturer, during the trial period. State laws and regulations regarding hearing aid dispensers, and hearing aid sales practices (including the availability of trial periods) vary; practitioners and consumers should be familiar with the policies in effect in their communities.

At the time of hearing aid dispensing, sometimes referred to as **hearing aid orientation,** the goal of the session is to provide new hearing aid users with the tools that will enable them to go forward with the hearing aid trial fitting and practice using amplification in their daily routine. These tools include information and certain skills that must be acquired for hearing aid use to be successful. In addition to being provided with written information, the new hearing aid user must be able to do the following: (1) insert and remove the hearing aids, (2) operate any nonautomatic controls or features, (3) change the batteries, (4) use a telephone, and (5) perform basic maintenance tasks.

The hearing aid dispenser should also have certain tools and accessories available for hearing aid users. These vary depending on the style of the hearing aid(s) and may include wax loops, brushes, forced-air blowers, dri-aid kits, battery testers, and devices to hold hearing aids in place (e.g., "Huggies" for children or athletes). Provided in Figure 12.25 are photos of some of these tools.

Hearing aid troubleshooting is another topic that is discussed with new hearing aid users during the dispensing visit and/or trial period. The ability to perform basic troubleshooting is important for clients, audiologists, and speech–language pathologists. Because of the large numbers of speech–language pathologists employed by school districts, nursing homes, and hospitals, where clients with hearing loss may not be able to troubleshoot their hearing aids independently, speech–language pathologists in particular should develop these skills.

During the dispensing visit, written information is usually provided to the user and to caregivers, if applicable. Many hearing aid users consult a professional when their hearing aid does not work as expected. Speech–language pathologists and related professionals may find the following information on hearing aid troubleshooting particularly useful if they serve clients with hearing aids in settings where audiologists are not readily available. It is helpful to have the basic tools discussed earlier, a supply of different sizes of batteries, and a **hearing aid stethoset,** pictured in Figure 12.26 (page 464), available to assist with troubleshooting.

Table 12.1 (page 465) summarizes general information about hearing aid maintenance and troubleshooting for each of the major categories of hearing aids, in-the-ear, and behind-the-ear models. Information for behind-the-ear models can be applied to body-worn and eyeglass hearing aids, which both involve the use of an earmold. For each type of hearing aid, the problems of feedback, intermittent hearing aid function, and no hearing aid function are addressed.

FIGURE **12.25** **Hearing aid maintenance tools: wax loop, brush, air blower, dehumidifier, and battery tester.**

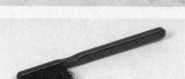

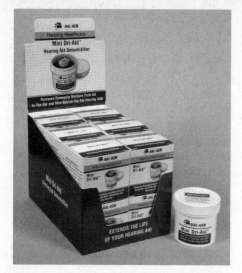

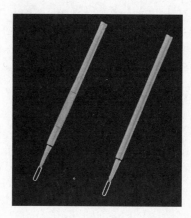

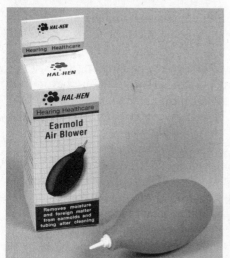

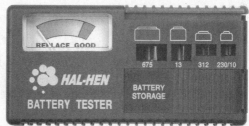

Source: Photos courtesy of Hal-Hen.

Suggested Schedule for Periodic Reevaluation

Once the hearing aid trial period is successfully concluded and the hearing aid(s) are purchased, periodic rechecks will be needed to ensure that the client's hearing sensitivity is stable and that the hearing aids are providing optimal function. For very young children, audiological reevaluations and hearing aid checkups usually occur frequently,

FIGURE 12.26   **Hearing aid stethoset.**

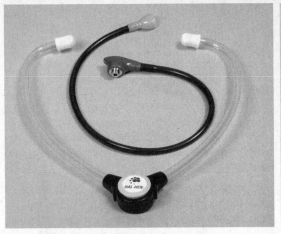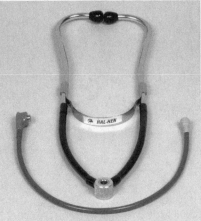

Source: Photos courtesy of Hal-Hen.

possibly on a 3- or 6-month basis. School-age children are typically seen at least annually for audiological reevaluations and hearing aid/amplification checkups, or more often if concerns arise regarding their hearing or hearing aids. For adult hearing aid users, a suggested follow-up schedule includes a recheck of hearing and hearing aids at 1 year after the initial hearing aid fitting. The schedule for periodic follow-up beyond this point should be agreed on with the dispenser based on the client's individual needs.

Assistive Devices

While hearing aids are central to audiological (aural) rehabilitation, they are not the only assistive technology that may benefit individuals with hearing loss and their families. Clinicians should be aware of a wider array of assistive devices that can be used in conjunction with hearing aids or separately. Some devices are "hardwired" (a wire connects the sound source to the listener); others use wireless technology such as infrared or frequency-modulated (FM) waves to conduct the signal from its source to the receiver. Consider the following definition of **assistive devices,** adapted from Wayner (1998), to get an idea of the possibilities: any non-hearing aid device designed to improve the ability of an individual with a hearing loss to communicate and to function more independently despite his or her hearing loss, either by transmitting amplified sound more directly from its source or by transforming it into a tactile or visual signal.

These devices may be classified in several ways. For example, Compton (1995) classifies assistive devices according to their intended purpose: enhancing face-to-face communication, enhancing reception of broadcast media, and enhancing the ability to be alerted by signals. Devices designed to enhance telephone use comprise another category that deserves special attention.

TABLE 12.1   Hearing Aid Maintenance and Troubleshooting

**General Hearing Aid Care
and Maintenance (all types)**

1. Keep hearing aids clean
2. Keep hearing aids dry
3. Keep hearing aids and earmolds in good repair
4. Be careful with hearing aid batteries (storage, use, and disposal)
5. Store hearing aids in a safe place. Avoid dropping hearing aid(s)
6. Keep hearing aids away from hair spray
7. Avoid opening the hearing aid case
8. Avoid exposing the hearing aid to extreme temperature changes

Notes:
3. This includes replacing earmold tubing on a regular basis
4. *Consumer safety information pertaining to batteries should be provided to all consumers.
5. This means away from children, pets, and moisture.
6. Hair spray can clog the microphone
7. This can void the manufacturer's warranty

Behind-the-Ear Hearing Aids

Problem	Possible Cause	Possible Solution
Feedback	Earmold is not inserted properly	Reinsert earmold, making sure it is seated properly in the ear canal
	Earmold tubing is cracked	Check tubing for cracks, especially near where the tubing connects with the earmold
	Vent too large	Contact dispenser to have vent size altered
	Earmold does not fit properly	Contact dispenser to have earmold replaced; this will be more frequent in young children, whose ears are growing, and for those with greater degrees of hearing loss and earmolds with soft material that may shrink over time
	Ear wax buildup in ear canals	Check with hearing aid dispenser or health care provider to determine whether excess ear wax needs to be removed
Intermittent Function	Weak battery	Replace battery
	Battery contacts are dirty	Clean battery contacts
	Moisture in earmold tubing or hearing aid	Remove moisture from earmold tubing with forced air blower; use dri-aid kit (drying agent) to store hearing aid when aid is not in use
	For body aids and FM systems with cords, broken cords may cause intermittent function	Replace cord(s)

(continued)

TABLE 12.1 (continued)

Problem	Possible Cause	Possible Solution
No function	Battery dead	Replace battery
	Battery is upside down	Reinsert battery, making sure that the + on the battery matches the + on the hearing aid battery case
	Tubing and/or earhook clogged	Clean tubing and/or earhook
	Tubing is crimped	Check that tubing is not bent when hearing aid is inserted
	Hearing aid switches in wrong position	Check that the hearing aid is on ("M") Check that the telephone ("T") switch is not activated Change to proper setting
Discomfort	Earmold fits poorly or is inserted incorrectly	Consult with hearing aid dispenser promptly to avoid irritation of external ear/ear canal

In-the-Ear Hearing Aids

Problem	Possible Cause	Possible Solution
Feedback	Hearing aid is not inserted properly	Reinsert hearing aid, making sure it is seated properly in the ear canal
	Hearing aid does not fit properly	Contact hearing aid dispenser for modification or remaking of hearing aid; pay careful attention to this during the trial period/early in the hearing aid fitting
Intermittent function	Wax in receiver tube	Clean wax from receiver tube (located in the canal portion of the hearing aid, usually has soft rubber tubing lining) using wax loop; follow directions provided by hearing aid dispenser for keeping receiver clear.
	Microphone is clogged	Use brush to remove debris from microphone opening (on faceplate of hearing aid)
	Moisture may be affecting the hearing aid	Store the hearing aid with a drying agent (dri-aid kit) when not in use
No function	Battery is dead	Replace battery
	Receiver tube clogged	Follow steps outlined above
	Microphone clogged	Follow steps outlined above
	Check switches/settings	Be sure the hearing aid is in the "microphone" or "on" position and that the telephone coil ("T") switch, if applicable, is not activated
Discomfort	Hearing aid is not inserted properly	Reinsert hearing aid
	Hearing aid fits poorly or is rubbing, causing irritation	Consult hearing aid dispenser promptly so the hearing aid case can be modified or remade as necessary.

General note about feedback: If a hearing aid is in place and turned on, it is normal for feedback, or whistling, to occur in the following situations:

- If the user cups his hand around the hearing aid
- If the hearing aid comes into contact with another person (e.g., hugging someone)
- If the hearing aid comes into contact with another object (e.g., a pillow or a telephone receiver)

Feedback should *not* occur during normal hearing aid use that does not involve covering the microphone.

Face-to-face communication
- FM systems (may be individually tailored or generic)
- Stereo amplified listeners

Broadcast media (television and radio)
- Television decoders
- Radio with TV channels

Signal alerting
- Specialized alarm clocks with flashers or vibration
- Auxiliary telephone ringers or flashers
- Door knock signaler

Telephone
- Amplified handset
- Telecommunication device for the deaf (TDD)
- Telephones designed for individuals with hearing loss
- Telephone amplifiers (either portable or hardwired)

During the hearing aid selection process and discussion of the client's listening needs, the possibility of incorporating devices such as those above should be explored. If devices will be used in conjunction with the hearing aids, the hearing aid circuitry should include a telecoil ("T-coil") with "direct audio input" or DAI capability. DAI should be included in pediatric fittings so that other technologies may be added as the need arises.

For many of the above devices, specific ANSI standards for measurement and comparison purposes do not exist. Therefore, when these devices are recommended, the verification processes may be less formal, relying to a greater extent on client satisfaction and to a lesser extent on formalized testing. Individually tailored **FM systems,** such as those used in educational programs for students with hearing loss, are an exception. These systems are often used in educational settings so that students can benefit from the improved signal-to-noise ratio offered by FM technology, which overcomes the limitations imposed by the distance between the sound source and the hearing aid microphone.

Although ANSI standards for FM systems (also called auditory trainers) do not exist, fitting these devices for individuals with hearing loss is accomplished using generally accepted principles regarding prescription of gain, frequency response, and output parameters that are used during hearing aid fitting. Verifying the effectiveness of these fittings can be accomplished via aided sound field testing and through real ear measures. These verification measures should be conducted routinely and documented by a qualified audiologist to ensure that appropriate amounts of amplification are being delivered to the student/FM system wearer.

Another application of FM technology has been for students with auditory processing deficits. In these cases, the selection of appropriate device characteristics is particularly critical, so that the goals of improved signal reception (improved signal-to-noise ratio) without harm to peripheral hearing function, are accomplished. ASHA's position statement (The Use of FM Amplification Instruments for Infants and Preschool Children with Hearing Impairment, 1991) provides important information on this topic as does Guidelines for Fitting and Monitoring FM Systems (ASHA, 1994), which addresses the issues of fitting, monitoring, and determining the efficacy of these systems.

Lack of standardization in assistive devices makes it important for consumers to have an opportunity to try the devices before they make a final purchase. In some communities, centers exist, for example, within hearing and speech clinics or agencies, where a variety of devices are housed for this purpose.

The assessment process for assistive devices should take into account the client's listening needs, lifestyle, and abilities. How willing is the client to use an assistive device? Is the client willing to use a behind-the-ear hearing aid for the purpose of adding flexibility and adaptability? Is portability of the assistive device important? Can the client manipulate switches if these are necessary for use of the assistive technology? For example, one worker whose hearing aid telephone coils were not sufficiently powerful for her listening needs at work and who was required to use multiple telephones in the workplace was successful in using a portable telephone amplifier that was brought with her from station to station. An amplified handset for a single telephone, which solved listening problems at home, was not a suitable solution for the work setting.

Selection of devices flows from the assessment process. As with the selection of many devices or products, clinicians and consumers should take certain factors into account when assistive devices for those with hearing loss are under consideration. Compton's (1995) list of factors is summarized in Table 12.2.

Addressing these factors during the selection process will increase the likelihood that the selected device(s) will be of use to the consumer instead of relegated to a drawer or closet. Consumers should be given an opportunity to "try before you buy" and an opportunity to give feedback about how the device worked for them as part of an audiological rehabilitation program that incorporates assistive technology.

Adult Aural Rehabilitation

As we have noted, aural rehabilitation involves providing both devices and services to individuals with hearing loss, for the purpose of easing the communication difficulties associated with hearing loss. In clinical practice, the focus is on billable clinical activities, usually centered around the hearing aid dispensing/hearing aid orientation processes. These activities are critical to helping individuals with hearing loss achieve improved access to auditory signals. However, while these activities address the client's hearing ability, they do not necessarily address the client's ability to *listen*. While every client may not require or want to take part in individual or group aural rehabilitation, it is important to know the types of training that are available.

Sweetow (2005) has developed an aural rehabilitation tool called Listening and Communication Enhancement (LACE), which is an interactive, computer-based tool designed to provide listening retraining to clients in their homes. LACE provides both interactive and adaptive tasks. An adaptive task is one in which the user's responses determine the level of difficulty of the task. A correct response results in a more difficult stimulus item, whereas an incorrect response is followed by an easier stimulus item.

The three main areas addressed over this 20-day training program include degraded speech, cognitive skills, and communication strategies. Tasks in the degraded speech category are designed to help develop skills to hear better in noise and listen to fast speech.

TABLE 12.2 Factors to Consider When Choosing Assistive Devices

Effectiveness—to accomplish this, the client will require sufficient instruction in the use of the device

Affordability—whether the device is funded publicly or privately, the cost must be within the client's reach

Operability—the physical design must not be too complicated for the client to use

Reliability—the device should not break down or require frequent repairs

Portability—if the device will be used in more than one location, it should be easy to transport

Versatility—if necessary, the device should be able to be used in a variety of settings (e.g., indoors, outdoors) and for a variety of purposes

Mobility—may factor in to decisions about hardwired vs. wireless technology; distance between listener and sound source is a consideration here

Durability—the life expectancy of the device

Compatibility—ability of the device to be used with other devices and equipment the client has, including nonauditory devices

Cosmetics—client's personal preferences must be taken into account

Previous experience—may need to address prior negative experiences as a prerequisite for acceptance of newer devices

Need for nonauditory telecommunications systems—depending on the degree of hearing loss, some individuals may require a substitute for audition on the telephone, such as a telecommunication device for the deaf (TDD)

Need for alerting devices—consider safety issues, signal alerting/warning

Cultural issues—members of the Deaf community may consider some devices "hearing minded"

Source: Compton (1995).

The cognitive skills activities provide short- and long-term memory training and are designed to improve processing speed. Tasks related to communication strategies are designed to help clients develop skills to improve their performance in daily communication situations. For example, the program includes guidance on asking where to sit in a noisy restaurant and communication tips for clients and their communication partners.

There is some evidence that auditory training programs such as this make a difference that can be measured electrophysiologically. Tremblay et al. (2001) studied changes in the N1-P2 complex after speech sound training. Recall from Chapter 6 that the N1-P2 is a late evoked potential that occurs from 50 to 250 msec after the stimulus, and, unlike other types of auditory evoked potentials, depends on a response from the client. Tremblay et al. (2001) found the N1-P2 response to be a stable response that reflected training-induced changes in neural activity which are associated with improved speech perception. This work also suggests that the central auditory system is capable of change as a result of training, which could prove helpful in posttesting to verify the efficacy of LACE and other auditory training programs in the future.

Wayner (2005) and Hull (2005) reinforce the importance of providing aural rehabilitation services in addition to the hearing aid fitting. Ross (2004) makes the case that attention should also be paid to hearing assistance technology (HAT), including a variety of signal-alerting and other devices that can enhance the quality of life for clients with hearing loss. A central theme in these endeavors is treating clients as individuals, and considering the whole person when devising a treatment plan.

Wayner (2005) discusses aural rehabilitation classes provided at a hearing center over a nearly 25-year period. During that time, the hearing center's hearing aid return rate was 3 percent; this success was considered a result of a high participation rate in a series of three educational classes that took place during the hearing aid trial period.

Hull (2005) describes fourteen principles for providing effective aural rehabilitation. These include, among others:

- Providing an individualized aural rehabilitation plan that focuses on the specific needs of the client
- Making individual and group programs available to clients
- Helping clients develop assertive communication skills
- Exposing clients to additional hearing assistance technology, such as phone amplifiers, FM systems, and other devices for specific situations
- Involving the client's communication partners in aural rehabilitation

Clinicians have a responsibility to be aware of the various types of equipment that are available, and ensure that clients have access to appropriate devices and services.

Improving Classroom Listening

In Chapter 2 you learned about environmental acoustics and the effects of noise and reverberation on a child's ability to understand speech in the classroom. We also noted that ASHA has proposed guidelines for both noise and reverberation. Representatives of the Access Board, which developed the Americans with Disabilities Act (ADA) guidelines, the Acoustical Society of America (ASA), and the American National Standards Institute (ANSI) are working to develop standards for acoustics in classrooms.

How might the audiologist or speech–language pathologist bring about positive changes in the acoustic environment of a classroom? It is important to remember that changes will likely require the support of the school administration and that this support will likely require that administrators be educated about the relationship between the listening environment and learning. Because it is uncommon for professionals in other fields to make this connection, audiologists and speech–language pathologists must take on the important role of education through ongoing in-service and consultation. It may also be helpful to point out to administrators that the Americans with Disabilities Act of 1990 emphasizes removing barriers and improving accessibility for individuals who have a disability. As ASHA (1995) notes, these concepts must be expanded beyond structural barriers and physical accessibility and should include acoustical barriers to communication.

Experts in the area of noise control point out that unwanted noise can be generated from both within the classroom and from outside the classroom. The most common internal noise sources include students talking and movement of desks, chairs, and books. Use of rubber tips (or tennis balls) placed on the bottom of the legs of chairs and desks can reduce some of this noise, as can carpet.

External noise sources typically include noise from adjacent rooms, noise generated by heating/ventilation systems, and noise from outside traffic. These sources of noise may be addressed by modifications to the heating/ventilation system to make it quieter or by strategically placed landscaping to create noise barriers.

Reverberation, which is the continuation of sound as it bounces off hard surfaces, can be addressed by reducing the number of reflective surfaces in the environment. This can be accomplished by covering hard surfaces with sound-absorbing material. Acoustical tiles added to walls and ceilings are also effective. In addition, curtains (or even better, heavy drapes) often reduce reverberation, as does carpeting.

You may recall that the effect of distance on listening was also addressed in Chapter 2. As distance increases, the intensity of the signal decreases. In view of this, it is important in our discussions with teachers about environmental acoustics to emphasize the need to make every effort to limit the distance between speaker and listener. Because this is not easy to achieve, schools should be informed about the value of sound field amplification systems. Unlike personal amplification systems that require the listener to wear some type of receiver, **sound field amplification systems** are similar to public address systems in that the teacher wears a microphone and the signal is delivered to students in the classroom through speakers (usually two to four) that have been mounted on the ceiling or walls. One of the obvious advantages of this type of system is that all of the students in the classroom receive the teacher's speech information more clearly and no particular child is singled out by having to wear equipment. In addition, because these devices are less expensive than individual FM units and the entire class is being helped, this approach is cost-effective. Finally, use of a sound field device can decrease the likelihood that the teacher will develop vocal pathology, a condition that is common among teachers. Summarized in Table 12.3 are advantages and disadvantages of sound field amplification systems. It is important to note that for children who have hearing losses that are greater than mild in degree, a sound field unit is not recommended because the degree of amplification that it provides (approximately 10 dB) will not be sufficient. These students should make use of *individual* FM devices for classroom use.

Finally, Chermak and Musiek (1997) note that as new schools are being constructed, input should be provided during the planning stages to reduce the need later to address issues such as noise and reverberation in classrooms. For example, they recommend that new schools be located in relatively quiet sections of a community and that the location of instructional classrooms be away from the cafeteria, the gymnasium, and the playground. Also, the construction of the walls, doors, and windows should be such that they serve to minimize the amount of noise that can enter the classroom. Finally, heating/ventilation systems should be designed specifically to minimize noise.

Speech–language pathologists will inevitably be expected to be part of the decision-making process with respect to assistive devices in the classroom. Although it is the responsibility of the audiologist to select, evaluate, and fit prosthetic devices related to hearing loss, it is part of the scope of practice of the speech–language pathologist to

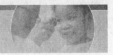

TABLE 12.3 Advantages and Disadvantages of Sound Field Amplification Systems

Advantages

Has been shown to improve academic performance

Provides amplification for *all* children in the classroom, not just one or two

Is cost-effective

Does not create a stigma for the child (or the parent)

Decreases the teacher's chances of developing vocal abuse

Has been shown to be well accepted by teachers

Can be coupled to other instructional equipment (VCR, cassette tape, etc.)

Disadvantages

If the classroom is small or very reverberant, feedback or an increase in reverberation may result.

If the speakers are not placed correctly, amplification can be distributed unevenly to the room

Improves the signal to noise ratio by only about 9 dB (vs. 20–30 dB for individual FM units)

May be too much amplification for children who have hyperacusis and is likely to be too little amplification for children who have moderate hearing loss or greater

Source: Crandell, C., & Smaldino, J. (1995). The importance of room acoustics. In R. Tyler & D. Schum (Eds.), *Assistive devices for persons with hearing impairment.* Published by Allyn and Bacon, Boston, MA. Copyright © 1996 by Pearson Education. Reprinted by permission of the publisher.

employ augmentative and alternative communication (AAC) techniques and strategies to assist their clients (ASHA, 1996b).

Assistive Technology in the Classroom

One type of wireless system that may be used in classrooms or large-group listening settings is the induction loop system. In this system, sound is converted to electrical signals, amplified, and then delivered as electromagnetic energy. This energy is picked up by use of the T switch on the student's hearing aid for all individuals who are seated within the loop of wire around the room that creates the electromagnetic field. Now that mainstreaming and inclusion are used regularly in schools, it is common to find only one or two students with hearing loss in a classroom. In such cases, the student may wear a personal loop around the neck, thus creating his or her own personal magnetic field.

Although an induction loop system can be inexpensive to use and is cosmetically appealing to students (who do not have to wear a separate receiver), disadvantages can include a weak signal and reception of unwanted signals due to interference from electrical wires or lights in the building. In cases of personal neck loop systems, intermittent reception can occur if the student moves his or her head outside of the loop.

The most common method of providing amplification to students in classroom settings is through use of FM technology. In this system, signals are changed into electrical signals and then transmitted to the listener by way of frequency-modulated radio waves. In the typical classroom use, these devices require that signals enter a teacher-worn microphone and are picked up by student-worn receivers. This can be accomplished in different ways. In the past it was common for students, on arriving at school, to remove their personal hearing aids and put on their FM receivers. These receivers allowed students to receive signals from the teacher's microphone (FM mode) or from the hearing aid microphones (HA mode) also located on the receivers. This HA setting allowed the student to hear information presented from fellow students in the classroom. Unlike signals directed to the teacher's microphone which will arrive at the students ear over a range of more than 100 feet, the HA microphones become less effective when information is more than approximately 6 feet away. Finally, the FM/HA mode allowed the student to receive signals from both microphones and in some cases, the audiologist is allowed to set these so that one microphone can be emphasized more than another.

In order to avoid removing the student's personal hearing aids to use an FM device, many school systems, speech–language pathologists, and audiologists now prefer to convert the child's personal hearing aids to FM receivers by attaching an "audio shoe" or "boot" to the aid, as depicted in Figure 12.27. With this approach, students leave their personal hearing aids on in school and receive information in the ways described above using FM, HA, and FM/HA.

There are numerous advantages to the use of FM technology, particularly the improved signal-to-noise ratio that is created for the student. However, these devices are expensive to purchase and maintain, and may also be vulnerable to interference from other radio signals.

Finally, based on information provided by Flexer (1999), a number of questions can be posed to the audiologist by speech–language pathologists, teachers, and parents as they learn about FM technology. Important themes raised include what settings are best for the child and what aspects of speech does the child have access to at these settings, how sound quality and equipment functioning will be monitored, and how outcomes will be measured. These questions highlight, once again, the importance of collaboration between audiologists and speech– language pathologists as they combine their expertise toward the common goal of enhancing speech understanding for children with hearing loss.

Cochlear Implants

Cochlear implants are a type of assistive technology for those with severe to profound hearing loss who do not benefit from conventional amplification. These devices are unique in that they require surgical intervention. They are similar to other types of assistive technology, however, in that clinicians and candidates for cochlear implants and their families must carefully consider the device (the implant itself) as well as the service (audiological rehabilitation) that will follow. As with other types of assistive technology, the cochlear implant (CI) device and the service to support its use are closely linked. Centers that provide cochlear implantation have a responsibility to see that

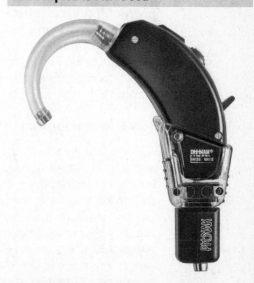

FIGURE 12.27 **Behind-the-ear hearing aid coupled to FM "boot."**

Source: Courtesy of Phonak Hearing Systems.

both technical expertise and audiological/speech–language (re)habilitation are made available to clients under their care.

Advances in technology have resulted in improved design and performance of cochlear implant devices. Developments in the criteria for cochlear implant candidacy, assessment tools used, strategies for programming these devices, and aural rehabilitation considerations following implantation have also occurred. Although most hearing and speech professionals do not work directly with cochlear implants, they are likely to encounter individuals who have implants, or who may be candidates for implants, so it is important to be aware of this technology.

History and Background

Cochlear implants work by providing electrical stimulation to the auditory nerve to give the recipient the sensation of sound. Allesandro Volta is credited with an early experiment using this type of electrical stimulation. In 1790 Volta, who had developed electrolytic cells, inserted metal rods connected to these cells into his ears. He reported a physical perception similar to being struck in the head and an auditory perception resembling the sound of boiling liquid. In 1957, two French surgeons placed an electrode on the auditory nerve of a deaf adult to provide electrical stimulation. In the 1980s Food and Drug Administration (FDA) approvals were granted for cochlear implants for adults, and in 1990 the FDA approved cochlear implants for children age 2 years and older. The FDA subsequently approved cochlear implants for children as young as 18 months of age. In special circumstances, or in certain hospitals where clinical trials are being conducted, implantation of children at 12 months of age is possible.

Cochlear Implant Systems

As Figure 12.28 shows, cochlear implants are composed of both external and internal parts. The externally worn parts include the microphone, the transmitter, and the speech processor. The implanted internal parts include the receiver/stimulator and the electrode array. The power source for a cochlear implant is a battery. Some models have a speech processor that is not worn at ear level (it is connected by a cord and resembles a body-worn hearing aid or a pager) and accommodates a AA-size battery, as shown in Figure 12.28. Other models that have been developed use a behind-the-ear processor that uses a smaller battery size.

How Cochlear Implant Systems Work

With a cochlear implant, the sound signal is picked up by the microphone, sent to the speech processor for coding, returned to the transmitter, sent to the receiver/stimulator and then to the electrode array. The electrodes are placed in the cochlea in close proximity to auditory nerve tissue, which receives the stimulation that is then transmitted to the user's auditory brainstem and auditory association areas in the brain for processing. The electrodes are programmed in a manner consistent with the tonotopic arrangement of the cochlea. That is, the electrodes closest to the base of the cochlea are tuned to receive and transmit high-frequency sounds, while those at the apical end of the cochlea are programmed for low-frequency sounds.

Manufacturers of cochlear implants use various speech coding strategies in the speech processor. If you think about the acoustic aspects of speech that are important for understanding spoken information, you will recall that consonants make the largest contribution to speech intelligibility. The speech processor of a cochlear implant must analyze and filter sound, and make frequency, intensity, and timing cues from speech available to the CI user. The three manufacturers of multichannel cochlear implants in the United States are Cochlear Corporation, Advanced Bionics Corporation, and Med El Corporation. A description and background information on each company are available in *The Parents' Guide to Cochlear Implants* by Chute and Nevins (2002).

The coding strategy used determines how the cochlear implant's speech processor will convert sound into patterns of electrical impulses that will stimulate the auditory nerve. Nie, Barco, and Zeng (2006) point out that, for implant users, consonant recognition is improved with a high rate of stimulation, while vowel recognition is critically dependent on the number of electrodes stimulated. They further indicate that consonant recognition is more dependent on temporal (timing) cues, while vowel recognition is more dependent on spectral cues.

Moore and Teagle (2002) describe CI coding strategies used by Cochlear Corporation as falling into three broad categories:

1. Speech processing strategies that focus more on accurate representation of the frequency components of speech (e.g., Speak—spectral peak)
2. Strategies designed to more faithfully represent the temporal or timing characteristics of speech (e.g., CIS—continuous interleaved sampling)

FIGURE **12.28**   **The Nucleus 3 system.**

The Nucleus 3 system works in the following manner:
1 . Sounds are picked up by the small, directional microphone at ear level.
2. The speech processor filters, analyzes, and digitizes the sound into coded signals.
3. The coded signals are sent from the speech processor to the transmitting coil.
4. The transmitting coil sends the coded signals as FM radio signals to the cochlear implant under the skin.
5. The cochlear implant delivers the appropriate electrical energy to the array of electrodes, which has been inserted into the cochlea.
6. The electrodes along the array stimulate the remaining auditory nerve fibers in the cochlea.
7. The resulting electrical sound information is sent through the auditory system to the brain for interpretation.

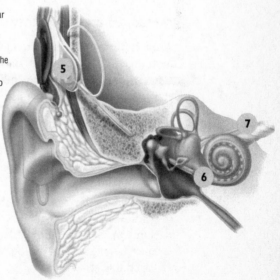

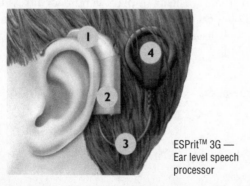

ESPrit™ 3G —
Ear level speech
processor

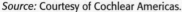

Source: Courtesy of Cochlear Americas.

3. Advanced, hybrid strategies that attempt to give the client the best features of both frequency emphasis and temporal emphasis systems (e.g., advanced combination encoder, or ACE, and n of m, which means the number of available stimulation sites or electrodes [n] out of the total number of sites or electrodes [m]).

These coding strategies are intended to provide the CI user with a speech processing mechanism that is as close to the speech processing that occurs in the normal cochlea as possible. Med El, another cochlear implant manufacturer, uses an advanced mathematic algrorithm to provide high-definition digital signal processing. While earlier coding strategies have focused on the "envelope" or overall intensity of the incoming signal, Wilson et al. (2005) describe emerging speech processor designs that attempt to represent the rapidly changing details in the frequency of the incoming signal (referred to as the fine frequency).

The purpose of developing advanced coding strategies is to provide CI users with improved speech recognition, both in quiet and in noisy settings. Another approach, called HiResolution—or HiRes—delivers electrical current through simultaneous stimulation of adjacent electrode contacts, allowing CI users to perceive additional spectral channels or frequencies. (Advanced Bionics Corporation, 2005). Dunn et al. (2006) compared three different Advanced Bionics coding strategies (CIS and two types of HiRes). Results of their clinical trial with bilateral CI users showed improvements in speech perception for five of the seven adults participating in the study.

In general, faster/higher stimulation rates are associated with improved speech understanding in adults with cochlear implants. There is a compromise between speech and the number of stimulation sites, and the audiologist works to find the optimal rate and speech processor strategy—the one that will result in the most comfortable and clear speech signal—for each cochlear implant user. For children, settings are refined as they mature and can provide feedback about the quality of sound they are receiving.

Assessment and Candidacy Considerations

As noted previously, the intended cochlear implant recipient is someone with a profound (age 12 to 24 months) or severe-profound (over age 2 years) sensorineural hearing loss with no benefit from conventional amplification. Table 12.4 provides additional details about cochlear implant candidacy.

Referral of clients for evaluation of their cochlear implant candidacy takes into account both audiological and nonaudiological factors. A team approach is critical to this process. Depending on the client's age, team members involved in cochlear implant assessment vary somewhat, and may include:

- The client
- The client's parents and/or family members
- Audiologist
- Surgeon (otolaryngologist)
- Speech–language pathologist
- Psychologist
- Social worker
- Educator

TABLE 12.4 Criteria for Cochlear Implant Candidacy

Young children: 12 months to 2 years
- Profound sensorineural hearing loss (nerve deafness) in both ears
- Lack of progress in development of auditory skill with hearing aid or other amplification
- High motivation and realistic expectations from family
- Other medical conditions, if present, do not interfere with cochlear implant procedure

Children: 2 to 17 years
- Severe-to-profound sensorineural hearing loss (nerve deafness) in both ears
- Receive little or no benefit from hearing aids
- Lack of progress in the development of auditory skills
- High motivation and realistic expectations from family

Adults: 18 years and over
- Severe-to-profound sensorineural hearing loss in both ears
- Receive little or no useful benefit from hearing aids
- Qualified candidates are those scoring, with a hearing aid, 50 percent or less on sentence recognition tests in the ear to be implanted and 60 percent or less in the nonimplanted ear or bilaterally.

Source: Courtesy of Cochlear Limited.

The majority of young children who may be cochlear implant candidates have parents who are hearing. Controversy over the decision to implant a young child instead of raising that child in the context of the Deaf community has been the subject of books, articles, and an award-winning documentary called *Sound and Fury*. Adults who may be candidates for implantation can face similar issues. These issues are among those that should be explored when cochlear implantation is under consideration.

Tye-Murray (2004) lists seven stages of the cochlear implant process, from the initial contact through aural rehabilitation. A comprehensive program will address all of these stages, which are summarized in Table 12.5.

Formal Cochlear Implant Evaluation

The formal evaluation process for cochlear implant candidates includes medical, hearing, speech, language, and psychological assessments. The medical evaluation will consider the candidate's general health and ability to undergo surgery. In addition, radiographic studies of the cochleas will be completed. Certain conditions, such as malformations affecting the inner ears/cochleas, can preclude implantation or make the process more difficult. Following meningitis, ossification (bony growth) can occur in the cochlea, which may make it advantageous for individuals who are postmeningitis to be implanted sooner rather than later once a decision to proceed with a cochlear implant has been reached.

Audiological Evaluation Components

A comprehensive evaluation of auditory capabilities is necessary when cochlear implantation is under consideration. In addition to the requirements regarding the degree

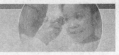

TABLE 12.5 Stages of Management of Cochlear Implants in Children

Stage	Professional(s)	Description
Initial contact	Clinical coordinator	Parent receives information about cochlear implants and candidacy; may be scheduled for an appointment at the cochlear implant center
Preimplant counseling	Speech and hearing professional (usually an audiologist)	Family and child (and educator) receive specific information about candidacy, benefits, commitments, and costs, and are asked to consider such issues as culture and communication mode
Formal evaluation	Audiologist, surgeon, speech–language pathologist, psychologist, educator	Perform medical, hearing, speech, language, and psychological evaluation to determine candidacy, and evaluate the educational environment and adequacy for support of auditory skill development
Surgery	Surgeon	The internal hardware of the cochlear implant is implanted
Fitting/tune-up	Audiologist	The device is fitted on the child and a map is created; parents (and child) receive instruction about care and maintenance
Follow-up	Audiologist and other members of the cochlear implant team	Any problems are explored, and new developments about cochlear implants are reviewed with the family
Aural rehabilitation	Speech and hearing professionals in both medical and educational centers and educators	The child receives long-term speech perception training and language therapy

Source: Foundations of Aural Rehabilitation; Children, Adults, and Their Family Members, 2nd edition, Tye-Murray. 2004. Reprinted with permission of Delmar Learning, a division of Thomson Learning: www.thomsonrights.com. Fax 800-730-2215.

of hearing loss (severe-profound for children over the age of 2 years, profound from 1 to 2 years), results should also demonstrate that the cochlear implant candidate receives little or no benefit from conventional amplification. The audiological test battery will depend on the child's age and ability to participate in the assessment. For very young children, a combination of electrophysiological (ABR), otoacoustic, and immittance testing (tympanometry and acoustic reflex testing) will be carried out, combined with behavioral testing. For somewhat older children, the test battery will include generating an audiogram and assessment of their speech perception skills, using age-appropriate speech audiometric techniques. Assessment will include word recognition testing in auditory only ("listen alone") conditions as well as auditory plus visual conditions, in which auditory and visual cues (speech reading) are provided. Depending on the age and language abilities of the child, closed-set or open-set materials (or both) may be used. A hearing aid evaluation and verification of benefit using objective (real ear measurements) and behavioral methods (aided sound field testing), and trial hearing aid fitting should also be completed.

The audiological test battery conducted prior to the cochlear implant will include generating an audiogram (air conduction, bone conduction, speech recognition thresholds, and word recognition scores), and immittance testing. Speech perception skills will be assessed using auditory only and auditory plus visual stimuli. Testing with amplification and a trial fitting with amplification will be completed in cases in which it is necessary to document lack of or minimal benefit from conventional hearing aids.

Assessing candidacy for a cochlear implant involves more than meeting audiological criteria. A Children's Implant Profile (CHIP) was developed by Hellman (1991) and includes the following eleven items for the cochlear implant team to consider:

Chronological age | Family support and structure
Duration of deafness | Expectations of family (parents and child)
Medical/radiological | Educational environment
Multiple handicapping conditions | Availability of support services
Functional hearing | Cognitive learning style
Speech and language abilities

The need to ensure that young infants identified with hearing loss through newborn hearing screening programs receive early and appropriate habilitation services has resulted in increased demand for assessment tools designed for use with very young infants. Cochlear implant teams, which include audiologists and speech–language pathologists, are responsible for assessing the skills of young infants before and after cochlear implantation. In a study of the PRoduction Infant Scale Evaluation (PRISE) and the Infant-Toddler Meaningful Auditory Integration Scale (IT-MAIS), Kishon-Rabin et al. (2005) found the PRISE to be a useful tool for implant team clinicians to assess prelinguistic skills of infants.

Kishon-Rabin et al. (2005) used two parent questionnaires to study the prelinguistic skills and early auditory skills of infants with hearing loss before and after cochlear implantation. The PRISE is a measure of vocal production that has eleven probes (questions). According to Kishon-Rabin et al. (2005), the design of the PRISE is consistent with developmental milestones for speech production in the first year of life in normally developing infants. The IT-MAIS has 10 probes and is also designed to reflect developmental milestones achieved in the first year of life for auditory skills. The IT-MAIS involves asking parents questions in three different areas of auditory development: (1) changes in vocalization associated with device use; (2) alertness to sounds in everyday environments; and (3) derivation of meaning from sound. This study found a correlation between results on the IT-MAIS and the PRISE, which reinforced the importance of early hearing ability to speech development found by other

TABLE 12.6   **Individual Questions of the PRISE**

1. Does the infant's voice sound pleasant?
2. Does the infant produce sounds other than crying?
3. Does the infant produce sounds in reaction to an auditory stimulus (not necessarily speech)?
4. Does the infant produce sounds of varying intonation?
5. Does the infant produce vowel-like sounds, such as /a/, /e/, /i/?
6. Does the infant produce different consonant-vowel combinations?
7. How often does the infant produce consonant-vowel combinations?
8. Does the infant reduplicate syllables?
9. Does the infant try to repeat the word she heard or a part of it?
10. Does the infant use a permanent sequence of sounds in relating to a certain object?
11. Does the infant use permanent sequences of sounds in relating to certain objects?

Source: Kishon-Rabin, Taitelbaum-Swead, Ezrati-Vinacour, and Hildescheimer (2005).

researchers, including Yoshinaga-Itano (1998). Table 12.6 contains the individual questions of the PRISE.

There are additional questions used by interviewers to solicit information from parents when administering the PRISE. These additional questions provide examples to clarify the type of information being sought. In addition to the correlation found between these parent questionnaires for auditory and speech skill development, these assessment tools have the practical advantage that they can be used in a nonclinical setting, such as the parents' home.

Decision Making

The overall goal of cochlear implant use is improved speech perception, so the client's existing speech perception ability without and with conventional amplification must be known. Although the criteria for cochlear implant candidacy appear straightforward, the process of deciding to use a CI can be complicated. Because surgery is involved, the risks inherent in undergoing an operation must be considered. Additional factors affecting the decision-making process for clients and clinicians include changes in technology and advances in surgical techniques, and the promise of new ways to treat hearing loss in the future. Some of the decisions that must be made involve the following:

- Should one ear or both ears be implanted?
- If one ear is implanted, will the ear with more (or less) residual hearing be implanted?
- Will a hearing aid be used in conjunction with a cochlear implant?
- If so, will the hearing aid be used in the same ear as the implant, or the opposite ear?
- Will other assistive technology be used along with the cochlear implant?

Dowell (2005) summarized issues facing potential CI candidates, noting that prospective CI users and their families need to make decisions based on best possible evidence available. Because improved speech perception is the goal of CI use, Dowell studied open-set speech perception ability in different groups of CI recipients. Their results showed that, at the 3-month postoperative evaluation, 75 percent of CI users score above 70 percent on open-set sentence testing. Given this finding, Dowell concluded that if a candidate's best open-set sentence perception score before implantation was below 70 percent, he would have a 75 percent chance of improvement with the implant. On the other hand, a client would also have a 25 percent chance of poorer performance following implant surgery. Dowell (2005) points to other data showing that 95 percent of CI users achieve an open-set sentence perception score of 40 percent or better. If the prospective CI user has sentence perception below 40 percent, he has only a 5 percent chance of a poorer outcome after implantation.

These data can be used in counseling potential adult CI candidates, as Dowell (2005) suggests. When a client achieves scores poorer than 70 percent with optimally fit hearing aids, and performance for the ear to be implanted is less than 40 percent, the client can be informed that there is a 75 percent chance of improvement with a CI (and less than a 5 percent chance of poorer performance postimplant). This approach assumes that the ear to be implanted will be the one with the poorest speech perception ability.

The conventional approach to cochlear implantation has been to implant one ear, often the better hearing ear. Changes in this thinking are emerging with changing technology and criteria for cochlear implant candidacy. For example, Francis et al. (2005) found that, for postlingually deafened adults with *asymmetrical* hearing loss, there is no added benefit to implanting the better-hearing ear. Speech perception ability was compared across three groups: one with bilateral profound hearing loss, one with bilateral severe hearing loss, and one with asymmetrical losses (a severe hearing loss in one ear and a profound loss in the other ear). As you might expect, Francis et al. (2005) found that speech recognition scores were higher for individuals with severe hearing loss in one or both ears compared with individuals who had profound hearing loss in both ears. However, when comparisons were made between participants with similar amounts of residual hearing in the nonimplanted ear, no difference in speech perception was found among individuals whose implanted ear had a profound hearing loss versus those whose implanted ear had a severe hearing loss. The authors also discuss audiological advantages to implanting the poorer-hearing ear. These advantages include preserving the better-hearing ear for hearing aid use, which has the potential to improve access to auditory information both in quiet and noisy settings.

Besides which ear to implant, advances in CI research have led to changes in thinking about the use of bilateral cochlear implants and various CI–hearing aid combinations. Terms describing various options for cochlear implant/hearing aid arrangements are defined in Table 12.7.

Bimodal Listening

Broadening candidacy criteria for cochlear implantation to include severe degrees of hearing loss has changed the population of CI users. One consequence of this is that children with cochlear implants tend to have usable hearing in their nonimplanted ears. Holt and colleagues (2005) studied children using cochlear implants in one ear and hearing aids in the opposite ear. This arrangement is referred to as **bimodal listening** (Blamey 2005). Holt et al. (2005) discuss several potential benefits of stimulating the nonimplanted ear, including:

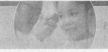

TABLE 12.7   Cochlear Implant or Cochlear Implant/Hearing Aid Arrangement Options

Term	Arrangement
Bimodal	• Use of a cochlear implant in one ear and a hearing aid in the *opposite* ear
Combined electric and acoustic stimulation (EAS)	• Use of a cochlear implant and a hearing aid in the *same* ear
Bilateral CI	• Use of a cochlear implant in *both* ears

• Helping to prevent neural degeneration associated with auditory deprivation
• Making use of bilateral listening advantages, such as binaural summation, localization, squelch effects, and head shadow
• Possibly improving access to finer spectral and temporal pitch cues that are not resolved well by cochlear implants.

Holt et al. (2005) also investigated whether children benefited from continuing to use a hearing aid in the ear opposite their cochlear implant and found that in the controlled laboratory setting, children with severe hearing loss in their nonimplanted ears did have improved word recognition skills through use of a hearing aid in the nonimplanted ear. It is important to note that this benefit was most apparent in noisy listening environments, and that the benefit emerged with experience. The authors also note that additional study is needed to determine the extent to which improved word recognition ability would extend to real-world settings, and whether the benefit would extend beyond improved word recognition skills to other auditory skills such as localization, attention, and academic achievement.

Although most hearing aid users are encouraged to use binaural amplification, Ching (2005) notes that the majority of CI users have not used another device in the nonimplanted ear. Ching (2005) speculates that some possible reasons for this are that CI candidates used to have limited residual hearing in the opposite ear, and/or that clinicians recommended that clients discontinue hearing aid use following cochlear implantation.

Ching (2005) analyzed speech perception benefits as a function of the hearing threshold at 500 Hz in the nonimplanted ear. Her findings showed that those with greater residual hearing at 500 Hz in the nonimplanted ear derive greater speech perception benefits than those with greater degrees of hearing loss. Based on this research, Ching recommends that bimodal fittings should be the management approach used for people who have residual hearing in their nonimplanted ear.

Electric/Acoustic Stimulation

Traditional cochlear implant surgery involves insertion of an electrode array into the 35-mm-long cochlea at a depth ranging from 17 to 25 mm. Dorman et al. (2005) discuss newer techniques, termed "soft surgery," in which an effort is made to preserve low-frequency residual hearing by using a shorter insertion depth (10 mm) for the electrode array. A shorter electrode depth results in less potential damage to the apical (low-frequency) end of the cochlea. This technique is called **EAS**, or **electric/acoustic stimulation,** which is the use of a cochlear implant and a hearing aid in the *same* ear. This procedure allows clients to make use of their low-frequency residual hearing acoustically, with amplification if necessary, while taking advantage of improved access to high-frequency sounds through electric stimulation from the cochlear implant.

Turner et al. (2005) indicate that combining acoustic stimulation with electrical stimulation helps to overcome some of the disadvantages that are a part of electrical stimulation via a cochlear implant. These disadvantages include:

- Limited frequency resolution by current electrode arrays (compared to more accurate frequency resolution with acoustic hearing)
- Destruction of any residual hearing from the implantation surgery

Turner et al. (2005) note that the consequence of limited frequency resolution provided by the electrode arrays that are now available is that speech can sound "fuzzy" to CI users. By preserving low-frequency residual hearing through EAS, this group has demonstrated improved speech understanding, particularly in the presence of noise. Another benefit of EAS was the perception of more natural sound quality, which resulted in greater appreciation for music. This group's multicenter FDA clinical trial has been expanded to include individuals with normal hearing up to 1,500 Hz and severe losses in the higher frequencies.

Speech-language pathologists and audiologists are familiar with the need to provide access to acoustic information in the "speech frequencies" to enhance the ability of an individual with hearing loss to hear and understand speech. Dorman et al. (2005) note that EAS—combining electric and acoustic stimulation in the same ear—creates a new set of questions about the frequency components in speech that are needed to achieve a high level of speech understanding. In addition to the placement of the electrode along the basilar membrane, the programming of the CI electrodes following implantation and subsequent listening experience/training are also important, according to work by Faulkner, Rosen, and Norman (2006). Continued exploration of EAS is under way, with the goal of finding the combination of electric and acoustic stimulation that results in the best speech perception scores for CI users.

Bilateral Cochlear Implants

We have seen that there are many questions about the CI characteristics (e.g., number of electrodes, electrode insertion depth, combination of acoustic and electrical stimulation) that will result in optimal speech perception for CI users. We have also discussed the work of Ching (2005) suggesting that CI users should make use of their nonimplanted ear with well-fit amplification. Audiologists are familiar with the benefits of binaural amplification, and regularly discuss these benefits with their clients. Commonly cited benefits of two-eared hearing for users of hearing aids are improved localization ability and enhanced ability to hear in noisy settings. Do these binaural benefits also apply to CI users? Are there any potential drawbacks to bilateral CI use?

Litovsky et al. (2006) studied **bilateral cochlear implants** in children. They point out that many adults have been implanted bilaterally and have improved ability to localize sounds, and note positive anecdotal reports about their hearing ability. Their preliminary work suggested that many children with bilateral cochlear implants perform better on measures of localization ability with two implants versus one. The researchers further noted that children with bilateral cochlear implants perform better than children using a *bimodal* arrangement (i.e., a CI in one ear and a hearing aid in the other). These researchers caution, however, that much more information is needed before the potential benefits of bilateral cochlear implants are fully understood. In addition, localization represents only one of a host of listening tasks that require study.

Whether we are looking at binaural benefits from cochlear implants or hearing aids, there is a need for clinical tools to assess these benefits in real-world environments. For example, many times each day we find ourselves listening to multiple speakers and/or overlapping conversations, yet hearing tests are most often done in a sound-treated test room. Noble et al. (2005) suggest that tests need to be developed to help discern the actual benefits of binaural amplification through implants or hearing aids in daily life. This is especially important because the benefits of listening with both ears tend to occur in challenging (versus quiet) listening situations. Therefore, there is a need to understand and assess the skills listeners use in everyday real-world environments.

Finally, the decision-making process for bilateral cochlear implants should include a discussion of potential future advances that might require the use of a nonimplanted ear. Litovsky et al. (2006) point out that potential advances in gene therapy, hair cell regeneration, stem cell research, or other possible treatments for hearing loss might not be viable options for children with bilateral CI.

Significant progress in stem cell research was announced in the summer of 2006. A research team at Stanford University, led by Stefan Heller, found that stem cells have the capacity to develop inner ear hair cells in the laboratory. Heller and his colleagues will try this experiment next in live animals, with the hope that it will result in eliminating deafness in animals and ultimately in humans in the future.

Based on these considerations, parents and caregivers may want to think seriously about conserving one ear for such future interventions when there is significant residual hearing. It should now be evident that there are no clear-cut guidelines for making these decisions and numerous technical and client factors that can affect CI decision making and performance. Among these factors are the use of one device or two, the insertion depth of the electrode array, the programming of the CI speech processor, the degree of hearing loss/residual hearing possessed by the client, the duration of the hearing loss, and the client's and family's motivation. Because of the complicated nature of these decisions, clinicians participating on CI teams must present evidence-based, current information to clients, parents, and caregivers as they help them determine the best course of action in each individual situation.

Implantation

According to the Food and Drug Administration 2005 data, nearly 100,000 people worldwide have received implants. This is an increase of 30,000 compared with a 2001 survey of cochlear implant vendors conducted by the National Institute on Deafness and Other Communication Disorders (NIDCD). According to the NIDCD, in the United States, roughly 22,000 adults and nearly 15,000 children have received them.

Candidates for cochlear implantation undergo medical evaluation to ascertain that they are fit to withstand surgery and the risks associated with general anesthesia. Implantation of the internal components of a cochlear implant takes 2 to 3 hours. An incision is made behind the ear and mastoid bone is removed to make a place for the internal receiver/stimulator coil. The electrode array is inserted into the cochlea and positioned in close proximity to neural structures, as shown in Figure 12.28. The hospital stay may range from 1 to 5 days.

Activation of the device generally takes place 1 month after surgery, to allow for healing of the incision site. At this time, the client returns for the fitting of the external components, the microphone, and the speech processor. The audiologist, using a computer, then works with the client to create an individual program for the speech processor. This individual program is called a **cochlear implant map,** and is created by determining comfortable levels of stimulation for the electrodes for an individual cochlear implant recipient. Adaptation to cochlear implant use will depend on the recipient. For children, a wearing schedule for the implant may be established, beginning in quieter environments for short time periods, working toward more challenging listening settings and gradually increasing the number of hours until full-time use is achieved. As with other assistive technology, periodic follow-up is needed for CI users. Cochlear implant users will be seen several times to achieve an optimum fitting, gradually decreasing to annual visits. Periodic tune-ups of the device may also be needed.

Parents of cochlear implant users and/or CI recipients will need training and instruction on the use of the device and basic troubleshooting. Topics for training include information about the batteries, how to work the controls on the device, how to test the device, how to obtain repair service, and warranty information. Cochlear implants should not get wet and can be affected by static electricity. Special care should also be taken to protect the implant when engaging in sports. This information should also be shared with the child's educators and therapists.

Rehabilitation Considerations

Factors that can affect outcomes for CI recipients included in the National Institutes of Health 1995 Consensus Statement are

- Etiology of the hearing loss
- Age of onset of deafness
- Age at implantation
- Duration of deafness
- Residual hearing
- Electrophysiological factors, including the need for viable nerve tissue (spiral ganglion cells) for stimulation
- Device factors, including the number of electrodes and the coding strategy used in the speech processor

In general, individuals who have lost their hearing postlingually will experience greater benefit from cochlear implantation than those with prelingual deafness, and benefits will be greater for those with a shorter duration of auditory deprivation. Some CI recipients communicate using sign language both before and after implantation. The development of listening skills and spoken language skills requires supportive home and educational environments. Individuals, particularly children, who receive cochlear implants should receive speech–language therapy that focuses on auditory skill development regardless of their primary communication mode. This requires commitment and hard work on the part of the family, the CI recipient, and the educational team. Close communication between the implant team and the child's educators is instrumental in this process.

Auditory Training Curriculum

In some cases implant procedures are carried out without adequate attention to the aural rehabilitation component of the process. In other words, the client moves thorough the steps outlined in Table 12.8 from initial contact to audiological mapping/follow-up, but is not provided with the necessary aural rehabilitation or is provided with inadequate aural rehabilitation.

One possible reason for this is that aural rehabilitation can be a time-consuming, long-term endeavor that may not be as cost-effective as other aspects of the implant process. Further, unlike the surgery and the mapping, which clearly fall in the domain of the surgeon and audiologist, respectively, aural rehabilitation is an area of expertise in which some audiologists and speech–language pathologists may have less experience and competence.

Consistent with the philosophy that audiology must be both a scientific and humanistic endeavor, the aural rehabilitation component of the CI process is as essential as the other components. Further, it is essential that both audiologists and speech–language pathologists be familiar with basic principles that guide the development of an auditory training program that would be appropriate for individuals following implant surgery.

Tye-Murray (2004) suggests four essential design principles of an auditory training curriculum, which are summarized in Table 12.8. It is important to note that this information is provided by Tye-Murray as a guide that should be modified depending on the specific needs of the client. Certainly, the auditory skills of a very young child with hearing loss will differ from those of a postlingually deafened adult. The clinical services that are provided to clients must be designed to meet their unique needs. It is also important to note that Tye-Murray's guidelines do not represent a strict sequence of events. In other words, the client does not have to completely master one skill level in order to move on to the next. In fact, aural rehabilitation is likely to be much more interesting and effective if a diversity of activities and difficulty levels are incorporated into the process. In general, when clients have achieved 80 percent mastery of a particular activity and difficulty level, movement to the next level of difficulty is appropriate. Conversely, when clients' performance is below 50 percent, it is appropriate to drop back to an easier level. Finally, this auditory training curriculum could be used for individuals using hearing aids or other types of assistive technology.

Ongoing Assessment of Auditory Skills

The Ling Six Sound Test (Ling, 1989) provides a way for clinicians working with individuals who have hearing loss to assess and monitor their clients' ability to hear and discriminate different speech sounds. As noted in Chapter 5, the Ling Six Sound Test consists of the sounds /a/, /u/, /i/, /sh/, /s/, and /m/. These sounds represent the sounds in the speech frequencies. This informative test is typically used for young clients with amplification, in the process of determining their candidacy for auditory training, and to establish a baseline for comparing pre- and posttherapy measures.

TABLE 12.8 Auditory Training Curriculum Outline

Auditory skills level

Sound awareness	This is the most basic of the auditory skills and refers to the degree to which the client is aware of the presence of sound. Playing "musical chairs" is an activity that can be used with young children.
Sound discrimination	This auditory skill involves determining whether two sounds are the same or different. Initial discrimination can involve nonspeech sounds that are grossly different and then gradually move to finer distinctions between sounds.
Identification	Labeling auditory stimuli is another basic skill. This does not mean that the client has to label the item expressively, but rather that he or she can identify it when the label is presented auditorily.
Comprehension	As language and auditory skills increase, the client is able to understand the meaning of spoken messages.

Stimulus units

Analytic activities	The focus here is on speech segments, such as phonemes or syllables. An emphasis is placed on reception of the acoustic cues for speech perception, such as the voiced vs. voicing distinction.
Synthetic activities	Activities of this type emphasize "top-down" processing, in which overall meaning is gained even if all of the individual components are not detected.

Nature of the activity

Formal	These activities are typically carried out in a more "traditional" therapeutic format, often involving structured activities and some drill.
Informal	These activities are contextualized; the auditory training occurs as part of everyday activities and by a number of people in the client's life.

Difficulty level of the activity (from easier to harder)

Closed vs. open set	Because a closed set of pictures or items is limited in number, it is easier than an open set.
Words vs. sentences	Single words or simple sentences are typically easier to process than more complex sentences.
Dissimilar vs. similar stimuli	Aural rehabilitation typically begins with dissimilar items so that the auditory contrast is great. Gradually, activities include more similar items.
High vs. low context	Contextual cues increase our ability to understand, so high context items are often used initially (e.g., talking about the "here and now" vs. abstract ideas, including visual images to enhance meaning).
Structured vs. spontaneous tasks	Structured listening activities are easier than understanding spontaneous speech due to numerous variables (e.g., rate, dialect) that can reduce the clarity of the message.
Favorable vs. unfavorable signal-to-noise ratio	The less favorable the signal-to-noise ratio, the more difficult speech perception becomes. Background noise can be problematic for cochlear implant users as well as hearing aid users. It is possible to couple an FM system to a cochlear implant system to improve the signal-to-noise ratio for a cochlear implant user in educational or other settings. Use of this additional technology should be explored if the cochlear implant user must contend with noisy environments.

Source: Tye-Murray (2004).

In administering the Six Sound Test, each of the sounds is presented at a normal conversational intensity level (50 dB) at a distance of 3 to 5 feet, without visual cues. The child is required to repeat the presented sound or raise a hand if the sound is heard. The sounds may also be presented at increasing distances. Individuals who have residual hearing up to 1,000 Hz should respond to the vowel sounds presented at a distance of 3 to 5 feet. This provides information about the client's ability to hear suprasegmental patterns. Those with residual hearing up to 2,000 Hz should detect the /sh/ sound. If this is accomplished, the implication is that the second formant of the /i/ sound is audible and that the client will be able to discriminate /i/ from /u/. Those with residual hearing up to 4,000 Hz should detect the /s/ sound. Once baseline results are established, use of the Six Sound Test allows the clinician to detect changes in the client's auditory function. Sanders (1993) points out that this is a way for speech–language pathologists to supplement audiological data.

Tinnitus

Tinnitus may be defined as a noise that is perceived in the ear or head that does not come from any external source. The word is derived from the Latin word *tinnire,* which means to ring or tinkle like a bell. Although the prevalence of tinnitus in the general population is difficult to measure, it has been estimated to be 35 percent, with approximately 17 percent reporting that their tinnitus is present all the time or nearly all the time. It has also been estimated that 12 million Americans are afflicted with tinnitus in its severest form.

Evaluation and treatment of tinnitus is complicated by several factors. First, a client's reaction to tinnitus is often related to the person's personality and psychological state. In fact, comparisons have been made between coping with tinnitus and coping with pain. Some people can tolerate significant pain and not be debilitated by it; others have difficulty coping with even minimal pain. Similarly, the same degree of tinnitus can produce very different degrees of upset in different clients. As will be discussed, some experts believe that the reason for this is that tinnitus involves certain brain centers responsible for emotional control and regulating stress.

Another factor that complicates the evaluation and treatment of tinnitus is the fact that there are currently no agreed-upon standardized recommended protocols for performing tinnitus assessment and treatment. Also, there is a lack of controlled research studies to document the effectiveness of various treatment methods. This results in various techniques being used, without guidance as to which might be best.

A third factor that makes work with tinnitus clients challenging is that audiology training programs tend to provide inconsistent tinnitus training to students. In fact, survey data collected from Au.D. programs reveal that slightly more than one-fourth of the programs provide a course dedicated to tinnitus management (Henry, Zaugg, & Schechter, 2005).

Tinnitus may result from sources involving a medical condition, such as a tumor or pathology in some part of the ear. It also may be generated from the central nervous system. It is the audiologist's responsibility to be familiar with situations that warrant medical referral due to tinnitus. These might include sudden onset tinnitus, tinnitus that worsens, or tinnitus that appears to occur in conjunction with the heartbeat. Also, tinnitus that occurs with a particular host of other symptoms, such as vertigo and hearing loss, would certainly warrant referral. Many of the clients who report tinnitus do not have unidentified medical conditions; their tinnitus simply accompanies their hearing loss.

Two Current Approaches

There are two main approaches that audiologists use to evaluate and treat clients whose tinnitus disrupts their lives. These are tinnitus masking (Vernon & Meikle, 1981) and tinnitus retraining (Jasterboff, 2000).

Tinnitus masking has been used by audiologists for 25 years. For many audiologists it is their main method of intervention for clients who have tinnitus. The goal of the tinnitus masking approach is to provide some relieve from the annoyance of tinnitus by "covering it" with an external stimuli. In addition to performing a complete hearing evaluation, the tinnitus assessment would also include collection of detailed case history. This history typically includes questions about the onset of the tinnitus and how it might have changed over time. Questions might also include a rating of the loudness and annoyance level of the tinnitus and the extent to which other sounds in the environment might "mask" it or distract the client from it. The client may also be asked whether her tinnitus is as much of a concern as her hearing ability and whether she has had previous treatment. Finally, questions about possible causes of the tinnitus are often posed, including questions about wax blockage or medications.

In addition to the tinnitus-oriented case history, the evaluation also often includes measures of tinnitus matching of pitch and loudness. These measures give the audiologist information about the client's perception of the tinnitus that can be used to plan management. Assessment of minimum masking level (MML) is also part of the tinnitus masking evaluation. MML is defined as "the level of broad-band sound that is required to make tinnitus inaudible." (Henry et al., 2002, p. 566). Insight into the potential effectiveness of masking can be gained by comparing the MML with the patient's perception of the loudness of the tinnitus. Prognosis may be better for those clients whose MML is less than or equal to their loudness match.

Regarding tinnitus intervention using masking, a number of clients who have both tinnitus and hearing loss will receive relief from their tinnitus by wearing hearing aids. If the client does not receive adequate tinnitus masking, tinnitus instruments can be used on a trial basis. Such devices amplify incoming sounds and deliver masking, usually by manipulating two separate volume controls. In addition, these clients are typically counseled to use a variety of everyday devices to produce sound in the environment. These devices include relaxation tapes that produce the sounds of nature, a fan, an air conditioner, or soft background music. Use of any of these is part of a process of creating a sound-rich environment to facilitate the masking of tinnitus.

Tinnitus retraining therapy (TRT; Jastenboff, 2000) has been employed by audiologists for the past decade and requires specific training. Based on a neurophysiologic model of tinnitus, TRT focuses less on the actual tinnitus and more on treating the client's emotional and stress response to the tinnitus. Specifically, treatment attempts to disconnect, through counseling, the negative emotional responses that have been tied to the tinnitus. In addition, through low-level auditory stimulation, attempts are made to facilitate habituation of the tinnitus.

In addition to performing a complete hearing evaluation, the assessment that precedes TRT includes collection of a detailed case history using the TRT initial interview. Many of the questions posed are the same as those noted in the previous section. In addition, TRT specifically includes questions regarding the presence of reduced tolerance to sound and a ranking of the importance of addressing problems with tinnitus, hearing abilities, and sound tolerance. Measurement of loudness discomfort levels are an important part of the evaluation, as is loudness and pitch matching. For TRT, tinnitus matching is used in the very important counseling process to demystify the tinnitus and decrease the associated negative emotions. Consider for a moment the client who finds that his tinnitus is actually only 3 dB more intense than his threshold. This reality could be an important step in helping the client to reframe his emotionally charged view of tinnitus.

Once the assessment has been completed, the client is assigned to a specific treatment category. As noted in Table 12.9, clients placed in category 0 have minimal problems and are typically treated successfully with counseling. You will note that clients in all other categories will be advised to use ear level sound generators. Importantly, only certain devices can be used for purposes of sound generation in TRT. These devices deliver low-level wide band noise in an open ear configuration. Unlike masking discussed in the previous section, the purpose of this noise is to "retrain" the brain so that the tinnitus will be habituated. This approach is based on the belief that if tinnitus detectability

TABLE 12.9 Summary of Categories Used in Tinnitus Retraining Therapy (TRT)

Category	Description	Treatment
0	Minimal problem with tinnitus	• Full treatment with TRT is not recommended • Basic counseling regarding TRT principles provided
1	Significant tinnitus At least one major life activity is affected	• Ear level sound generators
2	Significant problem with tinnitus and hearing loss	• Full treatment with TRT is recommended • Use of hearing aids to promote long-term habituation
3	Reduced sound tolerance	• Ear level sound generators specifically adjusted to promote desensitization
4	Sound exposure causes prolonged exacerbation of tinnitus or sound sensitivity	• Ear level sound generators specifically adjusted

Source: Henry et al. (2002).

can be reduced at subconscious levels, it can eventually be habituated at the conscious level. Also, in TRT the use of sound generators typically lasts for 1–2 years (8 hours per day) in order to achieve the desired habituation, compared to the immediate partial or complete relief sometimes reported with tinnitus masking.

As noted in Table 12.9, Category 1 clients have significant tinnitus and will be advised to use ear level sound generators. Clients assigned to category 2 have significant difficulties with both hearing ability and tinnitus. For these clients, a recommendation to use a combination unit would be made in order to facilitate habituation and improve speech understanding. Category 3 clients experience significant sound tolerance difficulties and category 4 clients experience exacerbation of tinnitus or hyperacusis in response to sound. Clients in these last two categories are fit with ear level sound generators with specific adjustments made based on the category.

Prevention

This chapter has focused on ways to help individuals who have hearing loss and the secondary impairments that can result from it. In addition to this important work, audiologists and speech–language pathologists must also assume the equally important role of preventing hearing loss, when possible. In cases where hearing loss cannot be prevented, clinicians must work collaboratively to minimize the secondary negative effects of hearing loss.

ASHA, in various documents (1982, 1988), has made it clear that prevention is one of our most important ethical and civic responsibilities because of the impact it can have in decreasing future rates of disability caused by communication disorders. Although prevention has often been viewed primarily as early identification of hearing loss aimed at reducing the negative impact of the loss on the person's life through early intervention, it is now viewed more broadly. In addition to early identification of existing hearing loss (referred to as secondary prevention), prevention also now includes "increased efforts to eliminate the onset of communication disorders and their causes (referred to as primary prevention) and to promote the development and maintenance of optimal communication" (ASHA, 1988). The term *tertiary prevention* is used in cases in which rehabilitation is carried out in an effort to reduce the disability caused by hearing loss.

Table 12.10, based on ASHA documents and clinical experience, provides some examples of the types of primary prevention activities that can be carried out collaboratively by audiologists and speech–language pathologists. This collaboration is justified because of the numerous relationships that exist between hearing, speech, and language. For example, in the case of the child who has a history of otitis media, one of the most likely negative consequences of this is delayed speech and language development. A prevention program that includes the professionals who can address these areas most effectively will be more useful than one that is more narrowly focused. Sometimes an individual who might be part of the "intended audience" of the prevention program will actually serve with the audiologist and speech–language pathologist in presenting the in-service activity. This becomes particularly valuable when a parent joins the audiologist and speech–language pathologist in presenting information to other parents.

Finally, audiologists can work toward prevention of hearing loss and reduction of the negative effects of hearing loss by becoming involved in organizations that affect public policy (ASHA, 1991). Local, state, and national organizations frequently recruit interested professionals to become active in the shaping of legislation that could ultimately affect a broad segment of the population of individuals who have hearing loss.

TABLE 12.10 **Sample Collaborative Prevention Activities for Audiologists and Speech–Language Pathologists**

Primary Theme of Prevention Activity	Intended Audience	Comments
Prenatal care	Women of child-bearing age and pregnant women; link with other programs when feasible (e.g., Women, Infants and Children Program [WIC])	Include the value of regular prenatal care, the potential consequences of drug and alcohol use and smoking. Stress the importance of good diet and the community supports that are in place to provide needed services.
Auditory-language stimulation with preschoolers who have a history of otitis media	Parents, day-care providers, preschool teachers, program administrators, early intervention program staff	Include information about effective ways to stimulate language development as well as ways to promote preliteracy skills through story reading, nursery rhymes and music.
Noise exposure among school-age and high school students	School-age and high school students, teachers, parents, physicians, school nurses, health educators	Include basic information regarding the anatomy and physiology of the auditory mechanism and the negative effects of noise on the cochlea. Also include common sources of noise and the associated decibel levels. Describe the effects of high-frequency hearing loss and use of custom and noncustom earplugs.
Head trauma among high school and college students	High school and college students, teachers, parents, physicians, school administrators	Include basic information regarding the anatomy and physiology of the brain and how this impacts speech, language and hearing and processing of auditory information. Stress the important role of the frontal lobe and how impairment here interferes with communication and behavior. Include information regarding drinking and driving, use of seat belts, and defensive driving.
Cerebral vascular accident (stroke) among elderly individuals	Elderly individuals, family members, rehabilitation specialists, adult day habilitation program staff, local senior citizen center staff	Include basic information regarding the anatomy and physiology of the brain and how this impacts speech, language, and hearing and processing of auditory information. Discuss risk factors for strokes, including smoking, excessive weight, and high blood pressure. Stress the value of maintaining overall health and regular exercise.

For additional information regarding the planning and implementation of prevention programs, refer to Appendixes A, B, and C of ASHA IV, 1991.

Traditionally, prevention of hearing loss has been done by providing informational counseling to individuals who might be at risk for developing hearing difficulties. Recently, researchers have begun to make breakthroughs in the prevention of hearing loss through investigation of various **otoprotective agents,** including medications and nutritional supplements. Campbell and Ryback (2007) have effectively summarized the current status of otoprotective agents. Their work serves as the foundation for the themes discussed in the following section.

Antioxidants are agents that prevent or reduce increases in the oxygen content of a substance and make up a major category of otoprotective agents. Antioxidants are useful to the body because they prevent excessive formulation of free radicals. This may be done either directly or indirectly. Direct antioxidants act to detoxify the free radicals; indirect antioxidants work by enhancing the body's internal antioxidant system. Antioxidants may also work to reduce cell death caused by ototoxins.

Three long-standing areas of concern for audiologists regarding protection of hearing are (1) the use of "micin" drugs, (2) the use of anticancer drugs, and (3) noise exposure. These are also areas under investigation by researchers interested in developing otoprotective agents.

Aminoglycoside Ototoxity

Aminoglycoside ototoxity refers to damage to the inner ear caused by a category of antibiotics that includes, gentamicin, neomycin, and kanamycin, among others. Campbell and Ryback note that D-methionine (D-met) is an otoprotective agent that is patented, licensed, and close to FDA-sponsored clinical trials for protection against this type of ototoxity. The drug has been shown to reduce impaired thresholds in animals who were injected with gentamicin. Importantly, research also suggests that the use of D-met does not interfere with the effectiveness of the "micin" drug. It is hypothesized that D-met is effective as an otoprotective agent because it functions as a free radical scavenger and also increases the body's internal antioxidant system.

Anticancer Drugs

Cisplatin (CDDP) is an anticancer drug that is commonly used to treat tumors and which, unfortunately, is ototoxic. D-met, discussed above, has been shown in animal studies to be very effective in protecting against hearing loss due to the use of this drug. Another compound, N-acetylcysteine (NAC), has been found to be an effective otoprotectant in rats who were administered CDDP. Concerns do exist, however, that NAC may interfere with the effectiveness of CDDP in destroying tumors.

Noise-Induced Hearing Loss

Currently, the FDA has not approved any otoprotective agent for use with clients who have noise-induced hearing loss. However, Campbell and Ryback believe that several agents are in good position to reach clinical trials. These include D-met, NAC, ebselen, and Acetyl-L-carnitine (ALCAR).

Studies involving noise-induced hearing loss in animals typically involve administering the otoprotective agent and then exposing that animals to several hours of intense noise. Auditory brainstem threshold and outer hair cell status are measured before and after the noise exposure. In such studies D-met, ebselen, and ALCAR have all shown excellent protective capabilities in animals. When NAC was used in humans exposed to 2 hours of loud music (Kramer et al., 2007), no statistically significant difference was noted between those who received NAC and those who did not. Finally, researchers are also studying the effectiveness of agents that can be taken shortly after exposure to noise in an effort to prevent permanent cochlear damage. Such agents are sometimes referred to as "rescue agents."

Hair Cell Regeneration

Hearing loss cannot always be prevented and this chapter discusses a variety of approaches for reducing the negative impact of hearing loss on communication. But imagine for a moment that cochlear hearing loss could be reversed. Exciting new research is under way on regeneration of hair cells and is summarized in this section of the chapter. The foundation of this material comes from Ryals, Matsui, and Cotanche (2007).

The discovery in the late 1980s that birds could regenerate hair cells after experiencing deafness led researchers to question whether this was possible in humans. When research on small mammals revealed no evidence of spontaneous hair cell restoration, researchers began studying the factors that might allow it to occur.

Before describing some of these factors, it is important to note that in birds, the primary manner in which new hair cells are formed occurs when supporting cells of the inner ear divide (through a process of mitosis) to become a supporting cell and hair cell. Supporting cells are **precursor cells,** meaning that they can become only a certain type of cell. This is unlike **stem cells,** for example, which can become any cell type in the human body. Researchers now believe that supporting cells in the inner ear of mammals can become hair cells, if induced to do so. Factors that might facilitate this process include proteins and enzymes essential to stimulating cells to leave their rest state and enter the cell cycle where mitosis can occur, growth factors such as hormones or vitamins that facilitate movement of the cell through the various stages of the cell cycle, and inhibitory agents, responsible for preventing overproduction of cells and proliferation of abnormal cells.

Counseling

When the authors of this text were in graduate school, the primary type of counseling that was carried out by audiologists involved providing information to clients. Although this type of informational or **content counseling** remains an important part of our work, there is now recognition that clients need much more than information and that audiologists and speech–language pathologists can and should provide it. This additional type of counseling is commonly referred to as **support counseling.**

A review of several definitions of **counseling** suggests that it is a process whereby an individual is helped to achieve greater self-understanding and understanding of others for purposes of solving some problem, resolving some conflict, or adjusting to some life event. Counseling often helps people to change in some way and typically leads them to more independent and self-directed behavior.

One of the primary reasons why audiologists and speech–language pathologists typically express a lack of confidence about performing support counseling is that many still think of counseling as a highly specialized activity carried out exclusively by trained counselors (psychologists, psychiatrists, social workers, school counselors, etc.) for individuals who have long-term intrapersonal conflicts. But counseling can certainly be viewed as something broader than this and something that is carried out routinely by many people, including clergy, parents, lawyers, teachers, speech–language pathologists, and audiologists. As Clark (1994) notes, in these cases the person receiving the counseling typically needs to find more productive ways to view some temporary life disruption. It is this second view of counseling that is most relevant to audiologists and speech–language pathologists and is therefore the focus of this chapter.

Let's think for a moment about why individuals who have hearing loss might be in need of counseling. First, hearing loss interferes with communication. Although the dictionary defines communication as the giving and receiving of information, those of us in this field understand that communication is much more. For most individuals oral communication is the means by which human beings manage their interactions with other people. When the close relationships that a person has developed with others are disrupted in some way, meaningful human interactions are threatened and the client's quality of life becomes reduced. It is for these reasons that research suggests that individuals who have hearing loss are more likely to be depressed, more likely to be less satisfied with their lives, and are more likely to have a reduced self-concept (Mulrow et al., 1990; Uhlmann et al., 1989).

In addition, for many people a hearing loss represents more global loss. For example, older people who find that they have a loss of hearing may be reminded that they are aging and that their physical health is at risk. It may cause them to think about what they will "lose" next. For parents whose child is diagnosed with hearing loss, this diagnosis can represent loss of the hopes and dreams that they had for their child. For a musician, hearing loss can mean the end of a career or the end of a source of great joy.

For these reasons, audiologists and speech–language pathologists must accept their role as counselors. In fact, ASHA's preferred practice patterns specifically include counseling as part of the responsibility of the audiologist (1997) and speech–language pathologist (1997). The preferred practice patterns for audiologists are included in Appendix C at the end of this chapter.

Bloom and Cooperman (1992) recommend use of the term **clinician-counselor** to designate the audiologist or speech–language pathologist who, in an effort to provide holistic care to the client, incorporates counseling into the overall management process. This term also highlights the fact that the clinician's primary role is not as counselor; rather, counseling is used as part of an overall plan to address personal issues stemming from the communication disorder. Bloom and Cooperman (1999) state that when counseling is included, individuals can make gains that are not solely related to their communication disorder. Specifically, they can also learn to view themselves and their environment more positively.

The Counseling Triangle

What, then, are the components that go into making one a good counselor? According to Bloom and Cooperman (1999), there are three components that make up the counseling triangle: skills, theories, and personal style. Skills in the counseling triangle are specific listening/attending activities that the clinician-counselor carries out in interactions with the client. Attending to the client, encouraging her to express her perception of the problem at hand, and communicating empathy are all skills that can help to establish rapport and create a climate of openness and trust.

The theories aspect of the counseling triangle refers to knowledge of specific counseling theories that can guide the clinician's interactions with the client. Perhaps the theory that has the broadest application to the work of professionals in communication disorders is **person-centered therapy,** developed by Carl Rogers (1980). The underlying principle of this approach is that clients not only have the ability to solve their own problems and move toward a more positive and healthy state, they also have the right to this. This also implies that clients are in charge of their recovery, with support from the clinician-counselor who helps the client draw from their own inner strengths. In order for person-centered therapy to be successful, audiologists must be willing and able to accept their role as nonexperts who provide answers and allow clients to direct their own management plan.

Audiologists must also view their clients with unconditional positive regard. This means that the clinician accepts clients as they are, regardless of the array of emotions they may be experiencing. It also means that even in the face of anger which may be directed to the clinician, or a lack of movement by the client toward stated goals, the client is still viewed as a person of dignity who deserves to reach a more positive emotional place.

Personal style is the third component of the counseling triangle and includes, among other things, the clinician-counselor's knowledge of self. Individuals choose helping professions for different reasons and sometimes those reasons are unhealthy. Is the helper seeking appreciation from their clients? Is the helper relying on the client to boost their own ego and to make them feel powerful? Does the helper judge his own self-worth based on the degree to which the client follows his advice? The audiologist who has self-awareness understands that it is not the role of the clinician-counselor to convince the client to take a certain course of action. Rather, the use of counseling is intended to guide the client to identify a solution or solutions that makes sense in his life. Finally, no plan of care should be predetermined without the active involvement of the client or, in the case of children, the parents. Remember that one of the goals of counseling is to help clients become more independent. This clearly cannot be achieved if they are not included in the decision-making process

Understanding Human Reactions

In addition to knowing about self, skills, and theories, an effective clinician-counselor also knows about human reactions to life's challenges. Although each client is unique and it is impossible to predict how a particular client or parent will react to a diagnosis of hearing loss, it is important for audiologists and speech–language pathologists to be aware of some of the patterns of behavior that have been noted when individuals are confronted with challenging life events.

One such reaction is grief, defined as "a pattern of physical and emotional responses to separation or loss . . . proceeding in stages from alarm to disbelief and denial, to anger and guilt, to finding a source of comfort, and finally to adjusting to the loss" (*Mosby Medical Encyclopedia,* 1996). Disbelief and denial are often noted in clients who cannot acknowledge that they have a hearing loss, even after it has been documented by the testing. Another example is the parent who, in an effort to find a more acceptable explanation for the test results indicating hearing loss, questions the audiologist's competence.

Anger is a second human reaction that can be encountered in our work, and although it can be a difficult stage for all those involved, it often signals movement away from denial. At this stage, the question that is typically raised is, Why did this have to happen to me (or to my child)? Van Hecke (1994) points out that the individual who has just been told that she has hearing loss may resent her peers who do not. She may also react to the news with a broader anger that "life is unfair to me" or "life is unjust." Often times, older individuals who have had some sense that life is fair find this mind-set severely challenged when personal difficulties arise. This can lead to anger, which is sometimes directed to the person who has delivered the unwelcome news. One client was furious with his audiologist because the factory at which he worked for 30 years did not educate him as to the dangers of noise exposure and the need to use ear protection. He was even more enraged to learn that the company did not fully cover the cost of his hearing aids.

Particularly for parents of children diagnosed with hearing loss, guilt can become an issue during this process. This may be manifested in the form of questions, such as What do you think could have caused my child's hearing loss? or Do you think the fact that I had some wine during my pregnancy could have caused this? The parent is attempting to receive reassurance that they did not do something to cause their child's loss.

It is important to make brief mention at this point of the questions that clients and parents ask. In the questions noted above, it should be very clear to the audiologist that the parent is seeking reassurance. But sometimes questions that appear to be simple content questions are, in fact, what Clark (1994) refers to as questions with an affective base. Unlike content questions, which typically are answered with factual information, affective, or emotionally based, questions require the clinician to understand the deeper issue that is being questioned and to respond in a humanistic manner.

Some clinician-counselors find it difficult to reassure clients and parents without providing them with false hope. For example, the mother of a child diagnosed with bilateral deafness who asks if you think everything will work out all right for her child, is clearly seeking reassurance. Although it is important to be as honest as possible with client and parents, it is also true that no one can predict the future and statistics about average performance of children with hearing loss may not apply to the particular child in question. In view of this, there is no reason to paint an unnecessarily bleak picture and there certainly are reasons to avoid doing so. There is value in pointing out that even though there will likely be challenging times ahead, the necessary support, guidance, and resources will also be available.

Anxiety, which is defined as a feeling of worry or fear due to some perceived threat, is another common reaction to receiving any medical diagnosis. With respect to hearing loss, anxiety can result from wondering if the loss will worsen or the extent to which the loss will interfere with the pursuit of individual goals and dreams.

In many cases, providing accurate factual information can be very effective in reducing a client's undue anxiety. In other words, when clients lack knowledge, they may "fill in" missing information with worst-case scenarios that, of course, create undue anxiety. Content counseling, in the form of reliable information, can reduce anxiety and facilitate the client's emotional health. Factual information can also help to reduce depression if the source of the depression is the client's unrealistic and catastrophic reaction to the diagnosis. It may be useful to summarize this discussion of counseling with a review of the essential themes involved in effective integration of counseling into the work of audiologists.

A Further Look at Diagnosis through Aural Rehabilitation—Five Sample Cases

Case #1—Joseph, Age 6 Months

Joe was "referred" after failing his initial newborn hearing screening and his follow-up screening. He was referred to the Part C (Early Intervention) Program for diagnostic audiological evaluation to rule out hearing loss at age 2 months. The diagnostic audiological evaluation consisted of brainstem auditory evoked response testing using clicks and tones and immittance measures. Test results revealed a bilateral sensorineural hearing loss of a moderate to severe degree. Recommendations made included an ENT consult to further investigate the etiology of the hearing loss and to obtain medical clearance for use of amplification; genetic counseling to further explore the cause of the hearing loss; hearing aid evaluation to select appropriate amplification devices and make earmold impressions; continued participation in the Part C early intervention program to pursue a multidisciplinary evaluation and services; this will link Joe and his parents/family with services to support the development of communication skills, including auditory, language, and speech skills. Appropriate counseling should also be provided to address the adjustment of parents and family to having a child with a hearing loss.

Based on the audiometric test data collected, Joe was fit with binaural behind-the-ear hearing aids with moderate gain and output not to exceed 120 dB SPL. The hearing aids should be equipped with tamper-resistant battery doors and direct audio input capability. Earmold characteristics include soft, shell-style earmolds using hypoallergenic material, long canal length, and relief vents. Verification of the fitting will be performed using real ear measures. Follow-up visits will be scheduled every 2 weeks for the duration of the trial period with follow-up every 1 to 3 months thereafter. Hearing aid orientation information will be reviewed with parents along with information regarding expectations for young children with new hearing aids using an instrument such as the DIAL.

A speech–language pathologist and/or teacher of the deaf and hard of hearing, provided by the early intervention program, will educate the family and caregivers about options for communication, including how to stimulate communication skill development, language and speech stimulation, auditory training, and development of listening skills.

Case #2—Markus, Age 3.5 Years

Markus was identified with hearing loss at age 13 months, after being referred to a hearing and speech center in his community. The reason for referral was parental concern that he had stopped babbling at about 9 months of age. In addition, he did not startle to sounds. Markus was diagnosed with a severe sensorineural hearing loss. Test techniques included sedated ABR testing, supplemented by behavioral testing using visual reinforcement audiometry and immittance testing. Markus has a history of occasional middle ear effusion. His history is also significant for anoxia at birth. Concerns about motor development have been raised by his preschool teachers. He currently attends a preschool program designed for children with hearing loss where a total communication approach is used.

Audiological reevaluation, scheduled to check the status of hearing levels and both the personal and classroom amplification systems, revealed a severe sensorineural hearing loss bilaterally, unchanged from the last evaluation 6 months ago. Middle ear function is within normal limits bilaterally. Markus's right personal hearing aid is working in accordance with manufacturer's specifications; however, he is experiencing feedback. The left-ear hearing aid is not working (dead) at this time. His FM system is functioning according to the manufacturer's specifications; however, earmolds are loose-fitting and feedback is occurring. Following the testing, earmold impressions were made. Recommendations included continued use of amplification as outlined above; repair of the left hearing aid; use of a loaner aid in the interim; new earmolds for personal and FM systems; real ear measures with both personal amplification and FM systems once the new earmolds are dispensed; and physical therapy evaluation in view of concerns regarding motor development.

Case #3—Kelly, Age 12 Years

Kelly has a moderate sensorineural hearing loss that was identified when she was 3 years old. She is in sixth grade and participates in the regular educational curriculum. In addition, she receives speech–language services 3 × 30 per week and resource room assistance three times per week including work on curriculum, written expression, and reading support. Kelly's IQ scores are in average range. She has reduced language, vocabulary, and pragmatic skills and is approximately 1 year behind in reading ability. Mild to moderate articulation errors were documented on the Goldman-Fristoe test of articulation. The resource room teacher also functions as overall case manager and contact person.

Kelly was seen for an annual audiological reevaluation at the beginning of the school year. Her family expressed concern about her hearing because she has been listening to her iPod through earphones at loud levels. Test results continue to support a moderate loss, unchanged from previous test results. Word recognition is good bilaterally when speech is presented at 80 dB HL. Immittance test results show normal middle ear pressure and compliance bilaterally. Acoustic reflexes are present at reduced sensation levels. Kelly's hearing aids are working according to the manufacturer's specifications and bring soft and average speech to appropriate targets on real ear measures. Kelly uses an ear-level FM system in the classroom. The FM system is also in working order and meets targets on real ear measures. Using the FM system, aided word recognition scores are good (88 percent) when speech is presented at 45 dB HL in the sound field.

Recommendations, designed to provide the audiological support necessary for successful functioning in the auditory-verbal environment of the classroom so that Kelly can continue to make progress in all academic areas, included annual reevaluation including audiological testing and assessment of personal amplification and classroom (FM) amplification systems; use of moderation when listening to music; consult with Kelly's classroom teacher to discuss strategies (see Appendix A) to assist her in school and to review audiological goals in Kelly's IEP.

Case #4—Bill, 48 Years

Bill works in a noisy factory setting. He has used disposable hearing protection sporadically for the past 5 years of his 25-year employment. He has a bilateral sensorineural hearing loss of mild sloping to moderate severe degree and reports tinnitus and difficulty hearing in noise. Bill is interested in improving his ability to hear his family at home. He also socializes in noisy settings and would like to hear better at these times. His wife would like the television to be at a comfortable listening level. Following the hearing assessment, a hearing aid evaluation took place. The first recommendation was medical clearance for amplification, using binaural mini-behind-the-ear aids in an open earmold configuration. The aids were digital and included directional microphones. Also recommended were use of custom hearing protection devices for on- and off-the-job noise exposure, counseling regarding the effects of noise, and information about the American Tinnitus Association.

Outcomes assessed at follow-up visits revealed that the television volume improved since Bill began using hearing aids. Bill also reported improved ability to hear the television and family/friends at home and in social settings. Bill also began using the custom hearing protection devices more consistently in the workplace due to improved comfort.

Case #5—Martha, Age 78 Years

Martha lives at home by herself. She has a moderate to severe sensorineural hearing loss bilaterally, which has progressed gradually over the past 8 to 10 years. Family members are concerned about her safety, noting that she has difficulty hearing the doorbell and the telephone ring. The telephone is an important link to Martha's sisters, children, and friends. In addition, Martha has been quiet and withdrawn at family gatherings, which she is beginning to avoid. Martha's family is interested in having her hear better to allow her to remain in her current living situation and to increase her ability to participate in family gatherings. Martha was initially somewhat resistant but agreed to go along with the hearing aid evaluation to appease her family.

Following the assessment, a hearing aid evaluation took place. During the hearing aid evaluation, a trial period with binaural in-the-ear digital hearing aids with an automatic telephone switch (on one ear) was urged. Also, Martha agreed to enroll in a 4-week aural rehabilitation group designed to teach members about hearing loss and hearing aid use. Participants also had an opportunity to practice communication skills in this setting. Martha adapted to hearing aid use after several visits to work on her ability to insert/remove the hearing aids, change the batteries independently, and clean/maintain the instruments. In addition to acquiring the technical skills needed to use hearing aids, Martha's confidence increased. Martha's family reported that she has begun to participate in family gatherings and can now hear the doorbell and the telephone ring.

Diagnosis of hearing loss is the foundation for audiological rehabilitation, which includes providing devices and services designed to assist individuals with hearing loss to improve their overall communicative function. It is important to recognize that amplification devices and other prosthetic devices do not restore hearing to "normal." In addition, the critical variable in successful provision of assistive technology is the delivery of services—client and family education, information and referral, counseling and support—designed to assist the client and the people they communicate with. Effective audiological rehabilitation requires willingness to listen to the client's concerns and hopes and facilitating for the client access to a wide array of resources that includes the clinician's individual technical expertise and that of colleagues within our own profession and across other disciplines.

This chapter provided an overview of the process of providing amplification to clients, including treatment planning, hearing aid selection, verification, and validation. Both conventional and advanced hearing aids were discussed. Issues related to the delivery of assistive technology were also addressed, as well as the use of surgical interventions, such as cochlear implants, bone anchored hearing aids, and middle ear implants. The responsibility of audiologists and speech–language pathologists to provide both content and support counseling was covered with specific techniques provided and case examples to illustrate.

QUESTIONS FOR DISCUSSION

1. Provide specific arguments in favor of the statement that aural rehabilitation is a combination of devices and services.
2. Compare and contrast technology used with traditional hearing aids versus technology available on programmable and digital aids.
3. Describe the contributions of case history, pure tone, and speech audiometry data for the fitting of hearing aids.
4. Describe the role of the speech–language pathologist in troubleshooting hearing aids. What specific tools should the speech–language pathologist have available to carry out troubleshooting?
5. What are cochlear implants, and what are the major steps that parents would be likely to go through in order to obtain this for their deaf child?
6. Define tinnitus and then describe various possible causes and corresponding treatments.
7. Describe the importance of room acoustics and FM technology in a classroom with two children with hearing loss.
8. What are three coding strategies used in the speech processor of a cochlear implant?
9. List three possible hearing aid/cochlear implant arrangements, and discuss the pros and cons of each arrangement.
10. What types of audiological tests are needed to measure benefits from various hearing aid/cochlear implant arrangements? Discuss testing in quiet versus noise and the information that can be derived from each.
11. What areas of research may have an impact on the future of cochlear implants?

RECOMMENDED READING

Abrahamson, J. (2000). Group audiologic rehabilitation. *Seminar in Hearing, 21*(3), 227–233.

American Tinnitus Association. (1997). *Information about tinnitus.* Portland, OR: Author.

Archbold, S., Nikolopoulos, T., Lutman, M., & O'Donoghue, G. (2002). The educational settings of profoundly deaf children with cochlear implants compared with age-matched peers with hearing aids: Implications for management. *International Journal of Audiology, 41,* 157–161.

Balmey, P., Barry, J., & Jacq, P. (2001). Phonetic inventory development in young cochlear implant users 6 years postoperation. *Journal of Speech, Language, and Hearing Research, 4,* 73–79.

Ching, T., Psarros, C., Hill, M., Dillon, H., & Incerti, P. (2001). Should children who use cochlear implants wear hearing aids in the opposite ear? *Ear and Hearing, 22*(5), 365–380.

Ching, T. Y. C., Britton, L., Dillon, H., & Agung, K. (2002). RECD, REAG, NAL-NL1: Accurate and practical methods for fitting nonlinear hearing aids to infants and children. *Hearing Review, 9*(8), 12–20, 52. Also available on-line at www.nal.gov.au, this article provides a detailed summary of methods for fitting hearing aids to infants and young children, including step-by-step information on using NAL-NL1 software.

Clark, J., & Martin, F. (1994). *Effective counseling in audiology: Perspectives and practice.* Englewood Cliffs, NJ: Prentice Hall.

DiSarno, N., Schowalter, M., & Grassa, P. (2002). Classroom amplification to enhance student performance. *Teaching Exceptional Children, 34*(6), 20–26.

Discolo, C., & Hirose, K. (2002). Pediatric cochlear implants. *American Journal of Audiology, 11,* 114–118.

English, K. (2001). *Counseling children with hearing impairments and their families.* Boston: Allyn & Bacon.

Hall, J., & Haynes, D. (2001). Audiological assessment and consultation of the tinnitus patient. *Seminar in Hearing, 22*(1), 37–49.

Humes, L. (2002). Changes in hearing benefit following 1 or 2 years of hearing aid use by older adults. *Journal of Speech, Language, and Hearing Research, 45,* 772–782.

Jastreboff, P. (2001). Tinnitus retraining therapy. *Seminars in Hearing, 22*(1), 51–63.

Jusczyk, P., & Luce, P. (2002). Speech perception and spoken word recognition: Past and present. *Ear and Hearing, 23*(1), 2–40.

Kricos, P., & Lesner, S. (2000). Evaluating the success of adult audiologic rehabilitation support programs. *Seminars in Hearing, 21*(3), 267–279.

Reich, G. (2001). The role of informal support and counseling in the management of tinnitus. *Seminars in Hearing, 22*(1), 7–13.

Rubenstein, T. (2002). Pediatric cochlear implantation: Prosthetic hearing and language development. *Lancet, 360,* 483–485.

Spitzer, J. (2000). Toward contemporary models of adult audiologic rehabilitation. *Seminars in Hearing, 21*(3), 205–212.

Spitzer, J., Ghossaini, S., & Wazen, J. (2002). Evolving application in the use of bone anchored hearing aids. *American Journal of Audiology, 11,* 96–103.

Tyler, R., & Schum, D. (1995). *Assistive devices for persons with hearing impairment.* Boston: Allyn & Bacon.

Valente, M., Goebel, J., Duddy, D., Sinks, B., & Peterein, J. (2000). Evaluation and treatment of severe hyperacusis. *Journal of the American Academy of Audiology,* 295–299.

Voll, L. (2000). Application of technology to improve signal to noise ratio. *Seminars in Hearing, 21*(2), 157–168.

Von Hapsburg, D., & Pena, E. (2002). Understanding bilingualism and its impact on speech audiometry. *Journal of Speech, Language, and Hearing Research, 45,* 202–213.

Waltzman, S., & Cohen, N. (2000). *Cochlear implants.* New York: Thieme.

Wayner, D. (2000). Audiologic rehabilitation for adults with cochlear implants. *Seminars in Hearing, 21*(3), 245–255.

Weber, P. (2002). Medical and surgical considerations for implantable hearing prosthetic devices. *American Journal of Audiology, 11,* 134–138.

Advanced Bionics Corporation. (2005, February). Increasing spectral channels through current steering in HiResolution Bionic Ear® users. Valencia, CA: Author.

Alpiner, J., Chevrette, W., Glascoe, G., Metz, M., & Olsen, B. (1974). *The Denver Scale of Communication Function.* Unpublished study, University of Denver.

American Speech-Language-Hearing Association (ASHA). (1982). Prevention of speech, language, and hearing problems: Committee on the prevention of speech, language, and hearing problems. *ASHA, 24,* 425–431.

American Speech-Language-Hearing Association (ASHA). (1988). Prevention of communication disorders: Committee on prevention of speech, language, and hearing disorders. *ASHA, 30,* 90.

American Speech-Language-Hearing Association (ASHA). (1991). The use of FM amplification instruments for infants and preschool children with hearing impairment. *ASHA, 33*(Suppl. 5), 1–2.

American Speech-Language-Hearing Association (ASHA). (1994, March). Guidelines for fitting and monitoring FM systems. *ASHA, 36*(Suppl. 12), 1–9.

American Speech-Language-Hearing Association (ASHA). (1995, March). Position statement and guidelines for acoustics in educational settings. *ASHA, 37*(Suppl. 14), 15–19.

American Speech-Language-Hearing Association (ASHA). (1996a, Spring). Scope of practice in audiology. *ASHA, 38*(Suppl. 16), 12–15.

American Speech-Language-Hearing Association (ASHA). (1996b, Spring). Scope of practice in speech-language pathology. *ASHA, 38*(Suppl. 16), 16–20.

American Speech-Language-Hearing Association (ASHA). (1997). *Preferred practice patterns for the profession of audiology.* Rockville, MD: Author.

American Speech-Language-Hearing Association (ASHA) Ad Hoc Committee on Hearing Aid Selection and Fitting. (1998). Guidelines for hearing aid fitting for adults. *American Journal of Audiology, 7,* 5–13.

American Speech-Language-Hearing Association. (2001). Scope of practice in speech-language pathology. Rockville, MD: Author.

American Speech-Language-Hearing Association. (2004). Scope of practice in audiology. *ASHA Supplement 24,* in press.

Assistive Technology Act of 1998. Public Law 105-394, 105th Congress.

Blamey, P. J. (2005). Sound processing in hearing aids and CIs is gradually converging. *The Hearing Journal, 58*(11), 44–52.

Bloom, C., & Cooperman, D. (1992). *The clinical interview: A guide for speech-language pathologists and audiologists* (2nd ed.). Rockville, MD: National Student Speech Language Hearing Association.

Bloom, C., & Cooperman, D. (1999). *Syngeristic stuttering therapy: A holistic approach.* Boston: Butterworth Heinemann.

Campbell, K., & Ryback, L. (2007). Otoprotective agents. In K. Campbell (Ed.), *Pharmacology and Ototoxicity for Audiologists* (pp. 287–300). Clifton Park, NY: Thomson Delmar Learning.

Chermak, G., & Musiek, F. (1997). *Central auditory processing disorders: New perspectives.* San Diego: Singular.

Ching, T. Y. C. (2005). The evidence calls for making binaural-bimodal fittings routine. *The Hearing Journal, 58*(11), 32–41.

Ching, T. Y. C., Hill, M., Dillon, H., & van Wanrooy, E. (2004). Fitting and evaluating a hearing aid for recipients of a unilateral cochlear implant: The NAL approach. Part 1. Hearing aid prescription, adjustment, and evaluation. *The Hearing Review,* 14–58.

Ching, T. Y. C., Incerti, P., & Hill, M. (2004). Binaural benefits for adults who use hearing aids and cochlear implants in opposite ears. *Ear and Hearing, 25*(1), 9–21.

Ching, T. Y. C., Incerti, P., & Hill, M., & Brew, J. (2004). Fitting and evaluating a hearing aid for recipients of a unilateral cochlear implant: The NAL approach. Part 2. Bimodal hearing should be standard for most cochlear implant users. *The Hearing Review,* 32–63.

Chute, P., & Masuda, A. (2000). The impact of middle ear implants. *Advance for Audiologists,* September/October, 27–29.

Chute, P. M., & Nevins, M. E. (2002). *The Parents' Guide to Cochlear Implants.* Washington, DC: Gallaudet University Press.

Clark, J. (1994). Audiologists' counseling purview. In J. Clark & F. Martin (Eds.), *Effective counseling in audiology: Perspectives and practice* (pp. 1–15). Englewood Cliffs, NJ: Prentice Hall.

Compton, C. (1995). Selecting what's best for the individual. In R. Tyler & D. Schum (Eds.), *Assistive devices for persons with hearing impairment.* Boston: Allyn & Bacon.

Cox, R., & Alexander, G. (1995). The abbreviated profile of hearing aid benefit. *Ear and Hearing, 16,* 176–186.

Custom Earmold Manual by Microsonic, Inc. (1994). Budapest, Hungary.

DeConde Johnson, C. (1994). Educational consultation: Talking with parents and school personnel. In J. Clark & F. Martin (Eds.), *Effective counseling in audiology: Perspectives and practice* (pp. 92–115). Englewood Cliffs, NJ: Prentice Hall.

Demorest, M., & Erdman, S. (1986). Scale composition and item analysis of the communication profile for the hearing impaired. *Journal of Speech and Hearing Research, 29,* 515–535.

Dillon, H., James, A., & Ginis, J. (1997). Client-oriented scale of improvements (COSI) and its relationship to several other measures of benefit and satisfaction provided by hearing aids. *Journal of the American Academy of Audiology, 8*(1), 27–43.

Dorman, M. F., Spahr, A. J., Loizou, P., Dana, C. J., & Schmide, J. S. (2005). Acoustic simulations of combined electric and acoustic hearing (EAS). *Ear and Hearing, 26*(4), 371–380.

Dowell, R. C. (2005). Evaluating cochlear implant candidacy: Recent developments. *The Hearing Journal, 58*(11), 9–23.

Dunn, C. C., Tyler, R. S., Witt, S. A., & Gantz, B. J. (2006). Effects of converting bilateral cochlear implant subjects to a strategy with increased rate and number of channels. *Annals of Otology, Rhinology, and Laryngology, 115*(6), 425–432.

Finitzo-Hieber, T., & Tillman, T. (1978). Room acoustics effects on monosyllabic word discrimination ability for normal and hearing-impaired children. *Journal of Speech and Hearing Research, 21,* 440–458.

Flexer, C. (1999). *Facilitating hearing and listening in young children.* San Diego: Singular.

Francis, H. W., Yeagle, J. D., Bowditch, S., & Niparko, J. K. (2005). Cochlear implant outcome is not influenced by the choice of ear. *Ear and Hearing, 26*(4), 7S–16S.

Gelfand, S. (2001) *Essentials of audiology* (2nd ed.). New York: Thieme.

Gollnick, D., & Chinn, P. (1994). *Multicultural education in a pluralistic society* (4th ed.). New York: Merrill.

Hellman, S. A. (1991). Selected topics of interest. *American Annals of the Deaf, 136*(2).

Henry, J., Zaugg, T., & Schecter, M. (2005). Clinical guide for audiologic tinnitus management I: Assessment. *American Journal of Audiology, 14*(1), 21–48.

Henry, J., Schechter, M., Nagler, S., & Fausti, S. (2002). Comparison of tinnitus masking and tinnitus retraining therapy. *Journal of the American Academy of Audiology, 13*(10), 559–581.

Holt, R. F., Kirk, K. I., Eisenberg, L. S., Martinez, A. S., & Campbell, W. (2005). Spoken word recognition development in children with residual hearing using cochlear implants and hearing aids in opposite ears. *Ear and Hearing, 26*(4), 82S–91S.

Hull, R. H. (2005). Fourteen principles for providing effective aural rehabilitation. *The Hearing Journal, 58*(2), 28–30.

Jastreboff, P. (1990). Phantom auditory perception (tinnitus): Mechanisms of generation and perception. *Neuroscience Research, 8,* 221–254.

Jasterboff P. J. (2000). Tinnitus habituation therapy (TRT) and tinnitus retraining therapy (TRT). In R. S. Tyler (Ed.), *Tinnitus Handbook* (pp. 357–376). San Diego: Singular.

Killion, M. (1997, December). SNR loss: "I can hear what people say but I can't understand them." *The Hearing Review.*

Kirkwood, D. (2005). Dispensers survey on what leads to patient satisfaction. *Hearing Journal, 58*(4), 19–26.

Kishon-Rabin, L., Taitelbaum-Swead, R., Ezrati-Vinacour, R., & Hildescheimer, M. (2005). Prelexical vocalization in normal hearing and hearing-impaired infants before and after cochlear implantation and its relation to early auditory skills. *Ear and Hearing, 26,* 17S–29S.

Kramer, S., Deisbach, L., Lockwood, J., Baldwin, K., Kopke, R., Scranton, S., & O'Leary, M. (2007). Efficacy of the Antioxidant N-acetylcysteine (NAC) in protecting ears exposed to loud music. *Journal of the American Academy of Audiology, 17*(4), 265–278.

Kuk, F. (1998). Hearing aid design considerations for optimally fitting the youngest patients. *The Hearing Journal, 52*(4), 55.

Kuk, F., & Keenan, D. (2005, February). Efficacy of an open-fitting hearing aid. *The Hearing Review,* 26–32.

Ling, D. (1989). *Foundations of spoken language for hearing impaired children.* Washington DC: Alexander Graham Bell Association for the Deaf.

Litovsky, R. Y., Johnstone, P. M., Godar, S., Agrawal, S., Parkinson, A., Peters, R., & Lake, J. (2006). Bilateral cochlear implants in children: Localization acuity measured with minimum audible angle. *Ear and Hearing, 27*(1), 43–59.

Loizou, P. C., Stickney, G., Mishra, L., & Assmann, P. (2003). Comparison of speech processing strategies used in the Clarion implant processor. *Ear and Hearing, 24*(1), 12–19.

Martin, F. (1994). Conveying diagnostic information. In J. Clark and F. Martin (Eds.), *Effective counseling in audiology: Perspectives and practice* (pp. 38–69). Englewood Cliffs, NJ: Prentice Hall.

Masuda, A. (2000, September/October). The impact of middle ear implants. *Advance for Audiologists,* 27–29.

Moore, J. A., & Teagle, H. F. B. (2002). An introduction to cochlear inplant technology, activation, and programming. *Language, Speech, and Hearing, Services in Schools, 33,* 153–161.

Mulrow, C., Aguilar, C., Endicott, J., Velez, R., Tuley, M., Charlie, W., & Hill, J. (1990). Association between hearing impairment and the quality of the life of elderly individuals. *Journal of the American Geriatric Society, 38,* 45–50.

Nabelek, A. (2005). Acceptance of background noise may be key to successful fittings. *The Hearing Journal, 54*(4), 19–15.

National Institutes of Health (NIH). (1995). Consensus Statement, Volume 13, Number 2, May 15–17, 1995.

National Institute on Deafness and Other Communication Disorders. (2002). Cochlear implants. Available at: www.nidcd.nih.gov/health/hearing/coch.asp

Newman, C., Weinstein, B., Jacobson, G., & Hug, G. (1991). Test-retest reliability of the hearing Handicap Inventory for Adults. *Ear and Hearing, 12*(5), 355–357.

Nie, K., Barco, A., & Zeng, F. (2006). Spectral and temporal cues in cochlear implant speech perception. *Ear and Hearing, 27*(2), 208–217.

Noble, W., Tyler, R., Dunn, C., & Witt, S. (2005). Binaural hearing has advantages for cochlear implant users also. *The Hearing Journal, 58*(11), 56–64.

Oliveira, R., Babcock, M., Venem, M., Hoeker, G., Parish, B., & Kolpe, V. (2005, February). The dynamic ear canal and its implications: The problem may be the ear, and not the impression. *The Hearing Review,* 18–82.

Pediatric Working Group of the Conference on Amplification for Children with Auditory Deficits. (1996). Amplification for infants and children with hearing loss. *American Journal of Audiology, 5*(1), 53–68.

Pirzanski, C. (2006, May). Earmolds and hearing aid shells: A tutorial. *Hearing Review,* 39–46.

Rogers, C. (1980). *A way of being.* Boston: Houghton Mifflin.

Ross, M. (2004). Hearing assistance technology: Making a world of difference. *The Hearing Journal, 57*(11), 12–17.

Ruggero, M., Rich, N., Recio, A., Narayan, S., & Robles, L. (1997). Basilar membrane responses to tones at the base of the chinchilla cochlea. *Journal of the Acoustical Society of America, 101,* 2151–2163.

Ryals, B., Matsui, J., & Cotanche, D. (2007). Regeneration of hair cells. In K. Campbell (Ed.), *Pharmacology and ototoxicity for audiologists* (pp. 301–319). Clifton Park, NY: Thomson Delmar Learning.

Sanders, D. (1993). *Management of hearing handicap: Infants to elderly.* Englewood Cliffs, NJ: Prentice Hall.

Schow, R., & Nerbonne, M. (1982). Communication screening profile; use with elderly clients. *Ear and Hearing, 3,* 135–147.

Seligman, M. (1975). *Helplessness: On depression, development, and death.* San Francisco: Freeman.

Signet Mosby medical encyclopedia. (1996). A Signet Book. St. Louis: Mosby.

Smirga, D. (2004, October). How to measure and demonstrate four key digital hearing aid performance features: Part I: The audibility window and precise recruitment accommodation. *The Hearing Review,* 30–38.

Spindel, J. (2001). An overview: Implantable hearing devices. *Audiology Today, 14*(1), 11–13.

Spindel, J. (2002). Middle ear implantable hearing devices. *American Journal of Audiology, 11*(2), 104–113.

Sweetow, R. W. (2005). Physical therapy for the ears: Maximizing patient benefit using a listening retraining program. *The Hearing Review, 56–58.*

Sweetow, R. W. (2005). Training the adult brain to listen. *The Hearing Journal, 58*(6), 10–16.

Tremblay, K., Kraus, N., McGee, T., Ponton, C., & Otis, B. (2001). Central auditory plasticity: Changes in the N1-P2 complex after speech-sound training. *Ear and Hearing, 22*(2), 79–90.

Turner, C., Gantz, B., Lowder, M., & Gfeller, K. (2005). Benefits seen in acoustic hearing + electric stimulation in same ear. *The Hearing Journal, 58*(11), 53–55.

Tye-Murray, N. (2004). *Foundations of aural rehabilitation: Children, adults, and their family members.* San Diego: Singular.

Uhlmann, R., Larson, E., Rees, T., Koepsell, T., & Dukert, L. (1989). Relationship of hearing impairment to dementia and cognitive dysfunction in older adults. *Journal of the American Medical Association, 261,* 1916–1919.

U.S. Census. (2000). Washington, DC: U.S. Department of Commerce.

Van Hecke, M. (1994). Emotional responses to hearing loss. In J. Clark & F. Martin (Eds.), *Effective counseling in audiology: Perspectives and practice* (pp. 92–115). Englewood Cliffs, NJ: Prentice Hall.

Venema, T. (2006). *Compression for clinicians.* Clifton Park, NY: Thomson Delmar Learning.

Vernon, J., & Meikle, M. (2000). Tinnitus masking. In R. Tyler (Ed.), *Tinnitus Handbook* (pp. 313–356). San Diego: Singular.

Vonlanthen, A., & Arndt, H. (2007). *Hearing instrument technology for the hearing health care professional* (3rd ed.). Clifton Park, NY: Thomson Delmar Learning.

Wayner, D. S. (1998). *Hear what you've been missing: How to cope with hearing loss* (pp. 77–100). Minneapolis, MN: Chronimed.

Wayner, D. S. (2005). Aural rehabilitation adds value, lifts satisfaction, cuts returns. *The Hearing Journal, 58*(12), 30–38.

Wazen, J., Caruso, M., & Tjellstrom, A. (1998). Long-term results with the titanium bone-anchored hearing aid: The U.S. experience. *American Journal of Otology, 19*(6), 734–741.

Wazen, J., Spitzer, J., Ghossaini, S., Kacker, A., & Zschommler, A. (2001). Results of bone-anchored hearing aid (BAHA) for unilateral hearing loss. *Laryngoscope, 111,* 955–958.

Wilson, B. S., Schatzer, R., Lopez-Poveda, E. A., Sun, X., Lawson, D. T., & Wolford, R. D. (2005). Two new directions in speech processor design for cochlear implants. *Ear and Hearing, 26*(4), Supplement, 73S–81S.

Wyatt, T. (2002). Assessing the communicative abilities of clients from diverse cultural and language backgrounds. In D. Battle (Ed.), *Communication disorders in multicultural populations* (3rd ed., pp. 415–459). Boston: Butterworth-Heinemann.

Yanz, J. (2005, May). A wearable Bluetooth device for hard of hearing people. *The Hearing Review, 38–41.*

Yates, G. (1995). Cochlear structure and function. In B. Moore (Ed.), *Hearing* (pp. 41–73). San Diego: Academic Press.

Yoshinaga-Itano, C., Sedey, A., Coulter, D., & Mehl, A. (1998). Language of early- and later-identified children with hearing loss. *Pediatrics, 102,* 1161–1171.

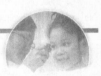

Appendix A
Educational Consultation: Talking with Parents and School Personnel

Suggested Implications and Recommendations

Consider the effects of the identified hearing impairment for each of the following skills when describing the implications of the hearing status in audiological reports to school personnel:

- Consistency of speech or auditory signal (due to fluctuating hearing levels)
- Speech recognition
- Hearing and speech recognition in presence of background noise
- Distance hearing
- Locating sound source
- Detection versus comprehension
- Speech reading
- Fatigue due to concentration required for listening
- Attention
- Language command (receptive, expressive)
- Use of amplification (hearing aids, FM systems, etc.)
- Cognition (thinking, reasoning)
- Social/emotional state
- Suspected or diagnosed auditory processing complications
- Primary language mode
- Academic achievement and school performance

Consider the following needs relative to the identified hearing impairment when making recommendations for a child or student:

Amplification Alternatives

- Personal (hearing aid, cochlear implant, tactile device)
- Personal FM system (hearing aid + FM)
- Auditory trainer (utilized without hearing aid)
- FM system only (Walkman-style)
- FM speaker system (sound field)

Communication Modifications

- Seating to facilitate hearing and listening (e.g., front row, end seat with better—right or left—ear to class and away from noise sources) that is flexible for different situations
- Attention obtained prior to speaking with child/student
- Limited auditory distractions
- Ease with which to see face and lips for speech-reading cues (avoid hands in front of face, mustaches well trimmed, no gum chewing)
- Information presented in simple, structured, sequential manner
- Teacher to check for understanding of information presented
- Clearly enunciated speech
- Extra time for processing information
- Limited visual distractions

Physical Environment Modifications

- Noise reduction (carpet room location, ventilation)
- Specialized lighting
- Room design specifications
- Flashing fire alarm

- Telecommunication device for the deaf (TDD) (more recently known as test telephone [TT])

Instruction/Material Modifications

- Visual supplements (overhead, chalkboard, charts, vocabulary lists, lecture outlines)
- Captioning or scripts for television, movies, filmstrips
- Buddy system for notes, extra explanations, directions
- Checking for understanding of information
- Down time/break from listening
- Extra time to complete assignments
- Materials at appropriate reading levels

Supplemental Services

- Instruction in speech, language, pragmatic skill development
- Instruction in auditory skill development
- Instruction in speech-reading skill development
- Interpreter (oral, manual)
- Tutor
- Note taker
- Instruction in hearing aid use, orientation, maintenance
- Instruction in social skills, responsibility, self-advocacy
- Instruction in sign language

Personal and Family Services

- Medical attention
- Financial assistance
- Counseling
- Community resources
- Vocational rehabilitation
- Ear protection
- Sign language instruction
- Family support
- Recreational opportunities
- Assistive devices
- Independent living skills
- Career/job exploration
- Deaf peer interaction opportunities

Source: John Greer Clark, Frederick N. Martin, Eds. *Effective Counseling in Audiology: Perspectives and Practice.*
Published by Allyn and Bacon, Boston, MA. Copyright © 1994 by Pearson Education. Reprinted by permission
of the publisher.

Glossary

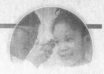

abscess: a collection of living and dead bacteria.

absolute wave latency: time, in milliseconds (msec), at which an individual wave elicited in auditory brainstem testing is identified; time between signal presentation and peak of wave.

acoustic feedback: sound resulting from reamplification of sound that leaks out from the hearing aid receiver and is picked up by the hearing aid microphone.

acoustic immittance: term used to refer collectively to acoustic impedence, acoustic admittance, or both.

acoustic reflex: response of the stapedius muscle to sound.

acoustic reflex decay: a reduction in the initial amplitude of the acoustic reflex; abnormal if the reduction is more than 50 percent of the initial amplitude within a 10-sec stimulation period when the ear is stimulated at an intensity 10 dB above the reflex threshold.

acoustic reflex threshold: softest intensity level at which the acoustic reflex is present.

acoustics: the study and science of sound and sound perception.

action potential (AP): change in nerve or muscle activity.

admittance: total energy flow through a system; unit of measure is the mmho.

ageism: generally negative view of the elderly.

air conduction hearing aid: most common type of hearing aid; directs amplified sound through the outer and middle ears to the cochlea by placing an earmold that is coupled to a hearing aid directly into the ear canal or by placing a custom-made hearing aid into the ear canal.

air conduction pathway: pathway of sound to the cochlea via the outer and middle ears.

Alzheimer's disease: a form of cortical dementia that can interfere with memory, language, and visual-spatial skills; progressive in nature, it can eventually result in cerebral atrophy and overall cognitive and mental deterioration.

ambient noise: any unwanted background noise.

American Sign Language (ASL; Ameslan): manual language system used by deaf individuals in the United States; considered by many deaf individuals to be their native language.

aminoglycoside ototoxity: damage to the inner ear caused by taking a category of antibiotics that includes gentamicin, neomycin, and kanamycin.

amplifier: see hearing aid amplifier.

ampulla: enlarged portion of semicircular canal containing sense organs for balance.

analog hearing aid: hearing aid in which the acoustic signal entering the hearing aid creates patterns of electrical currents that are similar to those of the acoustic input and then are converted back into acoustic energy.

ankylosis: joint stiffening; in audiology, typically refers to fixation of the stapes in otosclerosis

antioxidants: major category of otoprotective agent that prevents or reduces increases in the oxygen content of a substance, thereby preventing excessive formulation of free radicals.

anxiety: feeling of worry, upset, or fear, usually due to some perceived threat.

aphasia: language disorder resulting from damage to the brain.

apraxia: motor speech disorder characterized by the inability to execute a voluntary sequence of motor action; involuntary executions remain intact.

articulation index (AI): term once used to describe a method of quantifying the degree to which the speech signal is available to the listener; more current terms include *audibility index* and *speech intelligibility index*. Note: the speech intelligibility index involves different calculations than the audibility index.

ascending–descending approach: technique used to obtain threshold data in which responses to sound result in a decrease in the intensity of the next sound presented, and lack of response results in an increase in the intensity of the next sound presented.

Asperger's syndrome: disorder commonly viewed as a higher-functioning type of autism; IQ is typically normal; social language and affect are often impaired.

assistive device: any non-hearing aid device designed to improve the ability of an individual with a hearing loss to communicate and to function more independently, either by transmitting amplified sound more directly from its source or by transforming it into a tactile or visual signal.

assistive listening device: item, piece of equipment, or system used to enhance or improve an individual's functional hearing ability.

assistive technology device: item, piece of equipment, or system used to increase, maintain, or improve an individual's functional capabilities.

509

assistive technology service: service that directly assists an individual in selection, acquisition, or use of an assistive technology device.

asymmetrical hearing loss: bilateral hearing loss in which the degree of loss is different for each ear.

athetoid cerebral palsy: type of cerebral palsy characterized by extreme rigidity of the upper extremities.

atresia: congenital disease of the external auditory canal involving absence of the normal opening.

attenuator dial: part of an audiometer that allows for increasing and decreasing the decibel level of the signals.

attention deficit hyperactivity disorder (ADHD): developmental behavior disorder involving impulsivity, hyperactivity, and variability in task performance, resulting in academic, social, and emotional difficulties.

audibility index (AI): method of quantifying the degree to which the speech signal is available to the listener based on the energy of different speech sounds at different frequencies and the listener's hearing sensitivity; also referred to as speech intelligibility index and, formerly, articulation index.

audiogram: graphic display of an individual's hearing thresholds.

audiogram showing conductive hearing loss: abnormal air conduction thresholds and normal bone conduction thresholds.

audiogram showing mixed hearing loss: both air and bone conduction thresholds are abnormal, but air conduction thresholds are more impaired.

audiogram showing sensorineural hearing loss: both air and bone conduction thresholds are abnormal to an equal degree.

audiological screening: pass/refer procedure to identify individuals requiring further audiological assessment, treatment, and/or referral.

audiologist: professional who identifies, assesses, and manages disorders involving the auditory, balance, and other related systems; provides services across the age span, including hearing aid dispensing, rehabilitative audiology services, and auditory research.

audiology: professional discipline involving diagnosis, remediation, and prevention of disorders involving the auditory system.

audiometer: electronic instrument used to measure hearing sensitivity.

auditory brainstem implant (ABI): developed for individuals with Neurofibromatosis type II (NF2); uses an implanted electrode array and an external sound processor to send electrical simulation of the auditory neurons of the cochlear nucleus to improving ability to detect or understand speech information.

auditory brainstem response (ABR): brain wave or electrical potential that is generated when the ear is stimulated with sound; recorded through the use of surface electrodes.

auditory brainstem testing (ABR): electrophysiological assessment based on generation of wave patterns that reflect neural activity of the brainstem in response to sound; generated from cranial nerve VIII and brainstem; can be used to estimate hearing thresholds or to rule out retrocochlear pathology.

auditory evoked potentials: group of tests, all of which measure brain activity "evoked" by the introduction of auditory stimuli; tests include electrocochleography, auditory brainstem responses, middle latency responses, and late (cortical) auditory evoked responses.

auditory integration training (AIT): treatment approach to treating hyperacusis designed by G. Berard and intended to alter the functioning of the auditory and central nervous systems in an attempt to reduce behavior and cognitive problems that (theoretically) arise from peaks and valleys on an audiogram. Clients listen to modulated and filtered music presented from a specially designed device with various filter settings.

auditory middle latency response (AMLR): auditory evoked potential occurring from approximately 8 to 50 msec poststimulus; generated from auditory radiations and cortex.

auditory neuropathy: a condition in which the patient displays auditory characteristics supporting normal outer hair cell function and abnormal cranial nerve VIII (auditory) function; site of dysfunction lies somewhere between the outer hair cells and the brainstem; abnormal brainstem auditory evoked potentials with normal otoacoustic emissions is a common pattern.

auditory nuclei: site of a series of synapses involving transmission of auditory information and coding of auditory cues, including frequency, intensity, and time.

auditory perceptual skills: broad term encompassing a variety of auditory abilities, including sound awareness, auditory attention, auditory discrimination and auditory memory.

auditory processing disorders: deficits in processing of auditory signals not due to peripheral hearing loss or cognitive impairment.

auditory steady-state response (ASSR): an event-related evoked potential that is elicited using a steady-state tone versus a stimulus with a brief duration (e.g., a click).

augmentative alternative communication (AAC): communication approach used for individuals who do not have independent verbal communication skills.

aural rehabilitation: blend of device(s) and service(s) with the goal of improving overall communicative function; may include amplification, use of visual cues, and counseling; also, strategies and therapy provided to individuals with acquired hearing designed to improve speech understanding.

auricular hillocks: six hillocks, or growth centers, which appear as thickenings on the first branchial groove; form the external ear.

autism: disorder characterized by self-absorption, impaired social relationships, decreased responsiveness to others, and impaired language skills. Reduced cognitive skills are common, as are decreased eye contact and repetitive patterns of behavior; onset is prior to age 3 years.

automatic telephone switch: switch that can be added to a hearing aid to automatically change the circuit from the microphone position to the telephone position as the receiver of the telephone is placed near the hearing aid.

autosomal dominant: inheritance pattern in which a dominant gene creates a specific characteristic; the gene must be an autosome (i.e., non-sex-determining chromosome).

autosomal recessive: inheritance patterns in which two abnormal genes (one from each parent) are necessary for transmission; if both parents are carriers, each child has a 25 percent probability of inheritance.

autosome: any chromosome that is not an X-chromosome or a Y-chromosome (i.e., a chromosome other than a sex chromosome). Of the 23 pairs of chromosomes in humans, 22 pairs are autosomal and the remaining pair is X-linked.

barotrauma: trauma resulting from marked changes in atmospheric pressure that cannot be adequately equalized.

basal cell carcinoma: uncontrolled growth of the basal skin layer, often due to exposure to the sun.

basilar membrane: fibrous membrane separating the scala media from the scala tympani; has critical role in auditory perception of frequency.

behavioral observation audiometry (BOA): behavioral method of assessing children's hearing up to 4 months of age, involving careful observation of the infant's change in behavior (e.g., eye blinking, change in sucking activity, eye widening, searching) in response to auditory stimuli.

behavioral tests of hearing: tests that measure hearing sensitivity by observing a change in behavior on the part of the client in response to sound.

Bekesy audiometry: automatic method of audiometric testing in which the patient responds to pulsed and continuous tones, the patterns of which are recorded on a printout and interpreted as various sites of lesion.

benign paroxysmal positional vertigo (BPPV): common peripheral vestibular condition brought by changes in position.

binaural: both ears.

binaural integration: see tests of binaural integration.

binaural interaction: see tests of binaural interaction.

binaural separation: ability to process auditory information presented to one ear while simultaneously ignoring different stimuli presented to the opposite ear.

binaural squelch: improved understanding of speech in a background of noise that results from interaural phase and intensity cues that are available when listening with two ears.

binaural summation: improved threshold of hearing (by approximately 3 dB) that results from listening with two ears compared to listening with one ear.

Bluetooth technology: a short-range wireless digital communication standard used to carry audio information or data from one device to another; provides a clean, clear digital signal.

Bone anchored hearing aid (BAHA): implantable aid in which the receiver is surgically implanted in the temporal bone, behind the ear; appropriate in cases of chronic middle ear pathology with good bone conduction thresholds, or canal atresia.

bone conduction hearing aid: type of hearing aid that makes use of a vibrator placed on the mastoid area to route amplified sound directly to the cochlea, without involvement of the outer and middle ears.

bone conduction pathway: pathway of sound to the cochlea through vibration of the skull.

bone conduction vibrator: device used to stimulate the cochlea by vibrating the bones of the skull in bone conduction testing.

brain plasticity: ability of the brain to adapt to internal and external events; to change based on varying sensory input.

brainstem auditory evoked response testing: assessment of auditory evoked potentials generated from cranial nerve VIII and brainstem.

branchial arches: paired grooves that are formed at about the third week of fetal development, which come together at the midline to form arches.

Brownian motion: constant and random movement of air molecules.

Buffalo model: categorization system of various error patterns emerging on tests of auditory processing and the learning difficulties associated with each category; includes four categories of auditory processing results, speech–language evaluation findings, the associated learning difficulties, and remedial approaches to address the identified deficits; developed by Dr. Jack Katz.

calibration: checking the accuracy of the output of a measuring instrument.

caloric testing: part of the ENG battery involving heating and cooling endolymph of the vestibular system by directing temperature-controlled water or air into the ears in order to assess the relative sensitivity of the vestibular organs; provides separate right- and left-ear data regarding the horizontal semicircular canals.

canal atresia: absence of the ear canal opening.

carotid artery: one of two main sources of blood supply to the brain; carries oxygen and glucose to the scalp, face, and frontal lobe.

cellulitis: infection of the skin that does not involve nutritive connective tissue.

central auditory processing disorders: see auditory processing disorders.

central auditory system: part of the auditory system that extends from the auditory nerve to the auditory cortex; includes a complicated system of auditory relay stations that direct and code the auditory information.

central nervous system (CNS): portion of the nervous system that includes the cortex, brainstem, and spinal cord; involved in transmission of both sensory and motor impulses.

cerebral cortex: final auditory area in the process of auditory perception; includes Heschyl's gyrus, which is the primary area of auditory reception in the temporal lobe.

cerebral palsy: nonprogressive disorder involving movement and posture, due to brain damage early in life. Motor difficulties are the primary feature; may also include mental retardation, hearing loss, speech–language delays, and deficits in cognition, communication, and sensory function.

cerebrovascular accident (CVA): involves disruption of blood supply to the brain, commonly resulting in motor and brain function deficits; also referred to as a "stroke."

cerebrum: largest part of the brain; comprised of two halves, called cerebral hemispheres, which contain the lobes of the brain.

cerumen: waxy substance produced by the sebaceous glands of the external auditory canal.

cholesteatoma: invasive tumor of the middle ear resulting from the combination of skin, fatty tissue, and bacteria. More common in cases of repeated eardrum perforations or repeated sets of pressure equalization (PE) tubes.

chromosome: threadlike structure carrying genetic information; found in the cell nucleus.

cleft palate: division or crack in the roof of the mouth.

client-specific protocols: specific audiometric procedures developed for individual clients based on the presenting question(s) and the particular characteristics of the client.

clinician-counselor: term used to designate a clinician who incorporates counseling as part of an overall plan to address personal issues stemming from the communication disorder; aimed at providing holistic care and helping clients to view themselves and their environment more positively.

closed set: feature of speech audiometry test in which the client chooses the correct response from a given set of choices (e.g., WIPI test).

cochlea: snail-shaped sense organ of hearing that is carved into the temporal bone of the skull; consists of scala media, scala tympani, and scala vestibuli.

cochlear implant: unique, surgical type of assistive technology for those with severe to profound hearing loss who do not benefit from conventional amplification; includes externally worn parts (microphone, transmitter, and speech processor) and implanted internal parts (receiver/stimulator and electrode array).

cochlear implant map: individual program created for cochlear implant user based on determinations of threshold and suprathreshold needs of the client.

cochlear nuclei: bundles of nerves located on the brainstem at the junction of the pons and the medulla, forming the beginning of the central auditory system; all fibers from the eighth cranial nerve terminate here.

collapsing ear canal: either partial or complete closing of the ear canal during hearing testing, caused by the force of the headband of the earphones; often related to loss of elasticity in the cartilage of the ear; more common in older individuals.

communication mismatch: disparity created when two or more individuals communicating with each other use different languages or different communication systems (e.g., oral English and American Sign Language [ASL], ASL and Manually Coded English).

compensated measure: measure of acoustic admittance that have been corrected (compensated) so that the admittance of the ear canal is subtracted out and an estimate of the admittance at the lateral surface of the eardrum is obtained.

complex sound: a sound containing energy at more than one frequency.

compression: portion of the sound wave where molecules are close together.

compression limiting: method of output limiting in which the hearing aid's output is decreased as the strength of the input signal increases.

compression ratio: the relationship, in decibels, between the input signal and the resulting output signal.

computerized dynamic posturography (CDP): test to assess a client's ability to maintain balance under conditions similar to what might be encountered in his/her everyday life; consists of sensory organization and motor control tests.

conditioned play audiometry (CPA):   see play audiometry.

conditioning: technique used to shape a client's behavioral response to auditory stimuli, as in conditioned play audiometry.

conduct disorder: pervasive disorder in which conduct persistently disregards the rights of others, as well as age-appropriate norms and rules of society.

cone of light: reflection of light from the otoscope in the anterior and inferior quadrants of the eardrum.

content counseling: counseling that primarily involves providing the client with facts, details, or explanations about a topic.

continuous reinforcement: delivery of reinforcement after every demonstration of the desired behavior.

contralateral acoustic reflex: acoustic reflex obtained by stimulating the ear that is opposite the ear in which the tympanogram has been obtained; also referred to as crossed reflexes.

contralateral neural pathways: neural pathways that cross over (decussate) from one side of the brainstem to the opposite side.

corner audiogram: term used to denote an audiogram in which very limited pure tone responses (i.e., profound loss) are noted only in the low-frequency range, with no responses in the mid- to higher frequencies.

corpus callosum: structure connecting the cerebral hemispheres, responsible for inter-hemispheric transfer of neural information; largely comprised of myelin.

correction factors: values that are either added or subtracted to obtained thresholds based on the degree to which the audiometer is out of calibration.

cortico-spinal tract: "pyramidal tract fibers that descend from cortex to spinal cord and activate spinal motor neurons" (Bhatnagar & Andy, 1995, p. 339).

counseling: process by which an individual is helped to achieve greater self-understanding and understanding of others for purposes of resolving a problem, or conflict, or adjusting to some life event.

coupler, 2 cc: metal cavity used in measurement of electroacoustic characteristics of hearing aids, designed to simulate the average volume of air in an ear canal with an earmold.

craniofacial anomalies: malformations, typically present at birth, of the face and/or cranium.

Crib-o-gram: motion-sensitive device placed in an infant's crib to record responses to sound; not considered a reliable tool.

cristae: sense organs for balance contained in ampullae of semicircular canals.

cultural mismatch: disparity created when two or more individuals each have different cultural perspectives (e.g., white and nonwhite, hearing and Deaf).

cupula: "gelatinous substance of the cristae ampularis in which the kinocilia of the vestibular hair cells are embedded" (Stach, 2003, p. 73).

cycle of sound wave: air molecule movement from rest to maximum displacement in one direction, back to rest, and then to maximum displacement in the other direction; one compression and one rarefaction of a sound wave.

dB nHL: common unit of measure for denoting the intensity level of clicks used in auditory brainstem response (ABR) testing; based on the average softest level (of a group of individuals who have normal hearing) at which the click can be heard; mean click threshold is referred to as 0 dB nHL.

Deaf: (with a capital D) commonly used denotation among individuals who are born deaf and who believe that deafness is not a disability but rather a culture, with its own beliefs and customs.

deafness: hearing impairment that is 90 dB or greater on the audiogram; results in use of the visual modality as the primary means of communication (rather than the oral/aural modality).

decibel (dB):   commonly used unit of measure for intensity; one-tenth of a Bel.

decoding category of auditory processing: category of auditory processing associated with difficulties with reading and spelling (due to deficiencies in manipulating phonemes), increased time needed to process speech, receptive language difficulties, and sound discrimination errors.

dementia: term used to refer to a group of (usually acquired) disorders of the central nervous system that progressively interfere with a person's cognitive functioning.

depression: an emotional state involving extreme feelings of sadness, dejection, lack of worth, and emptiness.

developmental disability: severe, chronic disability of an individual 5 years of age or older, attributable to a mental or physical impairment or combination of mental and physical impairments; is manifested before the individual attains age 22 and is likely to continue indefinitely; substantial functional limitations are noted.

developmental/educational model of otitis media: view of otitis media that acknowledges both the short-term consequences (reduced access to speech sounds can interfere with speech and language development) as well as potential long-term consequences (difficulties with attending, understanding speech in background noise settings, and learning basic sound–symbol relationships) of the disease and associated hearing loss.

diabetes: a metabolic disease characterized by a deficiency in insulin production and abnormal utilization of glucose.

diagnostic audiometry: in-depth audiological assessment to determine the type and degree of hearing loss.

diagonal vent: type of vent in which the hollow channel runs diagonal to the sound bore until it intersects with it.

digital hearing aid: hearing aid in which an analog-to-digital converter changes the electrical current into a binary code using digits (0 and 1), before converting the input back to an analog, acoustic signal; associated with increased flexibility that is not typically possible with analog instruments.

digital noise reduction technology: allows the hearing aid circuit to monitor the incoming signal to determine whether it is speech or noise based on changes in signal amplitude.

direct audio input (DAI): direct input of a signal from a device (e.g., tape recorder, videotape) into a hearing aid by way of a hard-wired connection.

directional microphone: microphone that is more sensitive to sounds directed from the front, compared to sounds coming from other directions.

distortion product otoacoustic emissions: type of evoked OAE that is elicited by presenting two different tones to the ear; the tones have a relationship expressed as 2(f1 – f2); employed in clinical audiology for both diagnostic and screening purposes.

Dix-Hallpike maneuver: involves rapidly laying the client back so that his/her head hangs over one shoulder and simultaneously assessing possible nystagmus; client is then returned to a sitting position, the eyes are monitored again, and the procedure is repeated with the head hanging over the opposite shoulder; primary purpose is to assess for benign paroxysmal positional vertigo (BPPV).

Dizziness Handicap Inventory (DHI) assessment of the physical, functional, and psychological impact of balance issues on the patient; can be used as a way to measure improvements following vestibular rehabilitation.

dominantly inherited trait: inherited feature that can be passed on even if only one parent possesses it.

Down syndrome: genetic disorder commonly characterized by some degree of mental retardation, low muscle tone, and an increased incidence of middle ear pathology; associated speech–language delays are common.

durable hearing aid: nondisposable hearing aid.

dynamic range: decibel difference between the threshold of sensitivity and the loudness discomfort level; can be measured using speech or tones at discrete frequencies. It is often reduced in cases of cochlear hearing loss with abnormal loudness growth.

dyne: unit of force; the amount of power required to accelerate a weight of one gram a distance of one centimeter per second.

dysarthria: motor speech disorder resulting in inefficiency in the muscles used for respiration, phonation, articulation, and resonation.

early identification: diagnosis of hearing loss or other conditions as early in life as possible, to minimize negative effects on development.

early intervention: provision of services (audiological, medical, speech–language, developmental) as early in life as possible to minimize negative effects on development.

earmold acoustics: acoustic changes that occur to the output acoustic signal by the characteristics of the tube or channel through which the signal travels.

ectoderm: second and outer most of the three layers of cells in the embryo; makes up nervous system, eyes, ears, and skin.

effective masking (EM): the amount of masking noise necessary to just mask a signal; the decibel level to which a threshold is shifted given a level of masking noise.

effusion: fluid in a body space.

elasticity: a medium's ability to resist distortion to its original shape.

electroacoustic hearing aid characteristics: hearing aid output characteristics, including gain, frequency response, maximum output, and harmonic distortion.

electroacoustic verification: series of measures performed in a hearing aid test box to determine if a given device meets manufacturer's specifications.

electrocochleography: assessment/recording of auditory evoked potentials (compound action potentials) from the cochlea and eighth cranial nerve; also referred to as ECochG or ECoG, with the former being preferred; useful in monitoring auditory nerve function during surgery, and in diagnosis of Meniere's disease.

electroencecephalography (EEG): measurement of on-going electrical brain activity (in the form of electrical potentials) using scalp electrodes.

electronystagmogaphy: most commonly used test of balance; relies on electro-oculography to measure eye movement in order to gain information about the vestibular organs and their central vestibule-ocular pathways.

514

electro-oculography: This procedure involves attaching electrodes in specific arrangements around the eyes and then measuring and recording the resulting patterns with a chart recorder.

embryo: in humans, the time between implantation of the fertilized egg in the uterus and end of the seventh or eighth week of pregnancy.

embryology: study of the embryo or the very beginning stages of development.

emotional disorders: category of psychological disorder typically involving inwardly directed disturbances, such as anxiety, fear, extreme shyness, or depression.

endoderm: first and innermost of the of three layers of cells in the embryo; lines most of the internal organs and spaces.

endolymph: type of cochlear fluid found in the scala media.

ENG (electronystagmography): test using electro-oculography to measure eye movement and gain information about the vestibular organs and their central vestibulo-ocular pathways.

equivalent ear canal volume: acoustic admittance estimate of the volume between the probe tip and the eardrum.

Eustachian tube: structure extending from the naso-pharynx to the middle ear space; responsible for equalizing middle ear pressure.

Eustachian tube dysfunction: failure of the Eustachian tube to regulate middle ear pressure; usually due to failure of the Eustachian tube to open during yawning, chewing, sneezing, or swallowing.

Eustachian tube testing: tympanometric assessment of the Eustachian tube's ability to equalize air pressure.

evoked otoacoustic emissions: sounds generated by the cochlea and recorded in the ear canal that follow presentation of a stimulus; arise from activity of outer hair cells; evoked otoacoustic emissions may be transient, distortion product, or stimulus frequency.

external auditory canal: canal or tube that extends form the pinna to the tympanic membrane; also referred to as the ear canal or external auditory meatus.

external otitis: infection of the external ear characterized by thickened skin on the external ear and the ear canal.

extrinsic causes of hearing loss: external causes of hearing loss, including tumors, infections, injuries, metabolic disorders, and congenital causes that are nongenetic.

false negative rate: the total number of false negatives divided by the total number of abnormal individuals (based on the follow-up diagnostic test results) for the screening sample.

false negative screening result: the individual passes the screening, even though they are positive for the disorder or condition.

false positive rate: the number of false positives divided by the total number of normal individuals (based on follow-up diagnostic test results) for the screening sample.

false positive screening result: the individual fails the screening, even though he or she is negative for the disorder or condition.

far-field testing: measurement of evoked potentials from electrodes that are far from the generator site (of the potential); scalp electrodes are typically used.

fetal period: period from the end of the fetal stage (seven or eight weeks) to birth.

filtered speech: speech that is presented through a device that allows only certain energy through; with a high-pass filter, high-frequency speech information is audible; with a low-pass filter, low-frequency speech information is audible.

first level of response (FLR): obtained during screening by using an ascending approach (increasing intensity in 5-dB steps) for the purpose of determining the approximate hearing level at those frequencies at which the client failed the hearing screening.

fluent aphasia: type of aphasia characterized by vague, jargonlike language produced with good articulation and syntax; auditory comprehension deficits make understanding of self and others difficult.

FM (frequency-modulated) auditory trainer: assistive listening device that transmits information from speaker to listener via radio waves; components include a microphone worn by the speaker and a receiver worn by the listener; improves the signal-to-noise ratio and distance listening.

FM (frequency-modulated) device: an assistive listening device designed to improve the signal-to-noise ratio and improve distance listening by transmitting signals from a microphone worn by a speaker to an FM receiver worn by the listener.

FM (frequency-modulated) stimuli: pure tone that has been altered in such a way that its frequency is varied systematically; also referred to as warble tone.

FM (frequency-modulated) system: an assistive listening device designed to improve the signal-to-noise ratio and improve distance listening by transmitting signals from a microphone worn by a speaker to an FM receiver worn by the listener; includes personal and sound field types.

Frenzel lenses: special glasses, which are lighted on the patient's side, to prevent fixation as the eyes for observed for nystagmus.

frequency: number of cycles occurring in a designated time period, usually 1 sec.

frequency response: electroacoustic characteristic of hearing aids that specifies the gain delivered across frequency.

frequency–response graph: graph specifying the gain delivered by a hearing aid across frequencies, with frequency on the horizontal axis and gain on the vertical axis.

frontal lobe: lobe of the brain that plays an essential role in speech production; also involved in executive functions (e.g., memory, problem solving, inhibition, self-regulation, planning) that influence emotional mediation, personality, and pragmatic language abilities.

functional gain: comparison of aided versus unaided thresholds in the sound field.

functional hearing loss: synonymous term for non-organic hearing loss.

fundus tympani: thin plate of bone separating the middle ear cavity from the jugular bulb.

gain: the amount of amplification, measured in decibels.

gaze-evoken nystagmus: nystagmus occurring during "horizontal gaze to one or both sides of midline" (Stach, 2003, p. 190).

gene: functional unit of heredity; unit carrying physical characteristics from parent to child.

genetic counseling: provision of information by a genetic counselor regarding genetic factors causing hearing loss (or other conditions) for the purpose of helping families make informed decisions in the process of family planning.

genetic disorders: disorders that are caused by heredity.

gerontology: study of aging and the problems of the aged.

gestation: period between egg fertilization and birth.

glomus tumors: middle ear tumors that can occur on the jugular bulb (glomus jugulare tumors), in the middle ear (glomus tympanicum), or along the vagus nerve (glomus vagale).

gradient: part of the immittance battery; sensitive to the presence of middle ear fluid; calculations involve a ratio comparing the mean admittance values at two designated pressure points on the tympanogram with the overall admittance value.

grief: a pattern of physical and emotional responses to separation or loss; may include a series of stages, including alarm, disbelief, denial, anger, guilt, and hopefully, adjustment.

habituation: reductions in the strength and frequency of responses as the stimuli are repeated and lose their novelty.

hard of hearing: term used for hearing that is poorer than normal hearing, but not as impaired as in cases of deafness.

head-shadow effect: reduction in the energy of sound as it crosses from one ear to the other, due to attenuation by the head; as much as 12–16 dB may be lost in the higher frequencies.

hearing aid: electronic device consisting of a microphone, amplifier, and receiver used to amplify sound and deliver it to the user's ear.

hearing aid amplifier: hearing aid component that increases the intensity of the electric signal received from the microphone.

hearing aid microphone: hearing aid component that picks up acoustic energy (i.e., sound waves) in the air and converts it into electrical energy.

hearing aid orientation: component of overall aural rehabilitation program designed to provide new hearing aid users with information regarding use of amplification in their daily routine; includes insertion, removal, manipulation of controls, use with telephone, changing batteries, etc.

hearing aid receiver: hearing aid component that converts electrical signals received from the amplifier back into acoustic energy.

hearing aid selection: aspect of an overall aural rehabilitation program in which the electroacoustic and non-electroacoustic characteristics of the hearing aids are determined.

hearing aid specifications: data produced by hearing aid manufacturers regarding the electroacoustic characteristics of hearing aids, as measured using a 2-cc coupler; includes gain, frequency response, output, and harmonic distortion.

hearing aid stethoset: a stethoscope designed to allow a subjective listening check to be performed on a hearing aid in order to make judgments about its functioning.

hearing aid test box: sound-treated box in which measurements of electroacoustic characteristics of hearing aids are made.

hearing aid trial period: period of time, often mandated by state law, during which time the consumer is allowed to use a custom-made hearing aid with a return option if the hearing aid proves unsatisfactory; "terms" are often attached to the return.

hearing aid troubleshooting: process of identifying and, when possible, correcting problems that interfere with the functioning of a hearing aid.

hearing disability: degree to which hearing impairment interferes with a person's ability to engage in activities that are important to him or her.

hearing level (HL): designates use of audiometric zero as the referent for a particular decibel level (e.g., 50 dB HL means that the referent is audiometric zero).

hemotympanum: condition in which the tympanic membrane appears blue in color on otoscopy, due to the accumulation of blood in the middle ear space.

hertz (Hz): unit of measure for frequency; formerly cycles per second (cps).

Heschl's gyrus: also known as the superior temporal gyrus; believed to be the primary auditory reception area.

heterozygous: having two different genes at the same place on matched chromosomes; affected individuals transmit the condition to their offspring. All individuals with the condition will have one similarly affected parent; not all offspring will have the condition, since there is a 50 percent chance of its occurrence.

high-risk register: criteria that place a child at risk for hearing loss.

HI-PRO box: a commonly used interface that allows a hardware connection between the audiologist's personal computer and the hearing aid(s) being programmed.

homozygous: having two identical genes at the same place on matched chromosomes.

horn effect: modification of the frequency response of amplified sound by increasing the diameter of the earmold, usually at the exit point, for purposes of increasing high-frequency gain.

humanism: in audiological care, attitudes and actions that convey respect for and interest in the client's specific concerns and values.

immittance battery: group of objective measures of middle ear function.

impedance: total opposition or resistance to the flow of energy; unit of measure is the ohm.

implantable hearing aids: two broad classes of hearing aids that are surgically implanted, namely, bone-anchored hearing aids and middle ear implants.

Individuals with Disabilities Education Act (IDEA): PL 94-142 and 99-457; legislation requiring free and appropriate education for children over the age of 3 years who have disabilities.

inertia: tendency of an object to remain in its current state of motion.

inferior colliculus: the largest of the auditory structures of the brainstem, containing neurons that are sensitive to binaural stimulation.

inner hair cells: afferent, rounded or flask-shaped hair cells of the cochlea that are stimulated by incoming sounds of 40–60 dB.

input compression: type of compression in which the volume control is located after the automatic gain control (AGC) circuit and therefore affects both the gain and the output; typically used with individuals who have mild to moderate hearing losses and larger dynamic range.

insert earphones: earphones designed to be placed in the external auditory canal; components include a transducer connected through tubing to an expandable cuff.

intensity: objective measure of the strength of a sound; may be measured in various units, such as pressure or power.

intensity level (IL): designates the use of a power referent to measure sound energy (e.g., 10^{-16} W/cm^2).

interaural latency difference (ILD): time difference, in milliseconds (msec), between the absolute latency of wave V in each ear, in auditory brainstem response testing.

intermittent reinforcement: delivery of reinforcement on a variable schedule; not after every demonstration of the desired behavior.

interpeak latencies: time difference, in milliseconds (msec), between two waves (peaks) in auditory evoked response testing (e.g., the time between waves I and III, III and V, or I and V).

intrinsic causes of hearing loss: genetic disorders arising from chromosomal abnormalities; patterns of inheritance vary.

ipsilateral acoustic reflex: acoustic reflex obtained by stimulating the same ear in which the tympanogram has been measured; also referred to as uncrossed reflex.

Joint Committee on Infant Hearing 2000 Position Statement: a paper outlining principles and goals of universal newborn hearing screening programs, including follow-up and early intervention for infants with hearing loss.

jugular bulb: protrusion on the floor of the middle ear space.

kinocilium: the single long hair cell adjacent to the stereocilium; plays a role in balance.

kneepoint: point on the output curve representing the intensity level at which compression "kicks in"; the hearing aid is no longer functioning in a linear way.

labyrinth: term used to describe the inner ear because of its similarity to a maze of interconnecting caves.

late auditory evoked potentials: auditory evoked potentials occurring from 50 to 250 msec poststimulus; variability with subject's state of arousal limits clinical utility.

laser sintering: new process for scanning earmold impressions into 3D digital models.

latency–intensity function: graph that illustrates the changes in wave V latency associated with changes in intensity; used during latency–intensity testing to estimate hearing thresholds.

lateral lemniscus: considered by some to be the primary brainstem auditory pathway, receiving nerve fibers form the cochlear nuclei and superior olivary complex.

linear amplification: a hearing aid circuit that provides the same amount of gain for any and all input intensity levels; a one-to-one relationship between the output and the input signal is maintained until the amplifier is saturated.

localization: identification of the direction from which a sound is originating.

logarithmic scale: measurement scale based on exponents of a base number.

longitudinal waves: waves in which the air molecules move parallel to the direction of the wave motion (e.g., sound waves traveling in air).

loudness: subjective judgment regarding the intensity of a sound.

loudness discomfort level (LDL): formerly known as the uncomfortable level (UCL) for speech; the level at which the client perceives speech or other stimuli (e.g., pure tones) to be uncomfortable to listen to.

malingering: deliberate misrepresentation (e.g., exaggeration, feigning) of an impairment, illness, or condition.

malleus fixation: middle ear disorder involving fixation of the malleus head; may be total or partial.

Manually Coded English (MCE): manual form of oral English; unlike American Sign Language (ASL), MCE uses the same word order as oral English and many of the same grammatical structures.

manubrium: the handle of the malleus.

masking: noise of any kind that interferes with the audibility of another sound; in audiology, noise used to eliminate participation of the non-test ear while the test ear is assessed.

masking level difference (MLD): improved hearing sensitivity noted for binaural masked thresholds when the tone and noise are out of phase, compared to when they are in phase; an auditory test sensitive to retrocochlear (brainstem) involvement.

mastoid: part of the temporal bone of the skull, consists of pneumatized bone, located posterior to the pinna.

mastoiditis: infection of the mastoid bone; may be a complication of otitis media.

measurement plane tympanometry: tympanometric measure obtained at the probe tip; reflects acoustic admittance of the volume of air between the probe tip and the eardrum plus the admittance of the middle ear system.

medial geniculate body: the last subcortical auditory relay station, receiving most of its fibers from the inferior colliculus and lateral lemniscus.

medical model of otitis media: view of otitis media held by some professionals that focuses on the presence or absence of infection in the middle ear space.

melanoma: a high-mortality type of malignancy involving the pigment cells; can spread through the bloodstream.

Meniere's disease: a benign disorder of the inner ear that may result from increased endolymphatic fluid pressure. It is characterized by fluctuating hearing loss, vertigo, and tinnitus.

mental retardation: disorder characterized by subaverage intellectual abilities and deficits in adaptive behavior, impaired communication, and social skills.

mesoderm: middle of the three layers of cells in the embryo; gives rise to bone, connective tissue, muscle, blood vessels, lymph tissues, and parts of the heart and abdomen.

microphone: see hearing aid microphone.

microtia: abnormally small pinna; typically occurs with atresia.

middle ear effusion: fluid in the middle ear space.

middle ear implant (MEI): implantable aid in which the receiver is implanted in the middle ear cavity, usually on the ossicular chain, and an external coil is placed either behind or in the ear or in the ear canal; appropriate for individuals who have up to a severe sensorineural hearing loss.

millimho (mmho): unit of measure for admittance.

minimal sensorineural hearing loss: general term for hearing loss that is either unilateral or bilateral; bilateral is mild in degree and interferes with communication and educational performance.

minimum response levels: lowest levels at which very young children exhibit behavioral response to sound; in very young children these levels are typically above their true threshold; influenced by auditory responsiveness as well as hearing sensitivity.

mismatched negativity (MMN): a cortical event-related auditory evoked potential; reflects sensory processing within auditory cortex; a neuronal response to minimal changes in acoustic parameters such as frequency, intensity, location, and duration.

modiolus: central bony pillar of the cochlea through which auditory nerve fibers travel.

monaural: one ear.

monitored live voice testing: method of performing speech audiometry in which the audiologist presents words through the microphone of the audiometer; no longer the preferred option.

monosyllabic words: words containing only one syllable.

most comfortable level (MCL): intensity level at which the client perceives speech or other stimuli (e.g., pure tones) to be most comfortable.

motor control test: balance test that focuses on the muscles involved in maintaining posture; part of computerized dynamic posturography.

multichannel hearing aid: hearing aid that separates the input signal into separate frequency bands for purposes of independently manipulating the parameters (e.g., gain, output, compression).

multiple-memory hearing aid: hearing aid that provides more than one set of electroacoustic characteristics for use in different acoustic environments (e.g., quiet, noise, telephone).

multiple sclerosis: disease of the central nervous system characterized by destruction of the myelin sheath of nerve fibers.

myelinization: development of an insulating sheath (myelin) that covers nerves and enhances the speed with which neuronal communication occurs.

myringoplasty: surgical repair of the tympanic membrane (eardrum).

myringotomy: surgical procedure in which the eardrum is opened, typically to remove fluid.

narrow-band-noise: noise created by band-pass filtering that is centered at a specific audiometric frequency; most effective for pure tone masking.

negative finding: in medical terms, means that the person does not have the disease or condition.

neonatal hearing screening: use of physiological measures to identify hearing loss as early in life as possible; also called universal newborn hearing screening.

neonatal intensive care unit (NICU): a specialized unit in a hospital designed to provide support and monitoring for infants who are determined to be "at risk."

neurofibromatosis: a condition characterized by the occurrence of multiple tumors on the skin and spinal cord (neurofibromatosis type 1) or bilateral acoustic schwannoma (neurofibromatosis type 2).

neurogenic disorders: disorders resulting from damage to the peripheral or central nervous system.

neurophysiological immaturity: underdevelopment of the very young child's neurological system, which affects the ability to coordinate neuromotor responses to auditory signals that are presented at threshold levels.

noise: any unwanted sound.

noise-induced hearing loss: sensorineural hearing loss resulting from exposure to loud levels of sound; often characterized by a 4,000-Hz "notch."

nondiagnostic otoscopy: term used to denote otoscopy that is limited to identification of gross structural abnormalities, obvious drainage, or blockage, rather than to diagnose specific pathology (i.e., middle ear fluid).

nonelectroacoustic hearing aid characteristics: features of hearing aid fitting such as style, color, and level of technology.

nonfluent aphasia: type of aphasia characterized by sparse output and difficulties with prosody, articulation, and syntax; normal to near-normal understanding of spoken information is common.

nonoccluding earmold: an open earmold designed to avoid ear canal occlusion; commonly used in contralateral routing of signals (CROS) fittings and when low- to middle-frequency thresholds are normal.

nonorganic hearing loss: reported hearing loss (based on the responses given by the patient) that does not have any underlying organic basis; the terms pseudohypacusis and functional hearing loss are also used.

nonprogrammable hearing aid: hearing aid for which the audiologist manually adjusts the potentiometers (using a screwdriver).

notched tympanogram: tympanogram that contains more than one peak; may reflect additional mass in the middle ear system due to scar tissue on the eardrum or ossicular discontinuity; may be seen in clients who have normal middle ear systems; also referred to as multicomponent tympanogram.

nystagmus: particular pattern of eye movement involving a slow component in one direction and a fast component in the other direction resulting from the neural connections that exist between the vestibular and visual systems.

occlusion: a closing off or blockage.

occlusion effect: improvement (decrease) in the bone conduction threshold of tones of 1,000 Hz and below when the ears are tightly covered with an earphone.

ocular-motor testing: part of the ENG battery that includes assessment of the saccade, smooth pursuit, and optokinetic systems.

ohm: unit of measure for impedance.

omnidirectional: microphone that picks up sound coming from different directions (i.e., sounds coming from the sides, the back, and the front) with nearly equal sensitivity.

open set: feature of speech audiometry test in which the client chooses the correct response from the entire pool of options available in the language.

optokinetic system: visual system responsible for supporting stable visual images during head movement.

oral/aural: method of speech and language development that relies on use of spoken language for communication, avoiding the use of a formal sign language.

organ of Corti: the hearing organ, located in the scala media on basilar membrane.

osseocartilaginous junction: point where at which the osseous (bony) and cartilaginous portions of the ear canal meet.

ossicles: three middle ear bones (malleus, incus, stapes) that make up the ossicular chain, extending from the tympanic membrane to the oval window.

ossicular chain: see ossicles.

otalgia: ear pain.

otitis media (om): inflammation of the middle ear, usually due to Eustachian tube dysfunction, and often accompanied by accumulated fluid in the middle ear space.

otoacoustic emissions (OAEs): sounds generated in the cochlea that can be measured in the ear canal and arise from activity of the outer hair cells. One type is evoked and occurs in response to auditory stimuli; the other type is spontaneous, occurring without an external auditory stimulus.

otoconia: crystals of calcium carbonate of the otolithic membrane that increase the sensitivity of hair cells to linear acceleration and changes in gravity when the head is placed in different positions.

otolithic membrane: structure in the maculae containing otoconia into which stereocilia of the inner hair cells are embedded.

otoprotective agents: medications and nutritional supplements that can prevent or reduce the negative effects of ototoxic agents on hearing and balance.

otosclerosis: condition in which a layer of new bone is laid down, while older bone is resorbed; results in a spongy type of bone and conductive hearing loss; also called otospongiosis.

otoscope: instrument producing a light that can be directed into the ear canal for visual examination of the canal and eardrum.

otoscopy: process by which an otoscope is used to examine the ear canal and eardrum.

ototoxic: poison to the inner ear; can result in sensorineural hearing loss and/or problems with the balance mechanism.

outer hair cells: efferent, cylindrically shaped hair cells of the cochlea that respond to soft sounds.

output compression: compression circuit in which the volume control is located before the automatic gain control (AGC) circuit and therefore affects the gain of the aid but not the maximum output; typically used with individuals who have severe hearing loss and a reduced dynamic range.

output limiter: type of potentiometer used to restrict the maximum output of a hearing aid.

output limiting: electroacoustic characteristic of a hearing aid that restricts the maximum output of the aid, either by clipping the sound waves or by compressing them.

overmasking: occurs when the amount of masking delivered to the non-test ear crosses over to the test ear and elevates the threshold in the test ear, resulting in overestimation of the hearing loss in the test ear.

overreferral: unnecessarily referring a client for further testing or treatment due to a false positive result.

P-300 auditory evoked response: event-related auditory evoked potential affected by subject state and activity; recorded using an "oddball" paradigm; may be useful in studying higher-level auditory functions, such as those involved in auditory processing.

parallel vent: type of vent in which the hollow channel runs parallel to the sound bore; used to modify the low-frequency component of an amplification system.

pars flaccida: superior part of the eardrum that does not contain fibrous tissue.

pars tensa: stiff portion of the tympanic membrane making up the largest surface area of the eardrum.

patulous Eustachian tube: condition in which the Eustachian tube is abnormally opened.

peak amplitude: maximum displacement of the particles in a medium.

peak clipping: method of limiting the maximum output of a hearing aid by removing the amplitude peaks at specific levels; often criticized because of its negative effect on speech understanding.

peak compensated static acoustic admittance: the amplitude (height) of the tympanogram measured at the plane of the tympanic membrane.

penetrance: a measure of a gene's ability to produce its effect in an individual; a fully penetrant gene will produce the effect 100 percent of the time, while a gene with decreased penetrance will produce the effect in a lesser proportion of individuals.

perforated eardrum: an eardrum that has a hole or opening in it.

perforation: hole or opening in tissue of structure (e.g., eardrum perforation).

performance–intensity (PI) function: percentage of speech understood at a variety of intensity levels from near threshold to well above threshold.

perichondritis: infection of the skin characterized by swelling, redness, and pain.

perilymph: type of cochlear fluid found in the scala vestibuli and scala tympani.

period of sound wave: the time required to complete one cycle of vibration.

peripheral auditory system: part of the auditory system that includes the outer, middle and inner ears, as well as the auditory nerve.

peripheral nervous system: connects the central nervous system with other parts of the body via the spinal nerves and the cranial nerves; spinal nerves transmit sensory information to the higher brain centers and bring motor information from these higher centers to muscles; cranial nerves are closely related to production of speech (vagus, hypoglossal, facial, etc.).

person-centered therapy: therapeutic approach in which the clinician works to allow the client to direct themselves toward a more positive and healthy state.

pervasive developmental disorder, not otherwise specified (PDD-NOS): severe and pervasive impairment in the development of reciprocal social interaction or verbal and nonverbal communication skills; characteristics of autism may be noted, but not to a degree sufficient to meet the diagnostic criteria.

petrious: portion of temporal bone that houses the inner ear structures.

phase: location of an air molecule at a given point in time during displacement, based on degrees of a circle.

phonetically balanced word list: word list in which the sounds represented occur proportionally to their occurrence in spoken English.

phonophobia: fear of certain sounds.

physiological tests of hearing: tests that provide information regarding the integrity of structures that are important to the process of hearing; although information about hearing can be extrapolated, these tests are not direct measures of hearing.

PI rollover: phenomenon that occurs when increasing intensity results in decreasing word recognition; formula is PB Max – PB Min/PB Max; values of 0.25 to 0.45 can be significant for retrocochlear pathology.

pinna: part of the outer ear; external cartilaginous portion; also referred to as the auricle.

pitch: psychological and subjective correlate to frequency.

play audiometry: method of behavioral hearing testing in which responses to auditory signals are indicated by carrying out a predetermined play activity, for which the client has been conditioned.

polygenic: transmission pattern in which multiple genes contribute to the manifested condition.

positive finding: in medical terms, means that a person has the disease or condition.

postlingual deafness: deafness that occurs after the initial development of speech and language skills; 2 years of age is an often cited critical cutoff point.

potential: a change in nerve or muscle activity.

potentiometer: a resistor that allows changes to be made in the current delivered by a hearing aid.

preauricular pits: small depressions or holes located in front of the auricle; considered a craniofacial anomaly.

prelingual deafness: deafness that occurs prior to the development of speech and language skills; typically results in dramatic disruption in oral communication abilities.

presbycusis: hearing loss due to aging.

presbyopia: vision changes due to aging.

pressure equalization (PE) tube: tube inserted into the eardrum after myringotomy to equalize the middle ear pressure; also called a tympanostomy tube. Usually used because of inefficient Eustachian tube.

prevalence: of a disorder referring to the number of existing cases in the population.

probe assembly: part of immittance equipment that is positioned in the ear canal of the client during testing via a probe tip; includes loudspeaker, air pump, manometer, and microphone.

probe microphone testing: Insertion into the ear canal of a small probe tube attached to a microphone for purposes of measuring the amount of sound pressure delivered by a hearing aid to the tympanic membrane; takes into account individual ear canal size and resonance.

probe tone: acoustic signal emitted through the probe of the acoustic admittance device into the ear canal for purposes of measuring acoustic admittance.

programmable hearing aid: aid for which the parameters are adjusted either by a handheld programmer or computer.

pseudohypacusis: synonymous term for nonorganic hearing loss.

psychoacoustics: the combined study of psychology and acoustics; considers human auditory perception relative to acoustics.

psychogenic hearing loss: nonorganic hearing loss resulting from psychological factors.

psychometric standards: characteristics of screening and measurement instruments related to sensitivity, specificity, reliability, and validity.

pure tone average: usually, the average of the pure tone air conduction thresholds in one ear at 500, 1,000, and 2,000 Hz.

pure tones: signals consisting of only one frequency of vibration; typically produced by audiometers and tuning forks.

rarefaction: portion of the sound wave where molecules are far apart.

receiver: see hearing aid receiver.

receiver earmold: type of earmold that is similar to the shell mold but differs from other earmolds because it has a metal or plastic snap adapter inserted into it so that an external receiver, like that used in a body aid, can be coupled to it.

reflex: involuntary response to some external stimulus.

Rehabilitation Act of 1973: (amended in 1978); prohibits exclusion of individuals with disabilities in any federally funded programs of activities.

reinforcement: process of applying a reinforcer, which is any consequence that increases the frequency of a behavior.

reliability: consistency with which a tool measures whatever it is intended to measure; e.g., test–retest reliability is the consistency in results from one test session to the next.

residual hearing: the remaining or useable hearing of a person who has hearing loss.

residual inhibition: continued cessation of tinnitus even after a masking stimulus has been removed.

reticular formation: diffusely organized system of nuclei and tracts with connections to the spinal cord and cerebrum; may play a role in selective attention.

retrocochlear pathology: auditory dysfunction that is beyond the cochlea (e.g., at the auditory nerve or brainstem).

reverberation: persistence of sound in an environment after the original signal is terminated due to multiple reflections off hard surfaces.

reverberation time: the time required for the energy in a sound to decrease by 60 dB once the original signal is terminated.

rotational chair testing: assessment of the horizontal semicircular canals; involves movement of the head at various rates of oscillation and subsequent recording of horizontal eye movements.

saccade system: system of the eye movement involving a resetting eye movement that quickly brings the eyes back in the direction of the head turn.

saccule: endolymph-containing sac located in the vestibule of the ear that has a role in balance for linear movements.

scala media: middle of the three chambers of the cochlea containing endolymph and the basilar membrane and organ of Corti; also referred to as the cochlear duct.

schema: organized frameworks of connected ideas stored in memory.

scope of practice: official policy document that defines the role, responsibilities, and expectations for conduct for a professional discipline

screening: administration of a brief test for purposes of determining if an individual requires more extensive assessment; goal is to separate out those individuals who are most likely to have the condition from those who are not likely to have it.

Screening Instrument for Targeting Educational Risk (SIFTER): tool used in identifying students who may be at risk for hearing loss based on observations of classroom performance in the areas of academics, attention, communication, class participation, and school behavior.

screening tympanometer: tympanometer designed to determine rapidly whether further middle ear analysis is needed; algorithm results in a binary (pass/fail) outcome.

Section 504 of the Rehabilitation Act of 1973: portion of the Rehabilitation Act of 1973 that concerns provision of services to children in regular education programs.

select-a-vent system: system for both in-the-ear hearing aids and earmolds that allows the vent size to be changed based on the client's needs.

selective amplification: hearing aid gain that is distributed to particular frequency regions based on the client's audiometric threshold pattern.

semicircular canals: structures arising from the utricle that have a role in balance for angular changes.

sensation level: decibel referent based on the client's hearing threshold.

sensitivity: degree to which a screening tool identifies those individuals who have the disorder or condition.

sensory organization text: balance test designed to determine which input cues (e.g., vestibular, visual, proprioceptive) are being used to maintain balance; part of computerized dynamic posturography.

sex-linked or X-linked: a gene located on the X-chromosome; the X-chromosome occurs singly in the nucleus of a male, who also has a Y-chromosome, and occurs twice in the female nucleus, which has no Y-chromosome.

shell earmold: full earmold with no open space in the concha; appropriate for high-gain fittings where a good seal is needed.

short-term memory: memory storage system capable of holding small amounts of information for a few seconds; conscious thoughts at any given moment are being held in short-term memory.

signal-to-noise (S/N) ratio: the difference in decibels (dB) between the level of the signal and the level of the background noise.

signal-to-noise (S/N) ratio loss: the increase in signal-to-noise ratio (compared to that of people with normal hearing) for individuals with hearing loss in order for them to obtain 50 percent correct on a measure of word recognition.

simple harmonic motion: see sinusoidal motion.

simple sound: sound in which all of the energy is at one frequency; also referred to as pure tones.

sine wave: the wave created by sinusoidal motion.

sinusoidal motion: smooth and symmetrical movement of an object; also referred to as simple harmonic motion.

site-of-lesion tests: tests designed to determine the location of the anatomic site of dysfunction in the auditory system.

skeleton earmold: type of earmold that is characterized by an open space in the concha area; perhaps the most popular because of its effectiveness in sealing the ear canal for most hearing losses.

smooth pursuit system: system of oculo-motor control that allows a person to track a visual target with smooth, continuous eye movements.

somatosensory/proprioceptive system: supports balance during standing and walking; involves tactile cues, pressure sensors, and input to muscles regarding posture, movement, and position in space

sound: a type of vibratory energy resulting from pressure waves when force is applied to some object or system.

sound field amplification system: equipment consisting of strategically placed speakers and a talker-worn microphone used to improve the signal-to-noise ratio in a room.

sound field testing: audiometric assessment performed by presenting signals in a sound field through loudspeakers.

sound level meter: device used to measure the sound pressure level in an environment or for calibration of audiometric equipment.

sound pressure level (SPL): the amount of sound energy compared to a reference pressure (e.g., 0.0002 dyne/cm^2).

sound-treated test booth: room that has been modified in such a way that ambient noise levels are controlled sufficiently to allow reliable hearing assessment (i.e., meets the standard for permissible noise levels).

spastic cerebral palsy: type of cerebral palsy characterized by extreme limb rigidity followed by sudden release.

specificity: degree to which the screening tool identifies individuals who do not have the disorder or condition.

spectrogram: display generated by a sound spectrograph, depicting frequency, intensity, and time characteristics of a sound.

speech audiometry: assessment of a client's hearing using speech stimuli.

speech detection threshold (SDT): also referred to as the speech awareness threshold (SAT); the minimum hearing level for speech at which an individual can just discern the presence of speech material 50 percent.

speech noise: filtered broad-band noise designed to simulate the long-term average spectrum of conversational speech; used in masking during speech audiometry.

speech recognition threshold (SRT): formerly referred to as the speech reception threshold; the minimum hearing level for speech at which an individual can recognize 50 percent of the speech material.

speech–language pathologist: professional who identifies, assesses, and manages disorders involving speech, language, communication, voice, swallowing, and related disabilities; provides services across the age span, including selection and dispensing of augmentative and alternative communication devices.

spondee: two-syllable word with equal stress on each syllable (e.g., *airplane, baseball*); type of stimulus used in speech recognition threshold testing.

spontaneous nystagmus: nystagmus occurring without stimulation.

spontaneous otoacoustic emissions: sounds generated by the cochlea and recorded in the ear canal in the absence of sound stimulation; present in about half of individuals with normal hearing; clinical utility is limited.

squamous cell carcinoma: the most common malignant tumor of the pinna; can travel by blood vessels and the lymph system.

stacked auditory brainstem response: an attempt to record the sum of the neural activity across the entire frequency region of the cochlea in response to click stimulation.

standing wave: results from interaction of periodic waveforms (i.e., pure tones) of the same frequency produced in a closed sound field; the waves add and subtract to cause doubling of the amplitude at some points and zero amplitude at others.

stapedectomy: surgical procedure in which the stapes is removed and a synthetic prosthesis is inserted between the incus and oval window.

stapedius muscle: middle ear muscle that attaches to the neck of the stapes bone and is innervated by the facial nerve. It contracts in response to loud sound (as in the acoustic reflex).

steady-state evoked potential (SSEP): (40-Hz Response) auditory-evoked, event-related potential; involves some degree of processing of the stimulus; also referred to as the 40-Hz event-related potential, 40-Hz ERP, or steady-state evoked potential (SSEP); not yet used routinely in clinical settings.

Stenger principle: if two tones of the same frequency are presented to the two ears simultaneously, only the louder one will be perceived.

Stenger test: test based on the Stenger principle that is used to rule out nonorganic hearing loss in cases of unilateral loss.

stenosis of the ear canal: narrowing of the canal, often due to loss of elasticity of the muscle of the canal wall.

stereocilia: rows of hairs at the top of hair cells of the sensory receptors.

stimulus frequency otoacoustic emissions: type of evoked otoacoustic emission (OAE) that results when a single pure tone is presented to the ear; has limited clinical utility.

submucous cleft: abnormality of the palate in which surface tissues are intact and the underlying bone and muscle tissues are not.

superior olivary complex (SOC): auditory relay station that transmits information from the cochlear nucleus to the mid-brain; contributes to localization abilities by processing time and intensity cues. The SOC is the first point in the relay system where a signal delivered to one ear is represented on both sides of the central auditory system.

support counseling: counseling that involves acknowledging, exploring, and responding to the client's underlying emotional needs.

supra-aural earphones: earphones that are placed over the ear.

symmetrical hearing loss: hearing loss of the same degree in each ear.

synapse: point of communication between two neurons.

tactile responses: responses made, usually during bone conduction testing, to bone-conducted sounds, when vibrations of the bone vibrator are felt rather than heard.

tectorial membrane: gelatinous membrane that overhangs the organ of Corti; plays an important role in the shearing of cochlear hair cells.

tegmen tympani: thin layer of bone separating the middle ear cavity from the brain.

temperament: relatively stable, early-appearing combination of individual personality characteristics (e.g., social, emotional, activity level), likely to be genetically inherited.

temporal lobe: lobe of the brain which plays an essential role in our understanding of speech and language; contains Heschyl's gurus, the primary auditory reception area.

tensor tympani muscle: middle ear muscle that is attached to the manubrium of the malleus; contracts in response to nonauditory stimuli.

test sensitivity: degree to which a test identifies individuals who are positive for the disorder or condition.

tests of binaural integration: tests that involve fusion of different signals presented simultaneously to the two ears.

tests of binaural interaction: tests that involve presentation of stimuli to each ear in a sequential manner, or presentation of part of a total message to each ear, requiring the synthesis of the two parts.

tests of dichotic listening: tests that present different information simultaneously to each ear; binaural integration tasks involve repeating back everything that is presented; binaural separation involves repeating back information presented in one ear, while ignoring the information presented in the other ear.

tests of low-redundancy monaural speech: tests in which speech that has been altered so that the signal is less redundant than normal is delivered to one ear.

tests of temporal processes: tests that tap the listener's ability to correctly perceive the order or sequence of auditory stimuli, often using tones of varying frequency or duration.

threshold: level at which a stimulus is just barely audible; for pure tones, the lowest level at which a response to sound occurs in 50 percent of presented ascending trials.

tinnitus: a noise that is perceived in the ear or head that does not come from any external source; derived from the Latin word *tinnire*, which means to ring or tinkle like a bell. Client descriptions of the sound vary and include high-pitched ringing, buzzing, throbbing, hissing, and roaring.

tinnitus masker: electronic device that produces broad or narrow-band noise for purposes of masking tinnitus.

tinnitus retraining therapy: approach to tinnitus management based on habituation, involving use of broad-band stimuli to retrain the auditory system and counseling to reduce negative emotions attached to tinnitus.

tolerance-fading memory: category of auditory processing associated with decreased short-term auditory memory, reading comprehension, and auditory figure–ground skills. Expressive language weakness, reduced impulse control, poor motor planning, and poor handwriting are also noted.

tone control: type of potentiometer used to adjust the frequency response of a hearing aid.

tonotopicity: characteristic of the structures of the peripheral and central nervous systems pertaining to frequency transmission.

top-down processing skills: use of cognitive resources, such as prediction ability, prior knowledge, and/or contextual cues, to gain meaning from a message.

Total Communication: use of multiple modes of expression simultaneously for communication; often includes speech, speech reading, and sign language.

transducer: device that converts one form of energy to another.

transient evoked otoacoustic emissions: type of evoked otoacoustic emission (OAE) that is elicited using presentation of a brief stimulus such as a click; employed in clinical audiology for both diagnostic and screening purposes.

transverse waves: waves in which the air molecules move at right angles to the direction of the wave.

traumatic brain injury (TBI): traumatic insult to the brain that can result in impairment in physical, intellectual, emotional, social, or vocational functioning.

treatment planning: aspect of an overall aural rehabilitation program in which rehabilitation goals are determined and a plan for meeting those goals is designed.

tympanic membrane: three-layered vibrating structure serving as borderline between the outer and middle ears; transmits sound to malleus; also referred to as the eardrum.

tympanic membrane perforation: abnormal opening in the eardrum.

tympanometric peak pressure: middle ear pressure at which middle ear admittance is the greatest, as measured during tympanometry.

tympanometric width: measure of gradient; involves calculation of static admittance, dividing this value in half and then measuring down from the tympanometric peak by this amount to measure width.

tympanometry: measurement of eardrum compliance as a function of variations of air pressure in the external auditory canal; allows determination of the point (in pressure) at which the eardrum is most compliant.

tympanoplasty: reconstructive surgery of the middle ear.

undermasking: occurs when insufficient masking is placed in the non-test ear, allowing it to participate in the testing process; the response obtained in the test ear may be better than its actual threshold, resulting in underestimation of the hearing loss in the test ear.

underreferral: failure to refer a client for further testing or treatment due to a false negative result.

unilateral hearing loss: hearing loss only in one ear.

unilateral weakness: difference in the intensity of nystagmus between ears during caloric testing of the ENG.

universal newborn hearing screening programs: programs that use physiological measures to identify hearing loss as early in life as possible.

utricle: membranous sac located in the vestibule of the ear that has a role in balance for linear movements.

validation: aspect of overall rehabilitation program in which data are collected to ensure that the disability has been reduced and that established goals have been reached; often involves use of a hearing handicap scale or a specific postfitting measure.

validity: the degree to which a measuring instrument (e.g., a test or a screening) measures what it purports to measure.

velocity: the speed at which sound travels through a medium.

vent: opening or hollow channel in a hearing aid or earmold that allows sound and air into the ear; also allows reduction of low frequencies out of the ear canal.

verification: aspect of an overall aural rehabilitation program in which measures are made to determine that the hearing aids meet a set of standards; can include electroacoustics, cosmetic appeal, and comfort.

vertex negative: on auditory evoked response recordings, those waveforms that are plotted downward (below the horizontal axis); related to electrode placement.

vertex positive: on auditory evoked response recordings, those waveforms that are plotted upward (above the horizontal axis); related to electrode placement.

vertigo: perception of motion; the client experiences a sensation of spinning.

vestibular: pertaining to the vestibule, which is the portion of the inner ear related to balance.

vestibular compensation: a process in which the central nervous system recovers spontaneously after injury to the balance organs of the inner ear.

vestibular rehabilitation programs: designed to help individuals with balance disorders by facilitating habituation of the system's negative response (e.g., vertigo, nausea) to stimuli that evoke them (e.g., head movement); often requires performing the evoking activity repeatedly in order to reduce symptoms.

vestibular schwannoma: acoustic tumors that arise from the vestibular portion of the auditory nerve, specifically affecting the Schwann cells, which form the sheath covering the nerve.

vestibule: a cavity in the bony labyrinth of the cochlea; contains the utricle and the saccule; opens into the semicircular canals and cochlea.

vestibulo-ocular reflex (VOR): reflex that causes the eyes to move in the opposite direction as the head movement; also allows the eyes to remain still during head movement.

vibration: the to-and-fro motion of an object; also referred to as oscillation.

videonystagmography: method of balance testing that records images of eyeball movement and saves them to a computer.

visual reinforcement audiometry (VRA): behavioral test technique for children from approximately 5 months to 2 years of age; relies on the child's ability to localize by turning toward the source of the sound.

volume control: type of potentiometer used to vary the degree of resistance to the current of a hearing aid.

VU meter: display on the audiometer that provides information regarding the intensity of the input signal; typically has a range from −20 to +3 dB.

watt (W): unit of electrical power.

waveform: type of graph which displays sound, showing amplitude on the vertical axis and time on the horizontal axis.

wavelength: length of a sound wave, as measured from an arbitrary point on the wave to the same point on the next cycle of the wave.

wave morphology: shape or definition of the waves generated in auditory evoked testing.

white noise: broad spectrum noise sometimes used in masking during speech audiometry.

wide dynamic range compression (WDRC): type of compression using low kneepoints (e.g., 40 dB) and smaller compression ratios (e.g., 2:1 ratio) for purposes of increasing the gain for soft sounds.

WIPI test: closed-set, picture-pointing speech recognition task used when a verbal response mode is not possible.

word recognition score: formerly referred to as speech discrimination score; measure of speech audiometry that assesses a client's ability to identify one-syllable words presented at hearing levels that are above threshold. Other possible test stimuli include sentence or paragraph material.

Index

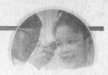

Bellis, T., 378–379, 383, 385, 387
Bell Laboratories, 45
Benign paroxysmal positional vertigo (BPPV), 272–273
Berlin, Charles I., 23, 69, 260
Bernstein, J., 244
Bess, F. H., 39, 171, 289
Biehler, R., 369–370
Bilateral cochlear implants, 483–484
Bimodal listening, 481–482
Binaural hearing, 437–439
Binaural integration, 382–384
Binaural interaction tests, 385
Binaural separation, 384
Binaural squelch, 438
Binaural summation, 437
Blamey, P. J., 481
Bloom, C., 495–496
Bluetooth technology, 454, 455
BOA (behavioral observation audiometry), 306, 405
Boettcher, F., 255
Bone-anchored hearing aids (BAHAs), 460–461
Bone conduction, 33–34
    relationship to air conduction, 34–37
    symbols for, 40–44, 45
Bone conduction hearing aids, 434, 435
Bone conduction pathway, 33–34
Bone conduction testing
    air conduction testing versus, 109
    masking for, 118–119, 121
    pure tone testing, 85–86, 89, 99–101
    recording masked test results for, 109
    threshold testing, 106–108
Bone conduction vibrator, 106
Botwinick, J., 341
BPPV (benign paroxysmal positional vertigo), 272–273
Brain plasticity, 376
Brainstem auditory evoked potentials (BAEP). *See* Auditory brainstem response (ABR) testing
Brainstem auditory evoked response testing (BAER). *See* Auditory brainstem response (ABR) testing
Brainstem evoked response (BSER). *See* Auditory brainstem response (ABR) testing
Branch, W., 6, 7
Branchial arches, 286, 287
Brandt, T., 277
Bray, P., 198, 199
Brimacombe, J., 148
Brownell, W., 68, 69
Brownian motion, 14
Brunt, M. A., 378

Buffalo model, 385, 386
Burch-Sims, P., 197

Cacace, A., 258–259, 377
Calibration, of audiometer, 86–91, 398–400
California Consonant Test (CCT), 147–148, 162
Caloric testing, 273–274
Campbell, K., 493
CAPD (central auditory processing disorder), 375–381
Carcinoma of the external ear, 235, 236
Carhart's notch, 242
Carotid artery, 357
Carrell, T., 226, 227
Carver, W. F., 314, 315
Case history
    form for, 92–93, 389–390
    masking, 104–108
    in pediatric audiology, 300–301, 302, 316–319
    sample cases, 498–500
Cellulitis, 234
Centers for Disease Control and Prevention (CDC), 413
Central auditory pathways, 74–76
Central auditory processing disorders (CAPD), 375–381
Central auditory system, 72–77, 375
    assessment of, 378–385
    central auditory pathways, 74–76
    disorders of, 258–262
    disrupted blood supply, 258
    in elderly persons, 340
    hereditary motor-sensory neuropathies, 258–259
    maturation of, 375, 376
    multiple sclerosis, 258
    plasticity of, 376
    summary, 76–77
Central nervous system (CNS), 72, 74, 357
Cerebral cortex, 75–76
Cerebral palsy (CP), 331, 352–354
Cerebrovascular accident (CVA), 356–357, 358–360
Cerebrum, 357
Cerumen buildup, 33, 34–36, 37, 58, 235–237, 437
Chaiklin, J. B., 132
Chambers, J., 150
Champlin, C., 150
Chermak, Gail D., 471
Chessman, M., 340
Children. *See* Pediatric audiology

Children's Auditory Performance Scale (CHAPS), 378, 379
Children's Implant Profile (CHIP), 479
Ching, T. Y., 482, 483
Chinn, P., 368
Cholesteatoma, 239
Chromosomes, 292
Chute, P. M., 475
CID Everyday Sentences, 146
CID W-22 lists, 135
Circumaural earphones, 99
Cisplatin (CDDP), 493
Clark, John Greer, 3, 17, 20, 56, 59, 65, 103, 149, 150, 168, 321, 495, 497, 506–508
Client Oriented Scale of Improvement (COSI), 459
Clients as individuals, 8
Client-specific protocols, 321–331
    communicating diagnostic information to parents, 328–329
    genetic counseling, 329
    model of, 322, 323–324
    for screening, 405–423, 415–417
Closed-set format, 146
Cochlea, 65–71
Cochlear damage, air-bone relationship due to history of, 36, 37
Cochlear hair cell regeneration, 494
Cochlear implant map, 485
Cochlear implants, 2, 473–488
    assessment and candidacy considerations, 476–477
    auditory training curriculum, 486, 487
    bilateral, 483–484
    bimodal listening, 481–482
    cochlear implant systems, 474
    decision making, 480–481
    electric/acoustic stimulation, 482–483
    formal evaluation, 477–480
    history and background, 474
    implantation, 484–485
    ongoing assessment of auditory skills, 486–488
    operation of, 474–476
    rehabilitation considerations, 485–486
    stages of management in children, 478
Cochlear microphonic (CM), 218–219
Cochlear nuclei, 73–74
Cognitive status, 348, 350–351
Collaboration, of audiologists, 9–11, 418, 492
Collapsing ear canals, 94, 110–111, 235, 340, 342
Communicated mismatch, 345–346, 348
Communication Probe for the Hearing Impaired (CPHI), 433

Hearing aid(s) (*continued*)
  implantable, 460–461
  maintenance and troubleshooting,
    462–463, 465–466
  maximum output, 447–450
  monaural versus binaural fitting,
    437–439
  noise and, 451–452
  open fittings, 452–453
  recent developments, 451–456
  schedule for reevaluation, 463–464
  selection of, 435–436, 469
  styles of, 436–437
  telephone use, 453
  treatment planning, 434
  validation, 459
  verification, 456–459
  wide dynamic range compression, 450
  wireless technology, 453–454
Hearing aid amplifier, 434
Hearing aid microphone, 434, 451–452
Hearing aid receiver, 434
Hearing aid stethoset, 462, 464
Hearing aid test box, 439, 440
Hearing disability, 420–421
Hearing Handicap Inventory for the
    Elderly—Screening Version, 422, 428
Hearing in Noise Test (HINT), 145
Hearing level (HL), 30
Hearing loss, 429–508. *See also* Assistive
    technology devices; Hearing aid(s);
    Individuals who are deaf
  asymmetrical, 102
  conductive, 40–41, 216
  consonant sounds in, 49–50
  counseling for, 494–500
  degrees of, 39–40
  early identification of, 283–284,
    405–414
  early intervention for, 283–284
  extrinsic causes of, 284
  genetic conditions related to, 289
  infant, incidence of, 410–411
  infant screening protocols, 405–414
  intrinsic causes of, 284
  mild, as confusing, 39–40
  mixed, 41–43
  model of aural rehabilitation,
    430–432
  multicultural issues in, 152, 346–347,
    368–370
  noise-induced, 36, 252–254, 493–494
  nonorganic. *See* Individuals with
    nonorganic hearing loss
  presbycusis, 80, 255–257, 340
  prevention, 491–494
  sensorineural, 41–43, 217, 441, 445

symmetrical, 102
tinnitus, 91, 488–491
Heller, Stefan, 484
Hellman, S. A., 479
Henry, J., 488, 489, 490
Hereditary motor-sensory neuropathies
    (HMSN), 258–259
Hersch's gyrus, 75
Hertz (Hz), 24, 29
Hertz, H. R., 24
Heterozygous, 291, 292
Hicks, A., 303
Hier, D., 221
High-risk register, 405
Hoeppner, J., 226, 227
Holmes, L., 290
Holt, R. F., 481–482
Homozygous, 292
Hood, L., 259, 260
Hood (plateau) method, 122, 123
Horn effect, 445–447
Hornsby, B., 47
Hosford-Dunn, H., 153
Howie, V., 245
Hughes, G., 274–275
Hull, R. N., 470
Human Genome Project, 288–292
Humanism, in audiology, 2–3, 6–11
Humes, L. E., 39, 171, 378
Hunter, L. L., 176
Hurley, R., 153
Hyde, M. L., 224, 225

IEP (Individualized Education
    Plan), 379
Immittance battery, 170, 421
Impedance, 170
Impedance-matching device, 61
Implantable hearing aids, 460–461
Incus, 60
Individualized Education Plan
    (IEP), 379
Individuals who are deaf, 343–351. *See
    also* Hearing loss
  age of onset, 347, 348
  audiological assessment, 347–350
  cognitive status, 348, 350–351
  communication mismatch and,
    345–346, 348
  cultural mismatch and, 346–347
  definitions, 343–345
  degree of residual hearing, 347–350
  other disabilities, 348, 350
  relevant features, 348
Individuals with developmental
    disabilities, 329–331, 351–356
  audiological assessment, 354–355

definitions, 351–355
management plans, 355–356
relevant features, 353
Individuals with Disabilities Education
    Act (IDEA), 297, 298, 414, 431
Individuals with neurogenic disorders,
    356–361
  stroke, 356–357, 358–360
  traumatic brain injury (TBI), 10,
    356–357
Individuals with nonorganic hearing
    loss, 362–368
  audiological assessment, 362–366
  definitions, 362
  management plans, 367
  patient counseling, 368
  pseudohypacusis, 362
  relevant features, 364
  report writing, 368
Inertia, 14
Infants. *See also* Pediatric audiology
  cochlear implant assessment, 477
  developmental stages, 282, 283
  language and articulation
    development, 293
  screening of, 182–184, 198, 300,
    405–414
Infant-Toddler Meaningful Auditory
    Integration Scale (IT-MAIS),
    479–480
Infection
  middle ear, 245–248, 415
  outer ear, 234–235
Inferior colliculus, 74
Informed questions, 338
Initial masking (IM)
  for air conduction testing, 117–118
  for bone conduction testing, 118–119
Injuries
  to inner ear, 257
  to outer ear, 235
Inner ear, 63–72
  cochlea, 65–71
  cochlear hair cells, 69, 494
  development of, 285, 286
  disorders of. *See* Inner ear disorders
  summary, 71–72
  vestibular system, 64–65, 262–263, 291
Inner ear disorders, 234, 248–257
  diabetes, 251
  in elderly persons, 340
  facial nerve disorders, 251–252
  fluid, 61
  Meniere's disease, 219, 252, 277, 278
  noise exposure, history of, 36
  noise-induced hearing loss, 36,
    252–254, 493–494

Pressure equalization (PE) tubes, 173, 245–248

Prevalence, 394

Prevention of hearing loss, 491–494

Prieve, B., 411

Primus, M. A., 39

Probe microphone testing, 456–459

Probe tone, 172

PRoduction Infant Scale Evaluation (PRISE), 479–480

Professional organizations, 4–5. *See also* American Academy of Audiology (AAA); American Speech-Language-Hearing Association (ASHA)

Pseudocysts, 236

Pseudohypacusis, 362
  audiological assessment, 362–366
  motivation for, 362

Psychoacoustics, 97

Psychogenic hearing loss, 362

Pure tone average, 98–99, 128

Pure tones, in pediatric audiology, 323

Pure tone testing, 79–124
  audiometer and, 84–86
  bone conduction testing, 85–86, 89, 99–101
  calibration in, 86–91
  cases, 97–98, 100, 104–108
  for hearing aids, 433
  masking in, 101–109, 117–124
  in pediatric audiology, 295, 323, 326, 327
  perception of speech sounds, 79–84
  potential pitfalls of, 110–112
  pre-testing steps, 91–94
  pure tone average, 98–99
  pure tones, defined, 79
  speech audiometry versus, 126, 128–130
  test process, 94–98
  traditional test protocols, 110

Raffin, M., 153, 155

Raggio, M. W., 148, 163–164

Ramkissoon, L., 369

Rarefaction, 14

Receiver earmold, 442

Reception threshold for sentences (RTS), 145

Rees, J., 341

Referrals
  forms for, 408
  overreferrals, 397, 400, 422

Reflexes, 184

Rehabilitation Act of 1973, Section 504, 297, 299

Reinforcement, 307

Reliability, 126, 377, 395, 399

Residual hearing, 347–350

Resonator tube, 58

Reticular formation, 75–76

Retrocochlear pathology, 136, 170

Reverberation, 471

Reverberation time, 50–52

Robinson, D., 3

Rogers, Carl, 496

Rosner, B., 415

Ross, M., 148, 314–315, 470

Rotational chair testing, 274–275

Runge, C., 153

Ryals, B., 494

Ryan, S., 198, 199

Ryback, L., 493

Saccade system, 263–264

Saccade testing of rapid eye movement, 267

Saccule, 65

Sanders, Derek, 488

Satya-Murti, S., 258–259

Scala media, 66, 69–70

SCAN test, 378, 380

Schechter, M., 488

School-age children. *See also* Pediatric audiology
  assistive technology in the classroom, 472–473
  auditory processing disorders (APD), 375
  cochlear implant assessment, 477
  cochlear implant management, 477
  developmental stages, 283
  educational consultations and, 506–508
  guidelines for classroom noise and reverberation, 50–52
  improving classroom listening, 470–473
  language and articulation development, 293
  screening, 417–420, 463–464

Schow, R., 422

Schrapnell's membrane, 58

Schubert, E. D., 147–148, 148, 163–164

Schuknecht, H., 255

Scope of practice, audiology, 1–2, 5–6, 391–392

Screening, 391–428
  administering, 404
  of adults, 420–423, 427
  audiological, 392
  for (central) auditory processing disorders, 378–381

costs of, 402–403
  defined, 392
  general components, 403–405
  of infants, 182–184, 198, 300, 405–414
  medical model versus educational model of, 9, 392–393
  pitfalls of, 421
  of preschool children, 182–184, 414–417
  protocol decisions, 395–403, 415–417
  protocols over life span, 405–423
  recommendations based on, 404–405
  reliability in, 395, 399
  reporting results, 425–428
  schedule for reevaluation, 463–464
  of school-age children, 417–420, 463–464
  sensitivity in, 393, 399, 400
  specificity in, 393–394, 399, 400
  speech-language pathologist role in, 380–381
  validity in, 394–395, 399

Screening Instrument for Targeting Educational Risk (SIFTER), 297, 379, 419

Screening Test for Auditory Processing Disorders (SCAN), 379

Sebaceous cysts, 236

Section 504 of Rehabilitation Act of 1973, 297, 299

Select-a-vent, 444

Selective amplification, 439

Selective Auditory Attention Test (SAAT), 379

Self Assessment of Communication Function (SAC), 433

Self-awareness, of audiologists, 8–9

Seligman, M., 370

Sells, J., 153

Semicircular canals, 65

Semont, A., 277

Sensitivity, 393, 399, 400

Sensorineural hearing loss, 41–43, 217, 441, 445

Sensory organization test (SOT), 275–277

Sentence tests, 146

Sex-linked, 292

Shanks, J. E., 179–180

Sharma, A., 226, 227

Shell earmold, 442, 443

Shepard, N., 267, 272

Short-term memory, 361

Signal-to-noise (S/N) ratio, 48–50, 145, 451–452

Significant differences, 153–155